Pharmacology in the Catheterization Laboratory

This book is dedicated to the contributors who worked hard to fulfill the task of bringing this book to production. To all former and current fellows trained in our program at Washington Hospital Center. To Andrew Ajani for his true friendship and contribution to the success of our program; he truly has emerged as a future leader in the field. To my partners, Lowell, Gus, Kenny, Bill, and Nelson, who allowed me to deviate from patient care and devote time to this educational effort. And finally to my parents, Bella and Mordechai, who have encouraged me throughout my career; and to my wife Tali and our children, Ori, Yarden, Jonathan, and Daniel, for supporting me amid the editorial process.

Ron Waksman, MD, FACC

I would like to dedicate this book to my co-editor, Professor Ron Waksman, who has been a principal mentor and inspiration for my career in cardiology. Professor Waksman remains a world leader in this field; his commitment, knowledge, and foresight continue to inspire us all.

Andrew E. Ajani, MBBS, MD, FJFICM, FRACP, FCSANZ

Pharmacology in the Catheterization Laboratory

EDITED BY

Ron Waksman MD, FACC

Associate Chief of Cardiology
Director of Experimental Angioplasty and New Technologies
Division of Cardiology
Washington Hospital Center
Washington, DC, USA

Andrew E. Ajani MBBS, MD, FJFICM, FRACP, FCSANZ

Associate Professor
Interventional Cardiologist
Director of Coronary Care Unit
Director of Physician Training
The Royal Melbourne Hospital
Melbourne, Victoria, Australia

WILEY-BLACKWELL
A John Wiley & Sons, Ltd., Publication

This edition first published 2010, © 2010 by Blackwell Publishing Ltd

Blackwell Publishing was acquired by John Wiley & Sons in February 2007. Blackwell's publishing program has been merged with Wiley's global Scientific, Technical and Medical business to form Wiley-Blackwell.

Registered office
John Wiley & Sons Ltd, The Atrium, Southern Gate, Chichester, West Sussex, PO19 8SQ, UK

Editorial offices
9600 Garsington Road, Oxford, OX4 2DQ, UK
The Atrium, Southern Gate, Chichester, West Sussex, PO19 8SQ, UK
111 River Street, Hoboken, NJ 07030-5774, USA

For details of our global editorial offices, for customer services and for information about how to apply for permission to reuse the copyright material in this book please see our website at www.wiley.com/wiley-blackwell

Library of Congress Cataloging-in-Publication Data
Pharmacology in the catheterization laboratory / [edited by] Ron Waksman, Andrew E. Ajani.
  p. ; cm.
 Includes bibliographical references and index.
 ISBN 978-1-4051-5704-9
  1. Cardiovascular agents. 2. Cardiac catheterization. I. Waksman, Ron. II. Ajani, Andrew E.
[DNLM: 1. Myocardial Revascularization. 2. Anticoagulants--therapeutic use. 3. Catheterization--methods. 4. Coronary Disease--drug therapy. 5. Fibrinolytic Agents--therapeutic use. 6. Platelet Aggregation Inhibitors--therapeutic use. WG 169 P536 2009]

RM345.P485 2009
615'.71--dc22   2009013415

A catalogue record for this book is available from the British Library.

Set in 9.5/12pt Minion by Newgen Imaging Systems Pvt. Ltd., Chennai, India
Printed and bound in Malaysia by Vivar Printing Sdn Bhd

1   2010

Contents

Contributors

JoEllyn M. Abraham, MD
Fellow, Division of Cardiovascular Medicine
Cleveland Clinic
Cleveland, OH, USA

Andrew E. Ajani, MBBS, MD, FRACP,
FJFICM, FCSANZ
Associate Professor
Interventional Cardiologist
Director of Coronary Care Unit
Director of Physician Training
The Royal Melbourne Hospital
Melbourne, Victoria, Australia

John A. Ambrose, MD, FACC
Chief of Cardiology
UCSF Fresno
Professor of Medicine
University of California
San Francisco, CA, USA

Alaeddin Ayyad, MD
Cardiology Fellow
Department of Cardiology
University of California San Diego
San Diego, CA, USA

Antonio L. Bartorelli, MD, FESC, FACC
Director, Interventional Cardiology
Department of Cardiovascular Sciences
Centro Cardiologico Monzino
I.R.C.C.S.
University of Milan
Milan, Italy

Eric R. Bates, MD
Professor of Medicine
Division of Cardiovascular Diseases
Department of Internal Medicine
University of Michigan
Ann Arbor, MI, USA

Richard C. Becker, MD
Professor of Medicine
Divisions of Cardiology and Hematology
Duke Clinical Research Institute
Duke University School of Medicine
Durham, NC, USA

Itsik Ben-Dor, MD
Professor
Cardiology Department
Interventional Cardiology Institute
Rabin Medical Center
Petach-Tikva, Israel;
Sackler Faculty of Medicine
Tel-Aviv University
Tel-Aviv, Israel

Michel E. Bertrand, MD, FRCP, FESC,
FACC, FAHA
Emeritus Professor of Cardiology
University of Lille
Lille Heart Institute
Lille, France

Deepak L. Bhatt, MD, MPH, FACC,
FAHA, FSCAI
Chief of Cardiology
VA Boston Healthcare System Director
Integrated Interventional Cardiovascular Program
Brigham and Women's Hospital and the VA Boston
Healthcare System
Senior Investigator, TIMI Study Group
Harvard Medical School
Boston, MA, USA

Bruce R. Brodie, MD
Clinical Professor of Medicine
University of North Carolina Teaching Service
Moses Cone Health System
Chairman, LeBauer Cardiovascular Research Foundation
Greensboro, NC, USA

Peter J. Casterella, MD
Interventional Cardiologist
Seattle Cardiology
Seattle, WA, USA

Mark W. Connolly, MD
Director, Cardiovascular and Thoracic Surgery
Heart and Vascular Institute
Department of Cardiovascular and Thoracic Surgery
St. Michael's Medical Center
Newark, NJ, USA

Ignacio Cruz-Gonzalez, MD, PhD
Associate Professor of Medicine
Harvard Medical School
Director, Cardiology Laboratory for Integrative Physiology
and Imaging
Interventional Cardiology Fellow
Cardiology Division
Massachusetts General Hospital
Boston, MA, USA

Bart Dawson, MD
Cardiovascular Medicine Fellow
Gill Heart Institute and
Division of Cardiovascular Medicine
University of Kentucky
Lexington, KY, USA

Neil P. Desai, PhD
Vice President, R&D
Abraxis Bioscience, LLC
Los Angeles, CA, USA

Pantelis Diamantouros, MD, FRCPC
Assistant Professor of Medicine
Division of Cardiology
Department of Internal Medicine
University of Western Ontario
London, ON, Canada

Germano Di Sciascio, MD, FACC, FESC
Assistant Professor of Cardiology
Director, Department of Cardiovascular Sciences
Campus Bio-Medico University of Rome
Rome, Italy

Zayd A. Eldadah, MD, PhD, FACC
Associate Director, Arrhythmia Research
Cardiac Arrhythmia Center
Division of Cardiology
Washington Hospital Center
Washington, DC, USA

Frederick Feit, MD, FACC
Associate Professor of Medicine
Division of Cardiology, Department of Medicine
New York University School of Medicine
New York, NY, USA

Valeria Ferrero, MD
Staff Cardiologist Catheterization Laboratory
Division of Cardiology, Università di Verona
Ospedale Civile Maggiore
Verona, Italy

Tim A. Fischell, MD, FACC, FSCAI
Director of Cardiovascular Research
Borgess Heart Institute
Professor of Medicine
Michigan State University
Kalamazoo, MI, USA

Shmuel Fuchs, MD, MACC, FSACI
Specialist in Cardiology and Internal Medicine, Head
Department of Internal Medicine B
Beilinson Hospital, Rabin Medical Center
Petach-Tikva, Israel

Anthony H. Gershlick, MD
Professor of Interventional Cardiology
Academic Department of Cardiology
University Hospitals of Leicester
Leicester, UK

Ziyad Ghazzal, MD, FACC, FSCAI
Professor of Medicine Cardiology/Interventional
Cardiology Deputy VP/Dean
Associate Dean for Clinical Affairs
American University of Beirut
Faculty of Medicine and Medical Center
Beirut, Lebanon

C. Michael Gibson, MS, MD
Associate Professor
Harvard Medical School
Director, TIMI Data Coordinating Center
Boston, MA, USA

Robert P. Giugliano, MD, SM
Senior Investigator
TIMI Study Group
Associate Physician
Cardiovascular Medicine
Brigham and Women's Hospital
Assistant Professor in Medicine
Harvard Medical School
Boston, MA, USA

Luis Gruberg, MD, FACC
Director, Cardiovascular Catheterization Laboratories
Professor of Medicine
Division of Cardiology
SUNY-Stony Brook University Medical Center
Health Science Center
Stony Brook, NY, USA

Saurabh Gupta, MD, FACC
Assistant Professor of Medicine
Division of Cardiovascular Medicine
Oregon Health and Science University
Portland, OR, USA

Ronen Gurvitch, MBBS, FRACP
Cardiologist
Interventional Cardiology Fellow
The Royal Melbourne Hospital
Melbourne, Victoria, Australia

Jan Holst, MD, PhD
Associate Professor
Vascular Centre
University Hospital MAS
Malmö, Sweden

Ik-Kyung Jang, MD, PhD
Associate Professor of Medicine
Harvard Medical School
Director, Cardiology Laboratory for Integrative Physiology
and Imaging, Cardiology Division
Massachusetts General Hospital
Boston, MA, USA

Allen Jeremias, MD, MSc
Director, Vascular Medicine and Peripheral Intervention
Division of Cardiovascular Medicine
SUNY-Stony Brook School of Medicine
Stony Brook, NY, USA

Pravin Kahale, MD, DM (Cardiology)
Interventional Cardiologist
Department of Invasive Cardiology
Adventist Wockhardt Hospital
Surat, India

Amir Kashani, MD, MS, CCDS, FACC
Section of Cardiology
Yale University School of Medicine
New Haven, CT, USA;
Clinical Instructor
Baylor College of Medicine
Houston, TX, USA

Damian J. Kelly, BSc, MRCP
Cardiologist Specialist Registrar
Department of Academic Cardiology
University Hospitals of Leicester, Glenfield Hospital
Leicester, UK

Ran Kornowski, MD, FACC, FESC
Director, Interventional Cardiology Institute
Cardiology Department
Rabin Medical Center
Petach-Tikva, Israel;
Sackler Faculty of Medicine
Tel-Aviv University
Tel-Aviv, Israel

Pramod Kumar Kuchulakanti,
MD, DM, FACC, FESC
Interventional Cardiologist
Director, Cardiac Catheterization Laboratory
Wockhardt Heart Center, Kamineni Hospitals
Hyderabad, India

David S. Kwon, MD, PhD
Cardiology Fellow
Cardiac Research Institute
Washington Hospital Center
Washington, DC, USA

Geoffrey Lee, MBCHB, FRACP
Cardiologist, Department of Cardiology
The Royal Melbourne Hospital
Melbourne, Victoria, Australia

Jeffrey Lefkovits, MBBS, FRACP, FCSANZ
Interventional Cardiologist
The Royal Melbourne Hospital
Melbourne, Victoria, Australia

Bengt Lindblad, MD, PhD
Associate Professor
Vascular Centre
University Hospital MAS
Malmö, Sweden

Joseph Lindsay, MD, FACC
Division Director Emeritus, Cardiology
Washington Hospital Center
Washington, DC, USA

Raj R. Makkar, MD, FACC, FSCAI
Director, Interventional Cardiology and Cardiac
Catheterization Laboratory
Cedars-Sinai Medical Center
Associate Professor
UCLA School of Medicine
Los Angeles, CA, USA

Tift Mann, MD, FACC
Interventional Cardiologist
Wake Heart Associates
Raleigh, NC, USA

Steven V. Manoukian, MD, FACC,
FSCAI
Director of Cardiovascular Research
Sarah Cannon Research Institute
Medical Director of Cardiology, Clinical Services Group
Hospital Corporation of America (HCA), Inc.
Interventional Cardiology
Centennial Heart
Nashville, TN, USA

Giancarlo Marenzi, MD, FESC
Director, Coronary Unit
Centro Cardiologico Monzino, I.R.C.C.S.
Department of Cardiovascular Sciences
University of Milan
Milan, Italy

Scott Martin, MD
Fellow, Division of Cardiovascular Medicine
Department of Medicine
SUNY-Stony Brook School of Medicine
Stony Brook, NY, USA

Dorinna D. Mendoza, MD
Cardiology Fellow
Division of Cardiology
Washington Hospital Center
Washington, DC, USA

David J. Moliterno, MD
Professor and Chief of Cardiology
Gill Heart Institute and Division of
Cardiovascular Medicine
University of Kentucky
Lexington, KY, USA

Debabrata Mukherjee, MD, FACC, FSCAI
Professor of Medicine
Director, Cardiac Catheterization Laboratory
Gill Heart Institute
Division of Cardiovascular Medicine
University of Kentucky
Lexington, KY, USA

Eugenia Nikolsky, MD, PhD
Director, Academic Affairs
Clinical Trial Center
Cardiovascular Research Foundation
New York, NY, USA

Julie H. Oestreich, PharmD, PhD
Post-Doctoral Fellow
Department of Pharmaceutical Sciences
University of Kentucky
Lexington, KY, USA

E. Magnus Ohman, MD, FRCPI, FESC, FACC, FSCAI
Professor of Medicine
Associate Director, Duke Heart Center
Director, Program for Advanced Coronary Disease
Duke Clinical Research Institute
Duke University Medical Center
Durham, NC, USA

Andrew T. L. Ong, MBBS, PhD, FRACP, FESC, FACC
Consultant and Interventional Cardiologist
Department of Cardiology
Westmead Hospital
Westmead, New South Wales, Australia

Nilesh U. Patel, MD
Chief, Minimally Invasive Robotic Cardiac Surgery
Department of Cardiovascular and Thoracic Surgery
St. Michael's Medical Center
Newark, NJ, USA

Giuseppe Patti, MD
Assistant Professor
Department of Cardiovascular Sciences
Campus Bio-Medico University of Rome
Rome, Italy

Khan Pohlel, MD, FACC
Interventional Cardiologist
Athens Cardiology Group
Athens, GA, USA

Yuri B. Pride, MD
Instructor in Medicine
Division of Cardiovascular Medicine
Beth Israel Deaconess Medical Center
Harvard Medical School
Boston, MA, USA

Flavio Ribichini, MD
Director, Catheterization Laboratory
Università di Verona
Ospedale Civile Maggiore
Verona, Italy

Alfredo E. Rodriguez, MD, PhD, FACC, FSCAI
Director, Cardiovascular Research Center (CECI)
Cardiac Unit, Otamendi Hospital
Buenos Aires School of Medicine
Buenos Aires, Argentina

Probal Roy, MD
Interventional Cardiologist
Australian School of Advanced Medicine
Macquarie University
Sydney, New South Wales, Australia

Maria Sanchez-Ledesma, MD
Fellow Research, Interventional Cardiology
Cardiology Division
Massachusetts General Hospital
Harvard Medical School
Boston, MA, USA

Mickey Scheinowitz, Phd, FACSM
Associate Professor
Department of Biomedical Engineering &
Neufeld Cardiac Research Institute
Tel-Aviv University
Ramat-Aviv, Israel

Sanjiv Sharma, MD, FACC, FSCAI
Clinical Instructor of Medicine
UCLA School of Medicine
Los Angeles, CA, USA;
Director, Research and Education
Bakersfield Heart Hospital
Bakersfield, CA, USA

Steven R. Steinhubl, MD
Global Vice-President, Thrombosis
The Medicines Company
Zurich, Switzerland
The Geisinger Clinic
Adjunct Research Faculty
Danville, PA, USA

Adam Strickberger, MD
Professor, Georgetown University School of Medicine
Cardiac Research Institute
Washington, DC, USA

Michele D. Voeltz, MD
Assistant Professor of Medicine
Division of Cardiology
Department of Medicine
Sarah Cannon Research Institute
Hospital Corporation of America
Nashville, TN, USA

Ron Waksman, MD, FACC
Associate Chief of Cardiology
Director of Experimental Angioplasty and
New Technologies
Division of Cardiology
Washington Hospital Center
Washington, DC, USA

Ralph Wessel, MD, FACC
Associate Professor of Medicine
Division of Cardiology
Department of Internal Medicine
UCSF Fresno
Fresno, CA, USA

Harvey D. White, DSc, FCSANZ
Director of Coronary Care and Green Lane
Cardiovascular Research Unit
Green Lane Cardiovascular Service
Auckland City Hospital
Auckland, New Zealand

Michael D. White, MD
Fellow, Interventional Cardiology Program
Division of Cardiology
Duke University Medical Center
Durham, NC, USA

Roswitha Wolfram, MD
Professor of Medicine
Department of Internal Medicine II
Vienna General Hospital
Vienna, Austria

Cheuk-Kit Wong, MD, FCSANZ
Consultant Cardiologist
Dunedin School of Medicine
Otago University
Dunedin, New Zealand

Bryan P. Yan, MBBS, FRACP
Assistant Professor
Chinese University of Hong Kong
Interventional Cardiologist
Prince of Wales Hospital
Hong Kong, China

Andrew Zinn, MD
Division of Cardiology
Department of Medicine
New York University School of Medicine
New York, NY, USA

Acknowledgements

The editors must acknowledge the commitment and support of Mr. Thomas Hartman, commissioning editor, and his dedicated staff at Wiley-Blackwell, including Ms. Kate Newell and Ms. Cathryn Gates, who helped bring this project to fruition. The editors are also grateful to Ms. Kathryn Coons for her coordination, management, and assistance in putting this book together.

Foreword

It is often stated that three "revolutions" in the last 30 years have resulted in percutaneous coronary intervention becoming the dominant revascularization modality for most patients with ischemic heart disease, namely the first balloon angioplasty by Andreas Gruentzig, the introduction of the bare metal stent, and more recently the emergence of drug-eluting stents. However, equally as important, but not as widely recognized, is the fact that evolutionary advances in adjunct pharmacotherapy have been the foundation for our subspecialty's progress. Without doubt, contemporary angioplasty could not have achieved its present day record of safety and efficacy without meticulous attention to antiplatelet and antithrombotic medication use in the catheterization laboratory. Recently it has been recognized that iatrogenic bleeding complications can seriously impair the early and late prognosis of patients undergoing percutaneous coronary intervention, mandating in-depth knowledge of the alternatives available to safely suppress the ischemic complications arising from coronary artery disease (or of the angioplasty itself) while minimizing hemorrhagic risk. Moreover, the interventionalist must be prepared and able to medically manage an unparalleled range of conditions, ranging from diabetes and chronic kidney disease to complications such as hypotension, arrhythmias, and anaphylaxis. Indeed, the modern interventional cardiologist must also be a hematologist, pharmacologist, endocrinologist, nephrologist, pulmonologist, and critical care specialist, a daunting task. Given the scope and impact of cardiovascular disease, we are blessed with an extraordinary amount of evidence-based medicine from which to draw to advantage our patients, but are simultaneously cursed with the professional and ethical responsibility to stay current with this vast quantity of information (which is constantly evolving). In this regard, the current book edited by Dr. Ron Waksman (with contributions from the world's authorities in this field) will prove of great value to all physicians and health care providers involved in the care of patients with coronary artery disease undergoing an invasive management strategy. Unlike other texts on percutaneous coronary intervention, the present work focuses on the appropriate utilization of adjunct pharmacotherapy, with a thorough discussion of the risk–benefit ratio for each condition and agent. Without doubt, a systematic understanding of the principles outlined in this book will allow the physician to individualize treatment decisions for each patient and condition, and optimize clinical outcomes for patients with coronary artery disease undergoing percutaneous coronary intervention.

Gregg W. Stone, MD
Professor of Medicine
Columbia University Medical Center
New York, NY, USA

Preface

The 'information age' is upon us and while an interested reader can easily locate information on anything from music to medicine, it is the *quality* of that information that's essential. Cardiovascular pharmacology and therapeutics have been subject to an enormous amount of change and evolution during the last decade. Cardiologists today prescribe medications that perhaps were not available to most of them during their training. These medications have complex mechanisms of action, pharmacokinetics, indications, contraindications, and drug–drug interactions. *Pharmacology in the Catheterization Laboratory* aims to meet the growing demand of medical professionals for complete, detailed, and accurate cardiac pharmacology information.

The editors have committed themselves to making the book a useful tool for those coping with the many changes inherent to modern medicine. It provides in-depth evaluation of the specific types of pharmacological agents utilized in the cardiac catheterization laboratory as well as those routinely prescribed for cardiac patients. Specifically, the book evaluates drugs with respect to their cellular and physiological actions, prescribed usage, dosages, adverse reactions, cautions and common routes of administration. Early chapters discuss anticoagulation therapies, such as low molecular weight heparin and fondaparinux, along with antiplatelet therapies such as clopidogrel and the novel prasugrel. Subsequent sections discuss percutaneous coronary intervention and its possible complications, post-procedure pharmacotherapy, and anticoagulation anomalies. In the book's index, emphasis is placed on drug classification, routes of administration, modes of action, indications and contraindications, treatments of adverse reactions, normal dosage, and drug effects on patient hemodynamics.

The strength of *Pharmacology in the Catheterization Laboratory* lies in the knowledge, experience, and judgment of its numerous contributors from around the world; and we would like to thank them all.

PART I

Elective PCI anticoagulation therapy/thrombin inhibitors

CHAPTER 1

Optimal antithrombotic therapy

Michel E. Bertrand
University of Lille, Lille, France

Over the last 25 years, percutaneous coronary intervention (PCI) has been shown to be a very effective method of myocardial revascularization in humans. Improvements in the design of the equipment and increased investigator experience have resulted in a high level of primary procedural success (~99%). However, PCI is inherently thrombogenic, and an optimal antithrombotic treatment is mandatory before, during, and after elective PCI.

Rationale for an optimal antithrombotic therapy

The primary mechanism of PCIs is related to endothelial denudation and extensive disruption of the media, leading to dissection and flaps. Subendothelial components (e.g., collagen, fibronectin, and von Willebrandt factor) are recognized by platelet surface receptors (e.g., GP Ib), and platelet adhesion occurs. This adhesion to the vessel wall activates the platelets, which are able to release from their alpha granules a number of substances, leading to vasoconstriction, chemotaxis, mitogenesis, and platelet aggregation. Aggregated platelets accelerate the production of thrombin by offering the surface for binding cofactors required for the conversion of prothrombin to thrombin, which ultimately catalyzes the conversion of fibrinogen to

fibrin. There is also an immediate release of tissue factor (extrinsic pathway) that is able to induce thrombin formation. Reciprocally, thrombin formation is also an important stimulus for platelet aggregation. The final consequence is a red-stabilized thrombus that is able to create an abrupt acute occlusion of the dilated vessel.

In the early stages of PCI , abrupt closure was not uncommon and occurred in 3.9–8.3% of the cases (1–3). Later, stent implantation resolved this shortcoming of PCI and the number of emergency bypass operations was markedly reduced to around 0.3%. Nevertheless, the metallic prosthesis is highly thrombogenic with a risk of acute and subacute stent thrombosis. Thus, it is mandatory to prescribe an optimal antithrombotic treatment that is based on antithrombinic and antiplatelet drugs.

Antithrombinic drugs

The group of antithrombinic drugs includes indirect antithrombins (unfractionated or low-molecular-weight heparin [LMWH]) and direct antithrombins (bivalirudin or pentasaccharide).

Unfractionated heparin (UHF)

Unfractionated heparin (UHF) needs an antithrombin III cofactor, may not inhibit clot-bound thrombin, and has an unpredictable antithrombin effect with nonlinear kinetics. In addition, UFH activates the platelet and is able to create heparin-induced thrombocytopenia (HIT). At the beginning

Pharmacology in the Catheterization Laboratory. Edited by Ron Waksman and Andrew E Ajani. © 2010 Blackwell Publishing, ISBN: 978-1-4051-5704-9.

of angioplasty, the use of UHF was empirical with a systematic injection of a standard dose (10,000 IU) at the beginning of the procedure. An additional dose of 5,000 IU was injected after each additional hour. Later, it was shown that 10–20% of patients were not adequately anticoagulated and that it was necessary to monitor the activated clotting time (ACT). The pooled data of six randomized, controlled trials (2), in which UHF was the control arm, showed that in 5,216 patients an ACT in the range of 350–375 s provided the lowest ischemic event rate. With an ACT ranging from 350 to 375 s, there was a 34% relative risk reduction in 7-day ischemic event when compared to ACT values of 171–295 s.

Low-molecular-weight heparin

Among numerous LMWH compounds, enoxaparin was the most often used compound in the catheterization laboratory. LWMH compounds have a selective anti-Xa activity and a predictable antithrombin effect with fixed dose–weight adjustment. In addition, monitoring is not necessary. Many small nonrandomized studies or registries have described the effects of decreasing doses (from 1 to 0.5 mg/kg) of IV enoxaparin during PCI. In addition, a meta-analysis (3) of randomized clinical trials including 2,005 patients have shown a similar efficacy of UFH and IV enoxaparin. The SYNERGY (4) trial compared enoxaparin to UFH in 10,027 high-risk patients with acute coronary syndromes (92% underwent catheterization and 46% were treated with PCIs). The results showed that enoxaparin was not superior but was at least as effective as UHF, but with the additional risk of significantly more bleedings. The results were distorted as a number of patients were admitted with a prior antithrombinic treatment and a meta-analysis (5) performed from several trials without prior. Antithrombotic treatment showed a small but significant benefit and that enoxaparin was as safe as UHF, at least on the basis of blood transfusion. The most important trial in the field of PCI is the STEEPLE trial (6). This is a randomized trial of 3,258 patients comparing three antithrombotic regimens during elective PCI performed via a femoral approach. The enoxaparin group included patients receiving 0.75 mg/kg IV and a second group receiving 0.5 mg/kg IV. They

were compared to a group of patients receiving 70–100 IU/kg of UFH if no GP IIb/IIIa was administered. On the contrary, the dose was reduced to 50–70 mg/kg when GP IIb/IIIa was given. The patients receiving UFH were monitored with a targeted ACT of 300–350 s in the first group and 200–300 s. In the case of GP IIb/IIIa administration. STEEPLE (6) was a safety trial and showed that 0.5 mg/kg of enoxaparin was safer than UFH with a significant 57% relative risk reduction of major bleedings from 2.8% to 1.2% ($p = 0.005$) (Figure 1.1). There was no significant difference in terms of ischemic complications but the trial did not address this issue. In addition, less than 20% of the patients receiving UFH reached the targeted ACT while 80% of the patients receiving enoxaparin reached the targeted anti-Xa activity.

Intravenous enoxaparin (0.5 mg/kg) is safer than UFH, is simpler to administer, does not require monitoring, and the same dose might be given when GP IIb/IIIa is also administered. The sheath can be removed at the end of the procedure. Radial approach combined with enoxaparin leads to very low level of major bleedings (0.8%).

Direct antithrombin inhibitors

Direct antithrombin inhibitors do not require a co-factor and are not inhibited by PF-4 or antiheparin proteins. They are effective against clot-bound thrombin without stimulation of platelet aggregation. Finally, they induce predictable anticoagulation without risk of thrombocytopenia. Among the different compounds (hirudin, desirudin, lepirudin, argatroban), bivalirudin was extensively studied in PCI and acute coronary syndromes. Bivalirudin is a polypeptide of 20 amino acids, inducing a reversible direct antithrombin effect, with a half-life of 25 min. The first trials (BAT (7), CACHET (8), REPLACE-1 (9)) suggested the interest of this drug during PCI and this was clearly established by the REPLACE-2 trial. This trial enrolled 6,000 patients undergoing urgent or elective PCI who were randomized in two groups: Bivalirudin (0.75 mg/kg bolus + 1.75 mg/kg/h of procedure) + provisional GP IIb/IIIa inhibitors (abciximab or eptifibatide). The second arm of the study included patients treated by UFH (65 IU/kg) plus GP IIb/IIIa receptor inhibitors (abciximab or eptifibatide). Both groups received aspirin + clopidogrel. Stent

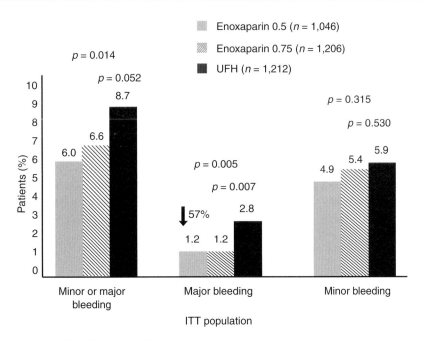

Figure 1.1 Results of the STEEPLE trial: non CABG related bleedings.

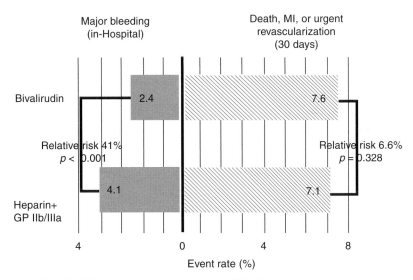

Figure 1.2 Results of the REPLACE-2 trial: net clinical outcome and bleedings.

implantation was performed in 85% of the study population. At 30 days, there were no significant differences between heparin + GPI and bivalirudin for a quadruple endpoint (including major ischemic complications [death, MI, urgent revascularization] and major bleeding). But there was a significant reduction in the rate of major bleeding (from 4.1% to 2.4%, $p < 0.001$) (Figure 1.2). All hemorrhagic endpoints (access site, major organ, and need for transfusion) were significantly reduced ($p < 0.001$). At 1 year of follow-up, the reduction in major bleedings has an impact on the net clinical outcome and particularly on the total mortality of high-risk (unstable angina and diabetics) or elderly patients. Thus this trial has validated bivalirudin as an alternative anticoagulant in PCI.

Fondaparinux

Fondaparinux is a synthetic selective inhibitor of factor Xa. It has been evaluated in two recent trials in patients presenting with acute coronary syndromes. It has never been studied in patients undergoing elective PCI and will be described in Chapter 4.

Antiplatelet drugs

These drugs include aspirin, thienoyridines, and GP IIb/IIIa receptor blockers.

Aspirin

Aspirin irreversibly blocks the cyclooxygenase activity. Since the early beginning of angioplasty, aspirin is advocated to be administered before the procedure, and Gruentzig recommended giving 160–325 mg p.o., at least 1–2 days prior to elective percutaneous transluminal coronary angioplasty (PTCA). Sometimes, interventional cardiologists use an IV injection of 300 mg immediately at the onset of the procedure.

ADP receptor antagonists

ADP receptor antagonists include ticlopidine and clopidogrel. Ticlopidine was shown to be superior to placebo in elective PCI (10,11) with a significant lower rate of acute complications after balloon angioplasty. Later, the combination of aspirin and ticlopidine was consistently superior to full anticoagulation with vitamin K antagonists or aspirin alone (12–15). Thus ticlopidine associated with aspirin became the standard of care in stented patients. However, ticlopidine induced a number of side effects with GI and skin problems and also severe leucopenia. Owing to a faster onset of action and a better safety demonstrated in the CLASSICS trial (16), clopidogrel has replaced ticlopidine and soon became the most frequently used thienopyridine. Initially, a loading dose of 300 mg was given at the moment of stent implantation followed by 75 mg/day during 1 month.

Later, the strategy for clopidogrel was implemented with the results of the CREDO (17) trial. This study of 2,116 patients (stable angina 44% of patients) compared aspirin 325 mg vs clopidogrel 300 mg LD/75 mg/day plus aspirin. The drugs were given 3–24 h before the elective procedure and pursued for 1 year. CREDO (17) was able to demonstrate two important points:

a The combination of aspirin and clopidogrel given for 1 year significantly decreases the rate of major complications (death, MI, and stroke) from 11.5% to 8.5% or a relative risk reduction of 22% ($p = 0.02$).

b In addition, CREDO (17) was able to arrive at the precise duration of the pre-PCI treatment: initially it was shown that patients receiving the dual antiplatelet treatment for more than 6 h before the procedure had a strong benefit with a 38.2% of relative reduction of MACE at 30 days (5.8% instead of 9.4%) ($p = 0.05$). Later it was shown that the cut-off was around 15 h.

Other trials conducted in nonelective procedures and in patients with acute coronary syndromes (ST or non-ST segment elevation ACS) have confirmed the importance of the dual antiplatelet treatment. Some trials conducted in high-risk patients have suggested a higher loading dose of 600 mg owing to a faster action and a higher level of platelet inhibition.

Glycoprotein IIb/IIIa receptor antagonists

Glycoprotein IIb/IIIa receptor is the most abundant integrin on the platelet surface. Platelet adhesion and aggregation determine conformational changes of these receptors, allowing ligand binding (fibrinogen, fibronectin, and von Willebrandt factor). Fibrinogen is the most potent ligand forming bridges between the platelets, leading to aggregation.

GPI can be divided into two main groups: (1) Small molecules (eptifibatide and tirofiban) with a low molecular weight (ranging from 500 to 800). They have a half-life of 2–2.5 h and the reversibility of the platelet inhibition is obtained 6–7 h after drug discontinuation. (2) Abciximab is a monoclonal antibody with a half-life of 10–15 min but the reversibility of platelet inhibition is achieved after 36 h.

Seven trials have been conducted with GP IIb/IIIa receptor inhibitors and the pooled data show a significant reduction of death or MI from 8.8% to 5.6% ($p < 0.000000001$). The TARGET (18) trial has compared, in patients undergoing elective stenting, a small molecule, namely tirofiban, to abciximab. This trial of 4,300 patients showed the superiority of abciximab over tirofiban at

30 days with a significant reduction of the primary endpoint (death, MI, and urgent target vessel revascularization [TVR]) but with similar results at 6 months (19). The rate of major bleeding was similar between the two groups although minor bleeding and thrombocytopenia occurred less frequently among tirofiban-treated patients.

Finally, a number of trials have demonstrated the benefits of GP IIb/IIIa receptor inhibitors in high-risk patients with acute coronary syndromes (non-ST-ACS). These data will be extensively described in the following chapters. Interestingly, a meta-analysis by Roffi (20) showed a great benefit even in terms of mortality rate reduction in diabetic patients. However, more recent, contemporary trials challenge this somewhat particular finding. A pooled analysis of GP IIb/IIIa and all PCI trials (17,793 patients) by Chew and Moliterno (21) demonstrated a 34% reduction of death and MI (from 8.5% to 5.6%).

Optimal antithrombotic strategy in elective PCI

This strategy has been defined in the ACC/AHHA (22) and European Society of Cardiology guidelines (23). Table 1.1 summarizes the main points.

However, special cases should be mentioned, particularly those of patients admitted with prior antithrombotic treatment (UFH, LMWH). In general, switching from one antithrombotic treatment to another is not recommended. Association of UHF and LMWH is not strongly recommended (higher risk of bleeding). However, a post hoc analysis of the ACUITY trial showed that switching from any heparin (either enoxaparin or UFH) to bivalirudin monotherapy was not associated with an increased risk for ischemic events. Furthermore, switch to bivalirudin provided to the patients the 50% bleeding advantage of bivalirudin when compared with consistent therapy on UFH or enoxaparin.

Table 1.1 Optimal antithrombotic–elective PCI.

	ESC Guidelines		ACC/AHA Guidelines	
Before an elective PCI procedure in CAD stable patients				
Aspirin				
Patients not chronically pretreated	500 mg before or 300 mg IV beginning	IB	300–325 mg	IA
Patients chronically pretreated			75–325 mg	IA
Clopidogrel	300 mg day before if not 600 mg, 2 h before	IC	300 mg at least 6 h before	IA
During the procedure				
Unfractionated heparin				IC
No injection of GP IIb/IIIa	100 IU/kg (ACT 250–300 s)			
If injection de GP IIb/IIIa	50–60 IU/kg (ACT 200–250 s)			
Enoxaparin	0.5 mg/kg	?		?
Bivalirudin: as an alternative to UFH				IB
Bivalirudin to treat HIT		IC		IB
GP IIb/IIIa				
Complex lesions, threatening/actual closure, no or slow reflow		IIaC		
Patients undergoing stent placement				IB
After the procedure				
Aspirin	for life (100 mg)	IB	for life	
Clopidogel 75 mg				
Bare metallic stent	1 month	IA	1 month	IB
Drug-eluting stents	6–12 months	IC	3 months (SES) 6 months (PES)	IB
Vascular brachytherapy	12 months	IC	12 months	IB

Conclusions

Optimal antithrombotic management in elective PCI has markedly changed over time. Since the empirical administration of a systematic standard dose of UFH as given at the beginning of angioplasty, the strategy has been considerably improved. This improvement is the result of trials demonstrating the benefit at the price of lower risk of bleeding. This is also based on a better assessment of bleeding risk following the identification of the predictive factors of this important complication. Nevertheless, this domain is rapidly evolving and changes might again occur in the near future.

References

1 Lincoff AM, Popma JJ, Ellis SG, Hacker JA, Topol EJ. Abrupt vessel closure complicating coronary angioplasty: clinical, angiographic and therapeutic profile. *J Am Coll Cardiol.* 1992;**19**:926–935.

2 Chew DP, Bhatt DL, Lincoff AM, *et al.* Defining the optimal activated clotting time during percutaneous coronary intervention: aggregate results from 6 randomized, controlled trials. *Circulation.* 2001;**103**:961–966.

3 Borentain M, Montalescot G, Bouzamondo A, Choussat R, Hulot JS, Lechat P. Low-molecular-weight heparin vs. unfractionated heparin in percutaneous coronary intervention: a combined analysis. *Catheter Cardiovasc Interv.* 2005;**65**:212–221.

4 Ferguson JJ, Califf RM, Antman EM, *et al.* Enoxaparin vs unfractionated heparin in high-risk patients with non-ST-segment elevation acute coronary syndromes managed with an intended early invasive strategy: primary results of the SYNERGY randomized trial. *JAMA.* 2004;**292**: 45–54.

5 Petersen JL, Mahaffey KW, Hasselblad V, *et al.* Efficacy and bleeding complications among patients randomized to enoxaparin or unfractionated heparin for antithrombin therapy in non-ST-Segment elevation acute coronary syndromes: a systematic overview. *JAMA.* 2004;**292**: 89–96.

6 Montalescot G, White HD, Gallo R, *et al.* Enoxaparin versus unfractionated heparin in elective percutaneous coronary intervention. *N Engl J Med.* 2006;**355**: 1006–1017.

7 Bittl JA, Chaitman BR, Feit F, Kimball W, Topol EJ. Bivalirudin versus heparin during coronary angioplasty for unstable or postinfarction angina: final report reanalysis of the Bivalirudin Angioplasty Study. *Am Heart J.* 2001;**142**:952–959.

8 Lincoff AM, Kleiman NS, Kottke-Marchant K, *et al.* Bivalirudin with planned or provisional abciximab versus low-dose heparin and abciximab during percutaneous coronary revascularization: results of the Comparison of Abciximab Complications with Hirulog for Ischemic Events Trial (CACHET). *Am Heart J.* 2002;**143**:847–853.

9 Lincoff AM, Bittl JA, Kleiman NS, *et al.* Comparison of bivalirudin versus heparin during percutaneous coronary intervention (the Randomized Evaluation of PCI Linking Angiomax to Reduced Clinical Events [REPLACE]-1 trial). *Am J Cardiol.* 2004;**93**:1092–1096.

10 Bertrand M, Allain H, Lablanche J. Results of a randomised trial of Ticlopidine versus placebo for prevention of acute closure and restenosis after coronary angioplasty (PTCA). The TACT study. *Circulation.* 1990;**82**(suppl III): III–190.

11 White C, Chaitman BR, Knudtson M, Chisholm R. Antiplatelet agents are effective in reducing the acute ischemic complications of angioplasty but do not prevent restenosis: results from the ticlopidine trial. *Coron Artery Dis.* 1991;**2**:757–767.

12 Schomig A, Neumann FJ, Kastrati A, *et al.* A randomized comparison of antiplatelet and anticoagulant therapy after the placement of coronary-artery stents [see comments]. *N Engl J Med.* 1996;**334**:1084–1089.

13 Bertrand M, Legrand V, Boland J, *et al.* Randomized multicenter comparison of conventional anticoagulation versus antiplatelet therapy in unplanned and elective coronary stenting. The full anticoagulation versus aspirin and ticlopidine (Fantastic) study. *Circulation.* 1998;**98**:1597–1603.

14 Leon M, Baim DS, Popma JJ, *et al.* A clinical trial comparing three antithrombotic-drug regimens after coronary-artery stenting. Stent Anticoagulation Restenosis Study Investigators. *N Engl J Med.* 1998;**339**:1665–1671.

15 Urban P, Macaya C, Rupprecht HJ, *et al.* Randomized evaluation of anticoagulation versus antiplatelet therapy after coronary stent implantation in high-risk patients: the multicenter aspirin and ticlopidine trial after intracoronary stenting (MATTIS). *Circulation.* 1998;**98**:2126–2132.

16 Bertrand ME, Rupprecht HJ, Urban P, Gershlick AH, Investigators, FT. Double-blind study of the safety of clopidogrel with and without a loading dose in combination with aspirin compared with ticlopidine in combination with aspirin after coronary stenting: the clopidogrel aspirin stent international cooperative study (CLASSICS). *Circulation.* 2000;**102**:624–629.

17 Steinhubl SR, Berger PB, Mann JT, 3rd, *et al.* Early and sustained dual oral antiplatelet therapy following percutaneous coronary intervention: a randomized controlled trial. *JAMA.* 2002;**288**:2411–2420.

18 Topol EJ, Moliterno DJ, Herrmann HC, *et al.* Comparison of two platelet glycoprotein IIb/IIIa inhibitors, tirofiban and abciximab, for the prevention of ischemic events with percutaneous coronary revascularization. *N Engl J Med.* 2001;**344**:1888–1894.

19 Moliterno DJ, Yakubov SJ, DiBattiste PM, *et al.* Outcomes at 6 months for the direct comparison of tirofiban and abciximab during percutaneous coronary revascularisation with stent placement: the TARGET follow-up study. *Lancet.* 2002;**360**:355–360.

20 Roffi M, Chew DP, Mukherjee D, *et al.* Platelet glyco-protein IIb/IIIa inhibitors reduce mortality in diabetic patients with non-ST-segment-elevation acute coronary syndromes. *Circulation.* 2001;**104**:2767–2771.

21 Chew DP, Moliterno DJ. A critical appraisal of plate-let glycoprotein IIb/IIIa inhibition. *J Am Coll Cardiol.* 2000;**36**:2028–2035.

22 Smith SC, Jr, Feldman TE, Hirshfeld JW, Jr, *et al.* ACC/AHA/SCAI 2005 guideline update for percutaneous cor-onary intervention: a report of the American College of Cardiology/American Heart Association Task Force on Practice Guidelines (ACC/AHA/SCAI Writing Committee to Update 2001 Guidelines for Percutaneous Coronary Intervention). *Circulation.* 2006;**113**:e166–e286.

23 Silber S, Albertsson P, Aviles FF, *et al.* Percutaneous coro-nary interventions. Guidelines of the European Society of Cardiology-ESC. *Kardiol Pol.* 2005;**63**:265–320; dis-cussion 321–323.

CHAPTER 2

Low molecular weight heparin in the catheterization laboratory

Yuri B. Pride[1], JoEllyn M. Abraham[2], &
C. Michael Gibson[1,3]

[1]Harvard Medical School, Boston, MA, USA
[2]Cleveland Clinic, Cleveland, OH, USA
[3]TIMI Data Coordinating Center, Boston, MA, USA

Low molecular weight heparin (LMWH) has become an important class of antithrombins that rivals unfractionated heparin (UFH) in the prevention and treatment of both arterial and venous thrombosis. There are currently three LMWHs approved for use in the United States as alternatives to UFH: enoxaparin, dalteparin, and tinzaparin. The efficacy of enoxaparin in the prevention of postoperative deep vein thrombosis (DVT) was first reported in 1982 (1,2) and its use began in Europe. Enoxaparin was approved in the United States in 1993, followed by dalteparin in 1994 and tinzaparin in 2000. Only enoxaparin and dalteparin have the approval of the Federal Drug Administration (FDA) for use in unstable angina and non-ST-segment elevation myocardial infarction (NSTEMI), and enoxaparin has a further indication for use in ST-segment elevation myocardial infarction (STEMI) as an adjunctive treatment during fibrinolytic therapy. Bemiparin, certoparin, nadroparin, and reviparin are other LMWHs that are not approved for use in the United States (Table 2.1). Globally, LMWHs are used approximately as frequently as UFH for acute coronary syndrome (ACS) but UFH is the most common antithrombin used in the United States, and LMWHs are the most common antithrombins used in Europe (3,4).

Table 2.1 Comparison of low-molecular-weight-heparin preparations.

	Mean molecular weight (Da)	Anti-Xa: anti-IIa ratio
Bemiparin	3,600	8.0
Certoparin	5,600	2.4
Dalteparin	6,000	2.7
Enoxaparin	4,200	3.8
Nadroparin	4,500	3.6
Reviparin	4,000	3.5
Tinzaparin	4,500	1.9

Structure and mechanisms of action

Like UFH, LMWHs are polysulfated glycosaminoglycans. LMWHs are produced by controlled enzymatic or chemical depolymerization of UFH to yield chains that have molecular weight between 2,000 and 9,000. UFH, by comparison, has polysaccharide chains that range in molecular weight from between 3,000 to 30,000. The LMWHs are not clinically interchangeable as they are prepared by different methods (5).

Both UFH and LMWH are considered to be indirect anticoagulants as they require the plasma cofactor antithrombin (AT) in order to function as anticoagulants (Figure 2.1). Both UFH and LMWH have a unique pentasaccharide sequence that is distributed along the heparin chains. This sequence binds to AT, causing a conformational change in

Pharmacology in the Catheterization Laboratory. Edited by Ron Waksman and Andrew E Ajani. © 2010 Blackwell Publishing, ISBN: 978-1-4051-5704-9.

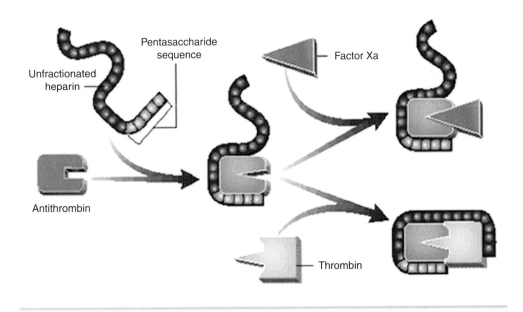

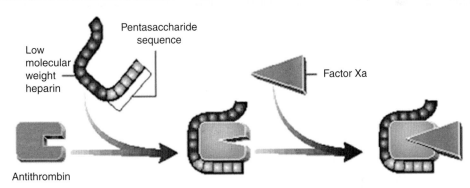

Figure 2.1 Unfractionated heparin and low-molecular-weight heparins catalyze antithrombin-mediated inactivation of thrombin and factor Xa. Reprinted with permission from Weitz (6). Copyright © 1997 Massachusetts Medical Society. All rights reserved.

AT that accelerates its interaction with thrombin and factor Xa (activated factor X). As shown in Figure 2.1, the mechanistic difference between UFH and LMWH is based on their relative ability to inhibit thrombin and factor Xa. While a pentasaccharide-containing heparin chain of any length can bind to AT and subsequently inactivate factor Xa, only a longer chain of at least 18 saccharide units can bind to both antithrombin and thrombin and create a ternary complex (6). Based on its relatively longer chain lengths, UFH has equivalent inhibition of factor Xa and thrombin, while LMWH has relatively shorter heparin chains and thus greater inhibition of factor Xa. The superior proximal Xa inhibition

of LMWH leads to decreased thrombin generation and a decrease in rebound thrombosis, which can be seen following the administration of UFH (7).

There are at least three additional potential pharmacological advantages of LMWH. First, LMWH is associated with less tissue factor pathway inhibitor depletion, which in the case of UFH has been shown to cause rebound hypercoagulability. Second, LMWH is associated with less platelet aggregation and platelet–endothelial interactions, leading to a lower incidence of heparin-induced thrombocytopenia and thrombosis syndrome (HITTS). Third, LMWH has been shown to cause superior attenuation of the increase of von Willebrand Factor (vWF) in ACS as compared to UFH, which can cause elevations in vWF in ACS and thus an increased potential for thrombosis (7).

Pharmacokinetics and metabolism

LMWH has minimal propensity to bind to plasma proteins, endothelial cells, and macrophages (8). Its bioavailability approaches 100% and its dose-independent clearance leads to a more predictable anticoagulant response than that of UFH (5). The plasma half-life of LMWH is 2–4 h after intravenous administration and 3–6 h after subcutaneous administration compared to the half-life of 1 to 2 h for UFH. This allows for intermittent intravenous or subcutaneous administration of LMWH without continuous infusion. It is renally cleared, as opposed to UFH, which is cleared by both hepatic and renal mechanisms.

Dosing

For ACS and STEMI, enoxaparin is dosed at 1 mg/kg (up to 100 mg per dose) given subcutaneously every 12 h. As an adjunctive treatment to fibrinolysis, enoxaparin is administered at 30 mg intravenously plus 1 mg/kg subcutaneously 15 min prior to or 30 min following fibrinolytic administration and then continued at 1 mg/kg subcutaneously every 12 h to be continued for 8 days or until hospital discharge. If given prior to percutaneous coronary intervention (PCI), the dosing is the same as for prior to fibrinolysis but the IV bolus is not given if the last enoxaparin dose was given <8 h prior to PCI and administered until the patient is stabilized. In patients >75 years old, the dosing is 0.75 mg/kg SC every 12 h (up to 75 mg per dose) and intravenous administration is not recommended as an adjunct to fibrinolysis. For patients with renal insufficiency who have a creatinine clearance of <30 mL/min, the dosing is 1 mg/kg subcutaneously daily.

Dalteparin has an indication for use in UA and NSTEMI but not for STEMI. The dosing is 120 U/kg subcutaneously every 12 h (up to 10,000 U per dose) to be given for 5–8 days. There are no manufacturer guidelines for modified dosing in elderly patients or those with underlying renal dysfunction. Both enoxaparin and dalteparin should be used in addition to aspirin unless there is a clear contraindication to its use.

Monitoring

Laboratory monitoring of LMWH is unnecessary except in high-risk patients, such as patients who are underweight or obese, patients who have renal insufficiency (which would cause prolongation of anti-Xa activity), and patients who are pregnant (who have been found to have lower than usual anti-Xa activity for the recommended dose) (7). LMWH does not significantly affect the partial thromboplastin time or activated clotting time and thus anti-Xa activity has been used as a surrogate for assessment of anticoagulation. For PCI, the therapeutic range for LMWH is anti-Xa 0.6–1.8 IU/mL. The recommended time for performing the assay is 4 h after administration as the anti-factor Xa activity peaks at approximately this time (5). In patients with severe renal insufficiency, UFH may be a safer choice than LMWH.

Side effects

As with any drug that interferes with the coagulation pathway, the major side effect of LMWH is bleeding. One limitation of the use of LMWH is that there is no antidote that has been consistently shown to neutralize its action in the case of bleeding. Protamine, which is used to reverse anticoagulation with heparin, has been shown to neutralize only 60% of the antifactor Xa activity of LMWH due to decreased protamine binding to lower-molecular-weight chains (5). Nonetheless, if reversal is necessary because of active bleeding and LMWH was administered within the previous 8 h, protamine can be administered at a dose of 1 mg per mg of enoxaparin administered. A second dose of protamine can be administered at 0.5 mg for every 1 mg of enoxaparin given if the bleeding persists. Smaller doses of protamine can be used if LMWH was administered more than 8 h prior to the event requiring anticoagulation reversal (5).

HITTS is less common with the use of LMWH as compared to UFH. The mechanism of HITTS with the use of UFH is that UFH causes platelet factor 4 (PF4) to be released from platelets. UFH then forms a complex with PF4 and in some patients antibodies are made to the complexes. The activity of these antibodies against platelets is the underlying mechanism in HITTS. LMWH has a lower affinity for both platelets and PF4, which results in the formation of fewer complexes. Nonetheless, some complexes are formed and HITTS has been reported following LMWH use. In addition, LMWH should not be used in patients with a history of HITTS (8).

While long-term treatment with heparin has been shown to cause osteoporosis as the result of heparin binding osteoblasts with subsequent osteoclast activation, the risk of osteoporosis is lower with LMWH. It is thought that this is reflective of the lower affinity of LMWH for osteoblasts (8).

Clinical evidence and current recommendations for use

LMWH for UA/NSTEMI

The American College of Cardiology/American Heart Association (ACC/AHA) 2007 guidelines for the management of patients with UA/NSTEMI suggest that UFH and LMWH are essentially equivalent except in the case of a patient in whom an initial conservative strategy is selected, in which case enoxaparin or fondaparinux are preferable to UFH (Class IIa, Level B) (9).

Early experience with LMWHs (10–12) led to two pivotal trials that examined the safety and efficacy of enoxaparin in patients presenting with UA/NSTEMI. The Efficacy and Safety of Subcutaneous Enoxaparin in Non-Q-Wave Coronary Events (ESSENCE) trial randomized 3,171 patients to UFH or enoxaparin for at least 48 h (13). At 14 days, the incidence of death, MI, or recurrent angina was significantly lower in patients randomized to enoxaparin than those receiving UFH (16.6% vs 19.8%, $p = 0.019$), and this difference remained significant at 30 days (19.8% vs 23.3%, $p = 0.016$). There was no significant difference in major bleeding (6.5% vs 7.0%, $p = $ NS), although the incidence of any bleeding event was significantly higher in the enoxaparin group (18.4% vs 14.2%, $p = 0.001$), primarily reflecting an increase in injection-site ecchymosis. The Thrombolysis

in Myocardial Infarction (TIMI) 11B trial randomized 3,910 patients to either UFH or enoxaparin and again showed that patients treated with enoxaparin had fewer adverse cardiovascular events (death, MI or urgent revascularization) at 8 days (12.4% vs 14.5%, $p = 0.048$) and 43 days (17.3% vs 19.7%, $p = 0.048$) with no difference in the incidence of major bleeding (14).

The Superior Yield of the New Strategy of Enoxaparin, Revascularization and GP IIb/IIIa Inhibitors (SYNERGY) trial randomized 10,027 patients presenting with NSTE-ACS and high-risk features undergoing an early invasive strategy to UFH or enoxaparin (15). More than half received a GP IIb/IIIa inhibitor and two-thirds received clopidogrel or ticlopidine. Patients randomized to enoxaparin were found to have equivalent incidence of death or nonfatal MI by 30 days compared to patients randomized to UFH (14.0% vs 14.5%, $p = $ NS). Rates of acute complications, including abrupt closure, threatened abrupt closure, unsuccessful PCI and emergency CABG surgery, were similar between groups. Unlike previous studies, a significantly higher incidence of major bleeding (9.1% vs 7.6%, $p = 0.008$) was reported in the enoxaparin group.

LMWH for STEMI

The 2004 ACC/AHA guidelines for the management of patients with STEMI suggest LMWH might be considered an acceptable alternative to UFH as ancillary therapy for patients aged <75 years undergoing fibrinolytic therapy provided they do not have underlying renal dysfunction (Class IIb, Level B) (16). There is still a paucity of data comparing UFH to LMWH in the context of PCI for STEMI.

It was not until 2001 that the first randomized trial comparing the use of enoxaparin to UFH as adjunctive treatment to fibrinolytic administration for STEMI was reported. The data comparing LMWH to UFH as adjunctive treatment to fibrinolysis is mixed. In the Second Trial of Heparin and Aspirin Reperfusion Therapy (HART II) trial, 400 consecutive patients with STEMI received aspirin and tissue t-PA and were randomized to enoxaparin or UFH for at least 3 days (17). There were no differences in arterial patency at 90 min (80.1% vs 75.1%), but a trend toward lower 1-week graft occlusion rates with enoxaparin (5.9% vs 9.8%, $p = 0.12$). In-hospital major bleeding and death at 30 days were equivalent between groups (3.6% vs 3.0% and 4.5% vs 5.0%, respectively).

The Assessment of the Safety and Efficacy of a New Thrombolytic Regimen (ASSENT)-3 trial radomized 6,095 patients with STEMI who were to undergo fibrinolytic therapy with tenecteplase to one of the three regimens: (1) full-dose tenecteplase plus enoxaparin, (2) full-dose tenecteplase plus UFH or half-dose tenecteplase plus low-dose UFH, and (3) a 12-h infusion of abciximab (18). In contrast to the HART II trial, the composite incidence of 30-day mortality, in-hospital reinfarction, and in-hospital refractory ischemia was significantly reduced with enoxaparin as compared to UFH (11.4% vs 15.4%, $p = 0.0002$), even when in-hospital major bleeding was added to the composite endpoint (13.7% vs 17.0%, $p = 0.0037$). Similarly, the Enoxaparin and Thrombolysis Reperfusion for Acute Myocardial Infarction Treatment (EXTRACT)-TIMI 25 study randomized 20,506 patients to enoxaparin or UFH following fibrinolytic therapy (19). The outcomes of this study also favored enoxaparin in terms of a composite of death or nonfatal recurrent MI within 30 days (9.9% vs 12.0%, $p < 0.001$) and nonfatal reinfarction alone (3.0% vs 4.5%, $p < 0.001$), and there was a trend toward decreased mortality (6.9% vs 7.5%, $p = 0.11$). However, major bleeding at 30 days was significantly higher in the enoxaparin group (2.1% vs 1.4%, $p < 0.001$).

LMWH for Elective PCI

To date, there are very few studies that have evaluated the relative safety and efficacy of LMWH, as compared to UFH, for elective PCI. One recent study prospectively compared enoxaparin to UFH in the setting of elective PCI and found that an intravenous bolus of 0.5 mg/kg of enoxaparin was associated with reduced rates of bleeding (5.9% vs 8.5%, $p = 0.01$) and an intravenous bolus of 0.75 mg/kg was associated with equivalent rates of bleeding (6.5% vs 8.5%, $p = 0.051$) compared to UFH (20). The study was not powered to evaluate efficacy, although interestingly the 0.5 mg/kg arm was terminated as the result of an increase in mortality in that group that was later found not to be

significant. Future studies are needed to evaluate the efficacy of LMWH for elective PCI.

Summary

LMWHs have specific advantages over UFH, including less induction of platelet aggregation, more consistent pharmacokinetics, ease of administration, and a lower incidence of HITTS. In the setting of NSTE-ACS, LMWHs appear to be slightly more efficacious in reducing ischemic outcomes, namely recurrent MI and urgent revascularization while being associated with a slight increase in the incidence of nonmajor bleeding. In STEMI patients undergoing fibrinolytic administration, enoxaparin has a similar efficacy advantage over UFH, but may be associated with an increase in major bleeding incidences. The use of LMWHs has not been rigorously evaluated in the setting of elective PCI.

References

1 Kakkar VV, Djazaeri B, Fok J, Fletcher M, Scully MF, Westwick J. Low-molecular-weight heparin and prevention of postoperative deep vein thrombosis. *Br Med J (Clinical Research Ed)*. 1982;**284**(6313):375–379.

2 Thomas DP, Merton RE, Lewis WE, Barrowcliffe TW. Studies in man and experimental animals of a low molecular weight heparin fraction. *Thromb Haemost.* 1981;**45**(3):214–218.

3 Klein W, Kraxner W, Hodl R, et al. Patterns of use of heparins in ACS. Correlates and hospital outcomes: the Global Registry of Acute Coronary Events (GRACE). *Thromb Haemost.* 2003;**90**(3):519–527.

4 Budaj A, Brieger D, Steg PG, et al. Global patterns of use of antithrombotic and antiplatelet therapies in patients with acute coronary syndromes: insights from the Global Registry of Acute Coronary Events (GRACE). *Am Heart J.* 2003;**146**(6):999–1006.

5 Hirsh J, Raschke R. Heparin and low-molecular-weight heparin: the Seventh ACCP Conference on Antithrombotic and Thrombolytic Therapy. *Chest.* 2004;**126**(3 Suppl):188S–203S.

6 Weitz JI. Low-molecular-weight heparins. *N Engl J Med.* 1997;**337**(10):688–698.

7 Wong GC, Giugliano RP, Antman EM. Use of low-molecular-weight heparins in the management of acute coronary artery syndromes and percutaneous coronary intervention. *JAMA.* 2003;**289**(3):331–342.

8 De Caterina R, Husted S, Wallentin L, et al. Anticoagulants in heart disease: current status and perspectives. *Eur Heart J.* 2007;**28**(7):880–913.

9 Anderson JL, Adams CD, Antman EM, *et al*. ACC/AHA 2007 guidelines for the management of patients with unstable angina/non-ST-Elevation myocardial infarction-executive summary a report of the American College of Cardiology/American Heart Association task force on practice guidelines (Writing Committee to Revise the 2002 Guidelines for the Management of Patients with Unstable Angina/Non-ST-Elevation Myocardial Infarction) developed in collaboration with the American College of Emergency Physicians, the Society for Cardiovascular Angiography and Interventions, and the Society of Thoracic Surgeons Endorsed by the American Association of Cardiovascular and Pulmonary Rehabilitation and the Society for Academic Emergency Medicine. *J Am Coll Cardiol.* 2007;**50**(7): 652–726.

10 Nurmohamed MT, Rosendaal FR, Buller HR, *et al*. Low-molecular-weight heparin versus standard heparin in general and orthopaedic surgery: a meta-analysis. *Lancet.* 1992;**340**(8812):152–156.

11 Gurfinkel EP, Manos EJ, Mejail RI, *et al*. Low molecular weight heparin versus regular heparin or aspirin in the treatment of unstable angina and silent ischemia. *J Am Coll Cardiol.* 1995;**26**(2):313–318.

12 Low-molecular-weight heparin during instability in coronary artery disease, Fragmin during Instability in Coronary Artery Disease (FRISC) study group. *Lancet.* 1996;**347**(9001):561–568.

13 Cohen M, Demers C, Gurfinkel EP, *et al*. A comparison of low-molecular-weight heparin with unfractionated heparin for unstable coronary artery disease. Efficacy and Safety of Subcutaneous Enoxaparin in Non-Q-Wave Coronary Events Study Group. *N Engl J Med.* 1997;**337**(7):447–452.

14 Antman EM, McCabe CH, Gurfinkel EP, *et al*. Enoxaparin prevents death and cardiac ischemic events in unstable angina/non-Q-wave myocardial infarction. Results of the thrombolysis in myocardial infarction (TIMI) 11B trial. *Circulation.* 1999;**100**(15):1593–1601.

15 Ferguson JJ, Califf RM, Antman EM, *et al*. Enoxaparin vs unfractionated heparin in high-risk patients with non-ST-segment elevation acute coronary syndromes managed with an intended early invasive strategy: primary results of the SYNERGY randomized trial. *JAMA.* 2004;**292**(1):45–54.

16 Antman EM, Anbe DT, Armstrong PW, *et al*. ACC/AHA guidelines for the management of patients with ST-elevation myocardial infarction: a report of the American College of Cardiology/American Heart Association Task Force on Practice Guidelines (Committee to Revise the 1999 Guidelines for the Management of Patients with Acute Myocardial Infarction). *Circulation.* 2004;**110**(9):e82–e292.

17 Ross AM, Molhoek P, Lundergan C, *et al*. Randomized comparison of enoxaparin, a low-molecular-weight heparin, with unfractionated heparin adjunctive to recombinant tissue plasminogen activator thrombolysis and aspirin: second trial of Heparin and Aspirin Reperfusion Therapy (HART II). *Circulation.* 2001;**104**(6):648–652.

18 Efficacy and safety of tenecteplase in combination with enoxaparin, abciximab, or unfractionated heparin: the ASSENT-3 randomised trial in acute myocardial infarction. *Lancet.* 2001;**358**(9282):605–613.

19 Antman EM, Morrow DA, McCabe CH, *et al*. Enoxaparin versus unfractionated heparin with fibrinolysis for ST-elevation myocardial infarction. *N Engl J Med.* 2006;**354**(14):1477–1488.

20 Montalescot G, White HD, Gallo R, *et al*. Enoxaparin versus unfractionated heparin in elective percutaneous coronary intervention. *N Engl J Med.* 2006;**355**(10):1006–1017.

CHAPTER 3

Direct thrombin inhibitor: Bivalirudin

Michele D. Voeltz & Steven V. Manoukian
Sarah Cannon Research Institute, Nashville, TN, USA

Introduction

Bivalirudin (Angiomax®; The Medicines Company, Parsippany, NJ), a direct thrombin inhibitor (DTI), was initially approved in the United States by the Food and Drug Administration (FDA) in December 2000 (1). Since that time, a number of clinical trials have confirmed the efficacy and safety of bivalirudin and its indications and clinical use in cardiovascular disease continue to expand. Because of its unique properties and mechanism of action, bivalirudin avoids many of the pitfalls of more traditional anticoagulant and antiplatelet therapies, including heparin (unfractionated and low molecular weight) and glycoprotein IIb/IIIa inhibitors (GPI). This chapter intends to review the pharmacology, clinical uses, and existing data for bivalirudin in cardiovascular disease.

Pharmacology

Thrombin (factor IIa), an essential component of the clotting cascade, is produced in response to vascular injury (2). It is derived from the proteolytic cleavage of prothrombin (factor II) following activation of both the intrinsic and extrinsic clotting cascades and leads to the conversion of fibrinogen to fibrin (3,4). Fibrin is then cross-linked to form

Pharmacology in the Catheterization Laboratory. Edited by Ron Waksman and Andrew E Ajani. © 2010 Blackwell Publishing, ISBN: 978-1-4051-5704-9.

the latticework of thrombus. In addition to its effect on fibrin conversion, thrombin increases leukocyte chemotaxis, vasoconstriction, and platelet aggregation (5–7).

There are three potential binding sites available for the inhibition of thrombin (3). The first is the active catalytic site, which binds to some DTIs. The second, exosite-1, ensures proper substrate orientation, and binds fibrinogen, fibrin, and some DTIs. Finally, exosite-2 binds indirect thrombin inhibitors, including heparin (both unfractionated and low-molecular-weight) (8,9).

DTIs are categorized based upon two important variables, their reversibility, and the number of thrombin sites to which they bind. Bivalirudin, as suggested by its name, is a reversible, bivalent inhibitor of thrombin, binding to both the catalytic site and exosite-1 (10,11). Bivalirudin is a synthetic, 20-amino acid peptide with a molecular weight of 2,180 Da, which, once bound to both circulating and clot-bound thrombin, is slowly cleaved at the active site, leading to restoration of normal thrombin function and a half-life of approximately 25 min among patients with normal renal function (1,12). Additionally, bivalirudin effectively inhibits the binding of thrombin to the protease-activated receptor on platelets, thus preventing platelet activation, secretion of granule contents (such as adenosine diphosphate, serotonin, and thromboxane α2), and activation of GPI receptors (13). When administered by intravenous infusion, bivalirudin demonstrates linear pharmacokinetics, limiting the need for repeated activated clotting time (ACT) measurements over time (12).

In contrast to bivalirudin, the inhibition of thrombin by heparins (both unfractionated and low molecular weight) is indirect and mediated by circulating antithrombin, rendering it less effective against clot-bound thrombin (14). Furthermore, unfractionated heparin binds plasma proteins and does not demonstrate linear pharmacokinetics, requiring repeated ACT measurements over time and providing an unreliable degree of anticoagulation per dose administered.

Clinical uses

Bivalirudin is currently approved for (1) patients undergoing percutaneous coronary intervention (PCI), (2) patients with non-ST-elevation acute coronary syndromes (ACS), and (3) patients with heparin-induced thrombocytopenia (HIT) undergoing PCI. In the ACC/AHA/SCAI 2005 guideline update for PCI, bivalirudin receives a Class IIa indication for use in low-risk patients undergoing elective PCI, and a Class I indication in PCI patients with a history of HIT (15). With regard to use in ACS in patients being treated with an early invasive strategy, bivalirudin as a primary anticoagulant receives a Level of Evidence B (16). In this group of patients, the omission of GPI receives a Class IIa indication when bivalirudin is selected as the antithrombotic therapy in PCI.

For PCI, the recommended dosing regimen for bivalirudin is a 0.75 mg/kg intravenous bolus, followed by an infusion of 1.75 mg/kg/h for the duration of the PCI procedure (12). An ACT is recommended at 5 min, with an additional 0.3 mg/kg bolus if required. Continuation of bivalirudin for 4 h postprocedure at the aforementioned infusion rate is optional. After 4 h, the dose should be decreased to 0.2 mg/kg/h for up to a total infusion time of 24 h as needed. These continued infusions of bivalirudin post-PCI as mentioned are rarely employed clinically. Because it is partially renally cleared, dose reduction of bivalirudin should be considered in patients with significant renal impairment as follows: 1.0 mg/kg/h in patients with creatinine clearance <30 cc/min and 0.25 mg/kg/h in patients on hemodialysis with no reduction in bolus dose. For initial medical treatment in patients with non-ST-elevation ACS, the recommended dose is 0.1 mg/kg bolus followed by 0.25 mg/kg/h infusion. Dosing during PCI (after initial medical treatment) is a 0.5 mg/kg bolus at the beginning of the PCI and an increase in infusion rate to 1.75 mg/kg/h for the duration of the procedure (16).

Clinical trials

Bivalirudin has been evaluated in more than 24,000 patients in a number of randomized, controlled trials. The following section will review recent clinical studies evaluating its efficacy and safety.

Bivalirudin in PCI

The Bivalirudin Angioplasty Trial (BAT), published in 2001, was a randomized, controlled, double-blind trial, which compared bivalirudin with heparin during and after percutaneous transluminal coronary angioplasty in 4,312 patients with unstable angina (17). Overall, the trial revealed a reduction in the rate of the composite end point of death, MI, or revascularization at 7 days among patients treated with bivalirudin vs heparin (6.2% vs 7.9%, $p = 0.039$). Major hemorrhagic events occurred significantly less frequently with bivalirudin vs heparin (3.5% vs 9.3%, $p < 0.001$). Furthermore, among post-MI patients with angina ($N = 741$), there was a 51% relative risk reduction in death, MI, or revascularization at 7 days ($p = 0.009$). The favorable performance of bivalirudin in this landmark study resulted in its FDA approval and sparked further evaluation.

Published in 2003, the Randomized Evaluation in PCI Linking Angiomax to Reduced Clinical Events-2 (REPLACE-2) Trial compared the use of bivalirudin with provisional GPI to heparin with planned GPI in 6,010 patients undergoing elective or urgent PCI (18). The primary end point was a composite of death, MI, urgent revascularization, and major bleeding at 30 days. This noninferiority trial revealed no difference in this composite end point between bivalirudin with provisional GPI and heparin with planned GPI (9.2% vs 10.0%, $p = $ ns). However, bivalirudin with provisional GPI exhibited a superior safety profile, with significantly lower rates of major (2.4% vs 4.1%, $p < 0.001$) and minor (13.4% vs 25.7%, $p < 0.001$) hemorrhage, blood transfusion (1.7% vs 2.5%, $p = 0.021$), and thrombocytopenia with platelet count <100 K/mm (0.7% vs 1.7%,

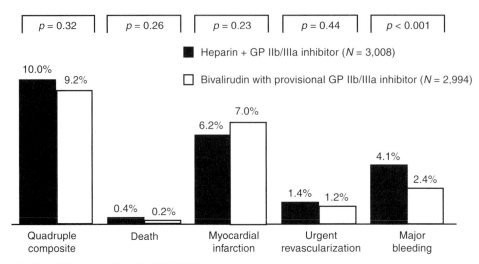

Figure 3.1 Overall 30-day results of the REPLACE-2 trial.

$p < 0.001$), compared to heparin with planned GPI. A summary of the 30-day results of REPLACE-2 is illustrated in Figure 3.1.

Several subgroup analyses have studied the efficacy and safety of bivalirudin in a variety of populations undergoing PCI in the REPLACE-2 trial. Chacko and colleagues evaluated outcomes in women and reported similar reductions in hemorrhagic events and equivalent ischemic end points among women treated with bivalirudin vs heparin plus GPI (19). Similarly, Chew *et al.* reported that patients with renal impairment demonstrated fewer hemorrhagic events and comparable rates of ischemic complications when treated with bivalirudin (20). Voeltz *et al.* reported a 44% relative reduction in the risk of major hemorrhage and similar ischemic event rates when bivalirudin was compared to heparin with GPI in the high-risk anemic population (21). Finally, an evaluation of 1,624 diabetic patients revealed no difference in the incidence of major bleeding or ischemic complications and a reduction in minor bleeding events for bivalirudin versus heparin plus GPI (22).

In REPLACE-2, major hemorrhage and blood transfusion were an independent predictors of mortality at 1 year (Odds Ratio [95% Confidence Interval], *p*-value; 2.66 [1.44–4.20], $p = 0.001$) and (4.26 [2.25–8.08], $p < 0.0001$) (23–25). An evaluation of hemorrhagic outcomes in REPLACE-2 by Feit *et al.* reported that treatment with a heparin plus GPI vs bivalirudin was an independent predictor

of major bleeding (1.97 [1.37–2.84], $p = 0.0003$) (26). With regard to the impact of bivalirudin on long-term mortality, an analysis performed by Lincoff and colleagues reported comparable 1-year outcomes with bivalirudin plus provisional GPI and heparin plus planned GPI with a nonsignificant trend toward decreased mortality in patients treated with bivalirudin (27). The REPLACE-2 trial emphasized the important role of bleeding and transfusion in mortality in patients undergoing PCI and confirmed that treatment with bivalirudin with provisional GPI results in significant reductions in major hemorrhage when compared to heparin with planned GPI.

Bivalirudin in acute coronary syndromes

The Acute Catheterization and Urgent Intervention Triage strategY (ACUITY) Trial enrolled 13,819 moderate- to high-risk patients with non-ST-elevation ACS and was performed at 450 centers in 17 countries. Patients with ACS were randomized to one of three treatment groups: (1) heparin (unfractionated or low molecular weight) plus GPI, (2) bivalirudin plus GPI, or (3) bivalirudin alone (28). The primary end points for the trial were a composite ischemia end point (death, MI, and unplanned revascularization for ischemia), major bleeding (noncoronary artery bypass graft surgery [CABG]-related), and the net clinical outcome (defined as the combination of composite ischemia or major bleeding) at 30 days. Overall, the frequency of the composite ischemic endpoint was similar when heparin plus GPI was compared to bivalirudin alone (7.3% vs 7.8%, *p* = ns) or compared to bivalirudin plus GPI (7.3% vs 7.7%, *p* = ns). In contrast, major bleeding complications were significantly less frequent with bivalirudin alone compared to heparin plus GPI (3.0% vs 5.7%, *p* < 0.001), but similar between the GPI-containing regimens. Significant reductions were also seen for

bivalirudin alone compared to heparin plus GPI in rates of major bleeding by the Thrombolysis in Myocardial Infarction (TIMI) bleeding criteria. Importantly, major bleeding was associated with higher rates of composite ischemia (23.1% vs 6.8%, *p* < 0.0001) and stent thrombosis (3.4% vs 0.6%, *p* < 0.0001), and was an independent predictor of mortality at 30 days (7.55 [4.68–12.18], *p* < 0.0001) (29). A summary of the 30-day results of ACUITY is illustrated in Figure 3.2.

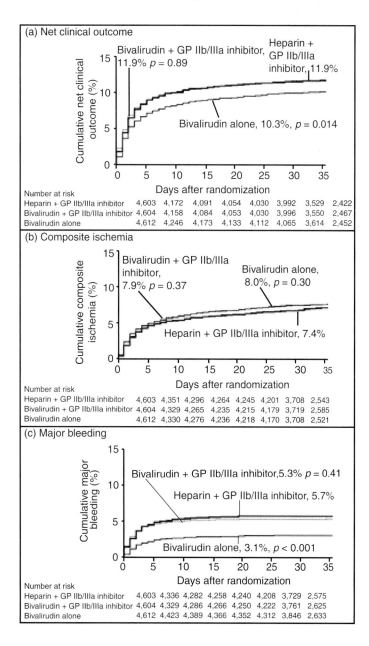

Figure 3.2 Overall 30-day results of the ACUITY trial.

In the 7,789 patients from the ACUITY trial undergoing PCI who were evaluated individually, the results were similar. Non-CABG-related major bleeding was significantly more common among patients treated with a heparin plus GPI compared with bivalirudin alone (6.8% vs 3.5%, $p < 0.0001$) (30). Among this subgroup, major bleeding was associated with a dramatic increase in the aforementioned ischemic composite end point as well as its individual components of death, MI, or urgent revascularization (31).

A recent evaluation of long-term outcomes in ACUITY revealed no significant difference in composite ischemia or mortality at 1 year in moderate- and high-risk ACS patients treated with any of the three therapies studied (32).

Bivalirudin in acute myocardial infarction

The Bivalirudin in the Management of Patients with ST-Segment Elevation Acute Myocardial Infarction Undergoing Primary PCI (BIAMI) Trial was a single-group pilot study evaluating the efficacy and safety of bivalirudin in 201 patients with STEMI treated with primary PCI. The primary composite end point of the study, which included death, MI, repeat revascularization, or disabling cerebrovascular event at 30 days, occurred in 4.1% of patients (33). At 6 months follow-up, the rate of major adverse cardiac events (MACE) was 8.9%.

Because of the favorable performance of bivalirudin in the BIAMI study, a randomized controlled trial evaluating the use of bivalirudin plus provisional GPI versus heparin plus planned GPI, the Harmonizing Outcomes with Revascularization and Stents (HORIZONS) Trial was launched. Stone and colleagues, at the Transcatheter Cardiovascular Therapeutics (TCT) 2007 meeting, reported a 24% reduction in net adverse clinical events, a composite of MACE and major hemorrhage (9.2% vs 12.1%, $p = 0.006$) and a 40% reduction in major hemorrhage (4.9% vs 8.3%, $p < 0.0001$) in patients treated with bivalirudin plus provisional GPI vs heparin plus GPI. Furthermore, mortality rates at 30 days were significantly lower for bivalirudin versus heparin plus GPI (2.1% vs 3.1%, $p < 0.05$). Although yet to be published, these preliminary data appear to indicate that bivalirudin is effective and safe among patients with acute ST-elevation MI.

Bivalirudin in peripheral vascular intervention

Several preliminary trials have evaluated the role of bivalirudin in percutaneous peripheral interventions. The largest of these, a 505-patient, multicenter, prospective study called the Angiomax Peripheral Procedure Registry of Vascular Events (APPROVE) Trial, enrolled patients undergoing renal, iliac, and femoral percutaneous transluminal angioplasty using bivalirudin alone (34). This trial reported a procedural success rate of 95%, with few ischemic events (1.4%), and a low rate of major and minor hemorrhage (2.2% and 0.4%, respectively). Overall, the evaluation reported favorable early results using bivalirudin in peripheral interventions; however, randomized, controlled data in this area are currently lacking.

Conclusion

Bivalirudin is a novel direct thrombin inhibitor, which is safe and effective in a number of clinical scenarios including PCI and non-ST-elevation ACS. Furthermore, preliminary data indicate that a role may exist for the use of bivalirudin in acute ST-elevation MI and percutaneous peripheral intervention. Because of its unique pharmacologic profile and reversible binding, bivalirudin offers an alternative to other antithrombotic agents, including heparins and GPI, while reducing rates of hemorrhagic complications while maintaining antiischemic efficacy.

References

1 *Angiomax Prescribing Information;* 2005.

2 Nawarskas JJ, Anderson JR. Bivalirudin: a new approach to anticoagulation. *Heart Dis.* 2001;**3**(2):131–137.

3 Weitz JI, Bates ER. Direct thrombin inhibitors in cardiac disease. *Cardiovasc Toxicol.* 2003;**3**(1):13–25.

4 White CM. Thrombin-directed inhibitors: pharmacology and clinical use. *Am Heart J.* 2005;**149**(1 Suppl): S54–S60.

5 Bar-Shavit R, Kahn A, Fenton JW, 2nd, Wilner GD. Chemotactic response of monocytes to thrombin. *J Cell Biol.* 1983;**96**(1):282–285.

6 Bar-Shavit R, Kahn A, Wilner GD, Fenton JW, 2nd. Monocyte chemotaxis: stimulation by specific exosite region in thrombin. *Science.* 1983;**220**(4598):728–731.

7 Gurm HS, Bhatt DL. Thrombin, an ideal target for pharmacological inhibition: a review of direct thrombin inhibitors. *Am Heart J*. 2005;**149**(1 Suppl):S43–S53.

8 Fortenberry YM, Whinna HC, Gentry HR, Myles T, Leung LL, Church FC. Molecular mapping of the thrombin-heparin cofactor II complex. *J Biol Chem*. 2004;**279**(41):43237–43244.

9 Sheehan JP, Wu Q, Tollefsen DM, Sadler JE. Mutagenesis of thrombin selectively modulates inhibition by serpins heparin cofactor II and antithrombin III. Interaction with the anion-binding exosite determines heparin cofactor II specificity. *J Biol Chem*. 1993;**268**(5):3639–3645.

10 Parry MA, Maraganore JM, Stone SR. Kinetic mechanism for the interaction of Hirulog with thrombin. *Biochemistry*. 1994;**33**(49):14807–14814.

11 Witting JI, Bourdon P, Brezniak DV, Maraganore JM, Fenton JW, 2nd. Thrombin-specific inhibition by and slow cleavage of hirulog-1. *Biochem J*. 1992;**283**(Pt 3): 737–743.

12 Moen MD, Keating GM, Wellington K. Bivalirudin: a review of its use in patients undergoing percutaneous coronary intervention. *Drugs*. 2005;**65**(13):1869–1891.

13 Coughlin SR. Thrombin signalling and protease-activated receptors. *Nature*. 2000;**407**(6801):258–264.

14 Carswell CI, Plosker GL. Bivalirudin: a review of its potential place in the management of acute coronary syndromes. *Drugs*. 2002;**62**(5):841–870.

15 Smith SC, Jr, Feldman TE, Hirshfeld JW, Jr, *et al*. ACC/AHA/SCAI 2005 guideline update for percutaneous coronary intervention: a report of the American College of Cardiology/American Heart Association Task Force on Practice Guidelines (ACC/AHA/SCAI Writing Committee to Update 2001 Guidelines for Percutaneous Coronary Intervention). *Circulation*. 2006;**113**(7):e166–e286.

16 Anderson JL, Adams CD, Antman EM, *et al*. ACC/AHA 2007 guidelines for the management of patients with unstable angina/non-ST-Elevation myocardial infarction: a report of the American College of Cardiology/American Heart Association Task Force on Practice Guidelines (Writing Committee to Revise the 2002 Guidelines for the Management of Patients with Unstable Angina/Non-ST-Elevation Myocardial Infarction) developed in collaboration with the American College of Emergency Physicians, the Society for Cardiovascular Angiography and Interventions, and the Society of Thoracic Surgeons endorsed by the American Association of Cardiovascular and Pulmonary Rehabilitation and the Society for Academic Emergency Medicine. *J Am Coll Cardiol*. 2007;**50**:e1–e157.

17 Bittl JA, Chaitman BR, Feit F, Kimball W, Topol EJ. Bivalirudin versus heparin during coronary angioplasty for unstable or postinfarction angina: Final report reanalysis of the Bivalirudin Angioplasty Study. *Am Heart J*. 2001;**142**(6):952–959.

18 Lincoff AM, Bittl JA, Harrington RA, *et al*. Bivalirudin and provisional glycoprotein IIb/IIIa blockade compared with heparin and planned glycoprotein IIb/IIIa blockade during percutaneous coronary intervention: REPLACE-2 randomized trial. *JAMA*. 2003;**289**(7): 853–863.

19 Chacko M, Lincoff AM, Wolski KE, *et al*. Ischemic and bleeding outcomes in women treated with bivalirudin during percutaneous coronary intervention: a subgroup analysis of the Randomized Evaluation in PCI Linking Angiomax to Reduced Clinical Events (REPLACE)-2 trial. *Am Heart J*. 2006;**151**(5):1032 e1–1032 e7.

20 Chew DP, Lincoff AM, Gurm H, *et al*. Bivalirudin versus heparin and glycoprotein IIb/IIIa inhibition among patients with renal impairment undergoing percutaneous coronary intervention (a subanalysis of the REPLACE-2 trial). *Am J Cardiol*. 2005;**95**(5):581–585.

21 Voeltz MD, Feit F, Stone GW, Manoukian SV. Anemia and outcomes in acute coronary syndromes. *Acute Coronary Syndromes*. 2005;**7**:47–55.

22 Gurm HS, Sarembock IJ, Kereiakes DJ, *et al*. Use of bivalirudin during percutaneous coronary intervention in patients with diabetes mellitus: an analysis from the randomized evaluation in percutaneous coronary intervention linking angiomax to reduced clinical events (REPLACE)-2 trial. *J Am Coll Cardiol*. 2005;**45**: 1932–1938.

23 Attubato MJ, Feit F, Bittl JA, *et al*. Major hemorrhage is an independent predictor of 1 year mortality following percutaneous coronary intervention: an analysis from REPLACE-2. *Am J Cardiol*. 2004;**94**(6 Suppl 1):39E.

24 Stone GW, Bertrand M, Colombo A, *et al*. Acute Catheterization and Urgent Intervention Triage strategY (ACUITY) trial: study design and rationale. *Am Heart J*. 2004;**148**(5):764–775.

25 Manoukian SV, Voeltz MD, Attubato MJ, *et al*. Bivalirudin reduces the risk of transfusion and associated mortality in patients undergoing percutaneous coronary intervention. *Cardiovascular Revascularization Therapies*. 2005.

26 Feit F, Voeltz MD, Attubato MJ, *et al*. Predictors and impact of major hemorrhage on mortality following percutaneous coronary intervention from the REPLACE-2 trial. *Am J Cardiol*. 2007;**100**:1364–1369.

27 Lincoff AM, Kleiman NS, Kereiakes DJ, *et al*. Long-term efficacy of bivalirudin and provisional glycoprotein IIb/IIIa blockade vs heparin and planned glycoprotein IIb/IIIa blockade during percutaneous coronary revascularization: REPLACE-2 randomized trial. *JAMA*. 2004;**292**(6):696–703.

28 Stone GW, McLaurin BT, Cox DA, *et al*. Bivalirudin for patients with acute coronary syndromes. *N Engl J Med*. 2006;**355**(21):2203–2216.

29 Manoukian SV, Feit F, Mehran R, *et al.* Impact of major bleeding on 30-day mortality and clinical outcomes in patients with acute coronary syndromes: an analysis from the ACUITY trial. *J Am Coll Cardiol.* 2007;**49**(12):1362–1368.

30 Stone GW, White HD, Ohman EM, *et al.* Bivalirudin in patients with acute coronary syndromes undergoing percutaneous coronary intervention: a subgroup analysis from the Acute Catheterization and Urgent Intervention Triage strategy (ACUITY) trial. *Lancet.* 2007;**369**(9565):907–919.

31 Manoukian S, Voeltz MD, Feit F, *et al.* Major bleeding is associated with increased 30-day mortality and ischemic complications in patients with non-ST elevation acute coronary syndromes undergoing percutaneous coronary intervention: the ACUITY trial. *Am J Cardiol.* 2006;**98**(Suppl A):45M.

32 Stone GW, Ware JH, Bertrand ME, *et al.* Antithrombotic strategies in patients with acute coronary syndromes undergoing early invasive management: one-year results from the ACUITY trial. *JAMA.* 2007;**298**:2497–2506.

33 Stella J, Stella R, Stella D, *et al.* The use of bivalirudin in the management of patients with ST-segment elevation acute myocardial infarction undergoing primary PCI (BIAMI) trial: in-hospital, 30-day, and 6-month results. *Cathet Cardiovasc Interv.* 2006;**67**:751(abstract A-34).

34 Allie DE, Hall P, Shammas NW, *et al.* The Angiomax Peripheral Procedure Registry of Vascular Events trial (APPROVE): in-hospital and 30-day results. *J Invasive Cardiol.* 2004;**16**(11):651–656.

CHAPTER 4

Fondaparinux in the cardiac catheterization laboratory

Michael D. White & Richard C. Becker
Duke University Medical Center, Durham, NC, USA

Anticoagulant therapy in the cardiac catheterization laboratory is of paramount importance to prevent the formation of thrombus on equipment and nonbiological surfaces that have been introduced into the coronary arterial circulation. The mainstay of therapy worldwide is unfractionated heparin due to a vast experience, clinician familiarity with monitoring, defined dosing and intensity of anticoagulation, ease of administration, and very low cost. Heparin interacts with antithrombin III through a specific pentasaccharide sequence, inducing a conformational change in the protein. Through this mechanism, antithrombin III becomes activated and its affinity for thrombin is enhanced by 1,000-fold. Antithrombin III and thrombin then form a complex, which is essentially irreversible and neutralizes the effects of factors IXa, Xa, XIa, and thrombin (Figure 4.1a) (1).

Fondaparinux, a highly sulfated and synthetic polysaccharide whose chemical structure, with the exception of the *O*-methyl group present on the reducing end, is identical to the pentasaccharide sequence isolated after the enzymatic cleavage of heparin (2). Fondaparinux does not bind to nor can it inactivate factor IIa (thrombin) directly (3). The 5-unit monosaccharide structure of the molecule is well short of the length required to form

a ternary complex that is able to bind both antithrombin III and thrombin. Accordingly, fondaparinux is considered an indirect, selective factor Xa inhibitor (4–6) (Figure 4.1b).

Pharmacology

Fondaparinux binds to antithrombin III with high affinity and increases its rate of factor Xa inhibition by 300-fold. The dissociation constant is 36 ± 11 nM in a 1:1 stoichiometric relationship (3,4). The interaction between factor Xa and antithrombin III is irreversible; however, this is not the case for antithrombin III and fondaparinux, in which each molecule of fondaparinux can bind to and activate antithrombin III, then dissociate, and activate other molecules. Endogenous circulating antithrombin III is the rate-limiting step for the factor Xa-inhibiting activity of fondaparinux. In addition, due to the synthetic and highly specialized structure of the molecule, fondaparinux does not interact with other endothelium-based cellular elements or plasma proteins, including platelet factor 4 (4,7).

After subcutaneous injection, fondaparinux is 100% bioavailable. The time for half-maximal and maximal serum concentrations is 25 min and 1.7 h, respectively (8) (Figure 4.2). The half-life of fondaparinux is between 17 and 21 h, which allows the drug to be dosed in a once daily fashion (9,10). The majority of drug is excreted unchanged in the urine; therefore, in vivo metabolism has not

Pharmacology in the Catheterization Laboratory. Edited by Ron Waksman and Andrew E Ajani. © 2010 Blackwell Publishing, ISBN: 978-1-4051-5704-9.

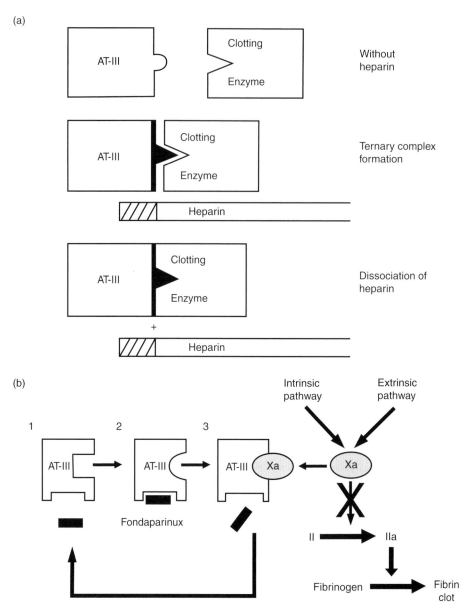

Figure 4.1 (a) Inactivation of clotting enzymes by heparin. Top: AT-III is a slow inhibitor without heparin. Middle: Heparin binds to AT-III through high-affinity pentasaccharide and induces a conformational change in AT-III, thereby converting AT-III from a slow to a very rapid inhibitor. Bottom: AT-III binds covalently to the clotting enzyme, and the heparin dissociates from the complex and can be reused (1). (b) Fondaparinux binds to antithrombin III. The formation of this complex allows for binding of factor Xa and a much higher affinity than thrombin, therefore inhibiting the conversion of factor II to IIa (5).

been studied extensively. In phase II and III clinical studies, fondaparinux was not given to patients with a serum creatinine greater than 1.8 mg/dL. It is contraindicated among patients with a creatinine clearance <30 mL per minute.

Fondaparinux, following either intravenous or subcutaneous administration, does not prolong the activated partial thromboplastin time, prothrombin time, or activated clotting time. Measuring anti-factor Xa levels with an assay calibrated using

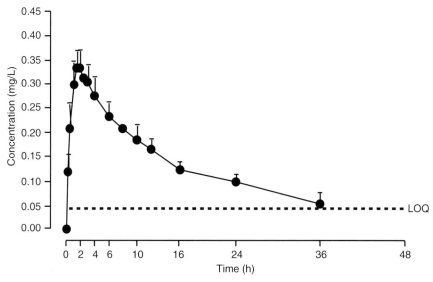

Figure 4.2 Plasma time–concentration profile of fondaparinux in healthy volunteers after a single subcutaneous dose of 2.5 mg (8).

fondaparinux as the reference standard can assess the drug's anticoagulant activity (11).

Clinical studies in coronary artery disease

The fondaparinux Phase II program in coronary artery disease included two studies. The PENTALYSE study compared unfractionated heparin and fondaparinux in patients with ST-segment elevation myocardial infarction (12). All patients received fibrinolytic therapy (tissue-plasminogen activator) and aspirin. They were than randomized, in an open-label fashion, to anticoagulant therapy. The fondaparinux treatment arms were divided into 4 mg (6 mg if >90 kg), 8 mg (6 mg if <60 kg or 10 mg if >90 kg), and 12 mg (10 mg if <60 kg). The standard treatment group received 5,000 units of unfractionated heparin, followed by an infusion of 1,000 units per hour during the first 48–72 h. A total of 81 patients were enrolled in the 4 mg arm, 77 patients in the 8 mg arm, 83 patients in the 12 mg arm, and 85 into the unfractionated heparin arm. According to the study design, fondaparinux was given once daily. On the first day, the dose was given intravenously and then subcutaneously for the remainder of the treatment course of 5–7 days. All the enrolled patients underwent coronary angiography at 90 min and at 5–7 days. Angiographic end points were defined as TIMI grade flow in the infarct-related artery. Clinical end points were all cause mortality, urgent target vessel revascularization, and the incidence of reinfarction. The primary safety end point was the incidence of intracranial hemorrhage or bleeding requiring blood transfusion. Secondary safety end points were any other causes of bleeding. TIMI grade 3 flow rates were similar in all 4 arms at 90 min, ranging from 60% to 68%. In the patients who had TIMI grade 3 flow on the initial angiogram and who did not undergo percutaneous intervention, there was a trend toward less reocclusion of the infarct-related artery in the combined fondaparinux groups (0.9%) as compared to those treated with unfractionated heparin (7.0%, $P = 0.065$). In addition, fewer revascularization procedures were performed during the 30-day follow-up period in patients receiving fondaparinux (39%) versus unfractionated heparin (51%, $P = 0.054$). The incidence of bleeding did not differ significantly across treatment arms.

The PENTUA (Pentasaccharide in Unstable Angina) study was a multicenter, randomized, double-blind dose-ranging study of fondaparinux in patients with unstable angina or non-ST segment myocardial infarction (13). Fondaparinux, administered once daily, was compared with enoxaparin given subcutaneously twice daily. The fondaparinux treatment groups included four dosing strategies (2.5, 4, 8, and 12 mg). Enoxaparin was given at a dose of 1 mg/kg. The primary efficacy end point was the combination of death, myocardial infarction, and recurrent ischemia at day 9. The treatment duration was from 2 to 8 days, with a median of 5 days. The rates of the combined endpoint were 27.9% in the 2.5 mg fondaparinux group, 35.9% in 4 mg group, 34.7% in the 8 mg group, and 30.3% in the 12 mg. The rate in the enoxaparin group was 35.7%. The study demonstrated a low combined event rate, driven primarily by a reduction in recurrent ischemia, in the 2.5 mg fondaparinux group—significantly lower than the enoxaparin group, as well as the 4 and 8 mg groups ($P < 0.05$). There was no difference in bleeding between groups. The observations made in phase II established the 2.5 mg fondaparinux dose as a foundation for phase III studies in acute coronary syndromes.

OASIS-5 (Organization to Assess Strategies in Acute Ischemic Syndromes Investigators-5) was a multicenter, randomized, double-blind, double dummy trial comparing fondaparinux and enoxaparin in patients with unstable angina or non-ST-segment myocardial infarction (14,15) in which 20,078 patients received either fondaparinux 2.5 mg daily or enoxaparin 1 mg/kg twice daily. Patients were included into the study if they met two of the following three criteria: (1) age of

60 years or greater, (2) an elevated level of troponin or creatine kinase MB isoenzyme, or (3) electrocardiographic changes indicating ischemia. The primary efficacy outcome, powered to establish noninferiority, was death, myocardial infarction, or refractory ischemia at 9 days. The primary safety outcome was to determine whether fondaparinux was superior to enoxaparin in the prevention of major bleeding. The primary outcome was reached in 579 of 10,057 patients (5.8%) treated with fondaparinux, and 573 of 10,021 patients (5.7%) receiving enoxaparin- hazard ratio 1.01 with a 95% confidence interval of 0.90–1.13; $P = 0.007$ for noninferiority. The fondaparinux group had a significantly lower rate of bleeding (2.1%) versus the enoxaparin group (4.1%) hazard ratio 0.52 with a 95% confidence interval of 0.44 to 0.61; $P = <0.001$ for superiority (Table 4.1).

The OASIS-6 trial was conducted to evaluate the effect of fondaparinux compared with standard of care treatment in patients with ST-segment elevation MI (16). The multicenter, randomized, double-blind, double dummy trial was divided into two different management stratae. Stratum 1 was fondaparinux compared with placebo for up to 8 days. Stratum 2 was fondaparinux compared with unfractionated heparin for 48 h. Stratum 2 was further subdivided into those patients who received primary percutaneous intervention as the initial treatment modality. The main outcome was a composite of death or reinfarction at 30 days. A total 12,092 patients were enrolled. In the control group

Table 4.1 Aggregate data from all percutaneous interventions performed using fondaparinux.

	Pilot	ASPIRE	ASPIRE	OASIS-5	OASIS-6
Number undergoing cardiac catheterization	61	118	115	3,134	1,890
Number lesions treated	73	162	152	4,417	2,228
Fondaparinux dose (mg IV)	12	2.5	5	2.5 mg SQ	2.5 mg SQ[a]
Total number of events	10	10	7	248	270
Abrubt closure	2	3	0	47	NA
Thrombus	0	6	5	28	NA
Threatened closure	0	0	0	166	NA
Dissection	8	0	0	0	NA
Side branch occlusion	0	1	2	0	NA

[a]OASIS-6 data is reported in totals and not fractionated between the dosing strategies. Only the total number of adverse events was reported.

(a combination of both the placebo and unfractionated heparin arms), 667 of 6,056 (11.2%) met the primary endpoint. In the fondaparinux group, 585 of 6,036 reached the primary endpoint—a statistically significant difference, hazard ratio 0.86; 95% confidence interval, 0.77–0.96; $P = 0.008$. This benefit was limited to patients who did not undergo primary percutaneous intervention. This observation requires further consideration.

Fondaparinux in the cardiac catheterization laboratory

A single, phase II study was performed using fondaparinux, given as an IV bolus of 12 mg, as the sole agent for anticoagulation in the cardiac catheterization laboratory. The outcome measure was acute vessel closure with 48 h of percutaneous coronary intervention. Heparin was contraindicated before, during, and for 24 h following the procedure. A total of 61 patients were enrolled in the pilot study. The primary endpoint was observed in two patients (3.3%). This was similar to the rates observed in patients treated with unfractionated heparin (17).

A larger, more contemporary trial using fondaparinux in the cardiac catheterization laboratory was the Arixtra Study in Percutaneous coronary Intervention: a Randomized Evaluation (ASPIRE) pilot study (18). A total of 350 patients undergoing percutaneous coronary intervention were randomized to receive unfractionated heparin, 2.5 mg fondaparinux, or 5 mg fondaparinux—all via the IV route. The primary efficacy endpoint was a combination of death, myocardial infarction, urgent revascularization, and "bailout" use of a GP IIb/IIIa antagonist. The primary safety outcome was a composite of major (as defined by intracranial, retroperitoneal, or intraocular hemorrhage or a fall in hemoglobin >3.0 g/dL or transfusion of >2 units of blood) and minor bleeding (all other bleeding episodes not categorized as major). One hundred and seventeen patients were randomized to receive unfractionated heparin, 118 received 2.5 mg of fondaparinux, and 115 received 5 mg of fondaparinux. The incidence of bleeding was 7.7% in the unfractionated heparin arm and 6.4% in the combined fondaparinux arms (hazard ratio, 0.81; $P = 0.061$). The overall risk of bleeding was less in the 2.5 mg fondaparinux group (3.4%) as compared with the 5 mg fondaparinux group (9.6%, $P = 0.06$). The combined efficacy outcome was 6.0% in the unfractionated heparin arm and 6.0% in the combined fondaparinux arms. The angiographic data revealed a higher rate of suspected angiographic thrombosis in patients treated with fondaparinux (5.1% in the 2.5 mg arm and 4.3% in the 5 mg arm) compared with those receiving unfractionated heparin (0.9%). This was the first hint of a potential problem with catheter/instrument thrombosis with fondaparinux in the cardiac catheterization laboratory. Despite the increase in angiographic thrombosis, no significant difference in efficacy between fondaparinux and unfractionated heparin were reported.

In both the OASIS-5 and -6 trials, a significant number of patients were brought to the cardiac catheterization laboratory while receiving fondaparinux (19). Of the original 20,078 patients enrolled into the trial, a total of 12,715 underwent cardiac catheterization. The dose of IV study drug administered was determined by the time since administration of the last subcutaneous dose of study, and drug by whether the primary operator provisionally planned a GP IIb/IIIa inhibitor. Reports of guiding catheter thrombosis led to a protocol amendment and investigators were permitted to give "open-label" unfractionated heparin prior to intervention (Table 4.2).

A total of 6,238 patients underwent percutaneous intervention—3,134 in the fondaparinux arm and 3,104 in the enoxaparin arm. The timing of intervention was within 24 h of randomization and up to 8 days following enrollment. The combination of fondaparinux/placebo was given for a mean of 2.4 ± 1.8 days prior to intervention, and enoxaparin/placebo was given for a mean of 2.6 ± 1.8 days prior to intervention. At day 9 in the fondaparinux treatment arm, 6.3% of patients had experienced death, myocardial infarction, or stroke, compared with 6.2% of patients receiving enoxaparin. At day 9, major bleeding occurred in 2.4% and 5.1% of patients, respectively ($P < 0.00001$). Considerable differences in bleeding were a primary determinant of clinical outcomes, including mortality, at later time points. The benefit of fondaparinux was observed irrespective of whether the study drug was resumed following intervention, patient age, renal function, and/or concomitant GP IIb/IIIa inhibitor use.

Table 4.2 PCI-Angiographic outcomes from the OASIS-5 Study.

	No UHF Before PCI		UHF Before PCI	
	Fondparinux	Enoxaparin	Fondaparinux	Enoxaparin
Number randomized	793	810	75	80
Angiographic variables				
Abrupt closure	15	13	1	0
Threatened closure	31	38	4	2
Catheter thrombosis	9	4	1	0

Source: Adapted from (19).

Patients enrolled in OASIS-5 trial experienced catheter thrombosis at a rate less than 1%. While guiding catheter thrombosis occurred in both groups, it was more common in the fondaparinux group with a rate of 0.9% compared with 0.4% in the enoxaparin group. In patients who had received a dose of enoxaparin greater than 6 h before intervention and received unfractionated heparin, the rate decreased to 0.2%, suggesting that additional anticoagulation may offer benefit with LMWH preparations as well. Abrupt closure and threatened abrupt closure occurred with greater frequency among patients given fondaparinux. Irrespective of treatment assignment, patients with catheter-related thrombus experienced higher rates of MI, stroke, and death than those without this complication.

Following the OASIS-5 protocol amendment, use of open-label unfractionated heparin was permitted in the final 1,758 patients who underwent percutaneous intervention. Additional unfractionated heparin was given to 75 patients who were randomized to fondaparinux and 80 patients who had received enoxaparin. The mean dose of unfractionated heparin in the fondaparinux group was 47 IU/kg. There were ten reported cases of guiding catheter thrombosis in the fondaparinux arm after the protocol amendment was initiated. In this cohort, nine patients did not receive any additional unfractionated heparin and one patient received a very low dose. Major hemorrhagic complications remained low even with supplemental heparin administration.

In the OASIS-6 trial a total of 3,788 patients underwent primary percutaneous intervention (13). There were 1,898 patients in the unfractionated heparin/placebo arm and 1,890 patients in the fondaparinux arm. During the percutaneous intervention, 20.8% of the patients in the fondaparinux arm received additional unfractionated heparin. The rates of death and myocardial infarction were not statistically different between the two groups at 30 days. The rate of major bleeding was also similar. However, there was a significantly higher rate of guiding catheter thrombosis (0 vs 22, $P < 0.001$) and coronary artery complications (225 vs 270; $p = 0.04$) with the use of fondaparinux alone. There were 496 patients who received additional unfractionated heparin prior to primary percutaneous intervention. It this subgroup, rates of coronary complications did not differ significantly.

The avoidance of catheter and equipment thrombosis during PCI is an absolute prerequisite for a successful outcome. *Ex vivo* flow models have shown a greater tendency toward catheter thrombus with fondaparinux (compared with enoxaparin and unfractionated heparin), even when combined with eptifibatide (see Schlitt *et al. In-vitro* comparison of fondaparinux, unfractionated heparin, and enoxaparin in preventing cardiac catheter-associated thrombus. *Coron Artery Dis.* 2008;**19**:279–284). The rate constant for factor XIIa inhibition by antithrombin III, in the presence of unfractionated heparin, is slow compared with factor Xa and thrombin. The ability of heparin compounds to prevent thrombosis on artificial surfaces may relate directly to locally achievable drug concentrations, the kinetics of thrombin inhibition, and their inhibitory effect on protein adsorption. The available data suggest, however, that anticoagulants that prevent contact-activated coagulation, including thrombin-mediated bioamplification, are the most effective in preventing thrombotic complications in the cardiac catheterization laboratory (20).

According to the recent update to the ACC/AHA Guidelines for the Treatment of ST-Elevation Myocardial Infarction for patients undergoing primary percutaneous intervention, fondaparinux has a class III indication for the sole anticoagulant used during the procedure. The guidelines recommend using an additional anticoagulant with anti-IIa activity for support during intervention (21).

Conclusion

The predictable pharmacological properties, efficacy, and safety of fondaparinux have made it an attractive treatment option for patients with non-ST segment elevation ACS, particularly for those not undergoing PCI. Patients who are scheduled to undergo percutaneous intervention should receive adjunctive, anticoagulation with unfractionated heparin to minimize the risk of catheter/equipment thrombotic complications (Table 4.1). At this time, there are no evidence-based guidelines for transitioning from fondaparinux to an alternative anticoagulant at the time of PCI, and the number of patients studied in OASIS-5 was modest. A trial, Switching from Fondaparinux to Bivalirudin or Unfractionated Heparin in ACS Patients Undergoing PCI (SWITCHIII) (22), is currently enrolling patients to answer this important question. For patients who present to the cardiac catheterization laboratory after receiving fondaparinux who need percutaneous intervention, unfractionated heparin should be given at doses required to achieve an ACT of at least 200 s. The attractive safety profile and potential efficacy of fondaparinux make it an attractive management option in the broad landscape of clinical practice. The optimal approach to managing patients who require PCI after an initial treatment with fondaparinux is most worthy of additional study.

References

1 Hirsh J, Warkentin TE, Shaughnessy SG, *et al.* Heparin and low- molecular-weight heparin: mechanisms of action, pharmacokinetics, dosing, monitoring, efficacy, and safety. *Chest.* 2001;**119**(1 suppl):64S–94S.

2 Prescribing information for Fondaparinux. Available at http://us.gsk.com/products/assets/us_arixtra.pdf. Accessed April 2, 2008.

3 Danielsson A, Raub E, Lindahl U, Bjork I. Role of ternary complexes, in which heparin binds both antithrombin and proteinase, in the acceleration of the reactions between antithrombin and thrombin or factor Xa. *J Biol Chem.* 1986;**261**:15467.

4 Olson, ST, Bjork, I, Sheffer, R, *et al.* Role of the anti-thrombin-binding pentasaccharide in heparin acceleration of antithrombin-proteinase reactions. Resolution of the antithrombin conformational change contribution to heparin rate enhancement. *J Biol Chem.* 1992;**267**: 12528.

5 Bauer KA. Fondaparinux sodium: a selective inhibitor of factor Xa. *Am J Health Syst Pharm.* 2001;**58**(Suppl 2):S14.

6 Comp PC. Selective factor Xa inhibition improves efficacy of venous thromboembolism prophylaxis in orthopedic surgery. *Pharmacotherapy.* 2003;**23**(6):772–787.

7 Gallus, AS, Coghlan, DW. Heparin pentasaccharide. *Curr Opin Hematol.* 2002;**9**:422.

8 Donat F, Duret JP, Santoni A, *et al.* The pharmacokinetics of fondaparinux sodium in healthy volunteers. *Clin Pharmacokinet.* 2002;**41**(12 suppl):1–9.

9 Bijsterveld NR, Moons AH, Boekholdt SM, *et al.* Ability of recombinant factor VIIa to reverse the anticoagulant effect of the pentasaccharide fondaparinux in healthy volunteers. *Circulation.* 2002;**106**:2550.

10 Bijsterveld NR, Vink R, van Aken BE, *et al.* Recombinant factor VIIa reverses the anticoagulant effect of the long-acting pentasaccharide idraparinux in healthy volunteers. *Br J Haematol.* 2004;**124**:653.

11 Paolucci F, Frasa H, Van Aarle F, *et al.* Two sensitive and rapid chromogenic assays of fondaparinux sodium (Arixtra) in human plasma and other biological matrices. *Clin Lab.* 2003;**124**:451.

12 Coussement PK, Bassand JP, Convens C, *et al.* A synthetic factor-Xa inhibitor (ORG31540/SR9017A) as an adjunct to fibrinolysis in acute myocardial infarction: the PENTALYSE study. *Eur Heart J.* 2001;**22**:1716–1724.

13 Simoons ML, Bobbink IWG, Boland J, *et al.* A dose-finding study of fondaparinux in patients with non-ST-segment elevation acute coronary syndromes: the Pentasaccharide in Unstable Angina (PENTUA) Study. *J Am Coll Cardiol.* 2004;**43**:2183–2190.

14 MICHELANGELO OASIS 5 Steering Committee. Design and rationale of the MICHELANGELO Organization to Assess Strategies in Acute Ischemic Syndromes (OASIS)-5 trial program evaluating fondaparinux, a synthetic factor Xa inhibitor, in patients with non-ST-segment elevation acute coronary syndromes. *Am Heart J.* 2005;**150**: 1107.e1–1107.e10.

15 Yusuf S, Mehta SR, Chrolavicius S, *et al.* Comparison of fondaparinux and enoxaparin in acute coronary syndromes. *N Engl J Med.* 2006;**354**:1464–1476.

16 Yusuf S, Mehta SR, Chrolavicius S, *et al.* Effects of fondaparinux on mortality and reinfarction in patients with acute ST-segment elevation myocardial infarction: the OASIS-6 randomized trial. *JAMA.* 2006;**295**:1519–1530.

17 Vuillemenot A, Schiele F, Meneveau N, *et al.* Efficacy of a synthetic pentasaccharide, a pure factor Xa inhibitor, as an antithrombotic agent. A pilot study in the setting of coronary angioplasty. *Thromb Haemost.* 1999;**81**: 214–220.

18 Mehta SR, Steg PG, Granger CB, *et al.* Randomized, blinded trial comparing fondaparinux with unfractionated heparin in patients undergoing contemporary percutaneous coronary intervention: Arixtra Study in Percutaneous Coronary Intervention: a Randomized Evaluation (ASPIRE) Pilot Trial. *Circulation.* 2005;**111**(11):1390–1397.

19 Mehta SR, Granger CB, Eikelboom JW, *et al.* Efficacy and safety of fondaparinux versus enoxaparin in patients with acute coronary syndromes undergoing percutaneous coronary intervention: results from the OASIS-5 trial. *J Am Coll Cardiol.* 2007;**50**: 1742–1751.

20 Mahaffey KW, Becker RC. The scientific community's quest to identify optimal targets for anticoagulant pharmacotherapy. *Circulation.* 2006;**114**:2313–2316.

21 Antman EM, Hand M, Armstrong PW, *et al.* 2007 focused update of the ACC/AHA 2004 guidelines for the management of patients with ST-elevation myocardial infarction. *J Am Coll Cardiol.* 2008;**51**:210–247.

22 Switching From Fondaparinux to Bivalirudin or Unfractionated Heparin in ACS Patients Undergoing PCI (SWITCHIII). Available at http://www.clinicaltrials.gov/ct2/show/NCT00464087?term=fondaparinux&rank=17. Accessed May 16, 2008.

PART II
Antiplatelet therapy

CHAPTER 5

Optimal antiplatelet therapy: Duration of antiplatelet therapy with drug-eluting and bare metal stents

Probal Roy[1] & Ron Waksman[2]
[1]Macquarie University, Sydney, Australia
[2]Washington Hospital Center, Washington, DC, USA

Introduction

Concurrent to technical advances, the evolution of adjunctive medical therapies has been critical in establishing the safety and efficacy of the percutaneous treatment of coronary artery disease (CAD). Adjunctive antiplatelet and anticoagulant therapy have reduced thrombotic complications associated with percutaneous coronary intervention (PCI). Though the focus of these therapies has been the reduction in postprocedural events, the benefit has been somewhat offset by an increased bleeding risk.

The use of dual antiplatelet therapy represented a significant advance in the evolution of medical therapy adjunctive to PCI. The addition of a thienopyridine to aspirin proved to be highly efficacious in reducing postprocedural thrombotic complications versus aspirin monotherapy or combination therapy with aspirin and coumadin (1–4). As a result of hematological toxicity (5) and potential reduced efficacy (6), ticlopidine has been replaced as the thienopyridine of choice. Currently, the combination of aspirin and clopidogrel pre- and post-PCI is the standard for care. Pretreatment with both aspirin and clopidogrel is well supported by large-scale randomized clinical trials (7,8). The optimal duration of dual antiplatelet therapy

Pharmacology in the Catheterization Laboratory. Edited by Ron Waksman and Andrew E Ajani. © 2010 Blackwell Publishing, ISBN: 978-1-4051-5704-9.

post-PCI remains unclear, particularly in the era of drug-eluting stents (DES). The beneficial effect of dual antiplatelet therapy post-PCI is twofold, each of which is fundamental when considering the optimal duration of therapy. As mentioned, dual antiplatelet therapy helps prevent thrombotic complications post-PCI, hence therapy is appropriate whilst patients remain at risk of these events. Secondly, dual antiplatelet therapy exerts further beneficial effects by preventing atherothrombotic events elsewhere in the coronary tree remote from the target lesion site. This chapter will examine the current available evidence pertaining to the optimal duration of antiplatelet therapy post-PCI. The emergence of DES has added further complexity to this issue and this will be addressed. Further issues arising from sustained dual antiplatelet utilization such as bleeding and cost will be examined. We will conclude with review of the current AHA/ACC/SCAI recommendations.

Antiplatelet therapy in the BMS era

Initially, the focus of dual antiplatelet therapy was the prevention of subacute stent thrombosis, a major limitation of PCI at the time. Stent thrombosis, a multifactorial process, results from the inherent thrombogenicity of the stent struts themselves, and also from the contribution of patient and procedural factors (9). Insertion of metallic stents impart considerable trauma to the vessel wall, which is followed by a healing response. Till complete endothelialization is achieved with total coverage of stent struts patients remain at increased risk of acute vessel closure secondary to thrombotic occlusion. Information on this healing response is sparse. Grewe *et al.* described the acute and chronic tissue response to stent implantation in a series of 21 autopsies. Acutely after stent implantation, complete endothelial destruction and covering of stent struts with thrombus was seen. In the ensuing weeks, invasion of smooth muscle and inflammatory cells initiated the healing response. The authors first found complete endothelialization as late as 12 weeks after stent insertion (10). Similar findings were reported in a coronary angioscopic study after Palmaz-Schatz stent implantation by Sakatani *et al.* Complete endothelial strut coverage was seen in 55% of 21 lesions at 1 month and 80% at 3 months (11). Despite these pathological and angioscopic findings, stent thrombosis beyond 30 days was a rare event. In the most robust series studying stent thrombosis in the BMS era, an incidence of 0.9% was reported, with events occurring beyond 30 days not reported (12). All large-scale randomized trials establishing the safety and efficacy of dual antiplatelet therapy over other antithrombotic strategies reported the primary end point at 30 days (1–4). Late stent thrombosis (>30 days) was a relative nonentity in the BMS era and hence based on the available randomized studies a recommendation for dual antiplatelet therapy for 4 weeks post–stent implantation was adopted.

Stent implantation represents the focal treatment of a systemic process. Treatment of an isolated lesion is insufficient to impact cardiac mortality in stable patients (13), which suggests that further events arise from disease progression remote to the target lesion site. Medical therapy is critical in targeting the systemic process of atherothrombosis, central to which is platelet aggregation. By inhibiting independent pathways of platelet aggregation, the combination of aspirin and clopidogrel provides a more potent platelet antiaggregatory strategy than aspirin alone. The hypothesis that dual antiplatelet therapy would be more protective of atherothrombotic events, providing rationale for sustained treatment, was tested in the CURE (The Clopidogrel in Unstable Angina

to Prevent Recurrent Events) trial. In this study, 12,562 patients presenting with non-ST elevation acute coronary syndromes were randomized to clopidogrel (300 mg loading dose, 75 mg maintenance dose) or placebo within 24 h of presentation. All patients were prescribed aspirin and 2,658 patients underwent PCI. Clopidogrel therapy was associated with a significant reduction in the primary end point (composite of cardiac death, myocardial infarction, and stroke) (9.3% vs 11.4%; RR, 0.8; CI, 0.72–0.90; $P < 0.001$) after a mean duration of 9 months (7). Analysis of patients undergoing PCI in this study was reported in the PCI-CURE study. Clopidogrel therapy (pre- and sustained treatment) was associated with a significant reduction in the composite end point of cardiac death, myocardial infarction, and revascularization after a mean follow-up period of 8 months. The advantage was primarily driven by a reduction in myocardial infarction (14) (Figure 5.1a). The benefit of sustained dual antiplatelet therapy in a less selected population was further illustrated in the Clopidogrel for the Reduction of Events During Observation (CREDO) trial. In this study 2,116 patients were randomized to either pre- and sustained treatment (12 months) with clopidogrel or to standard dual antiplatelet therapy for 4 weeks after stent implantation. Sustained treatment was associated with a relative risk reduction of 26.9% in the primary end point of death, myocardial infarction, and stroke (8) (Figure 5.1b). Though these studies do not specifically address the issue of stent thrombosis, they provide substantial evidence that prolonged dual antiplatelet therapy is protective of atherothrombotic events. In particular, the PCI-CURE and CREDO trials show improved patient outcomes with sustained treatment with aspirin and clopidogrel post-PCI, most likely related to the prevention of events arising remote to the target lesion. The impact of these studies on the duration of antiplatelet therapy post-PCI was somewhat diluted by the emergence of DES, which has further complicated the issue.

Antiplatelet therapy in the DES era

PCI in the BMS era remained limited by the problem of restenosis and the need for repeat intervention (15). DES, by allowing the local delivery

(a)

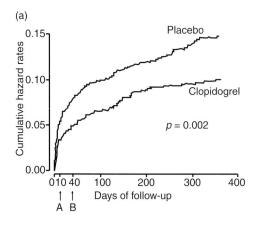

(b)

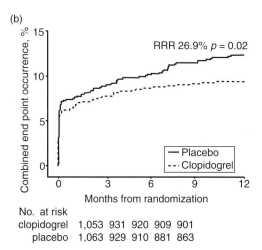

Figure 5.1 (a) Kaplan Meier cumulative hazard rates for cardiovascular death or myocardial infarction from randomization to end of follow-up in the PCI-CURE study. A = median time to PCI. B = 30 days after median time of PCI. (*Source*: Mehta SR, *et al. Lancet.* 2001;**358**(9281):527–533.) (b) Combined end point (death, myocardial infarction, or stroke at 1 year) Results at 1 year for clopidogrel vs placebo in the CREDO trial. (*Source*: Steinhubl SR, *et al. JAMA.* 2002;**288**(19): 2411–2420.)

of antiproliferative drugs, represented a critical advance in PCI. Short- and medium-term safety and efficacy for both sirolimus-eluting stent (SES) and paclitaxel-eluting stent (PES) was established in pivotal randomized trials (16,17), which subsequently led to their approval and routine use. Based on these pivotal trials an initial recommendation of dual antiplatelet therapy for 3 months after SES and 6 months after PES implantation was made. This has been superseded more recently by guidelines from the ACC/AHA/SCAI joint body, which recommend dual antiplatelet therapy for a minimum of 12 months after PCI for patients without increased bleeding risk (18).

The local delivery of antiproliferative drugs inhibit smooth muscle cell migration and proliferation hence reducing restenosis (19,20). As a consequence, healing, in particular endothelialization, is impaired with DES. This has been confirmed in autopsy series when compared with BMS. Healing has been shown to be further delayed in patients presenting with late stent thrombosis (21). Furthermore, impaired endothelialization was shown to be the strongest pathological predictor of late stent thrombosis with the ratio of uncovered to total stent struts correlating with the degree of endothelialization (22). The time required to achieve complete endothelialization after DES

implantation has not been established and remains critical when determining the optimal duration of antiplatelet therapy. In an angioscopic study of 15 lesions treated with SES implantation compared to BMS only 2 of the 15 (13.3%) lesions had complete endothelial coverage at 3–6 months (23). In contrast, all cases in the BMS control arm of this study had achieved endothelialization within this timeframe (Figure 5.2). Prior to DES, vascular brachytherapy (VBT) was the primary treatment for in-stent restenosis. Similar to DES, VBT inhibits cellular proliferation and retards healing. In animal models, endothelialization has been shown to be incomplete at 6 months after gamma radiation treatment and sustained antiplatelet therapy was thus recommended in patients receiving VBT (24). While dual antiplatelet therapy for 12 months after VBT was not associated with a significant reduction in late thrombosis, it was associated with major reductions in cardiac events and target lesion revascularization (25). DES have attenuated the problem of in-stent restenosis at the cost of impaired healing similar to that seen with VBT. Complete endothelialization after DES implantation is undoubtedly delayed but the time course remains uncertain. Patients will require dual antiplatelet therapy till endothelialization with complete stent strut coverage is achieved and this may hold the key

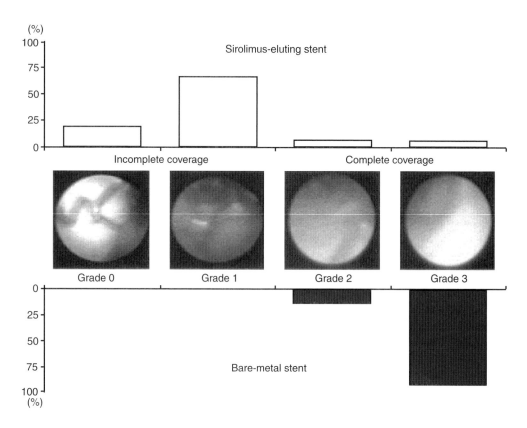

Figure 5.2 Grading for neointimal stent strut coverage on angioscopic imaging. Neointimal coverage was more complete with bare-metal stents compared with sirolimus-eluting stents at 3–6 months ($P < 0.0001$). (*Source*: Kotani J, *et al. J Am Coll Cardiol.* 2006;**47**(10):2108–2111.)

in determining the optimal duration of antiplatelet therapy post-PCI with DES.

The theoretical concerns of delayed endothelialization placing patients at risk for late stent thrombosis post-DES implantation have been realized. The first significant report consisted of a series of four patients presenting with late stent thrombosis after a minimum of 335 days after stent insertion. All patients discontinued both aspirin and clopidogrel (26). Ong *et al.* reported an incidence of late (>30 days) angiographic stent thrombosis of 0.35% (8 cases) occurring after a minimum of 2 months after DES insertion. In this series, no late events occurred in patients while taking both antiplatelet medications (27). More recently, reports have surfaced, suggesting an increased mortality and nonfatal MI rate with DES. Results from a meta-analysis by Camenzind (28) and BASKET-LATE (29) have suggested that late stent thrombosis with

DES after the cessation of clopidogrel is sufficient to unfavorably impact mortality and nonfatal MI. Whether DES is associated with increased rates of death and nonfatal MI has been refuted by a number of meta-analyses of randomized studies comparing DES with BMS with long-term follow-up (30–32). Though there remains a small but continual rise in late stent thrombosis with DES these studies did not show unfavorable morality and nonfatal MI outcomes in patients treated with DES. Despite the conflict in data regarding mortality and MI, most reports recognize the occurrence of late stent thrombosis beyond 12 months and the need for sustained dual antiplatelet therapy. The withdrawal of clopidogrel therapy has been established as a strong correlate of stent thrombosis in the DES era. The studies, which have shown this finding, have reported predictors of cumulative stent thrombosis at up to 9 months (33,34).

Conflicting data has been more recently reported from a two-institutional cohort study, which did not report clopidogrel cessation as a correlate of late stent thrombosis (>30 days) at long-term follow-up (35). However, the relative infrequency of late stent thrombosis makes identification of correlates of these events difficult. Unfortunately, it is difficult to derive strong conclusions regarding the optimal duration of dual antiplatelet therapy from these registry studies identifying correlates of stent thrombosis.

To date, there are no randomized studies addressing the issue of optimal antiplatelet therapy post-DES implantation. Recommendations for sustained dual antiplatelet therapy for 12 months and beyond have been supported by data from the Duke Heart Center registry. In this study, the sustained use of clopidogrel was associated with significant reductions in the adjusted rates of death and death or MI at 24 months post-DES implantation in patients who were event free at both 6 and 12 months. In contrast to the PCI-CURE and CREDO studies, the prolonged use of clopidogrel was not associated with reductions in death or MI in patients undergoing BMS implantation. Though the study was limited in that clopidogrel use was nonrandomized and self-reported, it stands as the only clinical evidence to support the use of dual antiplatelet therapy beyond 12 months (36).

The benefit of sustained dual antiplatelet therapy on cardiac outcomes seen in CURE, PCI-CURE, and CREDO is also an important consideration when determining the optimal duration of therapy post-DES implantation. As already discussed, the benefit of aspirin and clopidogrel in these studies was mostly due to the prevention of atherothrombotic events elsewhere in the coronary and cerebrovascular trees. This finding is independent of stent type and is expected to remain true in the DES era.

The optimal duration of dual antiplatelet therapy in the DES era remains uncertain. DES has clearly been shown to be associated with delayed endothelialization and an increased risk of late stent thrombosis versus BMS. Clopidogrel withdrawal has been identified as a strong predictor of stent thrombosis in many studies. The recommendation for dual antiplatelet therapy for 12 months or more

remains largely intuitive with a lack of robust data. There remains a need for randomized controlled trials with adequate power to detect differences in mortality, MI, and stent thrombosis to determine the optimal duration of dual antiplatelet therapy post-DES implantation.

Bleeding and cost

Though the use of dual antiplatelet therapy for 12 months or more may be protective of cardiac events related to both the target lesion and beyond, there remain considerable limitations. Prolonged therapy with aspirin and clopidogrel entails both safety and economic concerns. In the CURE study, clopidogrel therapy for a mean duration of 9 months was associated with significant increases in the incidences of major and minor bleeding. The increase in the rate of major bleeding (3.7% vs 2.7%; RR, 1.38; $P = 0.001$) was largely related to gastrointestinal and entry site bleeding. Minor hemorrhage, defined as bleeding other than major or life-threatening that required drug withdrawal, was also significantly increased (5.1% vs 2.4%; $P < 0.001$). There was no significant difference in life-threatening bleeding between clopidogrel and placebo groups (7). The PCI-CURE study showed no significant increase in the incidence of major bleeding with clopidogrel use. As in the CURE study, the incidence of minor bleeding was increased with clopidogrel use (14). The CREDO trial showed a nonsignificant rise in the rate of major bleeding (defined as intracranial hemorrhage or fall in hemoglobin greater than 5 g/dL) after sustained dual antiplatelet therapy for 12 months (8.8% vs 6.7%; $P = 0.07$). Approximately two-thirds of the incidence of all major bleeding in both groups occurred in the context of coronary bypass surgery (8). Bleeding remains a major limitation of prolonged dual antiplatelet therapy. Rates of major bleeding of up to 8.8%, as observed in the CREDO study, are not inconsiderable and need to be balanced against the reductions in cardiac events (Figure 5.3).

Coupled with the bleeding risk cost is the other major limitation of prolonged antiplatelet therapy. The average wholesale price for a monthly prescription of clopidogrel currently in the United States is $146.07; hence a 12-month-therapy will

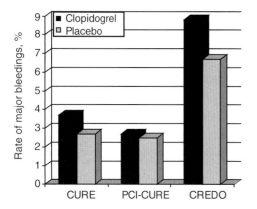

Figure 5.3 Rates of major bleeding in the pivotal randomized trials studying prolonged dual antiplatelet therapy. A significant difference was seen only in the CURE trial (3.7% vs 2.7%, *P* = 0.001).

cost in excess of $1700. Analyses from both CURE and CREDO have suggested that prolonged dual antiplatelet therapy is a cost-effective strategy (37,38). Though these studies show that prolonged therapy is cost-effective to the community, in the short term, it still entails increased cost. Increased cost to patients, which may influence compliance, remains an important consideration when recommending prolonged therapy.

Recommendations and conclusions

The current ACC/AHA/SCAI guidelines for antiplatelet therapy post-PCI state:

In patients who have undergone PCI, clopidogrel 75 mg daily should be given for at least 1 month after bare metal stent implantation (unless the patient is at increased risk of bleeding; then it should be given for a minimum of 2 weeks), 3 months after sirolimus stent implantation, and 6 months after paclitaxel stent implantation, and ideally up to 12 months in patients who are not at high risk of bleeding." (Level of evidence IB) (18). The recommendation for a minimum of one month clopidogrel post BMS is generally observed. However sustained therapy in patients receiving BMS, particularly in the acute coronary syndrome population, is supported by large randomized studies. The recommendation for 12 months of dual anti-platelet therapy post PCI with DES has been widely accepted and incorporated into routine clinical practice. Though the optimal duration of dual anti-platelet therapy post DES is uncertain, current data suggests that prolonged therapy (≥12 months)

is protective of cardiac events and thus supportive of the current guidelines. It remains to be determined if therapy beyond 12 months will be preventative of very late stent thrombosis in the DES era and whether the beneficial effects on atherothrombosis elsewhere in the vasculature remain.

References

1 Leon MB, Baim DS, Popma JJ, *et al.* A clinical trial comparing three antithrombotic-drug regimens after coronary-artery stenting. Stent Anticoagulation Restenosis Study Investigators. *N Engl J Med.* 1998;**339**(23):1665–1671.

2 Schomig A, Neumann FJ, Kastrati A, *et al.* A randomized comparison of antiplatelet and anticoagulant therapy after the placement of coronary-artery stents. *N Engl J Med.* 1996;**334**(17):1084–1089.

3 Bertrand ME, Legrand V, Boland J, *et al.* Randomized multicenter comparison of conventional anticoagulation versus antiplatelet therapy in unplanned and elective coronary stenting. The full anticoagulation versus aspirin and ticlopidine (fantastic) study. *Circulation.* 1998;**98**(16):1597–1603.

4 Urban P, Macaya C, Rupprecht HJ, *et al.* Randomized evaluation of anticoagulation versus antiplatelet therapy after coronary stent implantation in high-risk patients: the multicenter aspirin and ticlopidine trial after intracoronary stenting (MATTIS). *Circulation.* 1998;**98**(20):2126–2132.

5 Bertrand ME, Rupprecht HJ, Urban P, Gershlick AH, CLASSICS Investigators. Double-blind study of the safety of clopidogrel with and without a loading dose in combination with aspirin compared with ticlopidine in combination with aspirin after coronary stenting: the clopidogrel aspirin stent international cooperative study (CLASSICS). *Circulation.* 2000;**102**(6):624–629.

6 Bhatt DL, Bertrand ME, Berger PB, *et al.* Meta-analysis of randomized and registry comparisons of ticlopidine with clopidogrel after stenting. *J Am Coll Cardiol.* 2002;**39**(1):9–14.

7 Mehta SR, Yusuf S, Peters RJ, *et al.* Effects of pretreatment with clopidogrel and aspirin followed by long-term therapy in patients undergoing percutaneous coronary intervention: the PCI-CURE study. *Lancet.* 2001;**358**(9281):527–533.

8 Steinhubl SR, Berger PB, Mann JT, 3rd, *et al.* Clopidogrel for the reduction of events during observation. Early and sustained dual oral antiplatelet therapy following percutaneous coronary intervention: a randomized controlled trial. *JAMA.* 2002;**288**(19):2411–2420.

9 Zimarino M, Renda G, De Caterina R. Optimal duration of antiplatelet therapy in recipients of coronary drug-eluting stents. *Drugs.* 2005;**65**(6):725–732.

10 Grewe PH, Deneke T, Machraoui A, Barmeyer J, Muller KM Acute and chronic tissue response to coronary stent implantation: pathologic findings in human specimen. *J Am Coll Cardiol.* 2000; **35**(1):157–163.

11 Sakatani H, Degawa T, Nakamura M, Yamaguchi T. Intracoronary surface changes after Palmaz-Schatz stent implantation: serial observations with coronary angioscopy. *Am Heart J.* 1999;**138**(5 Pt 1): 962–967.

12 Cutlip DE, Baim DS, Ho KK, et al. Stent thrombosis in the modern era: a pooled analysis of multicenter coronary stent clinical trials. *Circulation.* 2001;**103**(15):1967–1971.

13 Boden WE, O'Rourke RA, Teo KK, et al. Optimal medical therapy with or without PCI for stable coronary disease. *N Engl J Med.* 2007;**356**(15):1503–1516.

14 Mehta SR, Yusuf S, Peters RJ, et al. Effects of pretreatment with clopidogrel and aspirin followed by long-term therapy in patients undergoing percutaneous coronary intervention: the PCI-CURE study. *Lancet.* 2001;**358**(9281):527–533.

15 Al Suwaidi J, Berger PB, Holmes DR, Jr. Coronary artery stents. *JAMA.* 2000;**284**:1828–1836.

16 Moses JW, Leon MB, Popma JJ, et al. Sirolimus-eluting stents versus standard stents in patients with stenosis in a native coronary artery. *N Engl J Med.* 2003;**349**:1315–1323.

17 Stone GW, Ellis SG, Cox DA, et al. A polymer-based, paclitaxel-eluting stent in patients with coronary artery disease. *N Engl J Med.* 2004;**350**:221–231.

18 Smith SC, Jr, Feldman TE, Hirshfeld JW, Jr, et al. ACC/AHA/SCAI 2005 Guideline Update for Percutaneous Coronary Intervention—summary article: a report of the American College of Cardiology/American Heart Association Task Force on Practice Guidelines (ACC/AHA/SCAI Writing Committee to Update the 2001 Guidelines for Percutaneous Coronary Intervention). *Circulation.* 2006;**113**(1):156–175.

19 Marx SO, Marks AR. Bench to bedside: the development of rapamycin and its application to stent restenosis. *Circulation.* 2001;**104**:852–855.

20 Rowinsky EK, Donehower RC. Paclitaxel (taxol). *N Engl J Med.* 1995;**332**:1004–1014.

21 Joner M, Finn AV, Farb A, et al. Pathology of drug-eluting stents in humans: delayed healing and late thrombotic risk. *J Am Coll Cardiol.* 2006;**48**(1):193–202.

22 Finn AV, Joner M, Nakazawa G, et al. Pathological correlates of late drug-eluting stent thrombosis. Strut coverage as a marker of endothelialization. *Circulation.* 2007;**115**(18):2435–2441.

23 Kotani J, Awata M, Nanto S, et al. Incomplete neointimal coverage of sirolimus-eluting stents: angioscopic findings. *J Am Coll Cardiol.* 2006;**47**(10):2108–2111.

24 Cheneau E, John MC, Fournadjiev J, et al. Time course of stent endothelialization after intravascular

radiation therapy in rabbit iliac arteries. *Circulation.* 2003;**107**(16):2153–2158.

25 Waksman R, Ajani AE, Pinnow E, et al. Twelve versus six months of clopidogrel to reduce major cardiac events in patients undergoing gamma-radiation therapy for in-stent restenosis: Washington Radiation for In-Stent restenosis Trial (WRIST) 12 versus WRIST PLUS. *Circulation.* 2002;**106**(7):776–778.

26 McFadden EP, Stabile E, Regar E, et al. Late thrombosis in drug-eluting coronary stents after discontinuation of antiplatelet therapy. *Lancet.* 2004;**364**(9444):1519–1521.

27 Ong AT, McFadden EP, Regar E, de Jaegere PP, van Domburg RT, Serruys PW. Late angiographic stent thrombosis (LAST) events with drug-eluting stents. *J Am Coll Cardiol.* 2005;**45**(12):2088–2092.

28 Camenzind E, Steg PG, Wijns W. Stent thrombosis late after implantation of first-generation drug-eluting stents: a cause for concern. *Circulation.* 2007;**115**(11):1440–1455; discussion 1455.

29 Pfisterer M, Brunner-La Rocca H, Buser P, et al. Late clinical events after clopidogrel discontinuation may limit the benefit of drug-eluting stents an observational study of drug-eluting versus bare-metal stents. *J Am Coll Cardiol.* 2006;**48**(12):2584–2591.

30 Spaulding C, Daemen J, Boersma E, Cutlip DE, Serruys PW. A pooled analysis of data comparing sirolimus-eluting stents with bare-metal stents. *N Engl J Med.* 2007;**356**(10):989–997.

31 Stone GW, Moses JW, Ellis SG, et al. Safety and efficacy of sirolimus- and paclitaxel-eluting coronary stents. *N Engl J Med.* 2007;**356**(10):998–1008.

32 Kastrati A, Mehilli J, Pache J, et al. Analysis of 14 trials comparing sirolimus-eluting stents with bare-metal stents. *N Engl J Med.* 2007;**356**(10):1030–1039.

33 Iakovou I, Schmidt T, Bonizzoni E, et al. Incidence, predictors, and outcome of thrombosis after successful implantation of drug-eluting stents. *JAMA.* 2005;**293**(17):2126–2130.

34 Kuchulakanti PK, Chu WW, Torguson R, et al. Correlates and long-term outcomes of angiographically proven stent thrombosis with sirolimus- and paclitaxel-eluting stents. *Circulation.* 2006;**113**(8):1108–1113.

35 Daemen J, Wenaweser P, Tsuchida K, et al. Early and late coronary stent thrombosis of sirolimus-eluting and paclitaxel-eluting stents in routine clinical practice: data from a large two-institutional cohort study. *Lancet.* 2007;**369**(9562):667–678.

36 Eisenstein EL, Anstrom KJ, Kong DF, et al. Clopidogrel use and long-term clinical outcomes after drug-eluting stent implantation. *JAMA.* 2007;**297**(2):159–168.

37 Weintraub WS, Mahoney EM, Lamy A, et al. Long-term cost-effectiveness of clopidogrel given for up to

one year in patients with acute coronary syndromes without ST-segment elevation. *J Am Coll Cardiol.* 2005;**45**(6):838–845.

38 Beinart SC, Kolm P, Veledar E, *et al.* Long-term cost effectiveness of early and sustained dual oral antiplatelet therapy with clopidogrel given for up to one year after percutaneous coronary intervention results: from the Clopidogrel for the Reduction of Events During Observation (CREDO) trial. *J Am Coll Cardiol.* 2005;**46**(5):761–769.

CHAPTER 6

Clopidogrel: How much, how soon, and how long

Alaeddin Ayyad[1] & Deepak L. Bhatt[2]
[1]University of California, San Diego, CA, USA
[2]VA Boston Healthcare System, Boston, USA

Introduction

Cardiovascular disease (CVD) remains the most common cause of mortality in the United States. According to the Centers for Disease (CDC), CVD accounted for more than 27% of all deaths in 2004. Antiplatelet therapy has been shown to decrease morbidity and mortality in patients with known CVD. Clopidogrel is a potent platelet aggregation inhibitor. It has been studied extensively and was shown to markedly decrease morbidity and mortality in patients presenting with acute coronary syndrome (ACS) or undergoing percutaneous coronary intervention (PCI). In this chapter, we review several clinical trials on clopidogrel and attempt to define the optimal timing, loading dose, and duration of clopidogrel therapy in patients with ACS or undergoing PCI.

Mechanism of action

Antiplatelet therapy works by inhibiting platelet activation, aggregation, and clot formation inside blood vessels, which is the primary mechanism by which myocardial ischemia and infarction develop (1). Adenosine diphosphate (ADP) is a potent platelet aggregating factor. It binds to a platelet surface receptor and causes a change in

Pharmacology in the Catheterization Laboratory. Edited by Ron Waksman and Andrew E Ajani. © 2010 Blackwell Publishing, ISBN: 978-1-4051-5704-9.

platelet conformation in such a fashion as to promote aggregation and clotting. Clopidogrel is a thienopyridine. Inactive *in vitro*, it is metabolized by the cytochrome P450 enzyme system in the liver to an active metabolite that irreversibly binds the ADP receptor thus inhibiting the activation of this receptor by its ADP ligand. By doing this, clopidogrel inhibits thrombus formation inside coronary arteries and decreases the likelihood of experiencing an ACS or dying of a myocardial infarction (MI) (2).

Timing and loading dose of Clopidogrel in patients presenting with ACS

The benefit of clopidogrel in ACS patients was demonstrated in the Clopidogrel in Unstable angina to Reduce recurrent Events (CURE) study. A total of 12,562 patients presenting with ACS without evidence of ST-elevation myocardial infarction (STEMI) were randomized to receive clopidogrel 300 mg loading dose then 75 mg daily or a matching placebo. All patients also received daily aspirin (75–325 mg). Patients were followed for a period of up to 12 months. At the end of follow-up, there was an overall 20% reduction in the primary outcome (defined as cardiovascular death, nonfatal MI, or stroke) in the clopidogrel group. A total of 2,658 patients underwent PCI. Analysis in the PCI substudy of the CURE trial (PCI-CURE) showed an overall 31% reduction in cardiovascular death or MI in patients randomized to receive clopidogrel (3). When the efficacy of the loading dose was analyzed, the greatest benefit was seen in patients undergoing PCI within 48 h after randomization to receive clopidogrel (RR 0.53 if PCI <48 h vs 0.72 after 48 h) (4). The CURE study has shown clopidogrel to significantly improve outcomes in patients with ACS regardless of when it is received or whether it is combined with a more invasive strategy. It did not investigate the optimal time and optimal loading dose at which clopidogrel should be given to achieve maximum benefit before proceeding with PCI.

The Clopidogrel for the Reduction of Events During Observation (CREDO) trial randomized 2,116 patients with symptomatic coronary artery disease who were either likely to undergo PCI to receive either clopidogrel 300 mg LD or placebo 3–24 h prior to PCI. At one year, there was 26.9% reduction in primary endpoint (death, MI, stroke) in the clopidogrel group. There was no significant reduction in primary endpoints (death, myocardial infarction (MI), or urgent target vessel revascularization (UTVR)) at 28 days in patients randomized to receive clopidogrel. However, in a post-hoc analysis of the results of CREDO, the 1,762 patients who underwent elective PCI were evaluated for the optimal timing of clopidogrel dosing prior to PCI. All patients received clopidogrel 75 mg for 28 days after PCI, 847 received 300 mg loading dose at intervals ranging from 3 to 24 h before PCI, and 915 received a matching dose of placebo at the same intervals. Primary outcomes were analyzed at 28 days after PCI. In the clopidogrel group, a trend toward reduction in primary outcome occurrence was noted only in patients treated >6 h prior to PCI (5,6).

Efficacy of pretreatment with clopidogrel was also analyzed in the Do Tirofiban and ReoPro Give Similar Efficacy Outcome Trial (TARGET) trial. Pretreatment with clopidogrel 300 mg significantly reduced death, MI, or UTVR at 30 days after PCI in all subgroups regardless of the pretreatment time. Subgroup analysis revealed no significant difference in efficacy among patients receiving their loading dose (LD) within 2 h compared with 2–6 h prior to PCI. However, significant additional benefit was seen in patients receiving their LD more than 6 h prior to PCI when compared to the <6 h group (7).

Thus based on the CREDO-Timing and TARGET studies a 300 mg dose of clopidogrel would likely provide a most significant benefit if given at least 6 h prior to PCI.

The Clopidogrel as Adjunctive Reperfusion Therapy (CLARITY)–Thrombolysis in Myocardial Infarction (TIMI) 28 was a randomized controlled trial of clopidogrel (300 mg LD plus 75 mg daily) vs placebo in 3,491 patients presenting within 12 h of experiencing STEMI and who were scheduled to undergo angiography 48–72 h after randomization. After 30 days, there was 36% relative reduction in the primary end point (death, MI, recurrent ischemia leading to urgent revascularization). The PCI substudy of CLARITY (PCI-CLARITY) analyzed the subgroup of 1,863 patients who underwent PCI. It confirmed the efficacy of clopidogrel 300 mg LD plus 75 mg daily prior to PCI in patients with STEMI but no time intervals were reported (Figure 6.1) (8,9).

To study whether a higher loading dose of clopidogrel would provide additional benefit or decrease the required time prior to PCI, the Intra-coronary Stenting and Anti-thrombotic Regimen–Rapid Early Action for Coronary Treatment (ISAR-REACT) study compared occurrence of primary outcomes (death, MI, or UTVR) within 30 days after PCI in 1,079 patients receiving abciximab and 1,080 patients receiving placebo. All patients undergoing elective PCI received a 600 mg (LD) of clopidogrel at least two hours prior to PCI. Primary outcome rates were similar in both groups at 4%. Study analysis placed participants into four subgroups, depending on the time at which they received their clopidogrel dose (2–3, 3–6, 6–12, and >12 h prior to PCI). In contrast to the CREDO-timing and TARGET findings, statistical analysis of these subgroups showed no significant difference in primary outcome occurrence at 30 days after PCI, suggesting that with a 600 mg LD no additional benefit is gained by increasing the treatment interval beyond 2–3 h prior to PCI (10,11).

The Anti-platelet therapy for Reduction of MYocardial Damage during Angioplasty (ARMYDA 2) study randomized 255 patients scheduled to undergo PCI to receive a LD of either 600 mg (126 patients) or 300 mg (129 patients). The LD was given 4–8 h before PCI and patients were followed for 30 days. The primary outcome

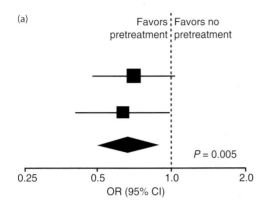

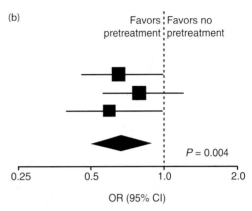

Figure 6.1 This figure comes from the PCI-CLARITY study and represents a meta-analysis of trials evaluating clopidogrel pretreatment (300 mg LD) vs placebo in patients undergoing PCI. (a) Occurrence of MI before PCI in PCI-CURE (top), PCI-CLARITY (middle), and meta-analysis of both (bottom). (b) Occurrence of death and MI in PCI-CURE (top), CREDO (middle), PCI-CLARITY (midbottom), and meta-analysis of all three (bottom) (8).

(death, MI, or target vessel revascularization) occurred in 4% of patients in the 600 mg group and in 12% in the 300 mg Group. All events were due to periprocedural MI (12).

If a high loading dose of clopidogrel obviates the need to wait a long time until PCI, would not even a higher dose provide additional benefit? Two studies attempted to answer this question. In the Intracoronary Stenting and Anti-thrombotic Regimen: Choose Between 3 High Oral Doses for Immediate Clopidogrel Effect (ISAR-CHOICE), aggregometry was used to study the pharmacodynamics of three different clopidogrel regimens (300, 600, and 900 mg) in 60 patients presenting for coronary angiography. Clopidogrel, its active metabolite, an inactive metabolite, and ADP-mediated inhibition were measured just before and 4 h after the clopidogrel dose was given. Although there was a significant increase in the concentration of the clopidogrel molecule, its active metabolite, and as a result more profound suppression of ADP mediated platelet aggregation when increasing the dose from 300 to 600 mg, no significant change in these parameters was seen when increasing the dose from 600 to 900 mg (13). The Assessment of the Best Loading Dose of Clopidogrel to Blunt Platelet Activation, Inflammation and Ongoing Necrosis Trial (ALBION trial) sought to answer the same question but with a slightly larger sample size (103 patients) and with more frequent blood sampling and analysis (8 vs 2 time points). In this study, higher LDs were associated with more rapid onset of action and incremental increase in platelet inhibition (PI), suggesting a dose–response effect. Peak PI occurred 5–6 h after the LDs were given in all groups (14).

The need for higher LD will be confirmed in a clinical trial investigating primary clinical outcomes. The Clopidogrel optimal Loading dose Usage to Reduce Recurrent EveNTs/Optimal Antiplatelet Strategy for InterventionS (CURRENT/OASIS 7) trial started recruiting patients in 2006. This trial will randomize close to 14,000 ACS patients, likely to undergo PCI within 24 h, to receive either 600 or 300 mg LD of clopidogrel. The results will likely be available in 2008 and should help determine whether a higher LD of clopidogrel is of more benefit to patients undergoing early invasive therapy for ACS. For now, the weight of clinical evidence supports the use of a LD of 600 mg in patients undergoing coronary angiography and PCI at least 2 h prior to the procedure, unless they are believed to be at very high bleeding risk.

Duration of clopidogrel treatment

The benefit of continued antiplatelet treatment in patients with ACS or undergoing PCI finds its rationale in the mechanism of disease leading to morbidity and mortality in patients with cardiovascular disease, namely, re-formation of thrombi within coronary arteries, a process highly dependent on platelet activation and aggregation, is inhibited by these agents. For this reason, aspirin was found to be highly efficacious in such patients. The American Heart Association (AHA) and the American College of Cardiology (ACC) now recommend indefinite use of aspirin in CVD patients and the addition of clopidogrel 75 mg for up to 1 year in patients with ACS.

The recommended duration of therapy also depends on the whether patients undergo PCI and on the type of stent they receive (15). Recent data suggest that patients who receive drug eluting stents are at higher risk of late stent thrombosis (16). Observational data seem to indicate that at least 1 and up to 2 years of dual antiplatelet therapy may be useful in these patients (17). Whether even longer duration of dual antiplatelet therapy is warranted in patients who have received drug-eluting stents is an area of ongoing controversy, as the risk of bleeding as well as the cost of therapy would need to be weighed against the small risk of late stent thrombosis. The drug-eluting stent experience is remarkably similar to the experience with brachytherapy, where 12 months of dual antiplatelet therapy was found to be superior to 6 months of therapy (18).

In many clinical trials, clopidogrel continued to reduce primary outcomes even at the conclusion of these trials. In the PCI-CURE study (3), dual antiplatelet treatment with clopidogrel and aspirin continued to significantly reduce the occurrence of myocardial infarction compared to aspirin alone up to 1 year of follow-up after PCI. Similar findings were reported in the CREDO trial with patients randomized to receive clopidogrel 75 mg daily for 1 year enjoying an additional 37.4% reduction in the combined primary outcome of death, MI, or stroke. The benefit of clopidogrel beyond the 1-year mark was not assessed in these studies (Figure 6.2) (6).

The Clopidogrel and Aspirin vs Aspirin Alone for the Prevention of Atherothrombotic Events (CHARISMA) trial randomized 15,603 patients at high risk for, or with known, CVD to either receive aspirin plus clopidogrel or aspirin plus placebo. Patients were followed for a median of 28 months. When the primary efficacy end point of death, MI, or stroke was analyzed, no significant difference was found between the study groups. Subgroup analysis did show a significant reduction ($P = 0.046$, RRR, 12.5%) in primary endpoint in patients with clinically

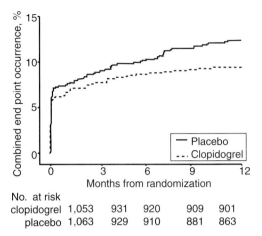

No. at risk

clopidogrel	1,053	931	920	909	901
placebo	1,063	929	910	881	863

Figure 6.2 This figure is reproduced from the CREDO trial. It suggests that the benefit of clopidogrel maintenance treatment (75 mg) in patients after PCI continues up to, and perhaps beyond, the 1 year study duration (6).

evident CVD (19). Unselected CVD patients might not enjoy the same benefit from clopidogrel therapy as patients with ACS or undergoing PCI. This might explain why patients in the CHARISMA study did not derive as much benefit as did patients in the CURE and CREDO trials. It is probably safe to assume that patients with ACS or requiring PCI are at higher risk for increased intracoronary thrombosis and therefore would most benefit from dual antiplatelet therapy. These patients might continue to benefit from such therapy beyond the 1-year limit studied in the CURE and CREDO trials, though such decisions need to be individualized based on the patient's ischemic and bleeding risks.

References

1 Libby P. Current concepts of the pathogenesis of the acute coronary syndromes. *Circulation*. July 17, 2001; **104**(3):365–372.

2 Richter T, Murdter TE, Heinkele G, *et al.* Potent mechanism-based inhibition of human CYP2B6 by clopidogrel and ticlopidine. *J Pharmacol Exp Ther*. October 16, 2003; **308**(1):189–197.

3 Mehta SR, Yusuf S, Peters RJ, *et al.* Clopidogrel in unstable angina to prevent Recurrent Events trial (CURE) investigators. Effects of pretreatment with clopidogrel and aspirin followed by long-term therapy in patients undergoing percutaneous coronary intervention: the PCI-CURE study [see comment]. *Lancet*. August 18, 2001; **358**(9281):527–533.

4 Lewis BS, Mehta SR, Fox KA, *et al.* Benefit of clopidogrel according to timing of percutaneous coronary intervention in patients with acute coronary syndromes: further results from the Clopidogrel in Unstable angina to prevent Recurrent Events (CURE) study. *Am Heart J.* December 2005;**150**(6):1177–1184.

5 Steinhubl SR, Berger PB, Brennan DM, Topol EJ, CREDO I. Optimal timing for the initiation of pretreatment with 300 mg clopidogrel before percutaneous coronary intervention. *J Am Coll Cardiol.* March 7, 2006;**47**(5):939–943.

6 Steinhubl SR, Berger PB, Mann JT, 3rd, *et al.* Early and sustained dual oral antiplatelet therapy following percutaneous coronary intervention: a randomized controlled trial [see comment] [erratum appears in *JAMA.* February 26, 2003;**289**(8):987]. *JAMA.* November 20, 2002;**288**(19):2411–2420.

7 Chan AW, Moliterno DJ, Berger PB, *et al.* Triple antiplatelet therapy during percutaneous coronary intervention is associated with improved outcomes including one-year survival: results from the Do Tirofiban and ReoProGive Similar Efficacy Outcome Trial (TARGET) [see comment]. *J Am Coll Cardiol.* October 1, 2003;**42**(7): 1188–1195.

8 Sabatine MS, Cannon CP, Gibson CM, *et al.* Clopidogrel as adjunctive reperfusion therapy (CLARITY)-thrombolysis in myocardial infarction (TIMI) 28 Investigators. Effect of clopidogrel pretreatment before percutaneous coronary intervention in patients with ST-elevation myocardial infarction treated with fibrinolytics: the PCI-CLARITY study [see comment]. *JAMA.* September 14, 2005;**294**(10):1224–1232.

9 Sabatine MS, Cannon CP, Gibson CM, *et al.* Addition of clopidogrel to aspirin and fibrinolytic therapy for myocardial infarction with ST-segment elevation [see comment]. *N Engl J Med.* March 24, 2005;**352**(12):1179–1189.

10 Kastrati A, Mehilli J, Schühlen H, *et al.* A clinical trial of abciximab in elective percutaneous coronary intervention after pretreatment with clopidogrel. *N Engl J Med.* 2004;**350**:232–238.

11 Kandzari DE, Berger PB, Kastrati A, *et al.* Influence of treatment duration with a 600-mg dose of clopidogrel before percutaneous coronary revascularization. *J Am Coll Cardiol.* 2004;**44**:2133–2136.

12 Patti G, Colonna G, Pasceri V, Pepe LL, Montinaro A, Di Sciascio G. Randomized trial of high loading dose of clopidogrel for reduction of periprocedural myocardial infarction in patients undergoing coronary intervention: results from the ARMYDA-2 (Antiplatelet therapy for Reduction of MYocardial Damage during Angioplasty) study [see comment]. *Circulation.* April 26, 2005;**111**(16):2099–2106.

13 von Beckerath N, Taubert D, Pogatsa-Murray G, Schömig E, Kastrati A, Schömig A. Stenting and antithrombotic regimen: choose between 3 high oral doses for loading doses of clopidogrel: results of the ISAR-CHOICE (Intracoronary Absorption, Metabolization, and Antiplatelet Effects of 300-, 600-, and 900-mg Immediate Clopidogrel Effect) trial. *Circulation.* 2005;**112**:2946–2950.

14 Montalescot G, Sideris G, Meuleman C, *et al.* A randomized comparison of high clopidogrel loading doses in patients with non-ST-segment elevation acute coronary syndromes: the ALBION (Assessment of the Best Loading Dose of Clopidogrel to Blunt Platelet Activation, Inflammation and Ongoing Necrosis) trial. *J Am Coll Cardiol.* September 5, 2006;**48**(5):931–938.

15 Smith SC, Jr, Allen J, Blair SN, *et al.* AHA/ACC guidelines for secondary prevention for patients with coronary and other atherosclerotic vascular disease: 2006 update: endorsed by the National Heart, Lung, and Blood Institute. [erratum appears in *Circulation.* June 6, 2006;**113**(22):e847]. *Circulation.* May 16, 2006;**113**(19): 2363–2372.

16 Bavry AA, Kumbhani DJ, Helton TJ, Borek PP, Mood GR, Bhatt DL. Late thrombosis of drug-eluting stents: a meta-analysis of randomized clinical trials. *Am J Med.* December 2006;**119**(12):1056–1061.

17 Eisenstein EL, Anstrom KJ, Kong DF, *et al.* Clopidogrel use and long-term clinical outcomes after drug-eluting stent implantation. *JAMA.* January 10, 2007;**297**(2):159–168.

18 Waksman R, Ajani AE, Pinnow E, *et al.* Twelve versus six months of clopidogrel to reduce major cardiac events in patients undergoing gamma-radiation therapy for in-stent restenosis: Washington Radiation for In-Stent restenosis Trial (WRIST) 12 versus WRIST PLUS. *Circulation.* August 13, 2002;**106**(7):776–778.

19 Bhatt DL, Fox KA, Hacke W, *et al.* Clopidogrel and aspirin versus aspirin alone for the prevention of atherothrombotic events [see comment]. *N Engl J Med.* April 20, 2006;**354**(16):1706–1717.

CHAPTER 7

Loading strategies of clopidogrel

Germano Di Sciascio & Giuseppe Patti
Campus Bio-Medico University of Rome, Rome, Italy

Percutaneous coronary intervention (PCI) with stenting is known to enhance platelet aggregation (1); thus, optimization of antiplatelet therapy has a pivotal role for the prevention of periprocedural acute ischemic complications and stent thrombosis in patients undergoing PCI (2,3). Dual antiplatelet treatment with aspirin and ticlopidine has dramatically reduced the occurrence of early cardiac events after coronary stenting, compared with aspirin alone or aspirin plus oral anticoagulants (3). Clopidogrel is an antiplatelet agent extensively used in clinical practice; it causes a nonreversible competitive inhibition of $P2Y_{12}$, the adenosine diphosphate (ADP) receptor present on platelet surface, affecting intracellular signaling events that modulate the ADP-induced platelet activation; use of clopidogrel has been associated with better safety profile than ticlopidine, with lower incidence of hematological and gastrointestinal side effects, as well as with a 49% risk reduction of cardiac events (death, myocardial infarction, and subacute thrombosis) at 30 days following coronary stenting (4) in a large meta-analysis due to better patient compliance and a more rapid onset of antiplatelet effect.

Clopidogrel loading pre-PCI

Prevention of periprocedural myocardial ischemic complications and reduction of early

Pharmacology in the Catheterization Laboratory. Edited by Ron Waksman and Andrew E Ajani. © 2010 Blackwell Publishing, ISBN: 978-1-4051-5704-9.

postprocedural platelet activation due to stent implantation represent the rationale for a pretreatment with clopidogrel in patients undergoing PCI (5). In the PCI-CURE study (6) (a subanalysis on 2,658 patients with acute coronary syndromes enrolled in the randomized CURE trial and receiving PCI), pretreatment with 300 mg clopidogrel loading dose at a median of 6 days before the procedure was associated, compared with placebo, with a significant risk reduction of death, myocardial infarction, and urgent repeat revascularization at one month (4.5% vs 6.4%; $P = 0.03$). Moreover, the randomized CREDO trial (7) on 2,116 patients undergoing elective or urgent PCI has shown that pretreatment with 300-mg loading dose of clopidogrel at least 6 h before the procedure is associated with 38% relative risk reduction of death, myocardial infarction, and target vessel revascularization at 28 days vs administration of clopidogrel, without loading dose, at the time of the procedure ($P = 0.05$). This is in agreement with previous data from optical aggregometry, demonstrating that a >40% platelet inhibition in patients receiving elective coronary stenting is achieved 12 h after the procedure in patients initiating clopidogrel with a 300 mg loading dose 3–24 h before PCI, as compared with after 2–5 days in those receiving clopidogrel, without loading dose, at the time of intervention (5). Furthermore, a post-hoc analysis on patients of the TARGET trial randomized to tirofiban or abciximab during PCI with stent (8), showed that pretreatment with a 300 mg loading dose of clopidogrel was associated with a better 30-day outcome, compared with a 300 mg loading dose given immediately after the procedure. This benefit was essentially driven by a significant reduction of postprocedural myocardial infarction (6% vs 9.5%, $P = 0.012$) and a lower 1-year mortality (1.7% vs 3.6%, $P = 0.011$); in particular, the outcome with >6 h pretreatment was more favorable than that of ≤6 h pretreatment. A recent randomized study (9) showed no benefit of 300 mg loading dose of clopidogrel given 3 days before the procedure compared with starting clopidogrel in the catheterization laboratory on the occurrence of periprocedural myocardial injury, defined as postprocedural elevation of Troponin-I or CK-MB (51% vs 43%, $P = 0.31$ and 7.4% vs 6.3%, $P = 0.78$, respectively); however, this study has included only patients with stable angina undergoing elective PCI and its results can probably be applied only to this low-risk population.

According to these studies, pretreatment with a 300-mg loading dose of clopidogrel (plus aspirin) at least 6 h before the procedure is a recommended antiplatelet therapy in patients undergoing PCI with stenting, especially in those at higher risk (for instance patients with acute coronary syndromes) (10,11). However, the rationale for using a 300-mg loading dose of clopidogrel derives from dose finding data on healthy volunteers (12); conversely, in patients with coronary artery disease there is an enhanced platelet reactivity as compared with healthy individuals (13), possibly requiring a more aggressive platelet inhibition.

What is the optimal loading dose of clopidogrel?

The degree of platelet inhibition at the time of the procedure correlates with early clinical outcome in patients undergoing coronary stenting (14). A higher loading dose with 600 mg of clopidogrel causes an earlier and stronger inhibition of ADP-induced platelet activation than does the 300 mg dose; in particular, the higher regimen in a study on patients undergoing PCI has been associated with approximately 30% of ADP-induced platelet aggregation rate at 6 h and 25% at 24 h vs 45% and 40% after conventional regimen (15) (Figure 7.1). After a 600 mg clopidogrel loading regimen a time-dependent increase in the level of platelet inhibition has been demonstrated during the first 2 h, with a maximal inhibition achieved at 2 h after drug administration and without time-dependent changes beyond this time point (16); moreover, 6 h after a 600 mg loading dose of clopidogrel a level of platelet aggregation similar to that of patients on chronic therapy has been demonstrated (17).

Thus, several loading issues with clopidogrel therapy have been raised (18) and a number of studies have explored the possibility that a loading regimen higher than the 300 mg dose may be associated with improved clinical outcome in the setting of PCI. A retrospective analysis on 1,734 patients undergoing coronary stenting have first indicated that pretreatment with 600 mg clopidogrel loading dose 2–4 h before the procedure is associated with a 35% risk reduction of 30-day adverse cardiac events, compared with pretreatment

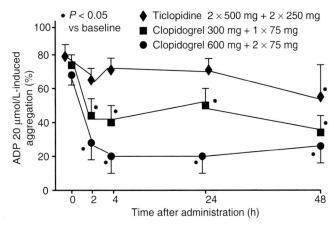

Figure 7.1 ADP-induced platelet aggregation after administration of ticlopidine and clopidogrel (at different loading doses) in patients undergoing coronary stenting. (*Source:* Modified from Müller *et al.* (15) with permission from BMJ Publishing Group Ltd.)

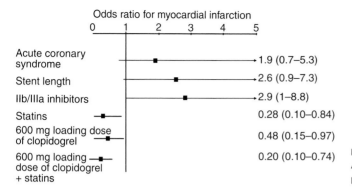

Odds ratio for myocardial infarction

Acute coronary syndrome	1.9 (0.7–5.3)
Stent length	2.6 (0.9–7.3)
IIb/IIIa inhibitors	2.9 (1–8.8)
Statins	0.28 (0.10–0.84)
600 mg loading dose of clopidogrel	0.48 (0.15–0.97)
600 mg loading dose of clopidogrel + statins	0.20 (0.10–0.74)

Figure 7.2 Multivariable analysis of the ARMYDA-2 evaluating independent predictors of outcome.

with ticlopidine 500 mg (19); this clinical benefit was evident in the first days following the procedure, was mainly observed in patients with acute coronary syndromes and was independent of use of GP IIb/IIIa inhibitors. More recently, a randomized trial (ISAR-REACT) (20) has utilized a 600 mg clopidogrel loading dose at least 2 h before PCI in patients with stable coronary artery disease and showed that this regimen may obviate the need for periprocedural use of abciximab, with similar occurrence of cardiac events (death, myocardial infarction, urgent target vessel revascularization) at 30 days: 4% both in the placebo and abciximab group. Similar results were obtained in the ISAR-DIABETES study (21), in which pretreatment with the same higher loading regimen of clopidogrel prevented an additive antiplatelet effect of abciximab in diabetic patients undergoing elective coronary interventions. Finally, in the CREDO trial, a time dependence in the clinical benefit of a 300-mg clopidogrel loading dose has been demonstrated, with 12–15 h of pretreatment required to significantly decrease adverse events (22); this is in agreement with data of optical aggregometry, indicating that at least 12 h are required after a 300 mg loading dose of clopidogrel to achieve a maximal platelet inhibition (5). Accordingly, in the ISAR-REACT study, in which all patients received a 600 mg loading dose in a nonrandomized fashion, no incremental clinical benefit was observed from durations of pretreatment longer than 2–3 h in patients undergoing PCI (23).

In order to explore the possible clinical advantage of higher loading regimens, the recent randomized, multicenter, ARMYDA-2 trial (24) first performed a head-to-head comparison between pretreatment with 600 vs 300 mg loading dose of clopidogrel in the setting of PCI. In particular, this study enrolled 255 patients with either stable or unstable angina and has evaluated the efficacy of this higher regimen given 6 h before the procedure and its effects on release of markers of cardiac injury (creatine kinase-MB, Troponin-I and myoglobin) and 30-day outcome after percutaneous revascularization. Primary end point was the 1-month occurrence of death, myocardial infarction, target vessel revascularization; this was reached by 4% of patients in the 600 mg loading dose group vs 12% of those in the 300 mg arm ($P = 0.041$) and it was entirely due to periprocedural myocardial infarction; at multivariable analysis (Figure 7.2), pretreatment with the higher loading regimen was associated with a 62% risk reduction of myocardial infarction (OR 0.48, 0.15–0.97; $P = 0.044$); the greatest clinical benefit was observed in patients of the 600 mg dose who were also receiving statins at the time of intervention (80% risk reduction; $P = 0.01$). Indeed, protective effect of the 600 mg dose was also expressed as a significant reduction of postprocedural peak levels of all markers of myocardial injury (creatine kinase-MB: 14% vs 26%, $P = 0.036$; Troponin-I 26% vs 44%, $P = 0.004$; myoglobin 30% vs 46%, $P = 0.015$) (Figure 7.3). Safety end points were similar in the two randomization arms of the ARMYDA-2 trial, with no increase in bleeding in patients randomized to the high dose of clopidogrel. These results strongly support the hypothesis that a more rapid and higher degree of platelet inhibition may reduce periprocedural myocardial injury in patients undergoing coronary interventions. Accordingly, ESC guidelines for percutaneous intervention (10) recommend, in order to

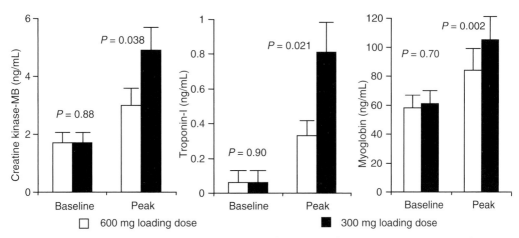

Figure 7.3 Significant reduction of postprocedural peak levels of all markers of myocardial injury in patients of the ARMYDA-2 trial randomized to 600 mg loading dose of clopidogrel.

ensure full antiplatelet activity, to initiate clopidogrel at least 6 h prior to the procedure with a loading dose of 300 mg, ideally administered the day before a planned PCI; if it is not possible, "a loading dose of 600 mg should be administered at least 2 hours before PCI."

The ability to reach maximal antiplatelet effect in a shorter time is likely to be the main factor explaining the beneficial effect of the high loading dose, but other mechanisms may be involved, that is, the higher regimen may reduce the rate of low-responders (8% vs 32% after the conventional 300 mg dose) (25,26), even though it does not significantly decrease interindividual variability (27). Moreover, clopidogrel may have anti-inflammatory effects, as suggested by a post-hoc analysis of the ARMYDA-2 trial, demonstrating a trend toward attenuation of postprocedural increase of C-reactive protein levels in the 600 vs 300 mg arm (28) and by a study from Angiolillo's group showing an increase (rebound?) of inflammatory markers after withdrawal of clopidogrel therapy in patients with diabetes mellitus (29). Clopidogrel may also influence linking mechanisms between thrombosis and inflammation by reducing platelet–leucocyte and platelet–endothelial interactions (30): in the ARMYDA-2 study, clinical benefit of the 600 mg loading was paralleled by a significant reduction of P-selectin levels at the time of intervention (31). Finally, as lipophilic statins and clopidogrel are competitive substrates at the site of CYP 3A4 enzyme system, platelet response after clopidogrel doses of 75–300 mg may be reduced by these statins

in a dose-dependent manner, whereas use of a 600 mg dose may overcome this inhibition (16).

Higher risk patients

Although patients enrolled in the ARMYDA-2 Trial (as well as the original ISAR-REACT Trial) can be classified as "moderate risk," a subanalysis of 175 patients (69% of the patients enrolled) who had clinical/angiographic features of elevated risk (age >70 years, diabetes, non-ST-segment elevation acute coronary syndrome or multivessel intervention) showed a 80% risk reduction of 30-day adverse events in the 600 vs 300 mg loading group (3.4% vs 12.6%; OR, 0.20; 95% CI, 0.04–1.0; $P = 0.05$). A recent randomized study (32) has enrolled patients with unstable angina or non-ST-segment elevation myocardial infarction and has demonstrated that pretreatment with 600 mg of clopidogrel at least 12 h before PCI with stenting is associated with significantly lower 30-day incidence of cardiovascular events, compared with the 300 mg dose (5% vs 12%, $P = 0.02$). Finally, the ISAR-REACT 2 trial (33), addressing patients with acute coronary syndromes undergoing PCI with routine pretreatment with 600 mg of clopidogrel at least 2 h before the procedure, revealed that abciximab confers additional clinical benefit only to patients with elevated baseline Troponin levels.

The value of an even higher clopidogrel loading (i.e., 900 mg) in unstable patients has also been explored: in the ALBION Trial a 900 mg regimen, despite a more pronounced antiplatelet effect vs the 300 mg dose, was not shown to provide an additional clinical benefit in the setting of PCI (34); the ISAR-CHOICE Trial has probably put the issue to rest, demonstrating no difference in platelet aggregation parameters (35) with a loading dose of 900 vs 600 mg, due to lack of further intestinal absorption, limiting bioavailability of the active thiol metabolite.

Contemporary issues in clopidogrel therapy

We can thus conclude that current optimal clopidogrel loading dose, leading to improved outcome and demonstrated by randomized trials, appears to be 600 mg; loading regimens of 900 mg are probably not proven. In the future, it will probably be advisable to apply methods of "point of care testing" to verify the degree of platelet aggregation that best correlate to clinical outcome in the individual patient in order to better manage dosing of powerful antiplatelet drugs in the catheterization laboratory (both Clopidogrel and GP IIb-IIIa antagonists).

To the question of whether GP IIb-IIIa Antagonists provide additional benefit when 600 mg clopidopgrel loading is given, we can reasonably answer "no" for low to moderate risk patients, as shown by ISAR-REACT, and "yes" for patients with Acute Coronary Syndromes with positive markers (ISAR-REACT 2).

As loading strategies get more clarified, other issues in clopidogrel therapy peri-PCI are being investigated and will need to be answered in the near future:

1 Is a further loading dose preintervention required in patients already receiving clopidogrel? Can we achieve additional benefit on outcome with 600 mg clopidogrel load in the increasing number of patients on chronic therapy?

2 Can clopidogrel loading (600 mg) be given in-lab immediately before PCI but after coronary angiography, when the anatomy is known and revascularization indications are more clear, without hours of preloading and without untoward effects on outcome?

3 What is the role of early high clopidogrel loading in patients with acute coronary syndromes, including STEMI?

4 In the modern DES era, is a 150 mg chronic daily therapy with clopidogrel more appropriate in selected patients to obtain optimal antithrombotic effect?

5 What is the role of in-lab and ambulatory aggregometry determinations in order to detect response variability and plan effective dosing strategies during PCI and for the long term?

References

1 Gawaz M, Neumann FJ, Ott I, May A, Schomig A. Platelet activation and coronary stent implantation. Effect of antithrombotic therapy. *Circulation.* 1996;**94**: 279–285.

2 Karvouni E, Katritsis DG, Ioannidis JP. Intravenous glycoprotein IIb/IIIa receptor antagonists reduce mortality after percutaneous coronary interventions. *J Am Coll Cardiol.* 2003;**41**:26–32.

3 Schömig A, Neumann FJ, Kastrati A, *et al.* A randomized comparison of antiplatelet and anticoagulant therapy after the placement of coronary-artery stents. *N Engl J Med.* 1996;**334**:1084–1089.

4 Bhatt DL, Bertrand ME, Berger PB, *et al.* Meta-analysis of randomized and registry comparisons of ticlopidine with clopidogrel after stenting. *J Am Coll Cardiol.* 2002;**39**:9–14.

5 Gurbel PA, Cummings CC, Bell CR, *et al.* Onset and extent of platelet inhibition by clopidogrel loading in patients undergoing elective coronary stenting: the Plavix Reduction Of New Thrombus Occurrence (PRONTO) trial. *Am Heart J.* 2003;**145**:239–247.

6 Mehta SR, Yusuf S, Peters RJ, *et al.* Effects of pretreatment with clopidogrel and aspirin followed by long-term therapy in patients undergoing percutaneous coronary intervention: the PCI-CURE study. *Lancet.* 2001;**358**: 527–533.

7 Steinhubl SR, Berger PB, Mann JT, 3rd, *et al.* Clopidogrel for the Reduction of Events During Observation. Early and sustained dual oral antiplatelet therapy following percutaneous coronary intervention: a randomized controlled trial. *JAMA.* 2002;**288**:2411–2420.

8 Chan AW, Moliterno DJ, Berger PB, *et al.* Triple antiplatelet therapy during percutaneous coronary intervention is associated with improved outcomes including one-year survival: results from the Do Tirofiban and ReoProGive Similar Efficacy Outcome Trial (TARGET). *J Am Coll Cardiol.* 2003;**42**:1188–1195.

9 Van der Heijden DJ, Westendorp IC, Riezebos RL, *et al.* Lack of efficacy of clopidogrel pre-treatment in the prevention of myocardial damage after elective stent implantation. *J Am Coll Cardiol.* 2004;**44**:20–24.

10 Silber S, Albertsson P, Aviles FF, *et al.* Guidelines for percutaneous coronary interventions. The Task Force for Percutaneous Coronary Interventions of the European Society of Cardiology. *Eur Heart J.* 2005;**26**:804–847.

11 Braunwald E. Application of current guidelines to the management of unstable angina and non-ST-elevation myocardial infarction. *Circulation.* 2003;**108**(16 Suppl 1): III28–III37.

12 Cadroy Y, Bossavy JP, Thalamas C, Sagnard L, Sakariassen K, Boneu B. Early potent antithrombotic effect with combined aspirin and LD of clopidogrel on experimental arterial thrombogenesis in humans. *Circulation.* 2000;**101**:2823–2828.

13 Gorog P, Ridler CD, Rees GM, Kovacs IB. Evidence against hypercoagulability in coronary artery disease. *Thromb Res.* 1995;**79**:377–385.

14 Hochholzer W, Trenk D, Bestehorn HP, *et al.* Impact of the degree of peri-interventional platelet inhibition after loading with clopidogrel on early clinical outcome of elective coronary stent placement. *J Am Coll Cardiol.* 2006;**48**:1742–1750.

15 Müller I, Seyfarth M, Rudiger S, *et al.* Effect of a high loading dose of clopidogrel on platelet function in patients undergoing coronary stent placement. *Heart.* 2001;**85**:92–93.

16 Hochholzer W, Trenk D, Frundi D, *et al.* Time dependence of platelet inhibition after a 600-mg loading dose of clopidogrel in a large, unselected cohort of candidates for percutaneous coronary intervention. *Circulation.* 2005;**111**:2560–2564.

17 Kastrati A, von Beckerath N, Joost A, Pogatsa-Murray G, Gorchakova O, Schomig A. Loading with 600 mg clopidogrel in patients with coronary artery disease with and without chronic clopidogrel therapy. *Circulation.* 2004;**110**:1916–1919.

18 Williams DO. Clopidogrel pre-treatment for percutaneous coronary intervention. *Circulation.* 2005;**111**: 2019–2021.

19 Pache J, Kastrati A, Mehilli J, *et al.* Clopidogrel therapy in patients undergoing coronary stenting: value of a high-loading-dose regimen. *Cathet Cardiovasc Interv.* 2002;**55**:436–441.

20 Kastrati A, Mehilli J, Schuhlen H, *et al.* A clinical trial of abciximab in elective percutaneous coronary intervention after pretreatment with clopidogrel. *N Engl J Med.* 2004;**350**:232–238.

21 Mehilli J, Kastrati A, Schuhlen H, *et al.* Randomized clinical trial of abciximab in diabetic patients undergoing elective percutaneous coronary interventions after treatment with a high loading dose of clopidogrel. *Circulation.* 2004;**110**:3627–3635.

22 Steinhubl SR, Darrah S, Brennan D, McErlean E, Berger PB, Topol EJ. Optimal duration of pretreatment

with clopidogrel prior to PCI: data from the CREDO trial. *Circulation.* 2003;**108**(Suppl I):I1742.

23 Kandzari DE, Berger PB, Kastrati A, *et al.* Influence of treatment duration with a 600-mg dose of clopidogrel before percutaneous coronary revascularization. *J Am Coll Cardiol.* 2004;**44**:2133–2136.

24 Patti G, Colonna G, Pasceri V, Lassandro Pepe L, Montanaro A, Di Sciascio G. A randomized trial of high loading dose of clopidogrel for reduction of peri-procedural myocardial infarction in patients undergoing coronary intervention results from the ARMYDA-2 (Antiplatelet therapy for Reduction of MYocardial Damage during Angioplasty) Study. *Circulation.* 2005;**111**:2099–2106.

25 Gurbel PA, Bliden KP, Hayes KM, Yoho JA, Herzog WR, Tantry US. The relation of dosing to clopidogrel responsiveness and the incidence of high post-treatment platelet aggregation in patients undergoing coronary stenting. *J Am Coll Cardiol.* 2005;**45**:1392–1396.

26 Chew DP, Bhatt DL, Robbins MA, *et al.* Effect of clopidogrel added to aspirin before percutaneous coronary intervention on the risk associated with C-reactive protein. *Am J Cardiol.* 2001;**88**:672–674.

27 Angiolillo D, Fernàndez-Ortiz A, Bernardo E, *et al.* High clopidogrel loading dose during coronary stenting: effects on drug response and interindividual variability. *Eur Heart J.* 2004;**25**:1903–1910.

28 Angiolillo DJ, Fernandez-Ortiz A, Bernardo E, *et al.* Clopidogrel withdrawal is associated with proinflammatory and prothrombotic effects in patients with diabetes and coronary artery disease. *Diabetes.* 2006;**55**:780–784.

29 Patti G, Colonna G, Pasceri V, *et al.* A randomized trial of high loading dose of clopidogrel for reduction of peri-procedural myocardial infarction in patients undergoing coronary intervention. *Eur Heart J.* 2005, Abstract Suppl–P433.

30 Xiao Z, Théroux P. Clopidogrel inhibits platelet-leukocyte interactions and thrombin receptor agonist peptide-induced platelet activation in patients with an acute coronary syndrome. *J Am Coll Cardiol.* 2004;**43**: 1982–1988.

31 Patti G, Chello M, Colonna D, *et al.* Clinical benefit of pre-treatment with high dose of clopidogrel before percutaneous coronary intervention is associated with lower procedural levels of P-selectin. Results from the ARMYDA-2 (Antiplatelet therapy for Reduction of MYocardial Damage during Angioplasty) SELECT substudy. *J Am Coll Cardiol.* 2006;**47**(Suppl 2):18B.

32 Cuisset T, Frere C, Quilici J, *et al.* Benefit of a 600-mg loading dose of clopidogrel on platelet reactivity and clinical outcomes in patients with non-ST-segment elevation acute coronary syndrome undergoing coronary stenting. *J Am Coll Cardiol.* 2006;**48**:1339–1345.

33 Kastrati A, Mehilli J, Neumann FJ, *et al.* Abciximab in patients with acute coronary syndromes undergoing percutaneous coronary intervention after clopidogrel pretreatment: the ISAR-REACT 2 randomized trial. *JAMA.* 2006;**295**:1531–1538.

34 Montalescot G, Sideris G, Meuleman C, *et al.* A randomized comparison of high clopidogrel loading doses in patients with non-ST-segment elevation acute coronary syndromes: the ALBION (Assessment of the Best Loading Dose of Clopidogrel to Blunt Platelet Activation,

Inflammation and Ongoing Necrosis) trial. *J Am Coll Cardiol.* 2006;**48**:931–938.

35 von Beckerath N, Taubert D, Pogatsa-Murray G, Schomig E, Kastrati A, Schomig A. Absorption, metabolization, and antiplatelet effects of 300-, 600-, and 900-mg loading doses of clopidogrel: results of the ISAR-CHOICE (Intracoronary Stenting and Antithrombotic Regimen: Choose Between 3 High Oral Doses for Immediate Clopidogrel Effect) Trial. *Circulation.* 2005;**112**:2946–2950.

CHAPTER 8

Cangrelor

Julie H. Oestreich[1] & Steven R. Steinhubl[2,3]
[1]University of Kentucky, Lexington, KY, USA
[2]The Medicines Company, Zurich, Switzerland
[3]Geisinger Clinic, Danville, PA, USA

The P2Y$_{12}$ receptor in platelet function

Adenosine diphosphate (ADP) P2Y receptors are critical regulators of platelet function. Although ADP is considered a weak agonist, platelet activation by more potent agonists are dependent upon ADP secretion from platelet granules and subsequent binding to P2Y receptors. ADP is the endogenous ligand for both P2Y$_{12}$ and P2Y$_1$ receptors that stimulate platelet aggregation (Figure 8.1) (1). The ubiquitously expressed P2Y$_1$ receptor mediates transient platelet shape change and increased intracellular calcium, whereas binding of ADP to the Gi-coupled P2Y$_{12}$ receptor is required for complete and irreversible platelet activation (1–3). Unlike the widely distributed P2Y$_1$ receptor, the P2Y$_{12}$ receptor has only been found on platelets, glioma cells, and vascular smooth muscle cells and therefore serves as a favorable therapeutic target (2,4). Specifically, P2Y$_{12}$ activation causes granule secretion of ADP and other mediators, thromboxane A2 generation, platelet recruitment, and potentiation of aggregation and coagulation (3).

P2Y$_{12}$ receptor inhibition in PCI

The value of platelet P2Y$_{12}$ receptor inhibition has been established by the clinical utility of the thienopyridines ticlopidine (Ticlid®) and clopidogrel (Plavix®). Due to the unfavorable adverse event profile of ticlopidine, clopidogrel is the

Pharmacology in the Catheterization Laboratory. Edited by Ron Waksman and Andrew E Ajani. © 2010 Blackwell Publishing, ISBN: 978-1-4051-5704-9.

preferred agent for prevention of acute and long-term adverse coronary events in ischemic patients. For patients undergoing percutaneous coronary intervention (PCI), long-term clopidogrel therapy for one year in addition to aspirin reduced the combined primary outcome of death, myocardial infarction (MI), and stroke by 26.9% (relative risk reduction) (5). Additionally, treatment with a loading of dose clopidogrel prior to PCI resulted in a 58.8% relative risk reduction of the combined end points of death, MI, and urgent target vessel revascularization, albeit these results were dependent upon the dose and time of administration (5,6). For a 300 mg loading dose, adequate pretreatment of at least 15 h is required to achieve therapeutic benefit. A more rapid onset of action and maximal pharmacodynamic effect can be obtained with a 600 mg loading dose, yet further evidence clarifying the optimal dose and pretreatment window would be beneficial (5–7).

Despite the undisputed clinical benefit and widespread utilization of clopidogrel in PCI, there are significant shortcomings associated with its use. As with all thienopyridines, clopidogrel is a prodrug that requires hepatic conversion by the cytochrome P450 system to attain pharmacological activity (7). Consequently, clopidogrel has a slow onset of action, and its activity is susceptible to variations in metabolism. The short-lived active metabolite of the drug is believed to form a disulfide bridge with extracellular cysteines on the P2Y$_{12}$ receptor to cause incomplete and irreversible inhibition of ADP-mediated aggregation for the life of the platelet (7–10 days) (2,4,8). There is no pharmacological antidote, and a small

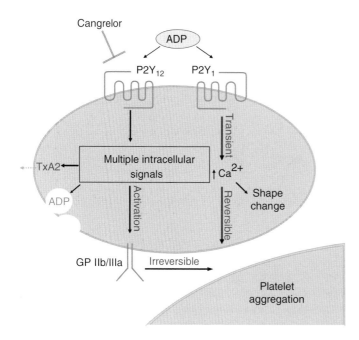

Figure 8.1 Effects of the ADP receptors P2Y$_1$ and P2Y$_{12}$ on platelet activation and aggregation. Cangrelor specifically and selectively inhibits the P2Y$_{12}$ receptor, one of two G protein-coupled platelet ADP receptors. Activation of the P2Y$_{12}$ receptor by ADP leads to thromboxane A2 generation, platelet granule release of ADP and other mediators of aggregation and coagulation, and increased expression and activation of the GP IIb/IIIa receptor. The P2Y$_{12}$ receptor causes irreversible and sustained platelet activation and aggregation. Conversely, the P2Y$_1$ receptor has transient and reversible effects on platelet shape change and aggregation mediated by calcium release. *Abbreviations*: ADP, adenosine diphosphate; TxA2, thromboxane A2; GP IIb/IIIa, glycoprotein IIb/IIIa.

percentage of patients undergoing PCI also require emergent coronary artery bypass graft (CABG) surgery (9). More importantly, in patients with an acute coronary syndrome, in whom ~15% will require CABG for revascularization (10), early initiation of clopidogrel can lead to either prolonged hospitalizations while awaiting surgery or an increased risk of bleeding if surgery is not delayed (11).

Furthermore, there is well-documented variability in the response to clopidogrel, as 4%–30% of patients do not obtain the expected degree of inhibition depending on the type of assay utilized and definition of nonresponsiveness employed (12,13). Evidence to support the clinical relevance of this variability is limited though nonresponders have shown a higher risk for thrombotic events in a few trials (14,15). The potential mechanisms of clopidogrel nonresponsiveness are diverse, yet several explanations relate to the intrinsic pharmacokinetic properties of the drug, including drug–drug interactions, bioavailability, and genetic variations in CYP450 enzymes (8). The newer thienopyridine, prasugrel, attempts to decrease variation in platelet response with increased receptor affinity, but is still plagued by required hepatic conversion to an active metabolite and irreversibility (2). These limitations have

spurred further development of novel P2Y$_{12}$ antagonists optimized for use in PCI.

Pharmacokinetics and pharmacodynamics of cangrelor

The novel antiplatelet agent cangrelor is a specific and potent antagonist of platelet activity (16). Cangrelor is an adenosine triphosphate (ATP) analogue (Figure 8.2) that competitively inhibits platelet activation and aggregation by reversibly binding the P2Y$_{12}$ receptor. The structure of ATP, an endogenous antagonist to the target receptor, was altered to produce a compound with increased stability, affinity, and potency (2).

Cangrelor is a rapid-acting and short-lived intravenous medication. Following a bolus dose and infusion regimen in healthy volunteers (15 µg/kg bolus plus 2 µg/kg/min or 30 µg/kg bolus plus 4 µg/kg/min), maximal and steady-state cangrelor concentrations are obtained within minutes of administration. The drug displays linear, dose-dependent pharmacokinetics at the studied range, and has a limited volume of distribution (~3.7 L) due to its polar nature and fast metabolism (17). Cangrelor levels return to baseline within 10 min after stopping the infusion because the drug is rapidly dephosphorylated by an ecto-ADPase

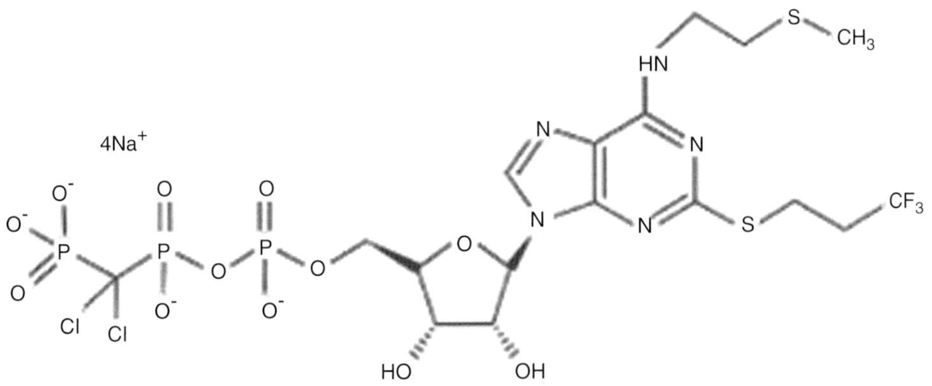

Figure 8.2 Structure of cangrelor, an ATP analogue and novel antiplatelet agent.

associated with vascular endothelial cells (17,18). In addition to the fast onset and reversible properties of the drug, its extremely short half-life (2.6–3.6 min) makes cangrelor an attractive option for patients undergoing PCI (17,19).

Similar to the pharmacokinetic data, the platelet pharmacodynamic response to cangrelor is rapid acting and quickly reversible following drug termination. *Ex vivo* testing of cangrelor-treated healthy volunteers demonstrates that platelet inhibition is obtained within minutes of initiating therapy as demonstrated by ADP-induced whole blood aggregometry and flow cytometric analysis of agonist-induced P-selectin expression. Fifty percent of platelet function is recovered within 10–30 min after stopping the infusion, and a complete return to baseline function is achieved within 60–90 min (17).

Cangrelor has been well tolerated in clinical trials alone and in combination with other agents including aspirin and heparin (20). Interestingly, the only reported drug interaction to date is a pharmacodynamic interaction with clopidogrel (21). Patients undergoing PCI, including those treated with cangrelor, will be expected to maintain long-term oral $P2Y_{12}$ inhibition to prevent adverse coronary events. A Phase II trial assessing the transition of patients from cangrelor to clopidogrel identified a probable competitive and time-dependent interaction between the drugs as assessed by whole blood electrical impedance aggregometry, light transmittance aggregometry, and flow cytometry. Healthy volunteers randomized to receive a 600 mg clopidogrel loading dose immediately following a cangrelor 30 μg/kg IV bolus and 1 h 4 μg/kg/min infusion obtained the expected degree of platelet inhibition for both antiplatelet agents (21). Cangrelor inhibited 80% of light transmittance platelet aggregation induced by 20 μM ADP, and clopidogrel inhibited 50–60% of the platelet response following a predicted delay of onset. Those randomized to receive the loading dose of clopidogrel simultaneously with cangrelor did not achieve the expected inhibition with clopidogrel as postinfusion pharmacodynamic measures returned and remained at baseline (Figure 8.3) (21). Most likely, there was a competitive interaction as the short-lived active metabolite of clopidogrel is unable to compete for receptor occupancy in the presence of reversible inhibitor cangrelor. Cangrelor's high affinity for the $P2Y_{12}$ receptor prevents clopidogrel's active metabolite from irreversibly binding the target receptor. The half-life of clopidogrel's unstable active metabolite is postulated to be very short, and evidence from this study also supports that no active metabolite remains 2 h after a 600 mg loading dose. The clinical relevance of this interaction in PCI patients is unknown, however, it is postulated that other non-thienopyridine, orally available $P2Y_{12}$ antagonists may avoid this interaction.

Clinical trials with cangrelor

The safety of cangrelor has been evaluated in healthy volunteers and patients with unstable angina, acute MI, and those undergoing PCI. Generally, the

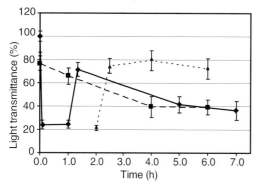

Figure legend:
- Clopidogrel at the end of cangrelor infusion
- Clopidogrel only
- Clopidogrel plus cangrelor

Figure 8.3 Clopidogrel inhibits ADP-induced platelet aggregation when administered immediately following a cangrelor infusion, but does not achieve the expected level of inhibition when administered simultaneously with cangrelor. The effect of cangrelor and clopidogrel on ADP-induced (20 µM) platelet aggregation was evaluated by light transmittance aggregometry. Subjects randomized to treatment arm 1 ($n = 10$) were administered a cangrelor 30 µg/kg IV bolus plus a 4 µg/kg/min infusion for 1 h immediately followed by oral administration of clopidogrel 600 mg at the end of the cangrelor infusion (solid line). Subjects in treatment arm 2 ($n = 10$) were first administered oral clopidogrel 600 mg followed by a 2-week washout period. After the washout period, subjects were readministered oral clopidogrel 600 mg simultaneous with a cangrelor 30 µg/kg IV bolus and a 4 µg/kg/min infusion for 2 h (dashed lines). Data are presented as mean ± SEM. Similar results were obtained with electrical impedance aggregometry and flow cytometry.

drug has been well tolerated, and the most common adverse effect, as expected, is prolongation of bleeding time (19).

In two separate Phase II multicenter trials (one open label and the other randomized, double-blinded and placebo controlled), 130 combined unstable angina and non-Q wave MI patients were administered an infusion of cangrelor or placebo in addition to aspirin and heparin or low-molecular-weight heparin. Both preliminary studies demonstrated that cangrelor infused up to 72 h was not accumulated nor associated with an increase in serious adverse events (22,23). Intravenous cangrelor has also been studied as adjunct therapy to fibrinolysis for acute myocardial infarction (24). One hundred and one patients were randomized

to receive one of three cangrelor doses in addition to 50 mg t-PA, cangrelor alone, or t-PA alone. Although the trial was stopped early, bleeding complications and major adverse clinical events were not different between combination therapy and standard t-PA, and a potential benefit could not be ruled out.

A phase II, multicenter, randomized, placebo and active-controlled trial was carried out to evaluate cangrelor in patients undergoing PCI (20). Patients in part 1 were randomized to placebo or a 1, 2, or 4 µg/kg/min cangrelor infusion starting before PCI in combination with aspirin and heparin. Part 2 compared the highest dose of cangrelor with abciximab. No statistically significant differences were obtained between cangrelor and either control group when comparing major and minor bleeding or comparing 30-day incidence of adverse cardiac events between cangrelor and abciximab. Although both cangrelor and abciximab completely inhibited ADP-stimulated platelet aggregation as measured by electrical impedance aggregometry, those treated with cangrelor returned to baseline platelet function more quickly after the infusion was terminated.

Two large-scale phase III clinical trials termed the CHAMPION Platform (cangrelor versus standard therapy to achieve optimal management of platelet inhibition) are ongoing to assess the safety and efficacy of cangrelor in patients with coronary atherosclerosis requiring PCI. Both prospective, randomized, double-blinded, and placebo-controlled studies are evaluating a composite primary endpoint of all-cause mortality, nonfatal MI, and ischemia-driven revascularization assessed 48 h after randomization. The first CHAMPION trial is expected to enroll 9,000 acute coronary syndrome patients who will be managed with PCI following randomization and administration of a clopidogrel 300 mg loading dose or cangrelor 30 µg/kg IV bolus and 4 µg/kg/min infusion. Subjects randomized to cangrelor will receive a clopidogrel loading dose following the infusion. Unlike the comparison between cangrelor and clopidogrel in the first trial, the other CHAMPION trial is investigating cangrelor to usual care in PCI subjects. Patients taking any thienopyridine in the previous 7 days or presenting with a ST-segment elevation MI within 48 h are not eligible for this study. Enrollment is expected to reach 4,400 subjects to assess the efficacy and tolerability of cangrelor added to standard treatment.

Summary

Cangrelor is a novel antagonist of the P2Y$_{12}$ receptor that reversibly and potently inhibits ADP-induced platelet aggregation. The intravenously administered cangrelor has a fast onset of action and is quickly reversible once the infusion is stopped. These unique characteristics provide advantages over currently available antiplatelet medications, supporting cangrelor as a promising option for patients undergoing PCI.

References

1 Hollopeter G, Jantzen HM, Vincent D, et al. Identification of the platelet ADP receptor targeted by antithrombotic drugs. Nature. 2001;**409**:202–207.

2 Kunapuli SP, Ding Z, Dorsam RT, Kim S, Murugappan S, Quinton TM. ADP receptors—targets for developing antithrombotic agents. Curr Pharm Des. 2003;**9**:303–2316.

3 Dorsam RT, Kunapuli SP. Central role of the P2Y12 receptor in platelet activation. J Clin Invest. 2004;**113**:340–345.

4 Ding Z, Kim S, Dorsam RT, Jin J, Kunapuli SP. Inactivation of the human P2Y12 receptor by thiol reagents requires interaction with both extracellular cysteine residues, Cys17 and Cys270. Blood. 2003;**101**:3908–3914.

5 Steinhubl SR, Berger PB, Mann JT, 3rd, et al. Early and sustained dual oral antiplatelet therapy following percutaneous coronary intervention: a randomized controlled trial. JAMA. 2002;**288**:2411–2420.

6 Steinhubl SR, Berger PB, Brennan DM, Topol EJ. Optimal timing for the initiation of pre-treatment with 300 mg clopidogrel before percutaneous coronary intervention. J Am Coll Cardiol. 2006;**47**:939–943.

7 von Beckerath N, Taubert D, Pogatsa-Murray G, Schomig E, Kastrati A, Schomig A. Absorption, metabolization, and antiplatelet effects of 300-, 600-, and 900-mg loading doses of clopidogrel: results of the ISAR-CHOICE (Intracoronary Stenting and Antithrombotic Regimen: Choose Between 3 High Oral Doses for Immediate Clopidogrel Effect) trial. Circulation. 2005;**112**:2946–2950.

8 Nguyen TA, Diodati JG, Pharand C. Resistance to clopidogrel: a review of the evidence. J Am Coll Cardiol. 2005;**45**:1157–1164.

9 Yang EH, Gumina RJ, Lennon RJ, Holmes DR, Jr, Rihal CS, Singh M. Emergency coronary artery bypass surgery for percutaneous coronary interventions: changes in the incidence, clinical characteristics, and indications from 1979 to 2003. J Am Coll Cardiol. 2005;**46**:2004–2009.

10 Mehta RH, Chen AY, Pollack CV, Jr, et al. Challenges in predicting the need for coronary artery bypass grafting at presentation in patients with non-ST-segment elevation acute coronary syndromes. Am J Cardiol. 2006;**98**:624–627.

11 The Clopidogrel in Unstable Angina to Prevent Recurrent Events Trial Investigators. Effects of clopidogrel in addition to aspirin in patients with acute coronary syndromes without ST-segment elevation. N Engl J Med. 2001;**345**:494–502.

12 Serebruany VL, Steinhubl SR, Berger PB, Malinin AI, Bhatt DL, Topol EJ. Variability in platelet responsiveness to clopidogrel among 544 individuals. J Am Coll Cardiol. 2005;**45**:246–251.

13 Mobley JE, Bresee SJ, Wortham DC, Craft RM, Snider CC, Carroll RC. Frequency of nonresponse antiplatelet activity of clopidogrel during pretreatment for cardiac catheterization. Am J Cardiol. 2004;**93**:456–458.

14 Barragan P, Bouvier JL, Roquebert PO, et al. Resistance to thienopyridines: clinical detection of coronary stent thrombosis by monitoring of vasodilator-stimulated phosphoprotein phosphorylation. Catheter Cardiovasc Interv. 2003;**59**:295–302.

15 Matetzky S, Shenkman B, Guetta V, et al. Clopidogrel resistance is associated with increased risk of recurrent atherothrombotic events in patients with acute myocardial infarction. Circulation. 2004;**109**:3171–3175.

16 van Giezen JJ, Humphries RG. Preclinical and clinical studies with selective reversible direct P2Y12 antagonists. Semin Thromb Hemost. 2005;**31**:195–204.

17 Akers WS, Oh JJ, Oestreich JH, Ferraris S, Wethington M, Steinhubl SR. Pharmacokinetics and pharmacodynamics of a bolus and infusion of cangrelor: a direct, parenteral P2Y12 receptor antagonist. J Clin Pharmacol. 2009 (in press).

18 Marcus AJ, Broekman MJ, Drosopoulos JH, et al. Metabolic control of excessive extracellular nucleotide accumulation by CD39/ecto-nucleotidase-1: implications for ischemic vascular diseases. J Pharmacol Exp Ther. 2003;**305**:9–16.

19 Fugate SE, Cudd LA. Cangrelor for treatment of coronary thrombosis. Ann Pharmacother. 2006;**40**:925–930.

20 Greenbaum AB, Grines CL, Bittl JA, et al. Initial experience with an intravenous P2Y12 platelet receptor antagonist in patients undergoing percutaneous coronary intervention: results from a 2-part, phase II, multicenter, randomized, placebo- and active-controlled trial. Am Heart J. 2006;**151**:689, e1–689 e10.

21 Steinhubl SR, Oh JJ, Oestreich JH, Ferraris S, Charnigo R, Akers WS. Transitioning patients from cangrelor to clopidogrel: pharmacodynamic evidence of a competitive effect. Thromb Res. 2008;**121**(4):527–534.

22 Jacobsson F, Swahn E, Wallentin L, Ellborg M. Safety profile and tolerability of intravenous AR-C69931MX, a new antiplatelet drug, in unstable angina pectoris and non-Q-wave myocardial infarction. *Clin Ther.* 2002; **24**:752–765.

23 Storey RF, Oldroyd KG, Wilcox RG. Open multicentre study of the P2T receptor antagonist AR-C69931MX assessing safety, tolerability and activity in patients with acute coronary syndromes. *Thromb Haemost.* 2001;**85**:401–407.

24 Greenbaum AB OE, Gibson MS, Borzak SL, *et al.* Intravenous adenosine diphosphate P2T platelet receptor antagonism as an adjunct to fibrinolysis for acute myocardial infarction. *Suppl J Am Coll Cardiol.* 2002;**39**:1002–1045.

CHAPTER 9

Prasugrel: A novel P2Y$_{12}$ receptor inhibitor

Itsik Ben-Dor[1,2], Mickey Scheinowitz[3], & Ron Waksman[4]
[1]Tel-Aviv University, Tel-Aviv, Israel
[2]Rabin Medical Center, Petach-Tikva, Israel
[3]Tel-Aviv University, Ramat-Aviv, Israel
[4]Washington Hospital Center, Washington, DC, USA

Clinical background

Dual antiplatelet therapy with aspirin and thienopyridines (clopidogrel) significantly reduces atherothrombotic events and improves long-term clinical outcomes in patients undergoing percutaneous coronary intervention (PCI) following acute coronary syndrome (ACS). Despite dual antiplatelet therapy with aspirin and clopidogrel, however, some patients still develop stent thrombosis and other recurrent cardiovascular ischemic events. These adverse clinical outcomes could result from hyporesponsivness to either aspirin or clopidogrel or from delayed onset of action of these agents. Although the prevalence of either aspirin or clopidogrel resistance may be reduced by increasing the dose of medication, it cannot be eliminated, and interindividual variability may still persist. A novel thienopyridine—prasugrel—is currently in clinical development and has pharmacologic properties that might overcome some of the limitations experienced with clopidogrel and aspirin therapy.

Thienopyridines

Thienopyridines are a class of ADP/P2Y12 receptor inhibitors. P2Y$_{12}$ is a family of G protein-coupled purinergic receptors known to be present on neuronal tissue and platelets. They possess four cysteine residues in the extracellular domain, which are likely to form two disulfide bridges with the N-terminal and the extracellular loop on the surface membrane (1). This receptor is involved in platelet aggregation via activation of GP IIb/IIIa pathway, and its inhibition results in antiplatelet activity. The previously used ticlopidine was shown to induce thrombotic thrombocytopenic purpura (TTP), however, it is no longer used and has been replaced by clopidogrel. Clopidogrel is a prodrug, which requires metabolism by the liver for its activation. The active metabolite has an elimination half-life of 8 h and acts by forming a disulfide bridge with the platelet ADP receptor.

Prasugrel (CS-747, LY640315), an investigational, third-generation thienopyridine with similar structure to first- and second-generation thienopyridines (ticlopidine and clopidogrel, respectively), is also a pro-drug necessitate hepatic metabolism to its active form. Cytochrome P-450 isoenzymes are required to achieve the active forms of these drugs. However, prasugrel requires one interaction with this enzyme while clopidogrel requires two interactions. Both result in oxidative steps that generate the active metabolite (R-138727), which irreversibly binds to the platelet P2Y$_{12}$ ADP receptor to achieve its inhibitory effect (Figure 9.1). It has been shown more recently that prasugrel interacts with the residues cystein 97 (upper portion of the transmembrane region) and cystein 175 (second extracellular loop) of the receptor (2). This inhibition is

Pharmacology in the Catheterization Laboratory. Edited by Ron Waksman and Andrew E Ajani. © 2010 Blackwell Publishing, ISBN: 978-1-4051-5704-9.

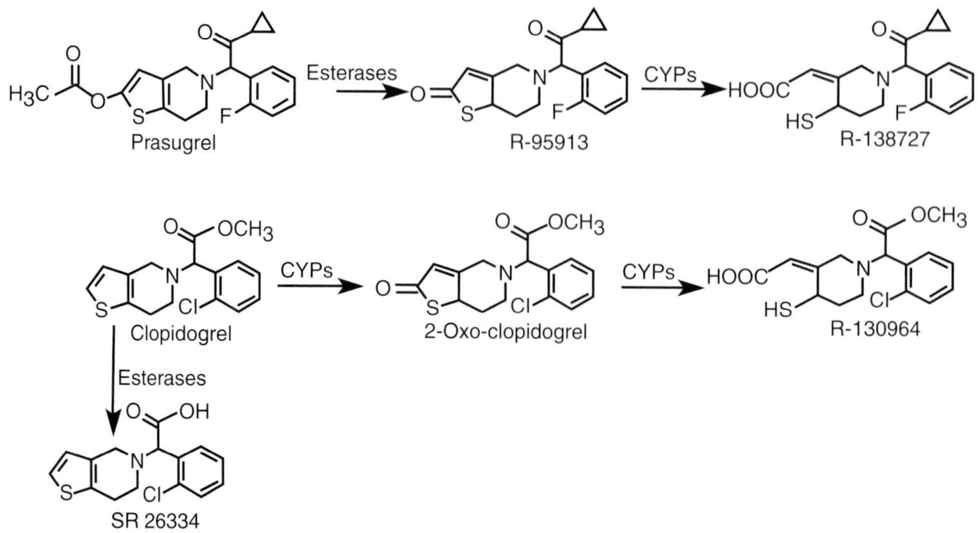

Figure 9.1 Structure and primary metabolic pathways for prasugrel and clopidogrel.

known to last for the life of the platelet. In addition, proton pump inhibition was found to delay the production of the active metabolite, however, with no effect on the inhibition of platelet activation (3). Prasugrel achieves plasma steady-state levels faster than clopidogrel (3 vs 5 days, respectively) (4) and maintains a higher platelet inhibition level *in vivo* (5). While renal excretion is the major route for prasugrel elimination (6), esterases act as the major carboxylic acid metabolite inactivators for clopidogrel (7). In rats, a single oral dose of prasugrel produced inhibition of platelet activation (IPA) by 10- and 100-fold more than clopidogrel or ticlopidine, respectively (5). Within 30 min of a single oral administration, 80% IPA was monitored. The active metabolite was also shown to inhibit platelet–leukocyte interaction, platelet procoagulant activity, and platelet thromboinflammatory markers (8).

Safety and tolerability of prasugrel in healthy volunteers

Antiplatelet effects, pharmacokinetics, safety, and tolerability were studied in a randomized, double-blind, double-dummy, placebo-controlled trial by Jakubowski *et al.* (4). Platelet aggregation was assessed with light transmission aggregometry and was measured pre-prasugrel, and at several time points post-prasugrel loading doses (40 and 60 mg) and maintenance doses (7.5 and 15 mg). At 24 h, IPA level was significantly increased following both loading doses of prasugrel: 65% with 60 mg and 74% with 40 mg. Peak IPA was achieved 60–90 min after prasugrel loading dose and this level was maintained for 24 h. At a maintenance dose, IPA was reduced to 37% 2 weeks following the loading regimen with no apparent differences between 7.5 and 15 mg of prasugrel. Prasugrel was well tolerated among these 30 healthy adults from both genders. No changes in liver enzymes were noted. The most common adverse events were headache, hematoma, and dizziness, though none required discontinuation of the medication. Two patients were dropped from the study due to untoward events: one placebo-controlled individual with pruritis and one individual on prasugrel who on day 17 developed hematoma.

In a more recent study, Payne *et al.* (9) studied the effect of switching from clopidogrel to prasugrel in healthy volunteers treated with aspirin. Forty subjects were randomized to either loading dose (60 mg) or maintenance dose (10 mg) of prasugrel for 11 days following 1 week of clopidogrel (600 + 75 mg). All subjects were on aspirin 81 mg throughout the study protocol (while on clopidogrel and prasugrel). Switching to prasugrel resulted in an additional 24% platelet inhibition within

4–5 days. Prasugrel was well tolerated among all participants. Bleeding-related adverse events were similar and were not dose-dependent. All other laboratory data were normal.

In a phase 1 study using healthy human subjects, inhibition of platelet aggregation was greater with a single 60-mg dose of prasugrel than with a single 300-mg dose of clopidogrel (10). Further, there was evidence that thienopyridine resistance may be less frequent in healthy volunteers with a loading dose of 60 mg of prasugrel than with 300 mg of clopidogrel. In a following phase 2 study, dose-ranging safety was carried out on patients undergoing elective or urgent PCI. The major end point included hemorrhagic events at 30 days (11). There were nonsignificantly higher rates of minor and minimal bleeding in patients treated with prasugrel, especially at the highest dose studied. In contrast, there were nonsignificantly lower rates of ischemic events after PCI when patients were treated with prasugrel compared with clopidogrel. Recently Frelinger *et al.* showed that prasugrel inhibited *in vivo* platelet activation to the same extent as clopidogrel but inhibited ADP-stimulated platelet–monocyte aggregates and platelet–neutrophil aggregates at a greater degree than clopidogrel (12). The poor, variable responses of clopidogrel were compared to prasugrel in 20 human liver microsomes showing that less clopidogrel thiolactone was generated with higher variability than prasugrel (13). And lastly, genetic variations of the cytochrome P450 enzymes, particularly CYP2C19, were shown to be associated with significantly higher risk of CV death, MI, or stroke, and for stent thrombosis among clopidogrel-treated patients but not for prasugrel (14). Thus, in healthy subjects, prasugrel has been well tolerated at a single loading dose of 80 mg or a maintenance dose of 15 mg/day for as long as 28 days. As with clopidogrel, the most frequently reported adverse events in healthy subjects were hematoma and minor bleeding.

Monitoring of antiplatelet therapy

Jakubowski *et al.* investigated the antiplatelet effect of prasugrel using the VerifyNow point of care assay with light transmission aggregometry (LTA). They found good correlation between the two assays among healthy subjects receiving aspirin and a prasugrel loading dose followed by a maintenance dose (15). Similar results ware demonstrated comparing IPA with LTA and vasodilator-stimulated phosphoprotein (VASP) in healthy subjects receiving aspirin and loading and maintaining doses of prasugrel for 7 days (16). In a clinical setup, IPA was measured and correlated among cardiac patients scheduled for PCI using LTA, VerifyNow, and VASP assays (17). There was agreement among all three IPA assays used both during loading dose and while on maintenance dose of prasugrel. In a more basic study, prasugrel active metabolite R-138727 effectively inhibited platelet procoagulant activity in whole blood following stimulation with ADP and or collagen (18). In addition, Li and colleagues have shown that the level of inhibition of platelet aggregation was faster and greater with prasugrel compared with clopidogrel (19). They used a 60-mg loading dose and a 10-mg maintenance dose of prasugrel and a 300-mg loading dose and a 75-mg maintenance dose of clopidogrel and measured IPA several hours following loading dose and up to 9 days while on maintenance dose. Inhibition of platelet aggregation was measured using turbidometric aggregometry under 5–20 μM ADP in 750 healthy individuals and patients with documented coronary artery disease. Thus, the results confirmed prior data demonstrating better pharmacokinetics of prasugrel over clopidogrel. Thus, due to the interpatient variability and tolerability, it should be recommended to monitor the level of inhibition of platelet activation even with prasugrel antiplatelet therapy.

Clinical benefits and risk of prasugrel compared to clopidogrel

Several studies reported that prasugrel has greater platelet inhibition compared to clopidogrel on patients with coronary disease (CAD). The first report was a dose ranging study of prasugrel at loading doses of 40 or 60 mg and maintenance doses of 5–15 mg compared to clopidogrel 300 mg loading dose and 75 mg maintenance dose for 4 weeks in 101 patients with stable CAD (20). At 4 hours after loading dose with 20 μM ADP, both prasugrel loading doses achieved significantly higher IPA levels (60.6% and 68.4% vs 30.0%, respectively; all $p < 0.0001$), and lower percentages (3% vs 52%,

$p < 0.0001$) of pharmacodynamic nonresponders (defined as IPA <20%) than clopidogrel. Prasugrel 10- and 15-mg maintenance doses achieved consistently higher IPA levels than clopidogrel 75 mg at day 28 (all $p < 0.0001$). On day 28, there were no nonresponders in the 10- and 15-mg prasugrel groups, compared with 45% in the clopidogrel group ($p = 0.0007$). Increasing the loading dose of clopidogrel to 600 mg did achieve improvement as reported in a recent study of aspirin-treated patients with coronary disease, however, a 60-mg loading dose of prasugrel and 10-mg/day maintenance dose achieved a faster onset of action and a greater level of IPA (PRI of 8.3% for 600 mg clopidogrel compared with 55.9% for 75 mg, $p < 0.0001$) (21).

Increasing the loading and maintenance doses of clopidogrel still resulted in better platelet inhibition with prasugrel as reported in PRINCIPLE-TIMI 44 randomized, double-blind study comparing prasugrel with high-dose clopidogrel in 201 patients undergoing elective PCI (17). A 60-mg prasugrel loading dose was compared with a 600-mg clopidogrel loading dose and 10-mg prasugrel and 150-mg clopidogrel maintenance doses were compared for 14 days, and were then crossed-over to the alternate treatment for an additional 14 days. IPA at 6 h was significantly higher in those who received prasugrel (74.8% ± 13.0%) compared with clopidogrel (31.8% ± 21.1%; $p < 0.0001$). During the maintenance-dose phase, IPA with 20 µmol ADP was higher in prasugrel patients (61.3% ± 17.8%) compared to clopidogrel (46.1% ± 21.3%; $p < 0.0001$). Overall, prasugrel was well tolerated with no Thrombolysis in Myocardial Infarction (TIMI) major bleeding and no subject discontinued therapy prematurely. Two subjects (2%) in the prasugrel group and no subject in the clopidogrel group experienced a TIMI minor bleeding episode.

Those trials showed consistent results of greater platelet inhibition of prasugrel compared with clopidogrel even at higher doses. Although no significant safety issues arose from those trials, this was not their main focus. The Joint Utilization of Medication to Block Platelets Optimally-Thrombolysis In Myocardial Infarction (JUMBO-TIMI) 26 trial (11), a large safety randomized controlled trial, compared prasugrel and clopidogrel in 904 patients undergoing elective or urgent PCI. Patients were randomized to one of three combinations of prasugrel loading and maintenance doses: 40 mg and 7.5 mg/day, 60 mg and 10 mg/day, and 60 mg and 15 mg/day, or standard dose clopidogrel of 300 mg and 75 mg/day. No significant differences were observed for the primary safety end point of non-CABG related TIMI major and minor bleeding between prasugrel and clopidogrel (1.7% vs 1.2%, $p = 0.59$ respectively). However, more TIMI minimal bleeding events were detected in the high-dose prasugrel group (3.6%) compared with the low-dose group (2.0%), intermediate dose group (1.5%), and clopidogrel group (2.4%). Patients receiving prasugrel showed a lower but not statistically significant MACE at 30 days—prasugrel group 7.2% compared with the clopidogrel group 9.4%; $p = 0.26$; HR, 0.76; 95% CI, 0.46 to 1.24—and significantly lower rates of target vessel thrombotic events (composite occurrence of stent thrombosis and urgent repeat target vessel revascularization)—0.6% in the prasugrel group vs 2.4% ($p = 0.02$) in the clopidogrel group.

A large phase III trial TRITON-TIMI 38 (TRial to Assess Improvement in Therapeutic Outcomes by Optimizing Platelet Inhibition with Prasugrel-Thrombolysis In Myocardial Infarction) (22) assessed the effectiveness of prasugrel compared to clopidogrel in 13,608 patients with moderate- to high-risk ACS scheduled to undergo PCI. Patients were randomized to treatment with either a prasugrel 60-mg loading dose followed by 10 mg/day maintenance dose or a clopidogrel 300-mg loading dose followed by a 75 mg/day maintenance dose for 6–15 months. A significant reduction in the composite clinical end point (death, MI, and stroke) was observed in the prasugrel group compared with the clopidogrel group (9.9% vs 12.1% with HR of 0.81, 95% CI 0.73–0.90, $p < 0.001$) (Figure 9.2). This difference was predominantly attributed to the decrease in ischemic episodes during the first 3 days after intervention. The prasugrel group also showed a significant reduction in the secondary end point of death, MI, or urgent target lesion revascularization at 30 and 90 days as well as in the end point of death, MI, stroke, or rehospitalization for ischemia. Definite stent thrombosis was significantly lower

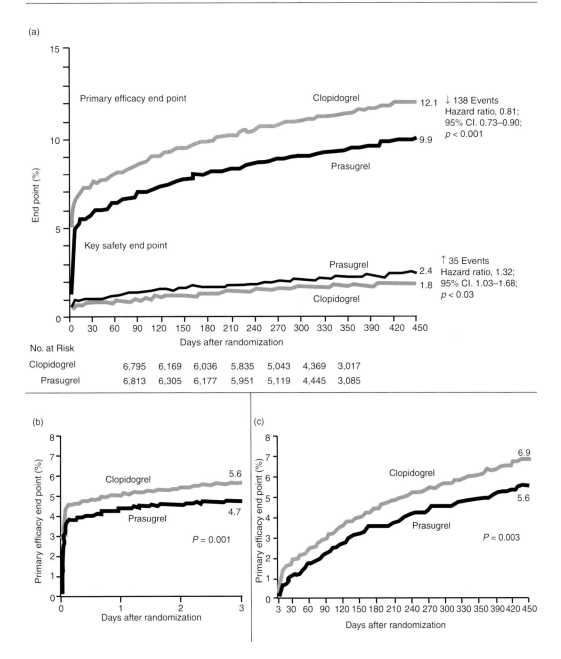

Figure 9.2 Cumulative Kaplan–Meier estimates of the rates of death from cardiovascular causes, nonfatal myocardial infarction, or nonfatal stroke during the follow-up period, and safety end point (Thrombolysis in Myocardial Infarction major bleeding not related to coronary artery bypass grafting) (Panel a) during the full follow-up period. Data for the primary efficacy end point are also shown from the time of randomization to day 3 (Panel b) and from 3 days to 15 months, with all end points occurring before day 3 censored (Panel c).

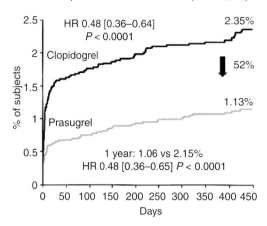

Definite/probable stent thrombosis (N = 12,844)

Figure 9.3 Reduction of definite stent thrombosis in the prasugrel group compared to the clopidogrel group.

in the prasugrel group (1.1% vs 2.4%, $p < 0.001$) (Figure 9.3). Similarly, the early and late stent thromboses were significantly lower in the prasugrel group compared to clopidogrel group (0.64% vs 1.6%, $p < 0.001$ and 0.49% vs 0.82%, $p = 0.03$, respectively) (23). The reduction in stent thrombosis was robust with respect to stent thrombosis definition, stent type (bare metal or drug-eluting stent), timing, and across several key clinical characteristics (24). TIMI major bleeding was observed in 2.4% of patients receiving prasugrel and 1.8% of patients receiving clopidogrel (HR 1.32, 95% CI 1.03–1.68, $p = 0.03$). The rates of life-threatening bleeding and fatal bleeding were greater in the prasugrel group than in the clopidogrel group (1.4% vs 0.9%, $p = 0.01$ and 0.4% vs 0.1%, $p = 0.002$). To weigh the benefits of improved ischemic outcomes against the risks of higher rates of bleeding, a net clinical outcome (net clinical benefit) was calculated using the prespecified definition of all cause death, nonfatal MI, nonfatal stroke, and nonfatal TIMI major bleed. This calculation favored prasugrel overall (12.9% vs 13.9% hazard ratio 0.81, $p = 0.004$), a finding that was robust to multiple net end points, including the addition of less severe bleeding. Diabetic patients showed the best clinical benefit. On the other hand, patients with a history of stroke or transient ischemic attack, elderly (>75 years), and patients with body weight <60 kg

demonstrated less net clinical benefit or clinical harm due to increased risk of bleeding.

Diabetic patients are known to have increased platelet reactivity with poor response to clopidogrel (25). In the TRITON-TIMI 38 trial, 3,146 patients had a preexisting history of diabetes mellitus (DM), of which 776 were receiving insulin. Stent thrombosis was significantly reduced while TIMI major bleeding was the same as clopidogrel. The net benefit of prasugrel over clopidogrel was 14.6% and 19.2%, respectively (HR 0.74 ranging between 0.62–0.89, $p = 0.001$). Thus, prasugrel is efficacious in patients with DM (26).

A landmark analysis investigating the short- (until 30 days) and long-term (>30 days) outcomes had shown a significant reduction in ischemic events using prasugrel during the first 30 days. However, over 30 days, TIMI major noncoronary artery bypass graft bleeding was similar to clopidogrel during the first 30 days but significantly greater from 30 days thereafter (27).

The increased risk of bleeding associated with prasugrel treatment was significant in the TRITON trial despite the exclusion of patients undergoing heart surgery and those with high bleeding risk or thrombocytopenia. The lack of increased bleeding with prasugrel compared with clopidogrel in the JUMBO trial may have resulted from the short (1 month) follow-up. In the TRITON study, the follow-up was substantially longer (6–15 months). Those observations strongly suggest that the majority of bleeding events occur later than 30 days after initiation of therapy. This raises concerns since prasugrel has been developed as an alternative to clopidogrel, implicating long-term use after PCI especially after drug-eluting stent implantation.

Ongoing trials such as the TRILOGY ACS trial (tArGETED Platelet Inhibition to cLarify the Optimal strategy to medically mange ACS) are currently underway in which patients with ACS will receive medical management without planned revascularization. This study will compare the safety and efficacy of prasugrel and clopidogrel in reducing the risk of cardiovascular death, MI, or stroke. The SWAP study will assess the impact of prasugrel after switching from clopidogrel to prasugrel on various parameters of platelet function. The ACAPULCO study will compare pharmacodynamic differences between high loading and maintenance doses of clopidogrel and standard doses of prasugrel in patients with ACS who are undergoing PCI. The OPTIMUS-3 study will compare standard doses of prasugrel with high loading doses and maintenance doses of clopidogrel in patients with type II diabetes and coronary artery disease.

Clinical implication

Patients who experience an ischemic event such as stent thrombosis despite treatment with clopidogrel may be hyporesponsive to this drug and may require more intensive P2Y$_{12}$ inhibition to prevent the occurrence of subsequent adverse thrombotic complications. Prasugrel, a more potent thienopyridine than clopidogrel, may be a good solution for such patients. In the future, when checking platelet responsiveness to clopidogrel becomes a routine practice, all patients with clopidogrel hyporesponsiveness will benefit from prasugrel regardless of the recurrence of clinical events.

Summary

Prasugrel, a potent novel thienopyridine, has been shown in preclinical and clinical studies to achieve faster onset of action, less interpatient variability, and greater potency of platelet inhibition compared with clopidogrel even when administered at high doses. Prasugrel is more efficacious in preventing ischemic events in patients with ACS undergoing PCI compared with clopidogrel, even in high-risk patients such as diabetics. However, the greater platelet inhibitory effects of prasugrel are also associated with an increased risk of bleeding. The net clinical benefit continues to favor prasugrel over clopidogrel.

References

1 von Kügelgen I. Pharmacological profiles of cloned mammalian P2Y-receptor subtypes. *Pharmacol Ther.* 2006;**110**:415–432.

2 Algaier I, Jakubowski JA, Asai F, von Kügelgen I. Interaction of the active metabolite of prasugrel, R-138727, with the residues cysteine97 and cysteine175 of the human P2Y(12)-receptor. *J Thromb Haemost.* 2008;**6**:1908–1914.

3 Small DS, Farid NA, Payne CD, et al. Effects of the proton pump inhibitor lansoprazole on the pharmacokinetics and pharmacodynamics of prasugrel and clopidogrel. *J Clin Pharmacol.* 2008;**48**:475–484.

4 Jakubowski JA, Payne CD, Brandt JT, et al. The platelet inhibitory effects and pharmacokinetics of prasugrel after administration of loading and maintenance doses in healthy subjects. *J Cardiovasc Pharmacol.* 2006;**47**:377–384.

5 Sugidachi A, Asai F, Ogawa T, Inoue T, Koike H. The *in vivo* pharmacological profile of CS-747, a novel antiplatelet agent with platelet ADP receptor antagonist properties. *Br J Pharmacol.* 2000;**129**:1439–1446.

6 Farid NA, Payne CD, Small DS, et al. Cytochrome P450 3A inhibition by ketoconazole affects prasugrel and clopidogrel pharmacokinetics and pharmacodynamics differently. *Clin Pharmacol Ther.* 2007;**81**:735–741.

7 Jakubowski JA, Winters KJ, Naganuma H, Wallentin L. Prasugrel: a novel thienopyridine antiplatelet agent. A review of preclinical and clinical studies and the mechanistic basis for its distinct antiplatelet profile. *Cardiovasc Drug Rev.* 2007;**25**:357–374.

8 Judge HM, Buckland RJ, Sugidachi A, Jakubowski JA, Storey RF. The active metabolite of prasugrel effectively blocks the platelet P2Y12 receptor and inhibits procoagulant and pro-inflammatory platelet responses. *Platelets.* 2008;**19**:125–133.

9 Payne CD, Li YG, Brandt JT, et al. Switching directly to prasugrel from clopidogrel results in greater inhibition of platelet aggregation in aspirin-treated subjects. *Platelets.* 2008;**19**:275–281.

10 Brandt JT, Payne CD, Weerakkody G, et al. Superior responder rate for inhibition of platelet aggregation with a 60 mg loading dose of prasugrel (CS-747, LY640315) compared with a 300 mg loading dose of clopidogrel. *J Am Coll Cardiol.* 2005;**45**(suppl A):87A.

11 Wiviott SD, Antman EM, Winters KJ, et al. Randomized comparison of prasugrel (CS-747, LY640315), a novel thienopyridine P2Y12 antagonist, with clopidogrel in percutaneous coronary intervention: results of the Joint Utilization of Medications to Block Platelets Optimally (JUMBO)-TIMI 26 trial. *Circulation.* 2005;**111**:3366–3373.

12 Frelinger AL, III, Michelson AD, Braunwald E, et al. Abstract 3995: comparison of the effects of prasugrel and high dose clopidogrel on in vivo and in vitro platelet activation: results from PRINCIPLE-TIMI 44. *Circulation.* 2008;**118**:S-814.

13 Hagihara K, Kazui M, Yoshiike M, Honda K, Farid NA, Kurihara A. A possible mechanism of poorer and more variable response to clopidogrel than prasugrel. *Circulation.* 2008;**118**:S-820.

14 Mega JL, Shen L, Wiviott SD, et al. Cytochrome P450 genetic variants predict cardiovascular outcomes following treatment with clopidogrel but not with prasugrel. *Circulation.* 2008;**118**:S-325–S-326.

15 Jakubowski JA, Payne CD, Li YG, *et al.* The use of the VerifyNow P2Y12 point-of-care device to monitor platelet function across a range of P2Y12 inhibition levels following prasugrel and clopidogrel administration. *Thromb Haemost.* 2008;**99**:409–415.

16 Jakubowski JA, Payne CD, Li YG, *et al.* A comparison of the antiplatelet effects of prasugrel and high-dose clopidogrel as assessed by VASP-phosphorylation and light transmission aggregometry. *Thromb Haemost.* 2008;**99**:215–222.

17 Wiviott SD, Trenk D, Frelinger AL, *et al.* Prasugrel compared with high loading- and maintenance-dose clopidogrel in patients with planned percutaneous coronary intervention: the prasugrel in comparison to clopidogrel for inhibition of platelet activation and aggregation-thrombolysis in myocardial infarction 44 trial. *Circulation.* 2007;**116**:2923–2932.

18 Frelinger AL, 3rd, Jakubowski JA, Li Y, *et al.* The active metabolite of prasugrel inhibits adenosine diphosphate- and collagen-stimulated platelet procoagulant activities. *J Thromb Haemost.* 2008;**6**:359–365.

19 Li GY, Ni L, Brandt JT, *et al.* Inhibition of platelet aggregation with prasugrel and clopidogrel: an integrated analysis in 750 subjects. *TCT.* 2008;abstract 174.

20 Jernberg T, Payne CD, Winters KJ, *et al.* Prasugrel achieves greater inhibition of platelet aggregation and a lower rate of non-responders compared with clopidogrel in aspirin-treated patients with stable coronary artery disease. *Eur Heart J.* 2006;**27**:1166–1173.

21 Wallentin L, Varenhorst C, James S, *et al.* Prasugrel achieves greater and faster P2Y12 receptor-mediated platelet inhibition than clopidogrel due to more efficient generation of its active metabolite in aspirin-treated patients with coronary artery disease. *Eur Heart J.* 2008;**29**:21–30.

22 Wiviott SD, Braunwald E, McCabe CH, *et al.* Prasugrel versus clopidogrel in patients with acute coronary syndromes. *N Engl J Med.* 2007;**357**:2001–2015.

23 Wiviott SD, Antman EM, Horvath I, *et al.* Prasugrel compared to clopidogrel in patients with acute coronary syndromes undergoing PCI with stenting: the TRITON—TIMI 38 stent analysis. *SCAI – ACCi2.* 2008; abstract.

24 Wiviott SD, Braunwald E, McCabe CH, *et al.* Intensive oral antiplatelet therapy for reduction of ischaemic events including stent thrombosis in patients with acute coronary syndromes treated with percutaneous coronary intervention and stenting in the TRITON-TIMI 38 trial: a subanalysis of a randomised trial. *Lancet.* 2008;**371**:1353–1363.

25 Angiolillo DJ, Shoemaker SB, Desai B, *et al.* Randomized comparison of a high clopidogrel maintenance dose in patients with diabetes mellitus and coronary artery disease: results of the Optimizing Antiplatelet Therapy in Diabetes Mellitus (OPTIMUS) study. *Circulation.* 2007;**115**:708–716.

26 Wiviott SD, Braunwald E, Angiolillo DJ, *et al.* Greater clinical benefit of more intensive oral antiplatelet therapy with prasugrel in patients with diabetes mellitus in the trial to assess improvement in therapeutic outcomes by optimizing platelet inhibition with prasugrel–thrombolysis in myocardial infarction 38. *Circulation.* 2008;**118**:1626–1636.

27 Kaul S, Shah PK, Diamond GA. Timing of benefit with prasugrel in patients with acute coronary syndromes undergoing percutaneous coronary intervention: reanalysis of TRITON-TIMI 38 results. *Circulation.* 2008;**118**: S-818–S-819.

CHAPTER 10

When to use glycoprotein IIb/IIIa inhibitors and which one to use: Abciximab, tirofiban, or eptifibatide?

Cheuk-Kit Wong[1] & Harvey D. White[2]
[1]Otago University, Dunedin, New Zealand
[2]Auckland City Hospital, Auckland, New Zealand

The glycoprotein IIb/IIIa inhibitors have been established for over a decade as effective potent antiplatelet agents during percutaneous coronary interventions (PCIs), with abciximab as the prototype, reducing complications and mortality in the early trials of standard PCI (1) and more recently in trials of primary PCI for acute myocardial infarction (2). However, recent advances have led to the need to reassess risk–benefit and cost-effectiveness. First, the current generation of coronary stents can seal dissections even in small vessels and residual dissections (with prothrombiotic potential) are less common. Second, the use of a 600 mg loading dose of clopidogrel results in high antiplatelet effects within 2 h (3) and may render glycoprotein inhibitors unnecessary in lower risk patients (4). Third, the routine use of abciximab in high-risk patients is common practice in some laboratories. However, in most trials that established the benefits of intravenous glycoprotein inhibitors, the control arm was placebo. The question as to whether routine intravenous glycoprotein inhibitors during PCI is better than bail-out *intracoronary* glycoprotein inhibitors has not been tested. Fourth, the use of glycoprotein inhibitors is associated with more bleeding complications from groin punctures (despite reducing ischemic complications). While

bleeding is clearly related to poor long-term outcome and mortality (5) the increasingly adopted radial approach and smaller catheters may reduce a large proportion of the major bleeding that is associated with the groin approach. Fifth, during PCI, not only does the plaque rupture by balloon dilatation activate platelets, but unfractionated heparin also activates platelets. Sixth, bivalirudin may have a major advantage over heparins because of its more potent inhibition of thrombin and its lack of platelet activation, and IIb/IIIa inhibitors may not add benefit by increasing antiplatelet inhibition but will increase bleeding complications.

Biology of the platelet glycoprotein receptor

The platelet GP IIb/IIIa receptor is an "integrin" $\alpha_{IIb}\beta_3$—adhesion receptor on the platelet membrane. Structurally, the receptor includes surface noncovalently linked α/β heterodimers with many cation-binding sites where adhesive ligands bind, and a cytoplasmic tail linked to the cytoskeletal apparatus (6). With platelet activation, the GP IIb/IIIa receptors ($\alpha_{IIb}\beta_3$ integrins) metamorphose into an active conformation binding the ligands fibrinogen, von Willebrand factor, and others. This constitutes the final common pathway of platelet aggregation. Clot formation and retraction ensues, the latter secondary to the linkage of the occupied GP IIb/IIIa receptors to the platelet cytoskeleton (6).

Pharmacology in the Catheterization Laboratory. Edited by Ron Waksman and Andrew E Ajani. © 2010 Blackwell Publishing, ISBN: 978-1-4051-5704-9.

Mechanisms of benefits of glycoprotein IIb/IIIa inhibitors

Abciximab is the Fab fragment of a monoclonal antibody to $\alpha_{IIb}\beta_3$, which cross-reacts with vitronectin and possibly other β_3 integrin receptors on endothelial cells, white blood cells, and smooth muscle cells. Eptifibatide is a peptide containing an analogous sequence with fibrinogen, and is specific for $\alpha_{IIb}\beta_3$, while Tirofiban is a small non-peptide molecule containing a $\alpha_{IIb}\beta_3$ recognition sequence, -Arg-Gly-Asp- (RGD), which is found in fibrinogen, von Willebrand factor, and other $\alpha_{IIb}\beta_3$

ligands. Of note, all three GP IIb/IIIa inhibitors react with resting and activated platelets, but abciximab has a longer half-life and potentially other actions by binding to other β_3 integrin receptors (Table 10.1).

During PCI, a correlation has been shown between >80% of platelet inhibition by these inhibitors and greater efficacy. In the AU-Assessing Ultegra (GOLD) study, which related the degree of inhibition after an abciximab bolus and 12-h infusion to ischemic outcome after PCI, platelet inhibition below 95% at 10 min, 80% at 1 h, or 70% at 8 h was associated with a marked increase in

Table 10.1 Comparison of GP IIb/IIIa inhibitors.

	Abciximab	Eptifibatide	Tirofiban
Nature	Monoclonal Fab antibody	Synthetic cyclic heptapeptide	Nonpeptide small molecule
Dosage	0.25 mg/kg iv bolus + infusion of 0.125 µg/kg/min up to 10 µg/min up to 12 h	Double 0.18 mg/kg iv boluses 10 min apart + infusion of 2 µg/kg/min up to 18–24 h	For PCI in the TARGET trial (7): 10 µg/kg iv bolus +0.15 µg/kg/min infusion for 18–24 h. Standard recommendation is for ACS: Initial 30-min iv infusion of 0.4 µg/kg/min + 0.1 µg/kg/min infusion (also used in ACUITY trial (8). In STRATEGY trial for PCI (9), 25 µg/kg iv bolus + 0.15 µg/kg/min infusion for 18–24 h
Renal failure		If GFR <50 mL/min reduce infusion to 10 µg/kg/min	If GFR <30 mL/min or bolus and infusion should be halved.
When there is clinical bleeding or need for emergency surgery	Bleeding time generally returns to 12 min within 12 h of stopping drug. Fresh platelet transfusion but transfused platelets may still be bound by abciximab displaced from endogenous platelet (with 10 units transfusion, receptor blockade may drop to 60–70%).	Short half-life (2–3 h) with <50% platelet inhibition effects 4 h after stopping drug.	Short half-life <2 h with <50% platelet inhibition effects 4 h after stopping drug.
Trial evidence to support efficacy in PCI—in ST elevation AMI	EPIC, EPILOG, EPISTENT, TARGET, others. PRIMARY PCI trials (2)	ESPIRIT FACILITATED PCI trials (10)	RESTORE / TARGET FACILITATED PCI trials (10)

GFR = Glomerular filtration rate.

ischemic event rates (11). Of interest, exposure to a subthreshold level of platelet inhibition can paradoxically induce platelet activation (the occupation of the GP IIb/IIIa receptors, $\alpha_{IIb}\beta_3$ integrins, by the drugs induces weaker activation signals as compared to the occupation by fibrinogen or other ligands) and release of chemokines and proinflammatory mediator including CD40 ligand (1,12). These properties may explain why in the GUSTO-IV trial patients with acute coronary syndrome (ACS) abciximab did not result in reduction in death/MI during the 24–48 h infusion period (11,13).

Clinical role of glycoprotein IIb/IIIa inhibitors

For patients undergoing PCI, the relative role of GP IIb/IIIa inhibitors is dependent on the extent of platelet activation by the coronary pathology, the use of other antiplatelet drugs particularly "clopidogrel loading," the choice of conjunctive antithrombotic drug for PCI and the risk of bleeding at the puncture site and other areas. In elective PCI, death and MI are reduced by approximately 35% when IIb/IIIa inhibitors are administered in the catheterization laboratory (7,14–17). When the decision is made before coronary angiography to administer upstream IIb/IIIa inhibitors to patients with non-ST elevation ACS with either tirofiban or eptifibatide, (as in the earlier trials without use of clopidogrel), all patients gain a small benefit (9% relative reduction in death or nonfatal myocardial infarction at 30 days) (18). However, a much larger benefit is gained ($\approx$20% reduction in death and MI) in patients who undergo PCI (18,19), diabetic patients (20), patients with ST depression, patients with troponin elevation (21), and patients defined as high risk (22).

Resolution of thrombus and improved coronary flow and myocardial perfusion occur with infusion of tirofiban or abciximab (8,22,23). In ST elevation MI, GP IIb/IIIa inhibitors can also be given upstream to "facilitate" PCI but this does not improve clinical outcome (10).

Early administration of GP IIb/IIIa inhibitors in the emergency room prior to PCI has been shown to improve pre-PCI coronary flow. In the TITAN-TIMI 34 trial, which included

343 patients, the incidence of normal pre-PCI TIMI myocardial perfusion was 24% in patients who received IIb/IIIa inhibitors vs 14% in those who did not ($p = 0.026$) (24).

In a meta-analysis including 3,949 patients with stenting performed in ~40%, the use of periprocedural intravenous abciximab reduced 30-day mortality (2.4% vs 3.4%; OR, 0.68; 95% CI, 0.47–0.99) and 6–12 month mortality (4.4% vs 6.2%; OR, 0.69; 95% CI, 0.52–0.92). Bleeding was not increased (2).

In the TARGET (Tirofiban And ReoPro Give similar Efficacy Trial) trial in 5,308 patients undergoing either elective PCI or PCI with a NSTEACS, abciximab was superior to tirofiban in preventing early 30-day ischemic events (death 0.4% vs 0.5%, non-fatal MI 5.4% vs 6.9%, target vessel revascularization 0.7% vs 0.8%, and composite 6.5 vs 7.6%, $p = 0.038$) (25). The mortality advantage with abciximab was seen exclusively in diabetics but this did not translate to improved 1-year outcome (Figure 10.1) (26).

The tirofiban bolus (10 µg/kg) used in TARGET fails to achieve >80% platelet inhibition in the first 2 h (27–30) and a higher bolus dose of 25 µg/kg has been investigated in a number of studies. Unfortunately, the large Tirofiban Novel dosing vs Abciximab with Evaluation of Clopidogrel and Inhibition of Thrombin Study (TENACITY) trial in intermediate to high-risk PCI patients evaluating this regimen compared to abciximab was stopped early after randomization of 383 patients for commercial reasons. (Moliterno, D., Plenary session in Transcatheter Cardiovascular Therapeutics Washington 2006). The composite of death, MI, and urgent target revascularization at 30 days was nonsignificantly lower in the tirofiban patients (6.9% vs 8.8%, OR, 0.77, 0.37–1.64). Major bleeding occurred in 1.5% of both groups. A recent meta-analysis (9) of five studies comparing this regimen with abciximab showed comparable efficacy and safety but with wide confidence limits.

From low-risk elective patients to higher risk acute patients undergoing contemporary PCI

In the ISAR-REACT (Intracoronary Stenting and Antithrombotic Regimen Rapid Early Action

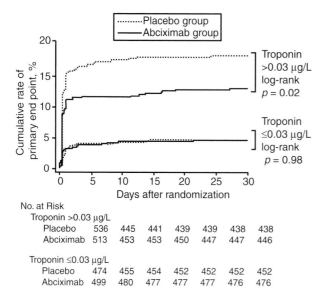

Figure 10.1 Kaplan–Meier analysis of cumulative incidence of death, myocardial infarction, or urgent target vessel revascularization for both treatment groups in the subsets with and without elevated troponin levels (>0.03 µg/L) in ISAR REACT-2. (*Source*: From Kastrati *et al.* (32) with permission. Copyright © 2006, American Medical Association. All Rights reserved.)

for Coronary Treatment) trial 2,159 low risk patients were pretreated with 600 mg of clopidogrel ≥ 2 h before elective PCI (4). Patients were randomized to receive either abciximab with low-dose heparin (70 µ/kg) or placebo with high-dose heparin (140 µ/kg). The abciximab group had more profound thrombocytopenia (1% vs 0%, *p* = 0.002) and transfusions (2% vs 1%, *p* = 0.007) while the primary 30-day end point of combined death, MI, or urgent target vessel revascularization (TVR) was identical in the two groups, as was the rate of any combined ischemic end points. Of note, patients with recent ACS (with positive troponin, or electrocardiographic changes), or angiographic evidence of thrombus were excluded. These results may be explained by the use of a 600 mg loading dose of clopidogrel, resulting in high antiplatelet effects (as assessed by platelet aggregation tests, surface expression of P-selectin and activated GP IIb/IIIa) within 2 h of administration (3).

The Intracoronary Stenting and Antithrombotic Regimen—Is Abciximab a Superior Way to Eliminate Elevated Thrombotic Risk in Diabetics (ISAR-SWEET) study was designed to specifically address whether the benefit of clopidogrel could be extended to diabetic patients with stable coronary disease, and had similar methodology to the two ISAR trials described above. The trial randomized

701 diabetic patients (29% requiring insulin and 51% oral hypoglycemic drugs) undergoing elective PCI, who were pretreated with 600 mg of clopidogrel, to receive abciximab or placebo (31). The primary end point of death or MI at 1 year was similar in the abciximab and placebo groups (8.3% vs 8.6%, *p* = 0.91). In this trial, 80% of patients were treated with bare metal stents (10% received DES and 10% PCI alone), and angiographic restenosis at 6 months was significantly reduced in the abciximab group (28.9% vs 37.8%, *p* = 0.01).

High-risk patients (*n* = 2,022, with >50% having troponin elevation) were randomized in the ISAR-REACT 2 trial (32) with similar design and end points as the above trials but more contemporary use of drug eluting stents (~50%). The primary 30-day end point of death and MI occurred in 8.9% of patients assigned to abciximab vs 11.9% assigned to placebo with a 25% relative risk reduction with abciximab (relative risk 0.75, 95% confidence interval 0.58–0.97, *p* = 0.03). Among patients without an elevated troponin level, there was no difference in the incidence of the primary end point events between the two groups, whereas among patients with an elevated troponin level, death, and MI was significantly reduced in the abciximab group (13.1% vs 18.3%, relative risk 0.71, 95% confidence interval 0.54–0.95, *p* = 0.02) (Figure 10.2).

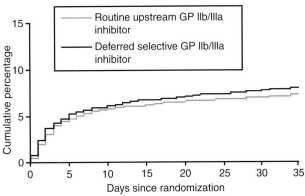

Figure 10.2 ACUITY Timing Trial: Time to event curves of routine upstream and deferred selective GP IIb/IIIa inhibitor administration for composite ischemia. (*Source*: From *Giugliano et al.* (39).) Kaplan–Meier estimates for routine upstream and deferred selective GP IIb/IIIa inhibitor use were 7.2% and 8.1%, respectively. Log-rank p value is for superiority. Thirty-five-day estimates based on time-to-event data and log-rank p value vary slightly from the binary event rate data and $\chi^2 p$ value.

No. at Risk								
Routine upstream GP IIb/IIIa inhibitor	4,605	4,347	4,287	4,261	4,241	4,202	3,694	2,559
Deferred selective GP IIb/IIIa inhibitor	4,602	4,333	4,274	4,238	4,219	4,178	3,733	2,569

Bivalirudin as the antithrombotic agent

Bivalirudin has mechanistic advantages over heparins, as bivalirudin acts directly on thrombin including clot-bound thrombin and, unlike unfractionated heparin and (to a lesser extent) enoxaparin, does not activate platelets (33). In the REPLACE-2 trial, 6,010 mostly stable patients who underwent elective or urgent PCI between October 2001 and August 2002, were randomized to bivalirudin with provisional GP IIb/IIIa (given in <10% of patients) or heparin plus planned GP IIb/IIIa inhibition. Major bleeding was reduced by 43% with bivalirudin. Although there was a statistically nonsignificant excess of myocardial infarction (mainly non-Q wave infarction) in the bivalirudin group of 0.8% at 30 days, mortality at 6 months and at 1 year both favored the bivalirudin group (1.0% vs 1.4%, $p = 0.15$ and 1.89% vs 2.46%, $p = 0.15$ respectively) (34).

The recent ACUITY trial recruited moderate and high-risk patients ($n = 13,819$) with ACS undergoing an invasive management strategy. Patients were randomized to five arms: (1) unfractionated heparin or LMWH + upstream GP IIb/IIIa inhibitors; (2) unfractionated heparin or LMWH + in-lab GP IIb/IIIa inhibitors; (3) bivalirudin + upstream GP IIb/IIIa inhibitors; (4) bivalirudin + in-lab GP IIb/IIIa inhibitors alone; or (5) bivalirudin alone (19,35).

The primary end point was a composite of death, MI, or unplanned revascularization for ischemia plus major bleeding. The time from drug administration to angiography was 5.3 h. Fifty six percent of patients underwent PCI, 32% had medical therapy and 12% had surgery. The primary end point showed noninferiority for the net clinical outcome; 11.7% heparin + IIb/IIIa groups vs 11.8% bivalirudin + IIb/IIIa groups, $p < 0.001$. The ischemic composite was 7.3% vs 7.7%, $p = 0.015$, for noninferiority and major bleeding was 5.7% vs 5.3% ($p < 0.001$) for noninferiority (19) for heparin + IIb/IIIa vs bivalirudin + IIb/IIIa.

The results for the bivalirudin alone group (with 9% provisional use of GP IIb/IIIa inhibitors) was 10.1% for the composite end point ($p < 0.015$); 7.8% for the ischemic end point ($p = 0.32$); and 3.0% for major bleeding ($p < 0.01$; all p values for superiority vs heparin + IIb/IIIa group). Major bleeding (which including groin hematomas >5 cm) was reduced by 47%. Notably, transfusions were less frequent with bivalirudin alone (1.6%) vs 2.7% with heparin + GP IIb/IIIa, $p < 0.001$. Thus the simpler regimen of bivalirudin alone resulted in significantly greater net clinical benefit (19). This benefit was consistent across all groups except in patients who did not receive pretreatment with thienopyridines, where there was no apparent effect, whereas in the 5,192 patients who also received thienopyridines there was an apparently larger effect (composite end point reduced from 12.2% with heparin + GP IIb/IIIa to 9.2% with bivalirudin alone, $p < 0.001$) (19), but the p-value for this treatment interaction was not statistically significant ($p = 0.054$).

The PROTECT TIMI-30 trial compared (36) eptifibatide (used in conjunction with low-dose unfractionated heparin or low-dose enoxaparin) and bivalirudin monotherapy in patients with moderate to high-risk PCI for NSTEACS using angiographic end points in 754 patients. Dose adjustment for eptifibatide (half-dose 1 μg/kg/min maintenance infusion) was made for low creatinine clearance <50 mL/min. There were mixed results. The primary end point of post-PCI coronary flow reserve was significantly greater with bivalirudin (1.43 vs 1.33 for pooled eptifibatide arms, $p = 0.036$). However, Thrombolysis In Myocardial Infarction (TIMI) myocardial perfusion grade more often was normal with eptifibatide treatment compared with bivalirudin (57.9% vs 50.9%, $p = 0.048$). The duration of ischemia on continuous Holter monitoring after PCI was significantly longer among patients treated with bivalirudin (169 vs 36 min, $p = 0.013$). There was no excess of TIMI major bleeding among patients treated with eptifibatide compared with bivalirudin (0.7%, $n = 4$ vs 0%, $p = NS$), but TIMI minor bleeding was increased (2.5% vs 0.4%, $p = 0.027$) as was transfusion (4.4–0.4%, $p < 0.001$). It was found in PROTECT TIMI-30 that increasing age was the only factor correlating with bleeding (37).

Timing of glycoprotein IIb/IIIa inhibitor administration

In an analysis from 12,296 patients randomized in the Chimeric 7E3 Antiplatelet Therapy in Unstable Refractory Angina (CAPTURE), Platelet GP IIb/IIIa in Unstable Angina: Receptor Suppression Using Integrilin™ Therapy (PURSUIT) and Platelet Receptor Inhibition for ischemic Syndrome Management in Patients Limited to very Unstable Signs and symptoms (PRISM-PLUS) trials (38), administration of a IIb/IIIa inhibitor before PCI resulted in a 33% reduction in death and MI by 72 h (2.9% vs 4.3%, $p = 0.001$) (38). In the 2,754 patients who had PCI

there was a 39% reduction in death and MI in the 48 h after PCI (4.9% vs 8.0%, $p = 0.001$). The effect after PCI was bigger in relative and absolute terms than the effect for upstream treatment but applied only to approximately 50% of patients who had PCI.

In the Can Rapid Risk Stratification of Unstable Angina Patients Suppress ADverse Outcomes with Early Implementation of the ACC/AHA Guidelines (CRUSADE) registry patients who received a GP IIb/IIIa inhibitor within 24 h ($n = 26,594$) compared with patients who did not receive a IIb/IIIa inhibitor within 24 h ($n = 14,296$), had a 42% lower hospital mortality (2.59% vs 4.59%, $p < 0.0001$).

The ACUITY trial also tested the timing of GP IIb/IIIa inhibitor administration and patients were randomized to receive IIb/IIIa inhibitors either upstream or administered in the catheterization laboratory. IIb/IIIa inhibitors were used in 98.3% and 55.7% of patients in the routine upstream and deferred selective group respectively, and for a significantly longer duration in the upstream group (median 18.3 vs 13.1 h, $p < 0.001$). Deferred selective IIb/IIIa inhibitor administration compared to routine upstream use resulted in reduced 30-day rates of major bleeding (4.9% vs 6.1% respectively, $p = 0.009$, relative risk [95% confidence interval] = 0.80 [0.67–0.95]), with a nonsignificant difference in composite ischemia (7.9% vs 7.1%, $p = 0.13$, relative risk [95% confidence interval] = 1.12 [0.97–1.29]) and identical rates of net clinical outcomes (11.7% vs 11.7%, $p = 0.93$, relative risk [95% confidence interval] = 1.00 [0.89–1.11]) (Figures 10.2, 10.3, and 10.4).

Thus this study failed to show that in laboratory administration of IIb/IIIa inhibitors resulted in an increase of ischemic events of <25% with the upper boundary of the 95% confidence limits being 29% worse. Most of this difference was related to more late unplanned revascularization for ischemia (2.8% vs 2.1%, $p = 0.03$), which could relate to less "passivation" by the laboratory administration of IIb/IIIa inhibitors. There is thus a trade-off with giving upstream IIb/IIIa inhibitors with a 1.2% increase in major bleeding but a 0.8% decrease in ischemia.

Bivalirudin monotherapy compared to a IIb/IIIa inhibitor-based regimen resulted in significantly lower 30-day rates of major bleeding (3.0% vs 5.5%, $p < 0.001$, relative risk [95% confidence interval] = 0.55 [0.46–0.66]) with similar rates of composite ischemia (7.8% vs 7.5%, $p = 0.51$, relative risk [95% confidence interval] = 1.04 [0.92–1.18]), resulting in improved net clinical outcomes (10.1% vs 11.7%, $p = 0.0045$, relative risk [95% confidence interval] = 0.86 [0.78–0.96]) (39).

In the EARLY-ACS (Early GP IIb/IIIa Inhibition in Non-ST-segment Elevation Acute Coronary Syndrome) trial, (39) 9492 high-risk patients were randomly assigned to receive either early eptifibatide (two boluses, of 180 μg per kilogram of body weight, administered 10 minutes apart, and a standard infusion ≥12 hours before angiography) or a matching placebo infusion with provisional use of eptifibatide after angiography (delayed eptifibatide). The primary endpoint was a composite of death, MI, recurrent ischemia within 96 hours, and the use of thrombotic bail-out during PCI. Thrombotic bailout was defined as a thrombotic complication during PCI that required eptifibatide therapy and the bailout medication was the one opposite to the initial study-group assignment.

The mean time to angiography was 21.3 hours Overall, 59% of patients underwent PCI and 13% underwent CABG. The primary end point occurred in 9.3% of patients in the early-eptifibatide group and in 10.0% in the delayed-eptifibatide group (odds ratio, 0.92; 95% confidence interval [CI], 0.80 to 1.06; $P = 0.23$). At 30 days, the rate of death or myocardial infarction was 11.2% in the early-eptifibatide group, as compared with 12.3% in the delayed-eptifibatide group (odds ratio, 0.89; 95% CI, 0.79 to 1.01; $P = 0.08$). Patients in the early-eptifibatide group had significantly higher rates of bleeding and red-cell transfusion. There was no significant difference between the two groups in rates of severe bleeding or nonhemorrhagic serious adverse events.

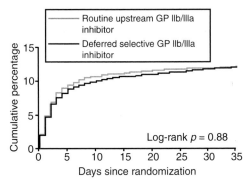

4,805 4,149 4,071 4,043 4,018 3,983 3,500 2,424
4,602 4,181 4,104 4,064 4,042 4,005 3,579 2,465

Figure 10.3 Results of the ACUITY trial. Time to event curves of routine upstream and deferred selective GP IIb/IIIa inhibitor administration and net clinical outcomes. (*Source*: From Stone et al. (39) with permission. Copyright © 2007, American Medical Association. All Rights reserved.) Kaplan–Meier estimates for routine upstream and deferred selective GP IIb/IIIa inhibitor use were 11.9% and 11.9%, respectively, for net clinical outcomes. Log-rank p values are for superiority.

Figure 10.4 Results of the ACUITY trial. Time to event curves of routine upstream and deferred selective GP IIb/IIIa inhibitor administration and major bleeding. (*Source*: From Stone et al. (39) with permission. Copyright © 2007, American Medical Association. All Rights reserved.) Kaplan–Meier estimates for routine upstream and deferred selective GP IIb/IIIa inhibitor use were 6.1% and 4.9%, respectively, for major bleeding. Log-rank p values are for superiority.

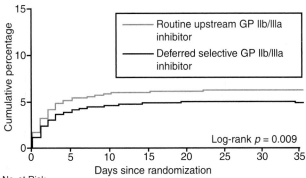

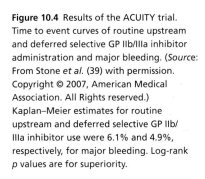

No. at Risk
Routine upstream   4,605 4,304 4,257 4,238 4,225 4,191 3,685 2,563
  GP IIb/IIIa
  inhibitor
Deferred selective   4,602 4,361 4,311 4,286 4,269 4,239 3,805 2,637
  GP IIb/IIIa
  inhibitor

The EARLY-ACS trial showed that the use of eptifibatide 12 hours or more before angiography was not superior to the provisional use of eptifibatide after angiography, but was associated with an increased risk of non–life-threatening bleeding and need for transfusion.

Thus it remains appropriate to give in laboratory IIb/IIIa antagonists based on the previous large data base but there is no need to give upstream therapy which offers no advantage and causes increased bleeding.

Intracoronary administration of IIb/IIIa inhibitors

The advantage of an intracoronary over an intravenous route of administration is the potential to achieve a higher concentration of GP IIb/IIIa inhibition at the site of the culprit lesion, a particularly achievable goal when coronary flow is impaired as in bail-out situations. A recent laboratory study demonstrated that GP IIb/IIIa inhibitors promote the disaggregation of platelet thrombi induced by collagen and shear *ex vivo*, reducing platelet thrombus volume by >75% (40). Previous studies have shown that abciximab as well as eptifibatide and tirofiban can reverse platelet aggregation and are capable of dispersing aggregates to single cells in a dose-dependent manner (41,42), in part by displacing fibrinogen from activated GP IIb/IIIa receptors and/or by altering fibrin exposure and susceptibility to plasmin-mediated fibrinolysis.

In vitro observations (41) indicate that complete dispersion of platelet aggregates back to single platelets (dethrombosis) requires a relatively high concentration of abciximab (6.25 μg/mL). While the intravenous standard bolus of 0.25 mg/kg achieves 80% blockade of all circulating platelets within 10 min, it will not achieve the local concentration required for dethrombosis, raising the need for local administration. A recent study in 403 consecutive patients with ST or non-ST elevation ACS undergoing PCI (~60% with total occlusion, ~60% with dissection and 5–7% with no reflow) examined whether intracoronary bolus administration of abciximab was associated with reduced major adverse event rates as compared to standard intravenous administration (43). At 30 days, death, MI,

and target vessel revascularization were significantly lower in patients receiving intracoronary abciximab (10.2% vs 20.2%, *p* < 0.008). Also a small study of 10 patients suggests that intracoronary administration of abciximab decreases angiographic thrombus and improves flow (44). Eptifibatide, which needs to be buffered because of its low pH, when given intracoronary, achieves higher levels of GP IIb/IIIa receptor occupancy in the coronary sinus compared to IV administration (45).

Is there a need for continuing glycoprotein IIb/IIIa inhibitors after successful PCI?

The EPIC trial showed the benefit of a continued 12-h abciximab infusion after PCI (7). However, with contemporary stenting techniques, residual dissections are uncommon and a continued infusion may not be necessary. The EASY (Same-Day Home Discharge After Transradial Coronary Stenting With a Single Abciximab Bolus) trial randomized 1,005 patients, who underwent transradial stent implantation with an abciximab bolus, to receive either a 12-h abciximab infusion and overnight hospitalization vs a bolus only and discharge 4–6 h after PCI (46). Clinical outcomes at 30 days and 6 months were similar between the two groups, and 88% of patients of the bolus-only group were safely discharged the same day.

Adverse effects of glycoprotein IIb/IIIa inhibitors

In addition to the bleeding risks described (above), thrombocytopenia is a less common but equally important complication. The reported incidence in abciximab trials has been higher than with eptifibatide or tirofiban. In the TARGET trial, abciximab was associated with a 2.4% incidence of thrombocytopenia (nadir platelet count <100 × 10^9 cells/L) within 24 h of administration, compared to 0.5% with tirofiban. Thrombocytopenia was associated with a higher incidence of severe bleeding (5.1% vs 0.7%), blood transfusions (6.1% vs 1.4%), and ischemic end points at 30-days (death 2.0% vs 0.4%, myocardial infarction 9.13% vs 6.11% and target vessel revascularization 6.07% vs 0.60%) (47).

The possible pathophysiological mechanisms causing thrombocytopenia include the presence of preexisting platelet surface antibodies, and the GP IIb/IIIa inhibitors inducing a conformational change in the GP IIb/IIIa receptors, leading to the expression of new epitopes recognized by these antibodies. Alternatively, the recognized epitope may be formed by the receptor–antagonist complex with a cross-reaction between the antibodies with the new epitopes, resulting in coating of the platelets with immunoglobulin and subsequent removal by the reticuloendothelial system.

The new epitopes generated are more frequent with abciximab. Previous treatment with abciximab (but not tirofiban) within 6 months was associated with a 4.4-fold increased incidence of thrombocytopenia (47). However, in the Reopro Readministration Registry of 500 consecutive patients with abciximab readministration (48), the overall rate of thrombocytopenia (4.6%) was similar to that seen after first-time exposure but profound thrombocytopenia (nadir platelet count $<20 \times 10^9$ cells/L) was more frequent after readministration (2.4%).

Conclusion

There are a number of unsettled questions in respect of the of administration of IIb/IIIa inhibitors. They appear to add little benefit in elective patients if 600 mg loading dose of clopidogrel is given. Upstream administration in patients with NSTEACS results in fewer ischemic events but more major bleeding than in laboratory administration. When abciximab is given in the laboratory in addition to a loading dose of 600 mg of clopidogrel in patients with NSTEACS who have elevated troponins, the incidence of MI is reduced. Upstream therapy should be with tirofiban or eptifibatide and in laboratory administration should be with eptifibatide or abciximab. Single bolus high-dose of tirofiban is promising but not approved for use.

IIb/IIIa inhibitors do not add to the anti-ischemic effects of bivalirudin except in bail-out situations and increase bleeding. The role of intracoronary administration of IIb/IIIa inhibitors deserves further study.

In NSTEACS will define further the relative benefits and risks of upstream treatment for greater than 12 h in conjunction with clopidogrel therapy as compared with treatment in the catheterization laboratory.

Acknowledgment

We are grateful to Barbara Semb for secretarial assistance.

References

1 Quinn MJ, Plow EF, Topol EJ. Platelet glycoprotein IIb/IIIa inhibitors: recognition of a two-edged sword? *Circulation.* 2002;**106**:379–385.

2 De Luca G, Suryapranata H, Stone GW, *et al.* Abciximab as adjunctive therapy to reperfusion in acute ST-segment elevation myocardial infarction: a meta-analysis of randomized trials. *JAMA.* 2005;**293**:1759–1765.

3 Hochholzer W, Trenk D, Frundi D, *et al.* Time dependence of platelet inhibition after a 600-mg loading dose of clopidogrel in a large, unselected cohort of candidates for percutaneous coronary intervention. *Circulation.* 2005;**111**:2560–2564.

4 Kastrati A, Mehilli J, Schühlen H, *et al.* A clinical trial of abciximab in elective percutaneous coronary intervention after pretreatment with clopidogrel. *N Engl J Med.* 2004;**350**:232–238.

5 Eikelboom JW, Mehta SR, Anand SS, Xie C, Fox KA, Yusuf S. Adverse impact of bleeding on prognosis in patients with acute coronary syndromes. *Circulation.* 2006;**114**:774–782.

6 Topol EJ, Byzova TV, Plow EF. Platelet GPIIb-IIIa blockers. *Lancet.* 1999;**353**:227–231.

7 The EPIC Investigators. Use of a monoclonal antibody directed against the platelet glycoprotein IIb/IIIa receptor in high-risk coronary angioplasty. *N Engl J Med.* 1994;**330**:956–961.

8 van den BM, Laarman GJ, Steg PG, *et al.* Assessment of coronary angiograms prior to and after treatment with abciximab, and the outcome of angioplasty in refractory unstable angina patients. Angiographic results from the CAPTURE trial. *Eur Heart J.* 1999;**20**:1572–1578.

9 Dawson CB, Mukherjee D, Vilgimigli Mea. Meta-analysis of high-dose single-bolus tirofiban versus abciximbab in patients undergoing percutaneous coronary intervention [abstract]. *Circulation.* 2006;**114**:II647.

10 Keeley EC, Boura JA, Grines CL. Comparison of primary and facilitated percutaneous coronary interventions for ST-elevation myocardial infarction: quantitative review of randomised trials. *Lancet.* 2006;**367**:579–588.

11 Steinhubl SR, Talley JD, Braden GA, *et al.* Point-of-care measured platelet inhibition correlates with a

reduced risk of an adverse cardiac event after percutaneous coronary intervention: results of the GOLD (AU-Assessing Ultegra) Multicenter Study. *Circulation.* 2001;**103**:2572–2578.

12 Peter K, Schwarz M, Ylanne J, *et al.* Induction of fibrinogen binding and platelet aggregation as a potential intrinsic property of various glycoprotein IIb/IIIa (alphaIIbbeta3) inhibitors. *Blood.* 1998;**92**:3240–3249.

13 The GUSTO V Investigators. Reperfusion therapy for acute myocardial infarction with fibrinolytic therapy or combination reduced fibrinolytic therapy and platelet glycoprotein IIb/IIIa inhibition: the GUSTO V randomized trial. *Lancet.* 2001;**357**:1905–1914.

14 The EPILOG Investigators. Platelet glycoprotein IIb/IIIa receptor blockade and low-dose heparin during percutaneous coronary revascularization. *N Engl J Med.* 1997;**336**:1689–1696.

15 The EPISTENT Investigators. Randomised placebo-controlled and balloon-angioplasty-controlled trial to assess safety of coronary stenting with use of platelet glycoprotein-IIb/IIIa blockade. *Lancet.* 1998;**352**:87–92.

16 The ESPRIT Investigators. Novel dosing regimen of eptifibatide in planned coronary stent implantation (ESPRIT): a randomised, placebo-controlled trial. *Lancet.* 2000;**356**:2037–2044.

17 Lincoff AM, Califf RM, Anderson KM, *et al.* Evidence for prevention of death and myocardial infarction with platelet membrane glycoprotein IIb/IIIa receptor blockade by abciximab (c7E3 Fab) among patients with unstable angina undergoing percutaneous coronary revascularization. *J Am Coll Cardiol.* 1997;**30**: 149–156.

18 Boersma E, Harrington RA, Moliterno DJ, *et al.* Platelet glycoprotein IIb/IIIa inhibitors in acute coronary syndromes: a meta-analysis of all major randomised clinical trials. *Lancet.* 2002;**359**:189–198.

19 Stone GW, McLaurin BT, Cox DA, *et al.* Bivalirudin for patients with acute coronary syndromes. *N Engl J Med.* 2006;**355**:2203–2216.

20 Roffi M, Chew DP, Mukherjee D, *et al.* Platelet glycoprotein IIb/IIIa inhibitors reduce mortality in diabetic patients with non-ST-segment elevation acute coronary syndromes. *Circulation.* 2001;**104**:2767–2771.

21 Boersma E, Harrington RA, Moliterno DJ, White H, Simoons ML, on behalf of all co-workers. Platelet glycoprotein IIb/IIIa inhibitors in acute coronary syndromes [letter]. *Lancet.* 2002;**360**:342–343.

22 Morrow DA, Antman EM, Snapinn SM, McCabe CH, Theroux P, Braunwald E. An integrated clinical approach to predicting the benefit of tirofiban in non-ST elevation acute coronary syndromes. Application of the TIMI Risk Score for UA/NSTEMI in PRISM-PLUS. *Eur Heart J.* 2002;**23**:223–229.

23 Zhao XQ, Théroux P, Snapinn SM, Sax FL, for the PRISM-PLUS Investigators. Intracoronary thrombus

and platelet glycoprotein IIb/IIIa receptor blockade with tirofiban in unstable angina or non-Q-wave myocardial infarction: angiographic results from the PRISM-PLUS trial (Platelet Receptor Inhibition for Ischemic Syndrome Management in Patients Limited by Unstable Signs and Symptoms). *Circulation.* 1999;**100**:1609–1615.

24 Gibson CM, Kirtane AJ, Murphy SA, *et al.* Early initiation of eptifibatide in the emergency department before primary percutaneous coronary intervention for ST-segment elevation myocardial infarction: results of the Time to Integrilin Therapy in Acute Myocardial Infarction (TITAN)-TIMI 34 trial. *Am Heart J.* 2006;**152**:668–675.

25 Topol EJ, Moliterno DJ, Herrmann HC, *et al.* Comparison of two platelet glycoprotein IIb/IIIa inhibitors, tirofiban and abciximab, for the prevention of ischemic events with percutaneous coronary revascularization. *N Engl J Med.* 2001;**344**:1888–1894.

26 Roffi M, Moliterno DJ, Meier B, *et al.* Impact of different platelet glycoprotein IIb/IIIa receptor inhibitors among diabetic patients undergoing percutaneous coronary intervention: do Tirofiban and ReoPro Give Similar Efficacy Outcomes Trial (TARGET) 1-year follow-up. *Circulation.* 2002;**105**:2730–2736.

27 Kabbani SS, Aggarwal A, Terrien EF, DiBattiste PM, Sobel BE, Schneider DJ. Suboptimal early inhibition of platelets by treatment with tirofiban and implications for coronary interventions. *Am J Cardiol.* 2002;**89**:647–650.

28 Schneider DJ, Herrmann HC, Lakkis N, *et al.* Enhanced early inhibition of platelet aggregation with an increased bolus of tirofiban. *Am J Cardiol.* 2002;**90**:1421–1423.

29 Herrmann HC, Swierkosz TA, Kapoor S, *et al.* Comparison of degree of platelet inhibition by abciximab versus tirofiban in patients with unstable angina pectoris and non-Q-wave myocardial infarction undergoing percutaneous coronary intervention. *Am J Cardiol.* 2002;**89**:1293–1297.

30 Schneider DJ, Herrmann HC, Lakkis N, *et al.* Increased concentrations of tirofiban in blood and their correlation with inhibition of platelet aggregation after greater bolus doses of tirofiban. *Am J Cardiol.* 2003;**91**:334–336.

31 Mehilli J, Kastrati A, Schuhlen H, *et al.* Randomized clinical trial of abciximab in diabetic patients undergoing elective percutaneous coronary interventions after treatment with a high loading dose of clopidogrel. *Circulation.* 2004;**110**:3627–3635.

32 Kastrati A, Mehilli J, Neumann FJ, *et al.* Abciximab in patients with acute coronary syndromes undergoing percutaneous coronary intervention after clopidogrel pretreatment: the ISAR-REACT 2 randomized trial. *JAMA.* 2006;**295**:1531–1538.

33 Xiao Z, Theroux P. Platelet activation with unfractionated heparin at therapeutic concentrations and comparisons with a low-molecular-weight heparin and with a direct thrombin inhibitor. *Circulation.* 1998;**97**: 251–256.

34 Lincoff AM, Bittl JA, Harrington RA, *et al.* Bivalirudin and provisional glycoprotein IIb/IIIa blockade compared with heparin and planned glycoprotein IIb/IIIa blockade during percutaneous coronary intervention: REPLACE-2 randomized trial. *JAMA.* 2003;**289**:853–863.

35 Stone GW, Bertrand ME, Moses JW, *et al.* Routine upstream initiation vs deferred selective use of glycoprotein IIb/IIIa inhibitors in acute coronary syndromes: the ACUITY Timing trial. *JAMA.* 2007;**297**:591–602.

36 Gibson CM, Kirtane AJ, Morrow DA, *et al.* Association between thrombolysis in myocardial infarction myocardial perfusion grade, biomarkers, and clinical outcomes among patients with moderate- to high-risk acute coronary syndromes: observations from the randomized trial to evaluate the relative PROTECTion against post-PCI microvascular dysfunction and post-PCI ischemia among antiplatelet and antithrombotic agents-Thrombolysis In Myocardial Infarction 30 (PROTECT-TIMI 30). *Am Heart J.* 2006;**152**:756–761.

37 Kirtane AJ, Piazza G, Murphy SA, *et al.* Correlates of bleeding events among moderate- to high-risk patients undergoing percutaneous coronary intervention and treated with eptifibatide: observations from the PROTECT-TIMI-30 trial. *J Am Coll Cardiol.* 2006;**47**:2374–2379.

38 Boersma E, Akkerhuis KM, Theroux P, Califf RM, Topol EJ, Simoons ML. Platelet glycoprotein IIb/IIIa receptor inhibition in non-ST-elevation acute coronary syndromes: early benefit during medical treatment only, with additional protection during percutaneous coronary intervention. *Circulation.* 1999;**100**:2045–2048.

39 Giugliano RP, White JA, Bode C, *et al.* Early versus delayed, provisional eptifibatide in acute coronary syndromes. *N Engl J Med.* 2009;360:2176–90.

40 Stone GW, Bertrand ME, Moses JW, *et al.* Routine upstream initiation vs deferred selective use of glycoprotein IIb/IIIa inhibitors in acute coronary syndromes: the ACUITY Timing trial. *JAMA.* 2007;**297**:591–602.

41 Goto S, Tamura N, Ishida H. Ability of anti-glycoprotein IIb/IIIa agents to dissolve platelet thrombi formed on a collagen surface under blood flow conditions. *J Am Coll Cardiol.* 2004;**44**:316–323.

42 Marciniak SJ, Jr, Mascelli MA, Furman MI, *et al.* An additional mechanism of action of abciximab: dispersal of newly formed platelet aggregates. *Thromb Haemost.* 2002;**87**:1020–1025.

43 Moser M, Bertram U, Peter K, Bode C, Ruef J. Abciximab, eptifibatide, and tirofiban exhibit dose-dependent potencies to dissolve platelet aggregates. *J Cardiovasc Pharmacol.* 2003;**41**:586–592.

44 Wohrle J, Grebe OC, Nusser T, *et al.* Reduction of major adverse cardiac events with intracoronary compared with intravenous bolus application of abciximab in patients with acute myocardial infarction or unstable angina undergoing coronary angioplasty. *Circulation.* 2003;**107**:1840–1843.

45 Burzotta F, Romagnoli E, Trani C, Crea F. Intracoronary administration of abciximab acutely increases flow through culprit vessels of patients with acute coronary syndromes undergoing percutaneous coronary intervention. *Circulation.* 2003;**108**:e138.

46 Deibele AJ, Jennings LK, Kirtane AJ, *et al.* Local platelet glycoprotein IIb/IIIa receptor occupancy with intracoronary eptifibatide during stenting; the ICE pilot trial [abstract]. *Am J Cardiol.* 2006;**98**:S45.

47 Bertrand OF. Same-day home discharge after transradial coronary stenting with a single abciximab bolus 6-month results of the EASY randomized trial [abstract]. *Circulation.* 2005;**112**:3362.

48 Tcheng JE, Kereiakes DJ, Lincoff AM, *et al.* Abciximab readministration: results of the ReoPro Readministration Registry. *Circulation.* 2001;**104**:870–875.

49 Neumann FJ, Kastrati A, Pogatsa-Murray G, *et al.* Evaluation of prolonged antithrombotic pretreatment ("cooling-off" strategy) before intervention in patients with unstable coronary syndromes: a randomized controlled trial. *JAMA.* 2003;**290**:1593–1599.

PART III

Acute coronary syndrome STEMI/ NSTEMI

CHAPTER 11

Antithrombotic therapy for non ST-elevation acute coronary syndromes

Andrew Zinn & Frederick Feit

New York University School of Medicine, New York, NY, USA

Introduction

There are 1.3 million admissions in the United States annually for unstable angina (UA) or non-ST-segment-elevation myocardial infarction (NSTEMI), together referred to as NSTE-acute coronary syndromes (ACS) (1). NSTE-ACS is typically due to rupture of an atherosclerotic plaque with platelet aggregation and thrombus deposition, leading to critical coronary artery obstruction. Treatment involves antithrombotic and anti-ischemic therapy, and early angiography with triage to an appropriate revascularization strategy. The probability of death is greatest in the first 30 days underlining the importance of in-patient management (2,3). Baseline predictors of mortality include elevated troponin, ST-segment depression, older age, diabetes, and impaired ventricular function (Table 11.1) (4–6).

Following angiography, most patients with NSTE-ACS are triaged to percutaneous coronary intervention (PCI). In the Superior Yield of the New Strategy of Enoxaparin, Revascularization and GlYcoprotein IIb/IIIa inhibitors and Acute Catheterization and Urgent Intervention Triage StrategY (ACUITY) trials; 92%, 47%, 18%, and 99%, 56% and 11%, underwent angiography, PCI and coronary artery bypass grafting, respectively (7,8). Among 35,897 patients with NSTE-ACS

Pharmacology in the Catheterization Laboratory. Edited by Ron Waksman and Andrew E Ajani. © 2010 Blackwell Publishing, ISBN: 978-1-4051-5704-9.

in the Can Rapid Risk Stratification of Unstable Angina Patients Suppress ADverse Outcomes with Early Implementation of the ACC/AHA guidelines (CRUSADE) registry, 82% underwent angiography, 52% PCI, and 12% CABG (9). Results of the ISAR-COOL trial indicate that there is no benefit for prolonged antithrombotic therapy prior to intervention (10). Thus, antithrombotic therapy for NSTE-ACS should be viewed as a temporizing measure prior to angiography and adjunctive therapy for PCI, and ideally be seamless from the emergency department to the catheterization laboratory.

Agents and regimens should be evaluated based upon their impact on mortality and/or established independent predictors of mortality; bleeding or in-hospital MI. When differing regimens result in similar rates of mortality, other issues including duration of therapy and cost become paramount. Periprocedural MI has been defined by CKMb elevation, although the magnitude predicting increased mortality is controversial, with thresholds of $\geq 3\times$ and $\geq 8\times$ normal proving significant in different analyses (11,12). There is now evidence that in-hospital bleeding complications also independently predict mortality in patients with NSTE-ACS (13–15). In the ACUITY trial, a liberal definition of major bleeding was as powerful a predictor of 1-year mortality as either TIMI major bleeding or in-hospital MI (with hazard ratios (HR) of 3.1, $p < 0.001$; HR = 3.0, $p < 0.0001$; and HR = 2.6, $p < 0.001$ respectively) (14,15). A comparison of older and contemporary definitions of bleeding is presented in Table 11.2 (7,16–18). An optimal antithrombotic

Table 11.1 Commonly used risk models in NSTE-ACS.

Risk model	Components and features of model
Thrombolysis in myocardial infarction (TIMI) risk score (1 point for each variable)	Age ≥65 years
	≥3 classic coronary artery disease risk factors
	Prior coronary stenosis ≥50%
	ST segment deviation on admission ECG
	≥2 anginal episodes in prior 24 h
	Elevated serum cardiac biomarkers
	Use of aspirin in prior 7 days
Independent predictors of in-hospital mortality in GRACE registry	Age
	Killip class
	Systolic blood pressure
	ST segment deviation
	Cardiac arrest during presentation
	Serum creatinine concentration
	Elevated serum cardiac biomarkers
	Heart rate
Independent predictors of 30-day mortality in the ACUITY trial	ACUITY major bleeding
	Age ≥75 years
	Left ventricular ejection fraction ≤50%
	Prior stroke
	ST segment deviation ≥1 mm
	Cardiac biomarker elevation
	Treatment strategy of CABG (vs PCI)
	Myocardial infarction

Table 11.2 Bleeding definitions used in clinical trials.

TIMI Major	≥5 g/dL decrease in hemoglobin or ≥15% point drop in hematocrit or intracranial hemorrhage
TIMI Minor	With source: ≥3 g/dL decrease in hemoglobin or ≥10% decrease in hematocrit. Without source: ≥4 g/dL decrease in hemoglobin or ≥12% decrease in hematocrit
GUSTO Severe	Intracranial hemorrhage or bleeding that causes hemodynamic compromise requiring intervention
GUSTO Moderate	Bleeding that necessitates blood transfusion but does not result in hemodynamic compromise
REPLACE Major	Intracranial, intraocular, or retroperitoneal hemorrhage or A decrease in hemoglobin ≥3 g/dL with a bleeding source or any decrease in hemoglobin ≥4 g/dL or Transfusion ≥2 units red blood cells
ACUITY Major	Intracranial, intraocular or retroperitoneal bleeding; access site bleeding requiring intervention or hematoma >5 cm or Hemoglobin drop >3 g/dL with a source or ≥4 g/dL without a source or Any blood product transfusion

regimen should provide maximal protection from both ischemic and bleeding complications.

Antiplatelet agents utilized for NSTE-ACS include aspirin, clopidogrel (Plavix), and three intravenous glycoprotein IIb/IIIa receptor inhibitors (GPIs); tirofiban (Aggrastat), eptifibatide (Integrillin), and abciximab (Reopro). Antithrombins include UFH, the low molecular weight heparin (LMWH) enoxaparin (Lovenox), the direct thrombin inhibitor (DTI) bivalirudin (Angiomax), and the factor Xa inhibitor fondaparinux (Arixtra). The sites of action and pharmacologic features of these agents are presented in Figure 11.1 and Table 11.3 (3,19,20).

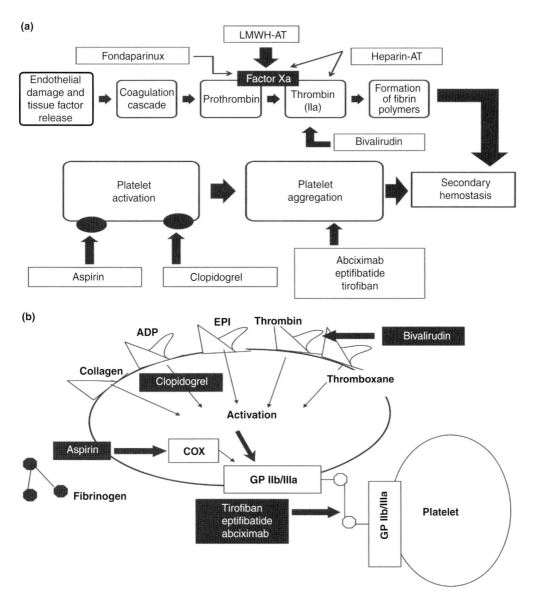

Figure 11.1 Sites of action of commonly used antiplatelets and antithrombins for NSTE-ACS (a). The coagulation cascade and the sites of action of antiplatelet and antithrombin medications are shown (see text). (b). Platelet receptors and sites of action of antiplatelet medications are shown (see text).

Specific agents

Aspirin

Aspirin is a nonsteroidal anti-inflammatory medication that irreversibly antagonizes cyclooxygenase-1, inhibiting breakdown of arachidonic acid to thromboxane A2 (a potent promoter of platelet aggregation) (19). In early ACS trials, aspirin resulted in absolute risk reductions for death or MI of 5–10% over periods from 5 days to 2 years (3). Subsequent ACS studies have universally employed aspirin as background therapy. Aspirin should be initiated at presentation and continued indefinitely unless contraindicated in all patients with ACS (2).

Table 11.3 Dosing, pharmacologic features, and side effects of commonly used medications.

Medication	NSTE-ACS dosing	Pharmacologic features	Major side effects
A. Oral Antiplatelet Agents			
Aspirin	Initial dose: 162–325 mg chewed	Enteric absorption (and via buccal mucosa when chewed) with metabolism to salicyluric acid in the liver	Bleeding
	After BMS implantation: 162–325 mg daily for 1 month		Allergic reactions
	After SES implantation: 162–325 mg daily for 3 months	Plasma half-life of 15 min but with irreversible platelet blockade for life of the blood cell (with normalization of platelet aggregation in 5 days)	
	After PES implantation: 162–325 mg daily for 6 months		
	Maintenance therapy with 75–162 mg daily for life	Renal excretion but no CKD dose adjustment	
	In patients already on aspirin therapy, the initial dose can be given orally		
Clopidogrel	Initial dose: 300–600 mg orally	Enteric absorption of the prodrug with metabolism to the active metabolite via a P450-dependant hepatic pathway	Bleeding
	After BMS: 75 mg daily for at least one month		Rash/allergic reaction
	After DES: 75 mg daily for at least 1 year	Plasma half-life of 8 h, but with irreversible platelet blockade for life of the blood cell	TTP (extremely rare)
	Maintenance therapy: 75 mg daily for at least 1 year		Neutropenia (rare)
	The degree and rapidity of platelet inhibition depends upon the dose, with 600 mg providing full antiplatelet effect in 2–4 h	50% excreted renally, 50% excreted via gastrointestinal tract	
B. GP IIb/IIIa Receptor Antagonists			
Abciximab	0.25 mg/kg intravenous bolus followed by 0.125 mcg/min intravenous infusion immediately prior to PCI	Plasma half life of ~30 min, but with persistence of platelet inhibition for 48 h after discontinuation	Bleeding and thrombocytopenia
	Infusion continued for 12 h following PCI	Effect can be reversed by platelet administration	

	Dosing	Pharmacokinetics	Adverse effects
Eptifibatide	180 mcg/kg intravenous double bolus followed by 2.0 mcg/kg/min infusion (reduced by 50% if creatinine clearance <50 cc/min) initiated either at presentation or at the time of PCI Infusion continued for 18–24 h after PCI	Plasma elimination half-life of ~2.5 h 50% elimination via renal excretion, necessitating a dose adjustment in CKD Effect cannot be reversed by administration of platelets	Bleeding, thrombocytopenia, and anaphylaxis
Tirofiban	Intravenous loading dose of 0.4 mcg/min for 30 min, followed by 0.1 mcg/kg/min infusion (reduced by 50% if creatinine clearance <50 cc/min) initiated either at presentation or at the time of PCI Infusion continued for 18–24 h after PCI	Plasma elimination half-life of ~2 h ~65% elimination via renal excretion, necessitating a dose adjustment in CKD Effect cannot be reversed by administration of platelets	Bleeding, thrombocytopenia and anaphylaxis
C. Heparins			
Unfractionated heparin	Intravenous loading dose of 60 units/kg (maximal bolus 4,000 units) followed by an infusion of 12 units/kg (maximal initial infusion 1,000 units/h) with titration to attain PTT 1.5–2 times ULN initiated at presentation During PCI: dosing titrated to achieve ACT of 200 s with concomitant GPI (60–70 units/kg if initiated in the laboratory) or 250–350 s without concomitant GPI (100–140 units/kg if initiated in the laboratory) Cessation of therapy upon completion of intervention	Plasma half-life varies depending upon dose (ranging from 30 to 150 min) Clearance is nonsaturable at low doses (via depolymerization by endothelial cells and macrophages) and saturable at higher doses (renal elimination) Can be reversed by administration of protamine sulfate (1 mg per 100 units of UFH)	Bleeding Thrombocytopenia HITTS Osteopenia
Enoxaparin	Initial dose of 1 mg/kg subcutaneously every 12 h (reduced to once every 24 h if creatinine clearance is <30 cc/min)[a] with an additional intravenous bolus administered during PCI if needed (0.3 mg/kg intravenously if last dose was >8 h prior, or 0.5–0.75 mg/kg bolus if initiated in the laboratory) Cessation of therapy upon completion of intervention	Can be administered subcutaneously or intravenously Plasma half life of ~4.5 h, but effects lasting ~12 h Metabolized by the liver and excreted via the kidney, necessitating dose adjustment in CKD Protamine sulfate does not adequately reverse the anti-coagulant effect	Bleeding Lower rates of thrombocytopenia, HITTS and osteopenia than UFH. Reversible elevation in liver enzymes

(Continued)

Table 11.3 Continued.

Medication	NSTE-ACS dosing	Pharmacologic features	Major side effects
D. Antithrombins			
Fondaparinux[b]	Initial treatment with 2.5 mg subcutaneously every 24 h, with UFH given during PCI	Elimination half life of 17–21 h	Bleeding
	Cessation of therapy upon completion of intervention	Primarily excreted unchanged via the kidney, necessitating a dose adjustment in CKD	Reversible elevation in liver enzymes
		No reversing agent	
Bivalirudin	Initial intravenous bolus of 0.1 mg/kg followed by 0.25 mg/kg/h infusion	Plasma half-life of 25 min	Bleeding
	During PCI: Additional bolus of 0.5 mg/kg with an increase in infusion to 1.75 mg/kg/h (if patients received prior therapy) or 0.75 mg/kg bolus followed by 1.75 mg/kg/h (if therapy initiated in the laboratory)	Excreted by the kidneys, with most clinicians adjusting dose in patients with advanced CKD	
	Infusion may be continued for 4 h at the operator's discretion	No reversing agent	

[a]The ACC/AHA guidelines allow for a loading dose of 30 mg intravenously, although this is often omitted.
[b]Fondaparinux use in patients with a creatinine clearance <30 cc/min is discouraged; BMS, Bare Metal Stent; SES, Sarolimus Eluting Stent (Cypher); PES, Paclitaxel Eluting Stent (Taxus); PCI, Percutaneous Intervention; PTT, Partial Thromboplastin Time; ULN, Upper limit of normal; ACT, Activated Clotting Time; UFH, Unfractionated heparin; CKD, Chronic Kidney Disease; TTP, Thrombotic Thrombocytopenic Purpura.

Clopidogrel

Clopidogrel is a thienopyridine whose active metabolite irreversibly inhibits the adenosine diphosphate (ADP) P2Y$_{12}$ receptor, preventing ADP-mediated GP IIb/IIIa receptor activation and platelet aggregation (19,20). It is indicated for NSTE-ACS based on the Clopidogrel in Unstable Angina to Prevent Recurrent Events (CURE) trial (21). In CURE, 12,562 patients with NSTE-ACS receiving aspirin were randomized to clopidogrel or placebo (21). At 12 months, the incidence of death, MI, or stroke was 9.3% vs 11.4% ($p < 0.001$) and among 2,658 patients who underwent PCI, the rate of death or MI at 8 months was 8.8% vs 12.6% ($p = 0.002$) (21,22). Clopidogrel has early benefit, demonstrated by a 35% reduction in the composite ischemic end point within 24 h (1.4% vs 2.1%; relative risk (RR) 0.66; 95% confidence interval (CI) 0.51–0.86) (21).

There has been concern regarding clopidogrel use prior to CABG. Among 901 patients in CURE who discontinued clopidogrel within 5 days of surgery, there was a trend toward increased bleeding (RR 1.53, $p = 0.06$) (21). However, in the larger ACUITY trial there was no increase in major bleeding among patients undergoing CABG who had received clopidogrel, although the best bleeding outcomes were in patients whose surgery was delayed (23). The incidence of ischemic complications was lower among clopidogrel-treated patients (23). Given these observations, the progressively decreasing minority of patients with NSTE-ACS undergoing surgery and the substantial early benefit of clopidogrel, the data favor early administration.

Unfractionated and low molecular weight heparin

UFH is a mixture of branched glycosaminoglycans derived from bovine or porcine tissue (24). One-third of heparin chains exert an anticoagulant effect by binding to lysine moieties on antithrombin (AT) via a pentasaccharide unit, producing a conformational change that accelerates AT's inhibition of serine proteases (3,24). Inhibition of factor IIa requires chains ≥3 polysaccharide units capable of forming a ternary complex between heparin, AT, and thrombin, while inhibition of factor Xa only requires heparin induced AT activation (24) (Figure 11.2). The heterogeneity of UFH, with chains ranging in molecular weight from 3,000 to 30,000 Da and nonspecific binding to plasma proteins, platelets, and endothelium result in unpredictable pharmacokinetics and platelet activation in ACS. The most serious complication of UFH is heparin-induced thrombocytopenia and thrombosis (HIT/HITTS), which results from autoantibodies to a complex of heparin and platelet factor 4, and occurs in up to 2.5% of patients receiving heparin (24,25). HITTS, which can be life- and limb-threatening, requires prolonged therapy with alternative anticoagulants (typically DTIs) (25). The evidence for utilizing UFH during NSTE-ACS results from a meta-analysis of six randomized comparisons of aspirin and UFH vs aspirin alone, in which UFH reduced the risk of

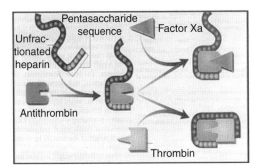

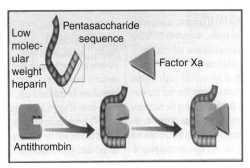

Figure 11.2 Comparison of unfractionated heparin and low molecular weight heparin interacting with coagulation proteases. Longer chain lengths of heparin are capable of forming a ternary complex with antithrombin and thrombin (factor IIa), resulting in an equal inhibition of factors Xa and IIa (left panel), while the shorter chain length of LMWH favors Xa inhibition (right panel). See text for details.

death or MI within 2–12 weeks (RR 0.67, 95% CI 0.44–1.02) (26).

LMWHs are derived from depolymerization of UFH, yielding shorter chains with less nonspecific binding (24). LMWH activates AT, but only 1/3 of LMWH-AT complexes can form the ternary complex required for IIa inhibition, resulting in a higher anti-Xa:anti-IIa ratio, from 2:1 to 4:1 for different LMWHs vs 1:1 for UFH (24) (Figure 11.2). Reduced nonspecific binding leads to more predictable pharmacokinetic properties and a lower incidence of HIT/HITTS than UFH (24). LMWH's reduced anti-IIA effect results in minimal elevation of the activated partial thromboplastin time making monitoring difficult, although anti-Xa levels can be measured. LMWH compounds differ in their characteristics, and a consistent utility in NSTE-ACS has been shown only for enoxaparin (3,24).

While the 2002 ACC/AHA guidelines favored enoxaparin over UFH based on the Efficacy and Safety of Subcutaneous Enoxaparin in Non-Q-Wave Coronary Events (ESSENCE) and TIMI-11B trials, these data are relevant in patients managed predominantly conservatively, which is no longer the standard of care (3,27,28). These trials showed a reduction in a composite ischemic end point, but no significant decrease in death or MI and increased TIMI minor bleeding with enoxaparin (27,28). Trials with a predominantly invasive strategy including the Aggrastat to Zocor (A to Z) and SYNERGY trials showed no difference in ischemic end points, but increased bleeding with enoxaparin vs UFH (8,29). The 2007 ACC/AHA guidelines give a class IA recommendation for either enoxaparin or UFH for NSTE-ACS treated with an early invasive approach (2). Such a strong endorsement of enoxaparin is inconsistent with the findings of A to Z, SYNERGY, and the Fifth Organization to Assess Strategies in Acute Ischemic Syndromes (OASIS-5) trial (see the section on "Fondaparinux"), each of which showed no benefit for enoxaparin compared with either UFH or fondaparinux on ischemic end points, unfavorable bleeding outcomes and a trend toward increased mortality in OASIS-5 (8,29,30). Furthermore, the use of enoxaparin in NSTE-ACS is problematic when patients undergo PCI within several hours of presentation or more than 6 h after their last dose, when there are conflicting recommendations for supplemental dosing.

Glycoprotein IIb/IIIa inhibitors

There are three GPIs available for use, each of which interferes with GP IIb/IIIa receptor binding via a fibrinogen bridge to a GP IIb/IIIa receptor on a neighboring platelet, thereby inhibiting aggregation (Figure 11.1b). Abciximab is the FAB fragment of a monoclonal antibody, while tirofiban and eptifibatide are smaller peptides, functioning by competitive inhibition (3). Both peptides contain an Arg-Gly-Asp recognition site that facilitates receptor binding (31). Major side effects include bleeding and thrombocytopenia. Abciximab has the longest duration of action, but unlike the competitive inhibitors, its effect can be mitigated by platelet transfusion, since it is administered in a lower ratio per receptor (31).

Six large trials and several meta-analyses of GPIs plus heparin in NSTE-ACS demonstrated a benefit in the prevention of ischemic outcomes compared with heparin monotherapy (3,32,33). Pooled analyses show a modest reduction in the composite of death and MI (RR 0.88, 95% CI 0.82–0.94, $p < 0.001$), however, there was no impact on mortality (RR 1.01, $p = 0.85$) (3,33). There was also excess bleeding, thrombocytopenia, and transfusion in patients receiving GPIs (32). As there are no positive data for "upstream" use of abciximab, this agent is indicated only during PCI (2).

In the ISAR-REACT 2 trial, in which 2,022 patients with NSTE-ACS received 600 mg of clopidogrel at least 3 h prior to PCI, death, MI, or target vessel revascularization was reduced from 12% to 8% with low-dose (70 units/kg) heparin plus abciximab compared to high-dose (140 units/kg) heparin alone (34). Thus, on a background of dual oral antiplatelet therapy high-dose heparin monotherapy is inferior to heparin/GPI in patients with NSTE-ACS undergoing PCI. Therefore, UFH/GPI administered either upstream or during PCI has been the established standard of care for patients with NSTE-ACS in whom an invasive strategy is planned. However, given the high rates and prognostic significance of bleeding and cost and complexity of GPI-based regimens, recent investigation has focused on developing simpler, less costly regimens that provide similar ischemic protection and survival with less bleeding.

Fondaparinux

Fondaparinux is a pentasaccharide analog of the AT-binding region of heparin that selectively inhibits factor Xa by binding to AT with a higher affinity than UFH. This causes a conformational change increasing AT's inactivation of factor Xa (30,35). Unlike heparin, fondaparinux cannot bind to thrombin, platelets, or other cellular elements (30,35). Potential advantages include predictable anticoagulation and absence of thrombocytopenia while limitations include use in chronic kidney disease and long half-life with no reversing agent (35). Fondaparinux and enoxaparin were compared in 21,000 patients with high-risk NSTE-ACS in the OASIS-5 trial (30). At 9 days, fondaparinux was noninferior to enoxaparin in the rate of death, MI, or refractory ischemia (5.8% vs 5.7%, $p_{ni} = 0.007$) with less major bleeding (2.2% vs 4.1%, $p < 0.001$) (30). Similar findings were observed in the 34% of patients who underwent PCI during hospitalization, with less major bleeding with fondaparinux (2.3% vs 5.1%, HR 0.45, 95% CI 0.34–0.5) (30). There was an increased rate of guiding catheter thrombus in the fondaparinux group (0.9% vs 0.4%, $p = 0.001$), which led to a recommendation that UFH be administered during PCI (2,30). In the overall population, 6-month mortality was lower in the fondaparinux group (5.8% vs 6.5%, HR 0.89, 95% CI 0.81–1.00) (30). Given the similar rates of MI in the two groups, OASIS-5 provides further evidence that bleeding contributes to mortality in NSTE-ACS. Fondaparinux is now endorsed by the ACC/AHA for treatment of NSTE-ACS (2), however, its long half-life, lack of a reversing agent, and risk of thrombus formation may limit its use with an early invasive strategy.

Bivalirudin

Like hirudin, which is synthesized by the medicinal leach, bivalirudin is a bivalent direct thrombin inhibitor. Bivalirudin has 20 amino acids (compared to 65 for hirudin), with identical binding regions. Unlike hirudin, which binds irreversibly to thrombin, bivalirudin is cleaved by thrombin at its arg-3/pro-4 bond, resulting in reversible binding. In combination with a shorter half-life, these differing pharmacological properties result in significantly lower rates of bleeding with bivalirudin (35–37) (Figure 11.3). In the ACUITY trial, bivalirudin plus routine GPI or bivalirudin plus

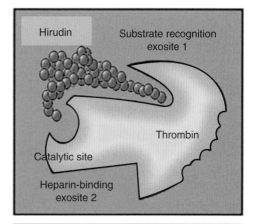

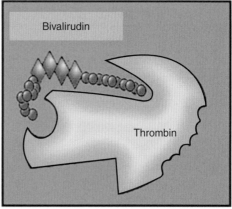

Figure 11.3 Comparison of hirudin and bivalirudin binding to thrombin. Bivalirudin is a bivalent 20–amino acid polypeptide comprised of a thrombin active site-directed peptide linked by a tetraglycine spacer to an analogue of the carboxy terminal of hirudin. Like hirudin, bivalirudin binds two thrombin moieties including the active site. Unlike hirudin, which remains bivalently bound to thrombin, thrombin will slowly cleave bivalirudin at its arginine$_3$-proline$_4$ bond, resulting in recovery of active site function, and limiting the drug's half-life to 25 min.

provisional GPI (bivalirudin monotherapy) were compared with an active control: heparin (either UFH or enoxaparin) plus routine GPI (7). In the bivalirudin monotherapy group, GPIs were used in <10% of patients. Bivalirudin monotherapy was superior to heparin plus routine GPI in the primary end point at 30 days (composite ischemia plus major bleeding, 10.1% vs 11.7%, $p = 0.015$), a finding that was driven by reduced major bleeding (3.0% vs 5.7%, $p < 0.0001$) with noninferiority on the ischemic composite (7). Similar outcomes were seen in the 7,780 patients undergoing PCI and the 3,852 diabetics (38,39). The total in-patient cost of care for bivalirudin monotherapy was significantly less than that for heparin/GPI (40).

Bivalirudin monotherapy is endorsed by the 2007 ACC/AHA guidelines for patients with NSTE-ACS undergoing an early invasive approach (2). These guidelines specify that bivalirudin monotherapy should be employed only with concomitant clopidogrel (2). This recommendation is derived from a borderline bivalirudin–clopidogrel interaction on the 30-day ischemic end point from ACUITY. Favorable 1-year results, published after the 2007 guidelines, have alleviated such concerns (14). Nonetheless, based on data presented earlier in this chapter, we strongly endorse early administration of clopidogrel for NSTE-ACS.

Conclusions

NSTE-ACS is a major health care concern. There is compelling evidence that both in-hospital MI and bleeding are independent predictors of mortality. Therefore, when comparing regimens, protection from both ischemic and bleeding complications is paramount. Factors such as ease of administration, economics, and seamless integration from presentation to the catheterization laboratory are desirable. Among currently available regimens, the combination of aspirin, bivalirudin, and clopidogrel comes closest to achieving these objectives. New antithrombotic agents including oral and intravenous platelet $P2Y_{12}$ antagonists, tissue factor pathway inhibitors and oral Xa inhibitors are being evaluated. The optimal antithrombotic regimen in NSTE-ACS will continue to evolve.

References

1 Rosamond W, Flegal K, Friday G, et al. Heart disease and stroke update: a report from the American heart association statistics committee and strokes statistics subcommittee. *Circulation.* 2007;**115**:e69–e171.

2 Anderson JL, Adams CD, Antman EM, et al. ACC/AHA 2007 guidelines for the management of patients with unstable angina/non–ST-elevation myocardial infarction: executive summary: a report of the American College of Cardiology/American Heart Association. Task Force on Practice Guidelines (Writing Committee to Revise the 2002 Guidelines for the Management of Patients With Unstable Angina/Non–ST-Elevation Myocardial Infarction). *Circulation.* 2007;**116**:803–877.

3 Braunwald E, Antman EM, Beasley JW, et al. ACC/AHA 2002 guideline update for the management of patients with unstable angina and non-ST-segment elevation myocardial infarction: a report of the American College of Cardiology/American Heart Association Task Force on Practice Guidelines (Committee on the Management of Patients With Unstable Angina). *J Am Coll Cardiol.* 2002;**40**(7):1366–1374.

4 Antman EM, Cohen M, Bernink PJ, et al. The TIMI risk score for unstable angina/non–ST elevation MI: a method for prognostication and therapeutic decision making. *JAMA.* 2000;**284**:835–842.

5 Manoukian SV, Feit F, Mehran R, et al. Impact of major bleeding on 30-day mortality and clinical outcomes in patients with acute coronary syndromes: an analysis from the ACUITY Trial. *J Am Coll Cardiol.* 2007;**49**(12):1362–1368.

6 Granger CB, Goldberg RJ, Dabbous O, et al. Predictors of hospital mortality in the global registry of acute coronary events. *Arch Intern Med.* 2003;**163**(19):2345–2353.

7 Stone GW, McLaurin BT, Cox DA, et al. ACUITY Investigators. Bivalirudin for patients with acute coronary syndromes. *N Engl J Med.* 2006;**355**:2203–2216.

8 Ferguson JJ, Califf RM, Antman EM, et al. Enoxaparin vs unfractionated heparin in high-risk patients with non-ST-segment elevation acute coronary syndromes managed with an intended early invasive strategy: primary results of the SYNERGY randomized trial. *JAMA.* 2004;**292**(1):45–54.

9 Stone GW. ACS management: state-of-the-art-and-science: addressing critical issues and controversies balancing bleeding risk with ischemic end point reduction – Where have we been and where are we heading? Proceedings of the Emergency Department and Interventional Cardiology Therapeutic Teams for Acute Coronary Syndromes 2007 Update; June 2, 2007; Philadelphia, Pennsylvania.

10 Neumann F, Kastrati A, Pogatsa-Murray G, et al. Evaluation of prolonged antithrombotic pretreatment ("cooling-off strategy") before intervention in patients with unstable coronary syndromes: a randomized controlled trial. *JAMA.* 2003;**290**:1593–1599.

11 Stone GW, Mehran R, Dangas G, et al. Differential impact on survival of electrocardiographic Q-wave versus enzymatic myocardial infarction after percutaneous intervention: a device-specific analysis of 7147 patients. *Circulation.* 2001;**104**(6):642–647.

12 Califf RM, Abdelmeguid AE, Kuntz RE, et al. Myonecrosis after revascularization procedures. *J Am Coll Cardiol.* 1998;**31**(2):241–251.

13 Moscuccia M, Fox A, Cannon C, et al. Predictors of major bleeding in acute coronary syndromes: the Global Registry of Acute Coronary Events (GRACE). *Eur Heart J.* 2003;**24**:1815–1823.

14 Stone GW, Ware JH, Bertrand M, *et al*. Anithrombotic strategies in patients with acute coronary syndromes undergoing early invasive management: one year results from the ACUITY trial. *JAMA*. 2007;298:2497–2506.

15 Manoukian SV, Feit F, Voeltz MD, *et al*. Incidence of major bleeding by the ACUITY and TIMI definitions and its impact on mortality in patients with acute coronary syndromes undergoing percutaneous intervention. *Circulation*. 2007;II-482.

16 Lincoff AM, Bittl JA, Harrington RA, *et al*. REPLACE-2 Investigators. Bivalirudin and provisional glycoprotein IIb/IIIa blockade compared with heparin and planned glycoprotein IIb/IIIa blockade during percutaneous coronary intervention: REPLACE-2 randomized trial. *JAMA*. 2003;**289**(7):853–863.

17 TIMI Study Group. The Thrombolysis in Myocardial Infarction (TIMI) trial. Phase I findings. *N Engl J Med*. 1985;**312**(14):932–936.

18 The GUSTO investigators. An international randomized trial comparing four thrombolytic strategies for acute myocardial infarction. *N Engl J Med*. 1993;**329**(10):673–682.

19 *Mosby's Drug Consult*, 16th Edition. Elsevier Mosby, 2006.

20 Steinhubl S, Roe MT. Optimizing platelet P2Y12 inhibition for patients undergoing PCI. *Cardiovasc Drug Rev*. 2007;**25**(2):188–203.

21 Yusuf S, Zhao F, Mehta SR, *et al*. Effects of clopidogrel in addition to aspirin in patients with acute coronary syndromes without ST-segment elevation. *N Engl J Med*. 2001;**345**(7):494–502.

22 Mehta SR, Yusuf S, Peters RJ, *et al*. Effects of pretreatment with clopidogrel and aspirin followed by long-term therapy in patients undergoing percutaneous coronary intervention: the PCI-CURE study. *Lancet*. 2001;**358**(9281):527–533.

23 Ebrahimi R, Manoukian SV, Feit F, *et al*. Implications of perioperative thienopyridine use prior to coronary artery bypass graft surgery—time for a paradigm shift? *Am J Cardiol*. 2006;**98**:31M.

24 Hirsh J, Raschke R. Heparin and low-molecular-weight heparin: the Seventh ACCP Conference on Antithrombotic and Thrombolytic Therapy. *Chest*. 2004;**126**(3 Suppl):188S–203S.

25 Ohman EM, Granger CB, Rice L, *et al*. Identification, diagnosis and treatment of heparin-induced thrombocytopenia and thrombosis: a registry of prolonged heparin use and thrombocytopenia among hospitalized patients with and without cardiovascular disease. The Complication After Thrombocytopenia Caused by Heparin (CATCH) registry steering committee. *J Thromb Thrombolysis*. 2005;**19**(1):11–19.

26 Oler A, Whooley MA, Oler J, *et al*. Adding heparin to aspirin reduces the incidence of myocardial infarction and death in patients with unstable angina. A meta-analysis. *JAMA*. 1996;**276**:811–815.

27 Cohen M, Demers C, Gurfinkel EP, *et al*. A comparison of low-molecular-weight heparin with unfractionated heparin for unstable coronary artery disease. Efficacy and Safety of Subcutaneous Enoxaparin in Non-Q-Wave Coronary Events Study Group. *N Engl J Med*. 1997;**337**:447–452.

28 Antman EM, McCabe CH, Gurfinkel EP, *et al*. Enoxaparin prevents death and cardiac ischemic events in unstable angina/non-Q-wave myocardial infarction: results of the Thrombolysis In Myocardial Infarction (TIMI) 11B trial. *Circulation*. 1999;**100**:1593–1601.

29 Blazing MA, de Lemos JA, White HD, *et al*. Safety and efficacy of enoxaparin vs unfractionated heparin in patients with non-ST-segment elevation acute coronary syndromes who receive tirofiban and aspirin: a randomized controlled trial. *JAMA*. 2004;**292**(1):55–64.

30 The Fifth Organization to Assess Strategies in Acute Ischemic Syndromes Investigators. Comparison of fondaparinux and enoxaparin in acute coronary syndromes. *N Engl J Med*. 2006;**354**:1464–1476.

31 Topol EJ, Byzova TV, Plow EF. Platelet GPIIb-IIIa blockers. *Lancet*. 1999;**353**:227–231.

32 Boersma E, Harrington RA, Moliterno DJ, *et al*. Platelet glycoprotein IIb/IIIa inhibitors in acute coronary syndromes: a meta-analysis of all major randomised clinical trials. *Lancet*. 2002;**359**(9302):189–198.

33 Roffi M, Chew DP, Mukherjee D, *et al*. Platelet glycoprotein IIb/IIIa inhibitors reduce mortality in diabetic patients with non-ST-segment-elevation acute coronary syndromes. *Circulation*. 2001;**104**(23):2767–2771.

34 Kastrati A, Mehilli J, Neumann FJ, *et al*. Abciximab in patients with acute coronary syndromes undergoing percutaneous coronary intervention after clopidogrel pretreatment: the ISARREACT 2 randomized trial. *JAMA*. 2006;**295**:1531–1538.

35 Dinwoodey D, Ansell JE. Heparins, low-molecular-weight heparins, and pentasaccharides. *Clin Geriatr Med*. 2006;**22**:1–15.

36 Carswell CI, Plokser GL. Bivalirudin: a review of its potential place in the management of acute coronary syndromes. *Drugs*. 2002;**62**(5):841–870.

37 Moen MD, Keating GM, Wellington K. Bivalirudin: a review of its use in patients undergoing percutaneous coronary intervention. *Drugs*. 2005;**65**(13):1869–1891.

38 Stone GW, White HD, Ohman EM, *et al*. Acute Catheterization and Urgent Intervention Triage strategy (ACUITY) trial investigators. Bivalirudin in patients with acute coronary syndromes undergoing percutaneous coronary intervention: a subgroup analysis from the Acute Catheterization and Urgent Intervention Triage strategy (ACUITY) trial. *Lancet*. 2007;**369**(9565):907–919.

39 Feit F, Ebrahimi R, Manoukian SV, *et al.* Bivalirudin monotherapy improves 30 day clinical outcomes in diabetes with acute coronary syndromes (ACS). Report from the ACUITY trial. *Circulation.* 2006;**114**:551.

40 Pinto D, Stone G, McLaurin B, *et al.* In hospital costs for patients managed with an early invasive strategy for NSTEMI/ACS: Preliminary results from the ACUITY study. *Am J Cardiol.* 2006;**98**:195M.

CHAPTER 12

Non antithrombotic postprocedural pharmacotherapy: The role of statins, beta-blockers, angiotension-converting enzyme, or aldosterone inhibitors in acute coronary syndromes and elective percutaneous coronary interventions

Itsik Ben-Dor[1,2], Ran Kornowski[1,2], & Shmuel Fuchs[1]

[1]Rabin Medical Center, Petach-Tikva, Israel
[2]Tel-Aviv University, Tel-Aviv, Israel

Percutaneous coronary intervention (PCI) is a potent therapeutic tool, which optimally should be used in conjunction with pharmacological adjunctive therapies. Of the latter, the most frequently used are antiplatelets and anticoagulation. Nevertheless, in patients with known and/or suspected coronary artery disease, a wide array of medications are consistently being used, both pre- and post-procedure. In this chapter, we attempted to summarize the role of this important pharmacotherapy, which included statins, beta-blockers, angiotensin-converting enzyme inhibitors (ACE-I), and aldosterone antagonist in patients who undergo PCI in elective procedures or during the course of acute coronary syndromes (ACS). This chapter provides a summary on no antithrombotic adjunctive pharmacotherapy used in chronic stable coronary patients and in those with ACS, whereas both groups may undergo elective or emergent PCI during the course of their disease.

Lipid-lowering statins therapy

Long-term treatment with statins has been shown to be beneficial in primary and secondary prevention studies (1–5). The landmark Scandinavian Simvastatin Survival Study Group (4S) study enrolled patients with angina or prior myocardial infarction (MI) and elevated cholesterol level. This study demonstrated that simvastatin therapy reduced total mortality by 30% and cardiovascular mortality by 42% (6). These results were extended to population of patients with established coronary artery disease (CAD) and average cholesterol levels in the Cholesterol and Recurrent Events (CARE) and the Long-Term Intervention with Pravastatin in Ischemic Disease Trial (LIPID) trials (7,8).

Pharmacology in the Catheterization Laboratory. Edited by Ron Waksman and Andrew E Ajani. © 2010 Blackwell Publishing, ISBN: 978-1-4051-5704-9.

Recent reports have also shown greater benefit for high-dose statins therapy compared with low dose in participants with stable CAD (9). However, this observation was not validated in the Incremental Decrease in End Points Through Aggressive Lipid Lowering (IDEAL) study, which assessed the impact of intensive lowering of LDL in patients with previous MI (10).

Following the established benefit of statin administration as a secondary prevention intervention in stable patients with CAD, a question was raised whether aggressive therapy, initiated early after ACS, will carry additive value. This question was recently examined in several clinical trials, which collectively evaluated the impact of dosages and timing of initiation of statins therapy among those patients. In the Myocardial Ischemia Reduction with Aggressive Cholesterol-Lowering (MIRACL) Study, high dose statins therapy (atrovastatin 80 mg), initiated within 24–96 h after hospital admission for ACS event, was compared with placebo. At 4 months, a significant reduction of 16% in the composite end point of death, MI, cardiac resuscitation, or recurrent myocardial ischemia was observed among patients who received high statin dose compared to placebo. This difference, however, was mostly due to the reduction in rehospitalization for angina (11). A second study, Pravastatin or Atorvastatin Evaluation and Infection Therapy: Thrombolysis in Myocardial Infarction 22 (PROVE IT/TIMI 22) trial, evaluated the role of similar intensive lipid-lowering (atrovastatin 80 mg) strategy but as compared to standard lipid therapy (pravastatin 40 mg), both initiated within 10 days following ACS event. The risk of death, MI, documented unstable angina, revascularization, or stroke was reduced by 16% ($p = 0.005$) among patients who received intensive lipid-lowering therapy. This benefit was observed as early as 30 days post-randomization, and continued throughout the 2.5 years of follow-up (12). Interestingly, the in the MIRACL trial, patients were excluded if coronary revascularization was planned or anticipated at the time of screening and thus, PCI during the 16 weeks of follow-up was performed in only 9.8% and 9.2% in the atrovastatin and placebo groups, respectively. By contrast, in the PROVE IT/TIMI 22 trial, 69% of the patients underwent PCI during the index hospitalization.

Thus, these trials support the initiation of intensive LDL-lowering strategy using high dose of statins very early after an ACS event, irrespective of the performance of early PCI. An additional question was subsequently raised, whether the beneficial effect of statins in ACS patients is due to the use of high dose or the early timing of administration. In the A to Z trial, patients with ACS were randomly assigned to aggressive statins therapy (simvastatin 40 mg/day for one month, then 80 mg/day) or to delayed conservative statins therapy (placebo for 4 months, then simvastatin 20 mg/day). At 1 and 4 months, there was no reduction in the incidence of the primary endpoint (cardiovascular death, MI, readmission for ACS, or stroke). Interestingly, aggressive simvastatin therapy was associated with a significant reduction in the primary end point from 4 months to the end of the study (13). This study, therefore, suggest that higher dose, rather than early in-hospital administration is the main contributing factor for the observed beneficial effects of statins in ACS patients. Further support to this observation was derived by a meta-analysis of placebo-controlled trials. This pooled analysis suggested that early initiation of statins therapy (within 14 days of an ACS) was not associated with reduction in death, MI, or stroke at 30-day and/or 4-month follow-up, although the frequency of unstable angina episodes at 4 months was lower (14).

In these ACS studies, there was a large heterogeneity in PCI performance during the ACS event. This variability limits the ability to assess the impact of early statin treatment on PCI outcomes. In the Lescol Intervention Prevention Study (LIPS), 1,669 patients with an averaged cholesterol levels were randomized to receive 80 mg fluvastatin or placebo, starting 2 days after PCI. At 3.9 years, the statin-treated group had significantly lower rates of clinical events (21.4%) compared to the placebo group (26.7%, $p = 0.01$). The need for any reintervention was also significantly lower among the statin-treated patients compared to placebo (32% vs 45.2% respectively, $p = 0.02$) (15). Importantly, a subanalysis of the LIPS study showed that fluvastatin reduced the risk of the overall adverse cardiac events in diabetic patients by 51% ($p = 0.0088$) (16).

Several recent angiographic studies assessed the impact of intense statin therapy on atherosclerosis progression. The Reversing Atherosclerosis with

Aggressive Lipid Lowering (REVERSAL) study found that patients with CAD who were treated with intensive statins therapy of atrovastatin 80 mg daily had no significant progression in median plaque volume (i.e., –0.4%) compared to baseline, while patients treated with standard statin therapy with pravastatin 40 mg daily had a 2.7% increase in median plaque volume over 18 months as measured by intravascular ultrasound (IVUS) (17). The possible atherosclerosis regression effect of statin therapy was also examined in the Study to Evaluate the Effect of Rosuvastatin on Intravascular Ultrasound-Derived Coronary Atheroma Burden (ASTEROID). In this open-label, uncontrolled study, the atherosclerosis regression effect of rosuvastatin 40 mg daily was evaluated in 507 patients who underwent coronary angiography but no PCI. Patients need to have mild CAD defined as <50% luminal narrowing. IVUS, performed at baseline and at 24 months revealed the median value of atheroma volume reduction to be 0.79% (18). Although these studies did not evaluate the impact of intense statin therapy on revascularization, the positive effect on halting atheroma progression and the encouraging data regarding atheroma regression (although of very mild magnitude) suggest a potential "proof of concept" mechanism by which statin therapy may reduce the need for coronary reintervention. This hypothesis was recently examined in a meta-analysis of 14 randomized trials (90,056 patients), which demonstrated that in addition to reduced major coronary events and stroke, and statin therapy also reduced by 24%. The benefit was more pronounced in high-risk patients and was directly correlated to the absolute reduction in LDL levels (19).

The pleiotropic effects of statins may also play a major role in reduction of acute coronary events and progression of atherosclerosis. Among these are anti-inflammatory effects with the accompanied reduction of CRP levels (20), reduced thrombus formation (21), restoration of endothelial function via increase of nitric oxide, and reduce oxidized LDL levels (22,23) and favorable affects on atheroma composition including increase in collagen and reduction in inflammatory components (24). The latter effects are associated with a reduction in atherosclerotic plaque vulnerability (25).

Interestingly, despite their prominent favorable effects on atherosclerosis formation and wide pleiotropic effects, lipid-lowering therapy seems to have no impact on the rate of restenosis. This dichotomy was demonstrated in early statin therapy studies, whereas the benefit of statins after PCI was mainly due to plaque stabilization and reduction in MI at remote coronary sites rather than halting restenosis (26–32).

Although subsequent study reported beneficial effects of pravastatin on clinical and angiographic restenosis (33), the increased use of drug-eluting stents with reduced rates of restenosis makes this therapeutic target almost impossible to be reassessed.

In response to the recent results, the NCEP has recently recommended lowering of the LDL target goals to <70 mg/dL for high-risk individuals, such as those with coronary disease and/or diabetes (34). Accordingly, LDL levels in patients who undergo PCI should be targeted to those "optimal" levels.

Angiotensin-converting enzyme inhibitor and angiotensin I receptor blocker

Angiotensin-converting enzyme inhibitor

Substantial data support the routine use of agents that block the rennin–angiotensin aldosterone (RAAS) system in various cardiac patient populations. Of note, the observed reduction in cardiovascular events is independent of their effects on blood pressure.

The potential benefit of ACE-I in patients without heart failure was examined in several studies. In the Heart Outcomes Prevention Evaluation (HOPE) trial, a primary prevention study in patients with established or risk factors for CAD, the primary end point of combined risk of CV death, MI, or stroke in was significantly reduced by ramipril (14.0% vs 17.8%, relative risk [RR] 0.78, $p < 0.001$). Interestingly, the rate of revascularization was also lower among patients who received ramipril (16.0% vs 18.3%, RR 0.85, $p = 0.002$) (35). Similar beneficial effects were observed in other, but not all studies (36,37). This inconsistency may reflect different patient populations. Nevertheless, in a very recent combined analysis of those three trials, ACE-I significantly reduced all cause mortality (7.8% vs

8.9%, $p = 0.0004$), cardiovascular mortality (4.3% vs 5.2%, $p = 0.0002$), nonfatal MI (5.3% vs 6.4%, $p = 0.0001$), all strokes (2.2% vs 2.8%, $p = 0.0004$), heart failure (2.1% vs 2.7%, $p = 0.0007$), coronary artery bypass surgery (6.0% vs 6.9%, $p = 0.003$), but not PCI (7.4% vs 7.6%, $p = 0.48$) (38).

The effects of ACE-I in patients presented with ACS were subsequently studied systematically. There is now unequivocal evidence derived from several randomized, placebo-controlled trials that ACE-I reduce mortality rate in patients admitted with acute ST elevation MI. Those trials can be subgrouped into two categories. The first consisted of high-risk MI patients with features indicative of increased mortality such as left ventricular ejection fraction less than 40%, clinical signs and symptoms of congestive heart failure (39,40), anterior location of infarction (41), and abnormal wall motion score index (42). In these high-risk patient studies, ACE-I was started between 3 and 16 days after the MI and was maintained for 1–4 years. A meta-analysis of six randomized, controlled trials suggests that long-term therapy with ACE-I reduces overall mortality by 18% and the risk of major clinical outcomes by 22% (43). Of note, the mortality reduction with ACE-I was correlated with the reduction in the rate of development of congestive heart failure. In addition, some data suggest that ischemic events, including recurrent infarction, and the need for coronary revascularization, can also be reduced by chronic administration of ACE-I after ST-elevation MI (44). This effect may contribute to the observed reduction in mortality.

The second group of studies assessed the potential benefit of ACE-I among all noncardiogenic-shock acute MI patients, provided they had a minimum systolic pressure of ~100 mmHg (45–47). ACE-I therapy was initiated early (within the first 24–36 h) and was maintained for short period of 4–6 weeks. Thus, these studies assessed the effect of early, short-term administration of ACE-I on mortality in all hemodynamically stable STEMI patients. On the other hand, studies, which included only high-risk AMI patients, evaluated the long-term benefit of ACE-I therapy initiated after the acute phase. All the post-MI short-term ACE I follow-up trials (with the exception of the Cooperative New Scandinavian Enalapril Survival Study II [CONSENSUS II] (48), in which

intravenous ACE-I was administered), consistently demonstrated a survival benefit. A meta-analysis of major placebo-controlled trials of >100,000 patients indicates a small, but significant 6.5% relative reduction in 30-day mortality when ACE-I were given early following STEMI (49). Since 40% of this survival advantage was due to reduction in mortality within the first 24 h and additional 45% of the mortality benefit was evident during days 2–7, very early administration of ACE-I is considered class I indication in high-risk STEMI patients and class IIa in patients without anterior infarction, pulmonary congestion, or LVEF less than 40% in the absence of hypotension (systolic blood pressure less than 100 mmHg or less than 30 mmHg below baseline) (50).

The role of ACE-I in preventing restenosis has been evaluated in several large randomized trials. None of the studies showed a reduction in restenosis rate following balloon angioplasty (51–53). The effect of ACE-I on stent restenosis was studied in relation to ACE gene polymorphism. In this regard, several studies (54,55) suggested a detrimental effect of ACE-I in patients with the D/D ACE allele, while others demonstrated no relation (56). One study suggested that ACE-I may reduce stent restenosis in type 2 diabetic patients with D allele (DD or ID) (57).

Angiotensin I receptor blocker

Inhibition of the RAAS system was with angiotensin receptor blocker (ARB) also evaluated in patients with acute MI. The Valsartan in Acute Myocardial Infarction Trial (VALIANT) (58) compared the efficacy and safety of long-term treatment with valsartan, captopril, and their combination in high-risk acute MI patients with impaired left ventricular function. This trial demonstrated that RAAS blocked with ARB did meet the primary end point of all cause mortality compared to captopril monotherapy for no inferiority. The combination of ACE-I and ARB was not superior to monotherapy and was associated with increased rate of adverse events (valsartan/captopril arm 34.8%, valsartan 29.4%, and captopril 28.4%). The Optimal Therapy in Myocardial Infarction with the Angiotensin II Antagonist Losartan (OPTIMAAL) study (59) compared the effects of the ARB losartan to that of ACE-I (captopril) in MI patients with clinical evidence of heart failure. There was a nonsignificant trend favoring captopril in terms of total mortality. The concern regarding potential increase in MI among ARB-treated patients (60,61) was disputed by a recent systematic review showing that ARB treatment is not associated with increased incidence of MI (62,63).

The effect of ARB on in-stent restenosis was not studied systematically. In an open-label study of 250 patients who were randomized to long-term administration of 80 mg of valsartan or placebo, in-stent restenosis was reduced by ~50% (19.2% compared to 38.6%, $p < 0.005$) (64). Nonetheless, those data have not been duplicated in another trial and with the rapid increase in utilization of drug-eluting stents, further evaluation of this potential benefit seems to be unlikely.

Aldosterone receptor antagonists

Eplerenone, a selective aldosterone inhibitor, has been evaluated in the Eplerenone Post-AMI Heart Failure Efficacy and Survival Study (EPHESUS). In this study, patients with left ventricular ejection fraction less than 40% were randomly assigned 3–14 days after MI to eplerenone or placebo. During a mean follow-up of 16 months, eplerenone significantly reduced mortality by 15%. Cardiovascular mortality or hospitalization for cardiovascular events was also reduced (65). The specific impact of eplerenone on PCI-treated patients during the course of MI needs to be determined.

Beta-blocker

Beta-blockers (BB) have been studied in multiple patient populations with CAD. The spectrum of their beneficial effects is wide and their impacts on outcome mostly depend on the patient's risk profile.

Administration of BB in individuals with stable CAD is associated with improved exercise capacity, reduction in exercise-induced ST depression, angina episodes, and nitroglycerine use. In a recent retrospective observational study, BB treatment in patients with CAD but without MI or heart failure was associated with reduced death rate (66). This observation, however, was not yet studied in

a prospective manner and thus should be awaited further evaluation.

Administration of BB to higher risk patient populations such as those with unstable angina was shown to reduce subsequent MI and/or recurrent ischemia (67–69). A meta-analysis suggested that beta-blocker treatment in patients with unstable angina was associated with a 13% relative reduction in the risk of progression to acute MI (70).

The administration of BB in patients presented with STEMI has been shown to reduce morbidity and mortality in multiple trials (71–75). Clinical studies from the prethrombolysis era demonstrated a significant relative risk reduction of 15–35% in 30-day mortality (76–78). Those results have been subsequently confirmed in the reperfusion/revascularization era.

Similar to ACE-I, the effect of BB in patients with acute MI can be divided to early and late, depending on the timing of initiation of the treatment. Pooled data from controlled trials involving over 26,000 patients undergoing early short-term intravenous administration of BB suggested a ~13% relative reduction in in-hospital mortality rates (79), which was mainly related to reduction in malignant arrhythmia. However, other studies failed to show advantage of very early treatment. For example, in the large COMMIT/CCS trial, 46,000 patients (93% with ST elevation or left bundle branch block), of whom 50% received thrombolytic therapy, early intravenous BB therapy was associated with no reduction in mortality. Assessment of subgroups of patients, based on their hemodynamic status at the time of admission, suggested that very early administration of intravenous BB among unstable patients is associated with increased mortality rates, whereas hemodynamically stable patients may benefit (80).

In the Thrombolysis In Myocardial Infarction trial, phase II-B (TIMI 2B), which randomly assigned 1,434 patients who were treated with thrombolysis to either early intravenous BB therapy followed by oral treatment or delayed oral BB. There was significant benefit for early BB therapy with lower rate of the combined end point of recurrent MI or death with in 21 days. However, this benefit was not seen when early intravenous BB therapy was delayed to 2–4 h after the onset of symptoms (71). A large meta-analysis of 51 short-term and 31 long-term trials suggests a statistically significant 23% mortality reduction with long-term administration of oral BB while early intravenous administration resulted in no significant reduction in mortality (81). Furthermore, a post-hoc analysis of the use of atenolol in the GUSTO-I trial did not support the routine use of early intravenous use of beta-blocker (82).

In collective, the data suggest that the advantage of early intravenous treatment with BB is limited while the benefit of oral BB is well established in noncardiogenic shock AMI patients. Whether BB carry added value in STEMI patients who undergo primary PCI was evaluated in a post-hoc analysis of the CADILLAC study. In this study, 2,082 patients were randomized in 2 × 2 fashion to balloon angioplasty versus stent implantation, with and without administration of abciximab. Patients with cardiogenic shock were excluded. At 30 days, patients who had received a preprocedural BB had a significantly lower mortality than those who had not (1.5% vs 2.8 %). However, the reduction in mortality was limited to patients who had not been receiving an oral BB before admission (72,73).

Pooled analysis of 2,537 patients enrolled in the Primary Angioplasty in Myocardial Infarction (PAMI), PAMI-2, and Stent PAMI trials suggested that both intravenous and oral BB given before primary PCI were associated with reduced in-hospital mortality and a nonsignificant lower 1-year mortality (74).

Lower mortality was also reported among patients in whom BB therapy was initiated after primary PCI. This was illustrated in an analysis of 2,442 patients who underwent successful primary PCI. At 6 months, post-PCI BB administration was associated with a significant reduction in mortality (2.3% vs 6.6%) (75).

Given the overwhelming evidence of benefit of early BB treatment in ST-elevation MI, patients without a contraindication who can be treated with BB within 12 h of the onset of infarction should receive oral (class I indication) or intravenous BB (class IIa), irrespective of administration of concomitant thrombolytic therapy or performance of primary PCI (50).

The effect of BB among patients with non-ST elevation MI was examined in the BB Heart Attack Trial (BHAT). In this study, mortality rates among patients with persistent electrocardiographic ST-segment depression who received nonselective BB was 7.6% compared to 13.6% among controls ($p = 0.012$) (83). This observation was confirmed in less selective non-ST elevation AMI patients including the Global Registry of Acute Coronary Events and the Worcester Heart Attack Study (84,85).

The benefit of BB in patients who undergo elective PCI was demonstrated in several trials. Large prospective registry, BB use was associated with a marked long-term survival benefit among patients undergoing successful elective percutaneous coronary revascularization. Of the 4,553 patients studied, 2,056 (45%) were treated with BB at the time of the procedure. BB therapy was associated with a mortality reduction from 1.3% to 0.8% at 30 days ($p = 0.13$), and a reduction from 6.0% to 3.9% at 1 year ($p = 0.0014$). Using propensity analysis, BB therapy remained an independent predictor for 1-year survival after PCI (hazard ratio, 0.63; 95% confidence interval, 0.46–0.87; $p = 0.0054$) (86). Also, the use of BB was associated with reduced rate of symptom-derived target vessel revascularization and MACE in a cohort of 4,840 patients (87).

Summary

Atherogenic risk factors continue to play a major role in the prognosis of CAD patients regardless of PCI performance. To prevent future cardiovascular complications and improve prognosis, numerous drugs have been developed to inhibit ischemic, hemodynamic and/or arrhythmogenic complications. The vast experience with pharmacotherapy that was shown to be beneficial in stable CAD patient population suggests similar benefit among unstable patients who present with ACS and also are candidates for PCI (Table 12.1). The main indications for using the above discussed cardiac medications relate to the presence of atherosclerotic CAD, modulation of atherogenic risk factors, and/or reduced LV function. An early administration ACE-I and BB and statin medication among hemodynamically stable ACS patients seems to be beneficial. The performance of PCI per se should not affect the decision regarding the type

Table 12.1 Beneficial effects of medical treatment in various coronary artery disease patient populations.

	Statins	ACE-I	ARB	Beta-blockers	Aldosterone antagonist
Stable CAD					
Mortality	Yes	Yes	Unknown	No	Unknown
MACE	Yes	Yes	Unknown	Yes	Unknown
Unstable angina					
Mortality	No	Unknown	Unknown	No	Unknown
MACE	Yes	Yes	Unknown	Yes	Unknown
Acute myocarial infarction					
Mortality	No	Yes	No	Yes	Yes[a]
MACE	Yes	Yes	Yes	Yes	Yes[a]
PCI					
Mortality	Unknown	Unknown	Unknown	Yes[b]	Unknown
MACE	Yes	Unknown	Unknown	Yes	Unknown
ISR	No	No	Yes[c]	Unknown[d]	Unknown

Abbreviations: CAD, coronary artery disease; ACE-I, angiotensin-converting enzyme inhibitors; ARB, angiotensin receptor blocker; PCI, percutaneous coronary intervention; MACE, major adverse cardiac events; ISR, in-stent restenosis.

[a]Only in patients with heart failure.
[b]Registry data.
[c]Limited experience (data derived from single small-randomized trial) (64).
[d]Only single trial showed benefit on clinical restenosis (87).

of medical therapy, which is primarily dictated by the patient's baseline characteristics and clinical status. Finally, at the era of drug-eluting stents, the restenosis end point may no longer dictate the clinical outcome of stable or unstable PCI-treated patients.

References

1 Colhoun HM, Thomason MJ, Mackness MI, *et al.* Collaborative AtoRvastatins Diabetes Study (CARDS). Design of the Collaborative AtoRvastatins Diabetes Study (CARDS) in patients with type 2 diabetes. *Diabet Med.* 2002;**19**:201–211.

2 Shepherd J, Cobbe SM, Ford I, *et al.* Prevention of coronary heart disease with pravastatins in men with hypercholesterolemia. West of Scotland Coronary Prevention Study Group. *N Engl J Med.* 1995;**16**(333): 1301–1307.

3 Heart Protection Study Collaborative Group. MRC/BHF Heart Protection Study of cholesterol lowering with simvastatins in 20,536 high-risk individuals: a randomised placebo-controlled trial. *Lancet.* 2002;**6**(360):7–22.

4 Gotto AM, Jr, Whitney E, Stein EA, *et al.* Relation between baseline and on-treatment lipid parameters and first acute major coronary events in the Air Force/Texas Coronary Atherosclerosis Prevention Study (AFCAPS/TexCAPS). *Circulation.* 2000;**8**(101):477–484.

5 Sever PS, Dahlof B, Poulter NR, *et al.* Prevention of coronary and stroke events with atorvastatins in hypertensive patients who have average or lower-than-average cholesterol concentrations, in the Anglo-Scandinavian Cardiac Outcomes Trial—Lipid Lowering Arm (ASCOT-LLA): a multicentre randomised controlled trial. *Lancet.* 2003;**5**(361):1149–1158.

6 Pedersen TR, Terje, Kjekshus J, *et al.* Randomised trial of cholesterol lowering in 4444 patients with coronary heart disease: the Scandinavian Simvastatins Survival Study (4S). *Lancet.* 1994;**19**(344):1383–1389.

7 Sacks FM, Pfeffer MA, Moye LA, *et al.* The effect of pravastatins on coronary events after myocardial infarction in patients with average cholesterol levels. Cholesterol and Recurrent Events Trial investigators. *N Engl J Med.* 1996;**3**(335):1001–1009.

8 Prevention of cardiovascular events and death with pravastatins in patients with coronary heart disease and a broad range of initial cholesterol levels. The Long-Term Intervention with Pravastatins in Ischaemic Disease (LIPID) Study Group. *N Engl J Med.* 1998;**5**(339):1349–1357.

9 LaRosa JC, Grundy SM, Waters DD, *et al.* Treating to New Targets (TNT) Investigators. Intensive lipid lowering with atorvastatins in patients with stable coronary disease. *N Engl J Med.* 2005;**7**(352):1425–1435.

10 Pedersen TR, Faergeman O, Kastelein JJ, *et al.* Incremental decrease in end points through aggressive lipid lowering (IDEAL) study group. *JAMA.* 2005;**16**(294):2437–2445.

11 Schwartz GG, Olsson AG, Ezekowitz MD, *et al.* Effects of atorvastatins on early recurrent ischemic events in acute coronary syndromes: the MIRACL study: a randomized controlled trial. *JAMA.* 2001;**4**(285):1711–1718.

12 Ray KK, Cannon CP, McCabe CH, *et al.* Early and late benefits of high-dose atorvastatins in patients with acute coronary syndromes: results from the PROVE IT-TIMI 22 trial. *J Am Coll Cardiol.* 2005;**18**(46):1405–1410.

13 de Lemos JA, Blazing MA, Wiviott SD, *et al.* Early intensive vs a delayed conservative simvastatins strategy in patients with acute coronary syndromes: phase Z of the A to Z trial. *JAMA.* 2004;**15**(292):1307–1316.

14 Briel M, Schwartz GG, Thompson PL, *et al.* Effects of early treatment with statins on short-term clinical outcomes in acute coronary syndromes: a meta-analysis of randomized controlled trials. *JAMA.* 2006;**3**(295):2046–2056.

15 Serruys PW, de Feyter P, Macaya C, *et al.* Fluvastatins for prevention of cardiac events following successful first percutaneous coronary intervention: a randomized controlled trial. *JAMA.* 2002;**26**(287):3215–3222.

16 Arampatzis CA, Goedhart D, Serruys PW, *et al.* Fluvastatin reduces the impact of diabetes on long-term outcome after coronary intervention—a Lescol Intervention Prevention Study (LIPS) substudy. *Am Heart J.* 2005;**149**:329–335.

17 Nissen SE, Tuzcu EM, Schoenhagen P, *et al.* Effect of intensive compared with moderate lipid-lowering therapy on progression of coronary atherosclerosis: a randomized controlled trial. *JAMA.* 2004;**3**(291):1071–1080.

18 Nissen SE, Nicholls SJ, Sipahi I, *et al.* Effect of very high-intensity statins therapy on regression of coronary atherosclerosis: the ASTEROID trial. *JAMA.* 2006;**5**(295):1556–1565.

19 Baigent C, Keech A, Kearney PM, *et al.* Efficacy and safety of cholesterol-lowering treatment: prospective meta-analysis of data from 90,056 participants in 14 randomised trials of statins. *Lancet.* 2005;**8**(366):1267–1278.

20 Ridker PM, Cannon CP, Morrow D, *et al.* C-reactive protein levels and outcomes after statins therapy. *N Engl J Med.* 2005;**6**(352):20–28.

21 Rosenson RS, Tangney CC. Antiatherothrombotic properties of statins: implications for cardiovascular event reduction. *JAMA.* 1998;**27**(279):1643–1650.

22 Dupuis J, Tardif JC, Cernacek P, Theroux P. Cholesterol reduction rapidly improves endothelial function after acute coronary syndromes. The RECIFE (reduction of cholesterol in ischemia and function of the endothelium) trial. *Circulation.* 1999;**29**(99):3227–3233.

23 Hernandez-Perera O, Perez-Sala D, Navarro-Antolin J, *et al.* Effects of the 3-hydroxy-3-methylglutaryl-CoA reductase inhibitors, atorvastatins and simvastatins, on the expression of endothelin-1 and endothelial nitric oxide synthase in vascular endothelial cells. *J Clin Invest.* 1998;**15**(101):2711–2719.

24 Crisby M, Nordin-Fredriksson G, Shah PK, Yano J, Zhu J, Nilsson J. Pravastatins treatment increases collagen content and decreases lipid content, inflammation, metalloproteinases, and cell death in human carotid plaques: implications for plaque stabilization. *Circulation.* 2001;**20**(103):926–933.

25 Williams JK, Sukhova GK, Herrington DM, Libby P. Pravastatins has cholesterol-lowering independent effects on the artery wall of atherosclerotic monkeys. *J Am Coll Cardiol.* 1998;**1**(31):684–691.

26 Weintraub WS, Pederson JP. Atherosclerosis and restenosis: reflections on the Lovastatins Restenosis Trial and Scandinavian Simvastatins Survival Study. *Am J Cardiol.* 1996;**1**(78):1036–1038.

27 Boccuzzi SJ, Weintraub WS, Kosinski AS, Roehm JB, Klein JL. Aggressive lipid lowering in postcoronary angioplasty patients with elevated cholesterol (the Lovastatins Restenosis Trial). *Am J Cardiol.* 1998;**1**(81):632–636.

28 Serruys PW, Foley DP, Jackson G, *et al.* A randomized placebo-controlled trial of fluvastatins for prevention of restenosis after successful coronary balloon angioplasty; final results of the fluvastatins angiographic restenosis (FLARE) trial. *Eur Heart J.* 1999;**20**:58–69.

29 Bunch TJ, Muhlestein JB, Anderson JL, *et al.* Effects of statins on six-month survival and clinical restenosis frequency after coronary stent deployment. *Am J Cardiol.* 2002;**1**(90):299–302.

30 Malik IS, Khan M, Beatt KJ. Effect of statins therapy on restenosis after coronary stent implantation. *Am J Cardiol.* 2000;**1**(86):810.

31 Kleemann A, Eckert S, von Eckardstein A, *et al.* Effects of lovastatins on progression of non-dilated and dilated coronary segments and on restenosis in patients after PTCA. The cholesterol lowering atherosclerosis PTCA trial (CLAPT). *Eur Heart J.* 1999;**20**:1393–1406.

32 Weintraub WS, Boccuzzi SJ, Klein JL, *et al.* Lack of effect of lovastatins on restenosis after coronary angioplasty. Lovastatins Restenosis Trial Study Group. *N Engl J Med.* 1994;**17**(331):1331–1337.

33 Mulder HJ, Bal ET, Jukema JW, *et al.* Pravastatins reduces restenosis two years after percutaneous transluminal coronary angioplasty (REGRESS trial). *Am J Cardiol.* 2000;**1**(86):742–746.

34 Grundy SM, Cleeman JI, Merz CN, *et al.* Coordinating Committee of the National Cholesterol Education Program. Implications of recent clinical trials for the National Cholesterol Education Program Adult Treatment Panel III Guidelines. *J Am Coll Cardiol.* 2004;**4**(44):720–732.

35 Yusuf S, Sleight P, Pogue J, Bosch J, Davies R, Dagenais G. Effects of an angiotensin-converting-enzyme inhibitor, ramipril, on cardiovascular events in high-risk patients. The Heart Outcomes Prevention Evaluation Study Investigators. *N Engl J Med.* 2000;**20**(342):145–153.

36 Fox KM, EURopean trial on reduction of cardiac events with Perindopril in stable coronary Artery disease Investigators. Efficacy of perindopril in reduction of cardiovascular events among patients with stable coronary artery disease: randomised, double-blind, placebo-controlled, multicentre trial (the EUROPA study). *Lancet.* 2003;**6**(362):782–788.

37 Braunwald E, Domanski MJ, Fowler SE, *et al.* Angiotensin-converting-enzyme inhibition in stable coronary artery disease. *N Engl J Med.* 2004;**11**(351):2058–2068.

38 Dagenais GR, Pogue J, Fox K, Simoons ML, Yusuf S. Angiotensin-converting-enzyme inhibitors in stable vascular disease without left ventricular systolic dysfunction or heart failure: a combined analysis of three trials. *Lancet.* 2006;**12**(368):581–588.

39 Pfeffer MA, Braunwald E, Moye LA, *et al.* Effect of captopril on mortality and morbidity in patients with left ventricular dysfunction after myocardial infarction. Results of the survival and ventricular enlargement trial. The SAVE Investigators. *N Engl J Med.* 1992;**3**(327):669–677.

40 Effect of ramipril on mortality and morbidity of survivors of acute myocardial infarction with clinical evidence of heart failure. The Acute Infarction Ramipril Efficacy (AIRE) Study Investigators. *Lancet.* 1993;**2**(342):821–828.

41 Ambrosioni E, Borghi C, Magnani B. The effect of the angiotensin-converting-enzyme inhibitor zofenopril on mortality and morbidity after anterior myocardial infarction. The Survival of Myocardial Infarction Long-Term Evaluation (SMILE) Study Investigators. *N Engl J Med.* 1995;**12**(332):80–85.

42 Kober L, Torp-Pedersen C, Carlsen JE, *et al.* A clinical trial of the angiotensin-converting-enzyme inhibitor trandolapril in patients with left ventricular dysfunction after myocardial infarction. Trandolapril Cardiac Evaluation (TRACE) Study Group. *N Engl J Med.* 1995;**21**(333):1670–1676.

43 Teo KK, Yusuf S, Pfeffer M, *et al.* Effects of long-term treatment with angiotensin-converting-enzyme inhibitors in the presence or absence of aspirin: a systematic review. *Lancet.* 2002;**5**(360):1037–1043.

44 Rutherford JD, Pfeffer MA, Moye LA, *et al.* Effects of captopril on ischemic events after myocardial infarction. Results of the Survival and Ventricular Enlargement trial. SAVE Investigators. *Circulation.* 1994;**90**:1731–1738.

45 Collins R, Peto R, Flather M, *et al.* ISIS-4: a randomised factorial trial assessing early oral captopril, oral mononitrate, and intravenous magnesium sulphate in 58,050 patients with suspected acute myocardial infarction. ISIS-4 (Fourth International Study of Infarct Survival) Collaborative Group. *Lancet.* 1995;**18**(345):669–685.

46 GISSI-3: effects of lisinopril and transdermal glyceryl trinitrate singly and together on 6-week mortality and ventricular function after acute myocardial infarction. Gruppo Italiano per lo Studio della Sopravvivenza nell'infarto Miocardico. *Lancet.* 1994;**7**(343):1115–1122.

47 Chinese Captopril Study. Oral captopril versus placebo among 13,634 patients with suspected acute myocardial infarction: interim report from the Chinese Cardiac Study (CCS-1). *Lancet.* 1995;**18**(345):686–687.

48 Swedberg K, Held P, Kjekshus J, Rasmussen K, Ryden L, Wedel H. Effects of the early administration of enalapril on mortality in patients with acute myocardial infarction. Results of the Cooperative New Scandinavian Enalapril Survival Study II (CONSENSUS II). *N Engl J Med.* 1992;**3**(327):678–684.

49 ACE Inhibitor Myocardial Infarction Collaborative Group. Indications for ACE inhibitors in the early treatment of acute myocardial infarction: systematic overview of individual data from 100,000 patients in randomized trials. *Circulation.* 1998;**9**(97):2202–2212.

50 Antman EM, Anbe DT, Armstrong PW, *et al.* American College of Cardiology; American Heart Association; Canadian Cardiovascular Society. ACC/AHA guidelines for the management of patients with ST-elevation myocardial infarction—executive summary. A report of the American College of Cardiology/American Heart Association Task Force on Practice Guidelines (Writing Committee to revise the 1999 guidelines for the management of patients with acute myocardial infarction). *J Am Coll Cardiol.* 2004;**4**(44):671–719.

51 Faxon DP. Effect of high dose angiotensin-converting enzyme inhibition on restenosis: final results of the MARCATOR Study, a multicenter, double-blind, placebo-controlled trial of cilazapril. The Multicenter American Research Trial With Cilazapril After Angioplasty to Prevent Transluminal Coronary Obstruction and Restenosis (MARCATOR) Study Group. *J Am Coll Cardiol.* 1995;**25**(2):362–369.

52 Kondo J, Sone T, Tsuboi H, *et al.* Effect of quinapril on intimal hyperplasia after coronary stenting as assessed by intravascularultrasound. *Am J Cardiol.* 2001;**15**(87):443–445.

53 Meurice T, Bauters C, Hermant X, *et al.* Effect of ACE inhibitors on angiographic restenosis after coronary stenting (PARIS): a randomised, double-blind, placebo-controlled trial. *Lancet.* 2001;**28**(357):1321–1324.

54 Ribichini F, Wijns W, Ferrero V, *et al.* Effect of angiotensin-converting enzyme inhibition on restenosis after coronary stenting. *Am J Cardiol.* 2003;**15**(91):154–158.

55 Jorgensen E, Kelbaek H, Helqvist S, *et al*. Predictors of coronary in-stent restenosis: importance of angiotensin-converting enzyme gene polymorphism and treatment with angiotensin-converting enzyme inhibitors. *J Am Coll Cardiol*. 2001;1(38):1434–1439.

56 Koch W, Mehilli J, von Beckerath N, Bottiger C, Schomig A, Kastrati A. Angiotensin I-converting enzyme (ACE) inhibitors and restenosis after coronary artery stenting in patients with the DD genotype of the ACE gene. *J Am Coll Cardiol*. 2003;4(41):1957–1961.

57 Guneri S, Baris N, Aytekin D, Akdeniz B, Pekel N, Bozdemir V. The relationship between angiotensin converting enzyme gene polymorphism, coronary artery disease, and stent restenosis: the role of angiotensin converting enzyme inhibitors in stent restenosis in patients with diabetes mellitus. *Int Heart J*. 2005;**46**:889–897.

58 Pfeffer MA, McMurray JJ, Velazquez EJ, *et al*. Valsartan, captopril, or both in myocardial infarction complicated by heart failure, left ventricular dysfunction, or both. *N Engl J Med*. 2003;13(349):1893–1906.

59 Dickstein K, Kjekshus J, OPTIMAAL Steering Committee of the OPTIMAAL Study Group. Effects of losartan and captopril on mortality and morbidity in high-risk patients after acute myocardial infarction: the OPTIMAAL randomised trial. Optimal Trial in Myocardial Infarction with Angiotensin II Antagonist Losartan. *Lancet*. 2002;7(360):752–760.

60 Verma S, Strauss M. Angiotensin receptor blockers and myocardial infarction. *BMJ*. 2004;27(329):1248–1249.

61 Strauss MH, Hall AS. Angiotensin receptor blockers may increase risk of myocardial infarction: unraveling the ARB-MI paradox. *Circulation*. 2006;22(114):838–854.

62 Tsuyuki RT, McDonald MA. Angiotensin receptor blockers do not increase risk of myocardial infarction. *Circulation*. 2006;22(114):855–860.

63 McDonald MA, Simpson SH, Ezekowitz JA, Gyenes G, Tsuyuki RT. Angiotensin receptor blockers and risk of myocardial infarction: systematic review. *BMJ*. 2005;15(331):873.

64 Peters S, Gotting B, Trummel M, Rust H, Brattstrom A. Valsartan for prevention of restenosis after stenting of type B2/C lesions: the VAL-PREST trial. Valsartan for prevention of restenosis after stenting of type B2/C lesions: the VAL-PREST trial. *J Invasive Cardiol*. 2001;13:93–97.

65 Pitt B, Remme W, Zannad F, *et al*. Eplerenone, a selective aldosterone blocker, in patients with left ventricular dysfunction after myocardial infarction. *N Engl J Med*. 2003;3(348):1309–1321.

66 Bunch TJ, Muhlestein JB, Bair TL, *et al*. Effect of beta-blocker therapy on mortality rates and future myocardial infarction rates in patients with coronary artery disease but no history of myocardial infarction or congestive heart failure. *Am J Cardiol*. 2005;1(95):827–831.

67 Gottlieb SO, Weisfeldt ML, Ouyang P, *et al*. Effect of the addition of propranolol to therapy with nifedipine for unstable angina pectoris: a randomized, double-blind, placebo-controlled trial. *Circulation*. 1986;**73**:331–337.

68 Early treatment of unstable angina in the coronary care unit: a randomised, double blind, placebo controlled comparison of recurrent ischaemia in patients treated with nifedipine or metoprolol or both. Report of The Holland Interuniversity Nifedipine/Metoprolol Trial (HINT) Research Group. *Br Heart J*. 1986;**56**: 400–413.

69 Theroux P, Taeymans Y, Morissette D, Bosch X, Pelletier GB, Waters DD. A randomized study comparing propranolol and diltiazem in the treatment of unstable angina. *J Am Coll Cardiol*. 1985;**5**:717–722.

70 Yusuf S, Wittes J, Friedman L. Overview of results of randomized clinical trials in heart disease. I. Treatments following myocardial infarction. *JAMA*. 1988;**14**(260):2088–2093.

71 Roberts R, Rogers WJ, Mueller HS, *et al*. Immediate versus deferred beta-blockade following thrombolytic therapy in patients with acute myocardial infarction. Results of the Thrombolysis in Myocardial Infarction (TIMI) II-B Study. *Circulation*. 1991;**83**:422–437.

72 Halkin A, Grines CL, Cox DA, *et al*. Impact of intravenous beta-blockade before primary angioplasty on survival in patients undergoing mechanical reperfusion therapy for acute myocardial infarction. *J Am Coll Cardiol*. 2004;**19**(43):1780–1787.

73 Faxon DP. Beta-blocker therapy and primary angioplasty: what is the controversy? *J Am Coll Cardiol*. 2004;**19**(43):1788–1790.

74 Harjai KJ, Stone GW, Boura J, *et al*. Effects of prior BB therapy on clinical outcomes after primary coronary angioplasty for acute myocardial infarction. *Am J Cardiol*. 2003;**15**(91):655–660.

75 Kernis SJ, Harjai KJ, Stone GW, *et al*. Does beta-blocker therapy improve clinical outcomes of acute myocardial infarction after successful primary angioplasty? *J Am Coll Cardiol*. 2004;**19**(43):1773–1779.

76 Randomised trial of intravenous atenolol among 16 027 cases of suspected acute myocardial infarction: ISIS-1. First International Study of Infarct Survival Collaborative Group. *Lancet*. 1986;**12**(2):57–66.

77 Hjalmarson A, Herlitz J, Holmberg S, *et al*. Effects on mortality and morbidity in acute myocardial infarction. *Circulation*. 1983;**67**:I26–I32.

78 Yusuf S, Sleight P, Rossi P, *et al*. Reduction in infarct size, arrhythmias and chest pain by early intravenous beta blockade in suspected acute myocardial infarction. *Circulation*. 1983;**67**:I32–I41.

79 Teo KK, Yusuf S, Furberg CD. Effects of prophylactic antiarrhythmic drug therapy in acute myocardial

infarction. An overview of results from randomized controlled trials. *JAMA*. 1993;**6**(270):1589–1595.

80 Chen ZM, Pan HC, Chen YP, *et al*. COMMIT (ClOpidogrel and Metoprolol in Myocardial Infarction Trial) collaborative group. Early intravenous then oral metoprolol in 45,852 patients with acute myocardial infarction: randomised placebo-controlled trial. *Lancet*. 2005;**5**(366):1622–1632.

81 Freemantle N, Cleland J, Young P, Mason J, Harrison J. Beta blockade after myocardial infarction: systematic review and meta regression analysis. *BMJ*. 1999;**26**(318):1730–1737.

82 Pfisterer M, Cox JL, Granger CB, *et al*. Atenolol use and clinical outcomes after thrombolysis for acute myocardial infarction: the GUSTO-I experience. Global Utilization of Streptokinase and TPA (alteplase) for Occluded Coronary Arteries. *J Am Coll Cardiol*. 1998;**32**:634–640.

83 Shivkumar K, Schultz L, Goldstein S, Gheorghiade M. Effects of propanolol in patients entered in the Beta-Blocker Heart Attack Trial with their first myocardial infarction and persistent electrocardiographic ST-segment depression. *Am Heart J*. 1998;**135**:261–267.

84 Emery M, Lopez-Sendon J, Steg PG, *et al*. Patterns of use and potential impact of early beta-blocker therapy in non-ST-elevation myocardial infarction with and without heart failure: the Global Registry of Acute Coronary Events. *Am Heart J*. 2006;**152**:1015–1021.

85 Silvet H, Spencer F, Yarzebski J, Lessard D, Gore JM, Goldberg RJ. Communitywide trends in the use and outcomes associated with beta-blockers in patients with acute myocardial infarction: the Worcester Heart Attack Study. *Arch Intern Med*. 2003;**13**(163):2175–2183.

86 Chan AW, Quinn MJ, Bhatt DL, *et al*. Mortality benefit of beta-blockade after successful elective percutaneous coronary intervention. *J Am Coll Cardiol*. 2002;**21**(40):669–675.

87 Jackson JD, Muhlestein JB, Bunch TJ, *et al*. Beta-blockers reduce the incidence of clinical restenosis: prospective study of 4840 patients undergoing percutaneous coronary revascularization. *Am Heart J*. 2003;**145**:875–881.

CHAPTER 13

Primary percutaneous coronary intervention for ST elevation myocardial infarction: Summary of optimal anticoagulation, glycoprotein IIb/IIIa platelet inhibitors, and other antiplatelet therapies

Bruce R. Brodie

LeBauer Cardiovascular Research Foundation, Greensboro, NC, USA

Primary angioplasty was introduced as an alternative reperfusion strategy for acute ST elevation myocardial infarction (STEMI) in the early 1980s and had potential advantages over fibrinolytic therapy in achieving greater rates of reperfusion with less bleeding. Following the publication of Keeley and Grines' meta-analysis of 22 randomized trials comparing primary percutaneous coronary intervention (PCI) with fibrinolytic therapy showing reduced mortality and reinfarction with less intracranial hemorrhage, primary PCI has become the preferred reperfusion strategy when it can be performed promptly by experienced personnel (1).

Since the early 1980s, adjunctive anticoagulant therapy and antiplatelet therapy with primary PCI have undergone considerable evolution. Initially, aspirin and unfractionated heparin were standard

treatment with primary PCI just as they were for fibrinolytic therapy. In the 1990s, platelet GP IIb/IIIa inhibitors were introduced as adjunctive therapy for elective PCI and were shown to be effective with primary PCI for STEMI, although the combination of unfractionated heparin and IIb/IIIa inhibitors was associated with a high frequency of bleeding (2–6). In the late 1990s, the thienopyridines, ticlopidine, and then clopidogrel were introduced as adjunctive antiplatelet therapy for PCI in addition to aspirin, and clopidogrel is now commonly used with primary PCI for STEMI. Bivalirudin, a direct thrombin inhibitor, has recently been shown to have some advantages over unfractionated heparin plus GP IIb/IIIa platelet inhibitors in the HORIZONS (Harmonizing Outcomes with RevascularIZatiON and Stents in Acute Myocardial Infarction) trial and could become standard care with primary PCI for STEMI (7). There are a host of new anticoagulant and antiplatelet therapies under investigation that could improve adjunctive pharmacologic therapy with primary PCI for STEMI in the future.

Pharmacology in the Catheterization Laboratory. Edited by Ron Waksman and Andrew E Ajani. © 2010 Blackwell Publishing, ISBN: 978-1-4051-5704-9.

Platelet inhibitors

Aspirin

Aspirin has been shown to provide survival benefit in early fibrinolytic trials and, based on these data, has been used with primary PCI since its introduction in the early 1980s. Aspirin inhibits platelet activation by reducing thromboxane A2 production. Aspirin has a Class I recommendation in the ACC/AHA guidelines for all patients with STEMI and should be administered 162–325 mg chewed as soon after the onset of symptoms as possible (8,9). Enteric coated aspirin is not recommended acutely because of variability of absorption.

Thienopyridines

The thienopyridines, ticlopidine and clopidogrel, inhibit platelet function by inhibiting the $P2Y_{12}$ receptor. Clopidogrel has been shown to be effective in reducing events in patients undergoing elective PCI with stenting and in patients with acute non-ST elevation acute coronary syndromes (ACS) undergoing PCI and stenting (10,11). Clopidogrel has also been shown in PCI-CLARITY (Clopidogrel as Adjunctive Reperfusion Therapy) to be effective in reducing the composite endpoint of death, reinfarction, and stroke with no increase in bleeding in patients with STEMI treated initially with fibrinolytic therapy followed by subsequent PCI (12). Dangas and colleagues recently reported from the HORIZONS Trial that a loading dose of 600 mg (which gives more rapid onset of platelet inhibition) vs 300 mg of clopidogrel before primary PCI was associated with lower 30-day MACE with no increased bleeding (13). Clopidogrel has not been studied in randomized comparisons with placebo with primary PCI for STEMI, but based on the above data has gained widespread use in this setting. Clopidogrel is generally given as soon as possible after the onset of STEMI and before angiography to maximize its benefit, since the chance of needing emergency bypass surgery in patients targeted for primary PCI is small.

Prasugrel is a novel thienopyridine that also inhibits platelet function by inhibiting the $P2Y_{12}$ receptor and provides much more rapid and complete platelet inhibition compared with clopidogrel. Prasugrel 60 mg was recently compared with clopidogrel 300 mg in patients with acute coronary syndromes including patients with STEMI in the TRITON-TIMI 38 (Trial to Assess Improvement in Therapeutic Outcomes by Optimizing Platelet Inhibition with Prasugrel) trial (14). Prasugrel resulted in a significant 19% reduction in death, myocardial infarction, or stroke at approximately 1 year but with an increased risk of major bleeding. In patients who were treated with stents, prasugrel resulted in a similar 19% reduction in death, myocardial infarction, or stroke and also resulted in a major 52% reduction in stent thrombosis (15). In a pre-specified subgroup of patients with STEMI targeted for primary PCI in the TRITON-TIMI 38 trial, prasugrel compared with 300 mg clopidogrel given prior to and following primary PCI was associated with a significant reduction in the primary endpoint at 15 months (cardiovascular death, myocardial infarction, or stroke) (HR 0.79 [0.65–0.97], $p = 0.022$) with no excess bleeding risk (15). As of this writing, prasugrel is awaiting Food and Drug Administration (FDA) approval for use in the United States.

Glycoprotein IIb/IIIa platelet inhibitors

There have been five large randomized trials evaluating abciximab with unfractionated heparin as adjunctive therapy with primary PCI for STEMI (Table 13.1) (2–6). All five trials have shown improved efficacy with abciximab with a reduction in major adverse cardiac events (MACE) driven primarily by a reduction in urgent target vessel revascularization (TVR). A meta-analysis of these five trials plus three smaller trials by De Luca and colleagues with a total of 3,949 patients treated with primary PCI found that abciximab reduced 30-day and 6- to 12-month mortality (2.4% vs 3.4%, OR 0.68 [0.47–0.99], $p = 0.047$ and 4.4% vs 6.2%, OR 0.69 [0.52–0.92], $p = 0.01$) and reduced 30-day reinfarction rates (1.0% vs 1.9%, OR 0.56 [0.22–0.94], $p = 0.03$) with no difference in bleeding (4.7% vs 4.1%, $p = 0.36$) (16). Based on these data, abciximab with unfractionated heparin has become standard adjunctive therapy with primary PCI for STEMI, and GP IIb/IIIa inhibitors are currently used in the great majority of patients treated with primary PCI. However, some of the trials were done before the use of stents and the widespread use of thienopyridines. The largest trial, CADILLAC, which had a 2 × 2 randomization

Table 13.1 Randomized trials comparing 30 day outcomes with abciximab vs placebo in STEMI treated with primary PCI.

	Abciximab (%)	Placebo (%)	p value
RAPPORT (2)	(n = 241)	(n = 242)	
Death	2.5	2.1	NS
Reinfarction	3.3	4.1	NS
Urgent TVR	1.7	6.6	0.006
Composite	5.8	11.2	0.03
ADMIRAL (3)	(n = 149)	(n = 151)	
Death	3.4	6.6	NS
Reinfarction	1.3	2.6	NS
Urgent TVR	1.3	6.6	0.02
Composite	6.0	14.6	0.01
ISAR-2 (4)	(n = 201)	(n = 200)	
Death	2.5	4.5	NS
Reinfarction	0.5	1.5	NS
Urgent TVR	3.0	5.0	NS
Composite	5.0	10.5	0.04
CADILLAC (5)	(n = 1,052)	(n = 1,030)	
Death	1.9	2.2	NS
Reinfarction	0.8	0.9	NS
Urgent TVR	2.5	4.4	0.02
Stroke	0.1	0.2	NS
Composite	4.6	7.0	0.01
ACE (6)	(n = 200)	(n = 200)	
Death	3.5	4.0	NS
Reinfarction	0.5	4.5	0.01
Urgent TVR	0.5	1.5	NS
Stroke	0.0	0.5	NS
Composite	4.5	10.5	0.02

Patients in the ADMIRAL, ISAR-2, and ACE Trials were treated with primary stenting. Half of CADILLAC patients were treated with stents.

Abbreviation: TVR, target vessel revascularization.

to abciximab vs placebo and stenting vs PTCA, found that abciximab reduced MACE in patients treated with PTCA but not in patients treated with stenting, although it did reduce the frequency of stent thrombosis (5). Consequently, there has no universal agreement about the importance of abciximab with primary PCI in the era of clopidogrel and stenting. The 2004 ACC/AHA guidelines for treatment of STEMI states that the use of abciximab with primary PCI for STEMI is reasonable (Class IIa indication) (8). This has not been changed in the recent 2007 update that antedated the HORIZONS (Harmonizing Outcomes with RevascularIZatiON and Stents in Acute Myocardial Infarction) trial results described below (9).

Eptifibatide and tirofiban have not been well studied with primary PCI for STEMI. There are data from small randomized trials and observational data from registries and randomized trials, suggesting similar outcomes with eptibibatide compared with abciximab (17,18). Eptibibatide has advantages of lower costs and shorter half-life, but it cannot be reversed with platelet transfusions and is not recommended in patients with severe renal insufficiency. Abciximab has a long half-life but can be reversed with platelet transfusions and is preferred in patients with severe renal insufficiency.

Other new platelet inhibitors

Cangrelor is a direct reversible anatagonist of the platelet $P2Y_{12}$ receptor (not a thienopyridine) that is currently under clinical investigation in the CHAMPION (Cangrelor vs standard tHerapy to Achieve optimal Management of Platelet InhibitiON) trial in patients with acute coronary syndromes (including STEMI) undergoing PCI (19). Given intravenously, it has a rapid onset of action, reaching steady state within 5 min of bolus injection, and rapid resolution of platelet inhibition within 60 min of discontinuation of the infusion. The rapid onset of action provides a real advantage in STEMI patients who usually can be treated only very shortly before intervention, and the very short half-life can minimize the risk of bleeding in situations requiring emergency bypass surgery. Unfortunately, the CHAMPION Trial was recently stopped due to lack of efficacy. Further analysis will be needed.

AZD 6140 is a oral reversible antagonist of the platelet $P2Y_{12}$ receptor (also not a thienopyridine) that provides rapid reversible platelet inhibition (19). AZD 6140 has potential advantages over clopidogrel in its rapid onset of action (does not require metabolic activation and achieves maximum platelet inhibition within 2 h), higher degree of platelet inhibition with less interpatient variability, and more rapid resolution of platelet inhibition (half-life of 12 h). In the phase II DISPERSE-2 (Dose Confirmation Study Assessing anti-Platelet Effects of AZD6140 vs Clopidogrel in NSTEMI) trial AZD 6140 showed a reduction in myocardial infarction with similar bleeding compared with clopidogrel (20). AZD 6140 (ticagrelor) is currently being studied in patients with acute coronary syndromes (including STEMI) in the PLATO (A Study of PLATelet Inhibition and Patient Outcomes) trial. Preliminary results suggest an efficacy benefit of ticagrelor over clopidogrel. The results will be presented at the European Society of Cardiology in August 2009.

Anticoagulants

Unfractionated heparin

Unfractionated heparin (UFH) has been the standard anticoagulant for all PCI, including primary PCI, since PCI was first performed. UFH has the advantage of familiarity, ease of monitoring in the catheterization laboratory with activated clotting times (ACT), the ability to be reversed with protamine, and relative safety in patients with renal insufficiency. UFH is a relatively nonselective anticoagulant, which inhibits factor Xa and thrombin and enhances activity of antithrombin III. UFH has several limitations, which include a variable dose response, potential to activate platelets, inability to act on clot bound thrombin, the risk of heparin-induced thrombocytopenia, and a relatively high incidence of bleeding complications. While UFH has been the standard anticoagulant for primary PCI, newer anticoagulants with potential advantages over UFH are finding increased use.

Low-molecular-weight heparin

Low-molecular-weight heparin (LMWH) inhibits factor Xa primarily and to a lesser extent thrombin and has advantages over UFH in that it has a more predictable effect, does not require monitoring, does not activate platelets, and has a lower frequency of heparin-induced thrombocytopenia (21). LMWH has been shown to have better efficacy than UFH when used with fibrinolysis for STEMI in the ExTRACT trial with less death and reinfarction at the expense of slightly more bleeding (22). It has not been well studied with primary PCI for STEMI, but a substudy of the FINESSE trial suggested that LMWH may be superior to UFH with primary PCI (23). The FINESSE trial randomized STEMI patients to primary PCI or facilitated PCI (abciximab or abciximab plus half dose reteplase) and found no clinical benefit with facilitated

PCI (24). Centers were prespecified to use either LMWH or UFH. Adjusted outcomes were significantly better with LMWH with less major bleeding, lower 30-day MACE, and lower 90-day mortality, and the findings were similar with both primary PCI and facilitated PCI (23). These results are very encouraging and further studies are planned.

Fondiparinux

Fondiparinux is a selective Xa inhibitor that was evaluated in patients with STEMI in the OASIS-6 Trial (Organization for the Assessment of Strategies for Ischemic Syndromes). Fondiparinux was associated with a reduction is death and reinfarction in patients treated with fibrinolytic therapy with no increased bleeding (25). However, there were mild trends toward worse outcomes with fondiparinux in patients treated with primary PCI and there was a significant increase in angiographic thrombus, no reflow, and guiding catheter thrombosis. These procedural complications appeared not to occur when UFH was added to fondiparinux for the PCI procedure. Based on these data, fondiparinux is not recommended for use with primary PCI.

Bivalirudin

Bivalirudin is a synthetic direct thrombin inhibitor that has potential advantages over UFH in that it has more predictable pharmokinetics, is not inhibited by plasma proteins, does not activate platelets, and is not associated with thrombocytopenia. Bivalirudin has been studied and compared with UFH plus platelet GP IIb/IIIa inhibitors with elective PCI in the REPLACE-2 Trial (Randomized Evaluation in PCI Linking Angiomax to Reduced Clinical Events) and with PCI for non-ST segment elevation acute coronary syndromes in the ACUITY Trial (Acute Catheterization and Urgent Intervention Triage Strategy) (26,27). In both REPLACE-2 and ACUITY, bivalirudin resulted in similar efficacy (MACE) with less bleeding, and in ACUITY, the composite end point of MACE or major bleeding was significantly less with bivalirudin (Table 13.2). The HORIZONS trial, which was recently published, evaluated bivalirudin in patients with STEMI treated with primary PCI (7). Bivalirudin, compared with UFH plus platelet GP IIb/IIIa inhibitors, resulted in similar 30-day MACE, less major bleeding, and a lower incidence of net adverse clinical events (MACE or major bleeding) (Figure 13.1, Table 13.2). Furthermore, 30-day mortality was significantly less with biva-lirudin (2.1% vs 3.1%, $p = 0.047$). And there was less thrombocytopenia (<50,000 cells/mm³) (0.5% vs 1.1%, $p = 0.02$). The frequency of stent thrombosis

in the first 24 h after PCI was greater in the biva-lirudin group (1.3% vs 0.3%, $p < 0.001$), although there was some catch-up from 24 h to 30 days such that at 30 days there were no significant differences between groups (2.5% vs 1.9%, $p = 0.30$).

HORIZONS is the first trial to show a significant reduction in mortality with any adjunctive therapy used with primary PCI for STEMI. Although mor-tality was not a primary end point and the trial was not powered to detect differences in mortality, there is physiological basis for the mortality reduction. Major bleeding in patients with acute coronary syndromes treated with PCI has been shown to be a strong predictor of subsequent stent thrombosis, other ischemic events, and death (28). Major bleed-ing was the strongest predictor of 30-day mortality in patients with acute coronary syndromes treated with an invasive strategy in the ACUITY Trial— stronger than periprocedural myocardial infarction (Figure 13.2) (28). Major bleeding can contribute to mortality due to mortality from the bleeding event itself, the need for transfusions, which carries an inherent risk, and the need for discontinuation of antiplatelet and anticoagulant therapy, which may predispose to stent thrombosis and other ischemic events. Thrombocytopenia is also associated with worse outcomes, and the reduction in thrombo-cytopenia with bivalirudin may also contribute to lower mortality.

Table 13.2 Randomized trials comparing 30 day outcomes with bivalirudin vs heparin + GP IIb/IIIa platelet inhibitors with PCI.

	Bivalirudin (%)	Heparin + IIb/IIIa (%)	p value
Replace-2 (26)	(n = 2,994)	(n = 3,008)	
Death	0.2	0.4	0.26
Myocardial infarction	7.0	6.2	0.23
Urgent TVR	1.2	1.4	0.44
MACE	7.6	7.1	0.40
Major bleeding	2.1	4.1	<0.001
NACE	9.2	10.0	0.32
Acuity (27)	(n = 4,612)	(n = 4,603)	
Death	1.6	1.3	0.31
Myocardial infarction	5.4	4.9	0.33
Urgent TVR	2.4	2.3	0.74
MACE	7.8	7.3	0.32
Major bleeding	3.0	5.7	<0.001
NACE	10.1	11.7	0.015
Horizons (7)	n = 1,800)	(n = 1,802)	
Death	2.1	3.1	0.047
Reinfarction	1.8	1.8	0.90
Ischemic TVR	2.6	1.9	0.18
Stroke	0.7	0.6	0.68
MACE	5.4	5.5	0.95
Major bleeding	4.9	8.3	<0.001
NACE	9.2	12.1	0.005

Abbreviations: TVR, target vessel revascularization; MACE, major adverse cardiac events; NACE, net adverse clinical events (MACE or major bleeding).

Current optimum antithrombotic therapy with primary PCI

The most recent ACC/AHA guidelines for man-agement of patients with STEMI were published in 2004 with a focused update in 2007 and include guidelines for antithrombotic therapy with primary

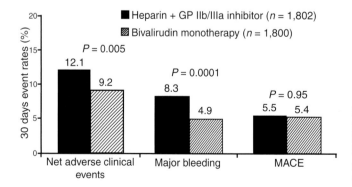

Figure 13.1 Outcomes (30-day) in patients with STEMI treated with primary PCI from the HORIZONS trial comparing bivalirudin with unfractionated heparin plus GP IIb/IIIa platelet inhibitors. (*Source*: Adapted from Stone *et al.* (7).)

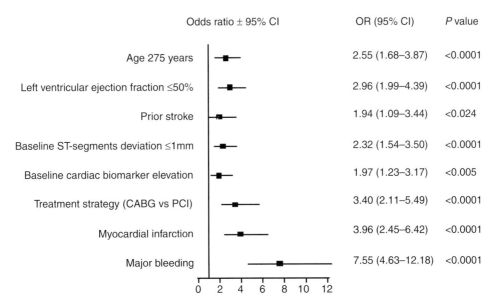

	Odds ratio ± 95% CI	OR (95% CI)	P value
Age 275 years		2.55 (1.68–3.87)	<0.0001
Left ventricular ejection fraction ≤50%		2.96 (1.99–4.39)	<0.0001
Prior stroke		1.94 (1.09–3.44)	<0.024
Baseline ST-segments deviation ≤1mm		2.32 (1.54–3.50)	<0.0001
Baseline cardiac biomarker elevation		1.97 (1.23–3.17)	<0.005
Treatment strategy (CABG vs PCI)		3.40 (2.11–5.49)	<0.0001
Myocardial infarction		3.96 (2.45–6.42)	<0.0001
Major bleeding		7.55 (4.63–12.18)	<0.0001

Figure 13.2 Independent predictors of 30-day mortality in patients with high-risk non-ST elevation acute coronary syndromes treated with bivalirudin or unfractionated heparin plus GP IIb/IIIa inhibitors from the ACUITY Trial. (*Source*: Reproduced from Manoukian *et al.* (28) with permission from Elsevier.)

PCI (8,9). These guidelines include aspirin 324 mg chewable as soon as possible after the onset of STEMI (Class I), unfractionated heparin, LMWH, or bivalirudin (Class I, 2007 update), and platelet GP IIb/IIIa inhibitors either up-front or immediately before PCI (abciximab Class IIa, eptifibatide, and tirofiban Class IIb, 2004). No guidelines are given for clopidogrel with primary PCI.

Recent data now support the use of clopidogrel 600 mg as soon as possible after the onset of STEMI in patients targeted for primary PCI. Clopidogrel has shown clear benefit in patients with non-ST elevation acute coronary syndromes treated with PCI and in patients with STEMI treated with fibrinolytic therapy, and clopidogrel 600 mg has been shown to result in better outcomes than 300 mg in patients treated with primary PCI in the HORIZONS trial (11–13).

Results with bivalirudin from HORIZONS Trial in STEMI, complemented by previous data with bivalirudin in patients with non-ST elevation acute coronary syndromes in the ACUITY trial support the use of bivalirudin (rather than UFH and GP IIb/IIIa inhibitors) in the majority of patients with acute coronary syndromes. Exceptions would be patients with very large thrombus burden, including patients with stent thrombosis, and

patients with refractory no-flow, who were either excluded from HORIZONS or were permitted bail-out IIb/IIIa use. Patients who receive UFH bolus can be transitioned to bivalirudin 30 min after heparin bolus. One concern with bivalirudin is the increased incidence of early (<24 h) stent thrombosis in the HORIZONS trial in the bivalirudin arm. New strategies to achieve more rapid platelet inhibition than is achieved with clopidogrel, perhaps with prasugrel or cangrelor, may help with this problem.

To summarize, current data support the following adjunctive antithrombotic therapy with primary PCI for STEMI:

1 Chewable aspirin 325 mg as soon as possible after the onset of STEMI.

2 Clopidogrel 600 mg as soon as possible after the onset of STEMI.

3 Bivalirudin 0.75 mg/kg IV bolus followed by an infusion of 0.25 mg/kg/h with the use of GP IIb/IIIa platelet inhibitors for large thrombus burden or refractory no reflow.

Bivalirudin can generally be discontinued at the end of the PCI procedure. Aspirin should be continued indefinitely and clopidogrel 75 mg/day should be continued for at least 1 year. As described above, there are a number of new anticoagulants and antiplatelet therapies under investigation, and the paradigm for adjunctive antithrombotic therapy with primary PCI continues to evolve rapidly.

References

1 Keeley EC, Boura JA, Grines CL. Primary angioplasty vs. intravenous thrombolytic therapy for acute myocardial infarction, a quantitative review of 23 randomized trials. *Lancet.* 2003;**361**:13–20.

2 Brener SJ, Barr LA, Burchenal JEB, *et al.* Randomized placebo-controlled trial of platelet glycoprotein IIb/IIIa blockade with primary angioplasty for acute myocardial infarction. *Circulation.* 1998;**98**:734–741.

3 Montalescot G, Barragan P, Wittenberg O, *et al.* Platelet glycoprotein IIb/IIIa inhibition with coronary stenting for acute myocardial infarction. *N Engl J Med.* 2001;**344**:1895–1903.

4 Neumann FJ, Kastrati A. Schmitt C, *et al.* Effect of glycoprotein IIb/IIIa receptor blockage with abciximab on clinical and angiographic restenosis rate after the placement of coronary stents following acute myocardial infraction. *J AM Coll Cardiol.* 2000;**35**:915–921.

5 Stone, GW, Grines CL, Cox DA, *et al.* Comparison of angioplasty with stenting with or without abciximab, in acute myocardial infarction. *N Engl J Med.* 2002;**346**:957–966.

6 Antoinucci D, Rodriquez A, Hempel A, *et al.* A randomized trial comparing primary infarct artery stenting with or without abciximab in acute myocardial infarction. *J Am Coll Cardiol.* 2003;**42**:1875–1879.

7 Stone GW, Witzenbichler B, Guagliumi G, *et al.* Bivalirudin during primary PCI in acute myocardial infarction. *N Engl J Med.* 2008;**358**:2218–2230.

8 Antman EM, Anbe DT, Armstrong PW, *et al.* ACC/AHA guidelines for the management of patients with ST-elevation myocardial infarction. *J Am Coll Cardiol.* 2004;**44**:671–719.

9 Antman EM, Hand M, Armstrong PW, *et al.* 2007 focused update of the ACC/AHA 2004 guidelines for the management of patients with ST-elevation myocardial infarction. *J Am Coll Cardiol.* 2008;**51**:210–247.

10 Steinhubl SR, Berger PB, Mann JT for the CREDO Investigators. Early and sustained dual oral antiplatelet therapy following percutaneous coronary intervention. A randomized controlled trial. *JAMA.* 2002; **288**:2411–2420.

11 Mehta SR, Usuf S, Peters RJ, *et al.* Effects pretreatment with clopidogrel and aspirin followed by long-term therapy in patients undergoing percutaneous coronary intervention: the PCI-CURE study. *Lancet.* 2001;**358**: 527–533.

12 Sabatine MS, Cannon CP, Gibson CM, *et al.* Effects of Clopidogrel pretreatment before percutaneous coronary intervention in patients with ST-elevation myocardial infarction treated with fibrinolytics. The PCI-CLARITY Study. *JAMA.* 2005;**294**:1224–1232.

13 Dangas G, Mehran R, Aoki J, *et al.* Loading with 600 mg versus 300 mg of clopidogrel in patients undergoing primary angioplasty for ST-segment elevation myocardial infarction: results from the HORIZONS-AMI Trial. *J Amer Coll Cardiol.* 2009 (in press).

14 Wiviott SD, Braunwald E, McCabe CH, *et al.* Prasugrel versus clopidogrel in patients with acute coronary syndromes. *N Engl J Med.* 2007;**357**:2001–2015.

15 Montalescot G, Wiviott SD, Braunwald E, *et al.* Prasugrel compared with clopidogrel in patients undergoing percutaneous coronary intervention for ST-elevation myocardial infarction (TRITON-TIMI 38): double-blind randomized controlled trial. *Lancet* 2009;373:723–31.

16 De Luca G, Suryapranata H, Stone GW, *et al.* Abciximab as adjunctive therapy to reperfusion in acute ST-segment elevation myocardial infarction. A meta-analysis of randomized trials. *JAMA.* 2005;**293**:1759–1767.

17 Srinivas VS, Skeif B, Negassa A, Bang JY, Shaqra H, Monrad S. Effectiveness of glycoprotein IIb/IIa inhibitor use during primary coronary angioplasty: Results of propensity analysis using the New York State percutaneous coronary intervention reporting system. *Am J Cardiol.* 2007;**99**:482–485.

18 Gurm HS, Smith DE, Collins JS, *et al.* The relative safety and efficacy of abciximab and eptifibatide in patients undergoing primary percutaneous coronary intervention. Insights from a large regional registry of contemporary percutaneous coronary intervention. *J Am Coll Cardiol.* 2008;**51**:529–535.

19 Kereiakes DJ, Gurbel PA. Peri-procedural platelet function and platelet inhibition in percutaneous coronary intervention. *J Am Coll Cardiol Interv.* 2008; **1**:111–121.

20 Cannon CP, Husted S, Harrington RA, *et al.* Safety, tolerability and initial efficacy of AZD6140, the first reversible oral adenosine diphosphate receptor antagonist, compared with clopidogrel, in patients with non-ST segment elevation acute coronary syndrome—primary results of the DESPERSE 2 trial. *J Am Coll Cardiol.* 2007;**50**:1844–1851.

21 Samana MM, Gerotziafes GT. C omparative pharmacokinetics of LMWHs. *Semin Thromb Hemost.* 2000;**26** (Suppl 1):31–38.

22 Gibson CM, Murphy SA, Montalescot G, *et al.* Percutaneous coronary intervention in patients receiving enoxaparin or unfractionated heparin after fibrinolytic therapy for ST-segment elevation myocardial infarction in the ExTRACT-TIMI 25 trial. *J Am Coll Cardiol.* 2007;**49**:2247–2248.

23 Montalescot G, Ellis SG, deBelder MA, *et al.* Enoxaparin in primary percutaneous coronary intervention: A formal

prospectdive substudy of the FINESSE Trial. Presented at Transcatheter Therapeutics, Washington, DC, 2007.

24 Ellis S, Tendera M, de Belder MA, *et al.* Facilitated PCI in patients with ST-elevation myocardial infarction. *N Engl J Med.* 2008;**358**:2205–2217.

25 Yusuf S, Mehta SR, Chrolavicius S, *et al.* Effects of fondaparinux on mortality and reinfarction in patients with acute ST-segment elevation myocardial infarction. The OASIS-6 Randomized Trial. *JAMA.* 2006;**295**:1519–1530.

26 Lincoff AM, Bittl JA, Harrington RA, *et al.* Bivalirudin and provisional glycoprotein IIb/IIIa blockade compared with heparin and planned glycoprotein IIb/IIIa blockade during percutaneous coronary intervention: REPLACE-2 randomized trial. *JAMA.* 2003;**289**:853–863.

27 Stone GW, McLaurin BT, Cox DA, *et al.* Bivalirudin for patients with acute coronary syndromes. *N Engl J Med.* 2006;**355**:2203–2216.

28 Manoukian SV, Feit F, Mehran R, *et al.* Impact of major bleeding on 30-day mortality and clinical outcomes in patients with acute coronary syndromes. An analysis from the ACUITY Trial. *J Am Coll Cardiol.* 2007;**49**:1362–1368.

CHAPTER 14

Rescue percutaneous coronary intervention

Damian J. Kelly & Anthony H. Gershlick
University Hospitals of Leicester, Leicester, UK

Evidence for rescue PCI

Contemporary management of acute ST-segment myocardial infarction (STEMI) aims to rapidly restore normal epicardial coronary flow in an attempt to limit infarct size and improve survival (1) While primary PCI for acute myocardial infarction is highly effective, fibrinolytic therapy remains the commonest reperfusion treatment worldwide with limited access to primary PCI in many regions. However, even with contemporary fibrinolytic agents, 30–50% of patients fail to achieve patency of the infarct-related artery at 90 min after the onset of lytic therapy (2). This group have been shown to have a poor prognosis compared to those patients treated successfully by fibrinolysis (3).

Meta-analysis of recent trials examining the role of "rescue" percutaneous coronary intervention (R-PCI) after failed fibrinolysis has demonstrated a mortality benefit in favor of R-PCI compared to conservative treatment (4,5). Collet and colleagues found a significant reduction in the combined end point of death or reinfarction in favor of rescue PCI (10.8% vs 16.8%; OR, 0.60; $p = 0.019$). There was an increase in nonfatal bleeding, mostly related to femoral artery sheaths and easily managed. Net benefit was largely driven by the Rescue Angioplasty

Pharmacology in the Catheterization Laboratory. Edited by Ron Waksman and Andrew E Ajani. © 2010 Blackwell Publishing, ISBN: 978-1-4051-5704-9.

vs Conservative Treatment or Repeat Thrombolysis (REACT) trial (6). This trial demonstrated that repeat fibrinolysis does not reduce mortality and should be considered inappropriate in most cases (Figure 14.1). Conversely the early benefits of R-PCI appear to persist during follow-up over a mean of 4.4 years (7). Current guidelines support the use of R-PCI following failed lytic therapy and in patients with STEMI who present with or develop cardiogenic shock (1). Unlike immediate R-PCI, delayed PCI to open an occluded coronary artery following myocardial infarction does not appear to be superior to conservative treatment if the patient remains asymptomatic (8).

R-PCI poses unique management challenges, quite distinct from primary PCI for STEMI. Antiplatelet and anticoagulant drugs are vital to ensure a successful outcome, but risk of bleeding is increased following administration of fibrinolytics.

Reasons for failure of initial fibrinolytic therapy

There are several theoretical reasons why repeated attempts at fibrinolysis might not restore vessel patency or improve outcomes. A stable "white-thrombus head" rapidly forms at the site of occlusion as activated platelets become enmeshed in cross-linked fibrin. Erythrocyte-rich thrombus predominates further downstream (9). Initial fibrinolysis often fails in the face of a large thrombus

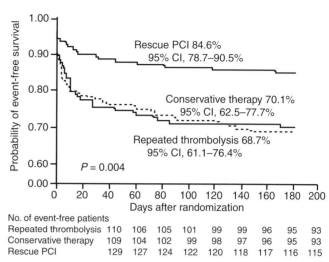

Figure 14.1 Kaplan–Meier estimates of the cumulative rate of the composite primary end point (death, recurrent myocardial infraction, severe heart failure, or cerebrovascular event) within 6 months. PCI, percutaneous coronary intervention; CI, confidence interval. (*Source*: Reproduced with permission from Gershlick *et al.* (6). Copyright © 2005 Massachusetts Medical Society. All rights reserved.)

No. of event-free patients									
Repeated thrombolysis	110	106	105	101	99	99	96	95	93
Conservative therapy	109	104	102	99	98	97	96	95	93
Rescue PCI		129	127	124	122	120	118	117	116	115

burden, or occlusive plaque. A "stump" occlusion may impair thrombolysis if there are no patent side-branches to allow distal perfusion of lytic. Coronary hypoperfusion, as occurs in the setting of cardiogenic shock, greatly reduces thrombolytic efficiency.

Thrombosis involves a balance between local thrombosis and endogenous fibrinolysis. Late administration of lytic (>4 h after symptom onset) substantially reduces the likelihood of reperfusion (10). Platelet-derived inhibitors of fibrinolysis such as platelet activator inhibitor 1 and thrombin activatable fibrinolysis inhibitor may be important where local levels of lytic within the thrombus are suboptimal (11). Observational data suggests that resistant fibrin structure may be promoted by high local thrombin levels and be associated with premature coronary artery disease and hyperhomocysteinemia (12).

Reasons for failure of repeated fibrinolysis

Following initial lytic failure, "white" platelet-rich thrombus predominates within the infarct-related coronary artery. White thrombi have been shown to be more resistant to lysis with tissue plasminogen activator (tPA) than erythrocyte-rich clots in a rabbit model of STEMI (13). Initial fibrinolysis may be paradoxically self-defeating by releasing trapped thrombin and enhancing platelet activation, while depleting endogenous fibrinogen stores and reducing the likelihood of further attempts at pharmacological thrombolysis being successful (14).

Clinical evidence for antiplatelet therapy in rescue PCI

Platelet inhibition helps tip the balance in favor of endogenous fibrinolysis and maintain arterial patency following rescue PCI. Sustained platelet activation is required to maintain thrombus integrity: thrombus stability appears to be dependant on continuous activation of the platelet GP IIb-IIIa receptor mediated by constant stimulation of the platelet $P2Y_1$ and $P2Y_{12}$ (adenosine diphosphate, ADP) receptors (15). Clopidogrel inhibits the platelet ADP receptor and acts synergistically with aspirin.

There is no efficacy data for clopidogrel specific to rescue PCI. However there is recent evidence for clopidogrel use as an adjunct to thrombolytic therapy for STEMI: the CLARITY-TIMI 28 trial demonstrated that addition of clopidogrel (at the licensed loading dose of 300 mg then 75 mg daily) to aspirin improved coronary artery patency rates following lytic therapy, with no significant increase in bleeding (16).

The optimal dose and duration of clopidogrel prior to rescue PCI is currently unknown. Laboratory tests of platelet aggregation suggest that maximal clopidogrel-induced platelet inhibition occurs around 2 h following a 600 mg loading dose (17). Studies in ACS patients have shown no excess of bleeding with 600 vs 300 mg, although there is no safety data following fibrinolysis (18). A 600 mg loading dose may be justified in patients at low risk of bleeding where clopidogrel was not given at the time of fibrinolysis and where R-PCI is imminent.

Clopidogrel should be given as early as possible before R-PCI. In the CREDO trial, there was an inverse relationship between adverse ischemic events and the duration of clopidogrel pretreatment prior to elective PCI, with benefit becoming significant only after 15 h of pretreatment (19). Similarly, pretreatment post-MI with clopidogrel for 2–8 days conferred a highly significant benefit in terms of reduction of ischemic complications in the PCI-CLARITY study (20). Patients diagnosed with failed fibrinolysis should receive clopidogrel prior to transfer to the PCI center.

Glycoprotein IIb-IIIa inhibitors

The "final common pathway" of platelet aggregation involves bridging of adjacent platelets by ligation of fibrinogen via the platelet GP IIb-IIIa receptor. Three inhibitors of the GP IIb-IIIa receptor are currently licensed in North America and Europe, namely abciximab, eptifibatide, and tirofiban. Of these, abciximab has the greatest body of evidence supporting its use during primary PCI for STEMI.

GP IIb-IIIa receptor inhibition may negate the antifibrinolytic effects of platelet activation and facilitate endogenous fibrinolysis (21). There is evidence from one study that abciximab use during primary PCI improves distal coronary flow velocity, an index of microvascular perfusion, and may help preserve ventricular function (22). Abciximab has been shown to attenuate capillary plugging by interfering with integrin receptors that mediate adherence of granulocytes to the injured vessel wall (23). Efforts to improve microvascular perfusion may be clinically relevant where a large thrombus burden is visible at angiography (24).

Clinical evidence for GP IIb-IIIa inhibitors during R-PCI

Unfortunately, there is limited data on GP IIb-IIIa inhibitor use in rescue PCI. We recommend GP IIb-IIIa inhibitor use during R-PCI in selected patients after careful assessment of each individual patient's bleeding risk.

Retrospective analysis of the Global Use of Strategies To Open occluded coronary arteries (GUSTO-III) trial demonstrated a significant reduction in ischemic events in 83 patients undergoing rescue PCI for failed fibrinolysis who received abciximab as adjunctive therapy in comparison to 309 patients undergoing rescue PCI who did not (3.6% vs 9.7%, $p = 0.042$ after correction for baseline characteristics). There was a trend toward increased severe bleeding, defined as bleeds causing hemodynamic compromise, in the abciximab group (3.6–1.0%, $p = 0.08$) with no reported intracranial hemorrhage (25). These groups were not, however, matched and follow-up was limited to 30 days.

The only prospective randomized trial to date, by Petronio and colleagues, focused on clinical outcomes following R-PCI. Eighty-nine patients were randomized to either abciximab (0.25 mg/kg bolus followed by 12 h infusion of 0.125 mcg/min) or placebo plus low-dose weight adjusted heparin (70 units/kg) during R-PCI at a mean of 8.5 h from symptom onset: the relatively long delay to R-PCI reflected the fact that all patients were referred from outside hospitals. At 6-month follow-up, the incidence of major adverse cardiac events was 11% in the abciximab group vs 34% in the placebo group ($p = 0.004$). There was a small but significant improvement in recovery of left ventricular wall motion scores at 30 days. The authors report no excess in bleeding with abciximab administration.

Concern over bleeding following full-dose fibrinolytic therapy has limited the use of GP IIb-IIIa inhibitors during R-PCI. Jong and colleagues looked at predictors of bleeding complications in 147 patients presenting for urgent or R-PCI within 48 h of thrombolysis. All received low-dose heparin and 83 received abciximab. The risk of major bleeding was fourfold with abciximab (12% vs 3%, $p = 0.04$). In multivariable analysis, abciximab use was the most powerful predictor of bleeding with a hazard ratio of 1.9 ($p = 0.04$), albeit with no associated excess mortality (26). In a further retrospective study, bleeding rates were compared between 22 patients undergoing R-PCI with abciximab within 15 h of failed fibrinolysis, and 36 matched patients undergoing elective PCI with abciximab

>15 h after successful thrombolysis. Major bleeding was observed in 23% of the R-PCI group, but in none of the patients undergoing delayed PCI >15 h following thrombolysis.

Recommendations for GP IIb-IIIa inhibitor use

GP IIb-IIIa inhibitors reduce ischemic events following R-PCI at the expense of increased bleeding. Benefit is likely achieved by a reduction in stent thrombosis and protection of the microcirculation from embolization of platelet aggregates, events more common following R-PCI than primary PCI.

We advise against the use of GP IIb-IIIa inhibitors in R-PCI if the thrombolytic agent used was streptokinase, or if the patient is older than 75 years. Rates of intracranial hemorrhage appear unacceptably high when GP IIb-IIIa inhibitors are used following streptokinase (27). Recent trials of "facilitated" fibrinolysis (GP IIb-IIIa inhibitors plus reduced-dose fibrinolytic compared to full-dose fibrinolysis) show a linear correlation between risk of intracranial hemorrhage and increasing age over 75 years, with no mortality benefit from facilitated fibrinolysis in this age group (28,29).

Reassuringly most periprocedural bleeds appear to be related to the femoral arterial sheath, with no fatalities due to bleeding in any of the rescue PCI trials (4). There is little safety data regarding use with intraaortic balloon pumps, or with radial artery access for R-PCI: the radial route can be expected to produce fewer access-site bleeding complications. Risk factors for bleeding with GP IIb-IIIa inhibitors are well established and broadly similar to those determined for thrombolytic agents (Table 14.1).

Anticoagulant therapy

Periprocedural heparin is used in rescue PCI on an empirical basis. Unfractionated heparin (UFH) should be weight adjusted (50–70 units/kg body weight) to maintain a periprocedural activated clotting time of >200 s. This recommendation is derived from the EPILOG trial with abciximab in elective PCI, where low-dose weight-adjusted heparin reduced bleeding compared to higher heparin bolus doses of 100 units/kg (30).

Table 14.1 Risk factors for bleeding in major clinical trials of GP IIb/IIIa inhibition during percutaneous coronary intervention. *Abbreviations*: ACT, activated clotting time; CABG, coronary artery bypass grafting. *Source*: Modified from Blankenship JC, *Am Heart J*. 1999;**138**:287–296, with permission from Elsevier.

Trial exclusion criteria
Bleeding diathesis
Recent stroke
Residential neurological deficit after stroke
Central nervous system mass or structural abnormality
Recent active bleeding
Recent major surgery
Baseline thrombocytopenia
Clinical risk factors
Female sex
Older age
Low- and high-weight groups
Acute myocardial infarction
Cardiogenic shock
Complex lesion morphology
Procedural risk factors
Procedural failure; repeat procedures
Long procedure duration
High periprocedural ACT
Concomitant fibrinolytic therapy
Large sheath sizes
Use of venous access sheath
Delay in sheath removal
Continued postprocedure heparin
CABG surgery

Consideration should be given to further reducing the UFH bolus dose in patients who are elderly or have low body weight (1). Following thrombolysis with tPA, heparin infusion is usually continued for 24 h. With concomitant abciximab infusion, a lower heparin infusion rate of 7 units/kg/h (max 800 units/h) may be used.

Low-molecular-weight heparins are unproven in R-PCI. Recent data however supports the use of enoxaparin as an adjunct to fibrinolysis in patients under the age of 75 years (31). Administration of LMWH within 12 h of randomization was an exclusion criterion in many rescue PCI trials: this should not preclude rescue PCI but will raise one's threshold for GP IIb-IIIa inhibitor use. The dose of UFH and particularly LMWH should be reduced in the face of severe renal impairment (Creatinine

Table 14.2 Summary of evidence-based treatment in rescue PCI.

Repeat administration of lytic agent following failure of thrombolysis has been shown to be clinically ineffective.

Rescue PCI limits infarct size and reduces mortality.

Aspirin plus clopidogrel (300–600 mg loading dose then 75 mg for at least 1 year).

GP IIb/IIIa receptor inhibitors reduce ischemic events, but increase bleeding. Use in selected patients <75 years following tPA thrombolysis. Risk of bleeding should be assessed on an individual patient basis.

Unfractionated heparin (50–70 units/kg) to maintain periprocedural ACT >200 s. The role of LMWH in R-PCI has not as yet been fully evaluated.

Newer agents such as prasugrel and the direct thrombin inhibitors (e.g., bivalirudin) require further evaluation in R-PCI.

---

clearance <30 mL/min): if prolonged LMWH use is anticipated, titration of dose relative to factor Xa activity is possible using commercial assays. The optimal dose of UFH in R-PCI following LMWH administration has not been established. Our practice is to use UFH during R-PCI as the anticoagulant effect can be reversed should major bleeding complications arise.

A summary of drug treatment in R-PCI is given in Table 14.2. Newer agents require further evaluation prior to use in R-PCI: these include the direct thrombin inhibitors (e.g., bivalirudin), and the thienopyridine antiplatelet drug, prasugrel.

Conclusions

Fibrinolysis is here to stay as a treatment for STEMI. When fibrinolysis fails, rescue PCI limits infarction and reduces mortality. Careful consideration of each individual patient's bleeding risk is required to guide adjuvant drug prescription and ensure good long-term outcomes.

References

1 Antman EM, Anbe DT, Armstrong PW, *et al.* ACC/AHA guidelines for the management of patients with ST-elevation myocardial infarction. *J Am Coll Cardiol.* 2004;**44**:E1–E211.

2 The effects of tissue plasminogen activator, streptokinase, or both on coronary-artery patency, ventricular function, and survival after acute myocardial infarction. The GUSTO Angiographic Investigators. *N Engl J Med.* 1993;**329**:1615–1622.

3 Indications for fibrinolytic therapy in suspected acute myocardial infarction: collaborative overview of early mortality and major morbidity results from all randomised trials of more than 1000 patients. Fibrinolytic Therapy Trialists' (FTT) Collaborative Group. *Lancet.* 1994;**343**:311–322.

4 Collet JP, Montalescot G, Le May M, Borentain M, Gershlick A. Percutaneous coronary intervention after fibrinolysis: a multiple meta-analyses approach. *J Am Coll Cardiol.* 2006;**48**:1326–1335.

5 Patel TN, Bavry AA, Kumbhani DJ, Ellis SG. A meta-analysis of randomized trials of rescue percutaneous coronary intervention after failed fibrinolysis. *Am J Cardiol.* 2006;**97**:1685–1690.

6 Gershlick AH, Stephens-Lloyd A, Hughes S, *et al.* Rescue angioplasty after failed thrombolytic therapy for acute myocardial infarction. *N Engl J Med.* 2005;**353**:2758–2768.

7 Carver A, Rafelt S, Gershlick A *et al.* Longer-term follow-up of patients recruited to the REACT (Rescue Angioplasty Versus Conservative Treatment or Repeat Thrombolysis) trial. *J Am Coll Cardiol.* 2009;**54**(2):118–26.

8 Hochman JS, Lamas GA, Buller CE, *et al.* Coronary intervention for persistent occlusion after myocardial infarction. The Occluded Artery Trial investigators. *N Engl J Med.* December 7, 2006;**355**(23):2395–3407.

9 Falk E. Coronary thrombosis: pathogenesis and clinical manifestations. *Am J Cardiol.* 1991;**68**:28B–35B.

10 Chesebro JH, Knatterud G, Roberts R, *et al.* Thrombolysis in myocardial infarction (TIMI) trial, Phase I. *Circulation.* 1987;**76**:142–154.

11 Guimaraes AH, Barrett-Bergshoeff MM, Criscuoli M, Evangelista S, Rijken DC. Fibrinolytic efficacy of Amediplase, Tenecteplase and scu-PA in different external plasma clot lysis models: sensitivity to the inhibitory action of thrombin activatable fibrinolysis inhibitor (TAFI). *Thromb Haemost.* 2006;**96**:325–330.

12 Collet JP, Allali Y, Lesty C, *et al.* Altered fibrin architecture is associated with hypofibrinolysis and premature coronary atherothrombosis. *Arterioscler Thromb Vasc Biol.* 2006;**26**:2567–2573.

13 Jang IK, Gold HK, Ziskind AA, *et al.* Differential sensitivity of erythrocyte-rich and platelet-rich arterial thrombi to lysis with recombinant tissue-type plasminogen activator. A possible explanation for resistance to coronary thrombolysis. *Circulation.* 1989;**79**:920–928.

14 Topol EJ. Early myocardial reperfusion: an assessment of current strategies in acute myocardial infarction. *Eur Heart J.* 1996;**17**(Suppl E):42–48.

15 Goto S, Tamura N, Ishida H, Ruggeri ZM. Dependence of platelet thrombus stability on sustained glycoprotein IIb/IIIa activation through adenosine 5'-diphosphate receptor stimulation and cyclic calcium signaling. *J Am Coll Cardiol.* 2006;**47**:155–162.

16 Sabatine MS, Cannon CP, Gibson CM, *et al.* Addition of clopidogrel to aspirin and fibrinolytic therapy for myocardial infarction with ST-segment elevation. *N Engl J Med.* 2005;**352**:1179–1189.

17 von Beckerath N, Taubert D, Pogatsa-Murray G, *et al.* Absorption, metabolization, and antiplatelet effects of 300-, 600-, and 900-mg loading doses of clopidogrel: results of the ISAR-CHOICE Trial. *Circulation.* 2005;**112**:2946–2950.

18 Montalescot G, Sideris G, Meuleman C, *et al.* A randomized comparison of high clopidogrel loading doses in patients with non-ST-segment elevation acute coronary syndromes: the ALBION trial. *J Am Coll Cardiol.* 2006;**48**:931–938.

19 Steinhubl SR, Darrah S, Berger PB, *et al.* Optimal duration of pretreatment with Clopidogrel prior to PCI: data from CREDO. *Circulation.* 2006;**108**(17 abstract suppl IV):374.

20 Sabatine MS, Cannon CP, Gibson CM, *et al.* Effect of clopidogrel pretreatment before percutaneous coronary intervention in patients with ST-elevation myocardial infarction treated with fibrinolytics: the PCI-CLARITY study. *JAMA.* 2005;**294**:1224–1232.

21 Collet JP, Montalescot G, Lesty C, *et al.* Effects of Abciximab on the architecture of platelet-rich clots in patients with acute myocardial infarction undergoing primary coronary intervention. *Circulation.* 2001; **103**:2328–2331.

22 Neumann FJ, Blasini R, Schmitt C, *et al.* Effect of glycoprotein IIb/IIIa receptor blockade on recovery of coronary flow and left ventricular function after the placement of coronary-artery stents in acute myocardial infarction. *Circulation.* 1998;**98**: 2695–2701.

23 Neumann FJ, Zohlnhofer D, Fakhoury L, *et al.* Effect of glycoprotein IIb/IIIa receptor blockade on platelet-leukocyte interaction and surface expression of the leukocyte integrin Mac-1 in acute myocardial infarction. *J Am Coll Cardiol.* 1999;**34**: 1420–1426.

24 Kirtane AJ, Vafai JJ, Murphy SA, *et al.* Angiographically evident thrombus following fibrinolytic therapy is associated with impaired myocardial perfusion in STEMI: a CLARITY-TIMI 28 substudy. *Eur Heart J.* 2006;**27**:2040–2045.

25 Miller JM, Smalling R, Ohman EM, *et al.* Effectiveness of early coronary angioplasty and abciximab for failed thrombolysis (reteplase or alteplase) during acute myocardial infarction (results from the GUSTO-III trial). *Am J Cardiol.* 1999;**84**:779–784.

26 Jong P, Cohen EA, Batchelor W, *et al.* Bleeding risks with abciximab after full-dose thrombolysis in rescue or urgent angioplasty for acute myocardial infarction. *Am Heart J.* 2001;**141**:218–225.

27 Antman EM, Giugliano RP, Gibson CM, *et al.* Abciximab facilitates the rate and extent of thrombolysis: results of the thrombolysis in myocardial infarction (TIMI) 14 trial. *Circulation.* 1999;**99**:2720–2732.

28 Savonitto S, Armstrong PW, Lincoff AM, *et al.* Risk of intracranial haemorrhage with combined fibrinolytic and glycoprotein IIb/IIIa inhibitor therapy in acute myocardial infarction. Dichotomous response as a function of age in the GUSTO V trial. *Eur Heart J.* 2003;**24**:1807–1814.

29 Sinnaeve PR, Huang Y, Bogaerts K, *et al.* Age, outcomes, and treatment effects of fibrinolytic and antithrombotic combinations: findings from Assessment of the Safety and Efficacy of a New Thrombolytic (ASSENT)-3 and ASSENT-3 PLUS. *Am Heart J.* 2006;**152**: 684–689.

30 Platelet glycoprotein IIb/IIIa receptor blockade and low-dose heparin during percutaneous coronary revascularization. The EPILOG Investigators. *N Engl J Med.* 1997;**336**:1689–1696.

31 Antman EM, Morrow DA, McCabe CH, *et al.* Enoxaparin versus unfractionated heparin with fibrinolysis for ST-elevation myocardial infarction. *N Engl J Med.* 2006;**354**:1477–1488.

CHAPTER 15

Facilitated primary percutaneous coronary intervention in acute ST-elevation myocardial infarction

Amir Kashani[1,2] & Robert P. Giugliano[3]

[1]Yale University School of Medicine, New Haven, CT, USA
[2]Baylor College of Medicine, Houston, TX, USA
[3]Brigham & Women's Hospital, Boston, MA, USA

Despite remarkable advances in the treatment of acute coronary syndromes, ST-elevation myocardial infarction (STEMI) remains a significant public health threat in both industrialized and developing countries (1). In the United States, the estimated incidence of myocardial infarctions is 565,000 new and 300,000 recurrent annual cases (2). Timely reperfusion of blood supply to the myocardial tissue is the main goal of therapy in these patients. The benefits of revascularization are directly related to the speed with which reperfusion is achieved after the onset of coronary occlusion. In the current era, primary percutaneous coronary intervention (PCI), when available, is the preferred reperfusion strategy (3,4). In the absence of primary PCI, however, rapid administration of fibrinolytic agents also results in excellent outcomes (5). The selection of the optimal combination of pharmacologic therapies before and during primary PCI is the topic of this chapter.

The use of fibrinolysis for myocardial reperfusion was first described by Fletcher *et al.* in 1958 (6). Soon thereafter, Boucek *et al.* utilized coronary angiography to assess the success of reperfusion after fibrinolysis (7). In subsequent years, significant advances were made in both pharmacologic therapies and mechanical techniques. The first successful

Pharmacology in the Catheterization Laboratory. Edited by Ron Waksman and Andrew E Ajani. © 2010 Blackwell Publishing, ISBN: 978-1-4051-5704-9.

percutaneous transluminal coronary angioplasty (PTCA) was performed in 1977 (8). Less than 2 years later, the first combined pharmacologic and mechanical approach to restoring perfusion in STEMI was reported (9). By the early 1980s, intracoronary streptokinase was shown to be safe and efficacious.

Over the next three decades, the use of primary PCI and pharmacologic therapy, alone, and the combination with one another was intensely studied. In the earlier years, primary PCI and pharmacologic therapy were considered equally appropriate alternatives for treatment of STEMI. However, as the two strategies matured, it became evident that primary PCI results in more rapid revascularization, optimization of the arterial lumen, reduction of recurrent ischemic events, and improved clinical outcomes (10,11). In a recent meta-analysis, the incidence of death (7% vs 9%; $P = 0.0002$), nonfatal myocardial infarction (MI) (3% vs 7%; $P < 0.0001$), stroke (1% vs 2%; $P = 0.0004$), the composite (8% vs 14%; $P < 0.0001$), and recurrent ischemia (6% vs 21%; $P < 0.0001$) were significantly lower (at 6 weeks) with primary PCI versus thrombolysis in 7,739 patients in 23 clinical trials (3). On the other hand, most patients with STEMI do not have access to 24-h primary PCI centers, hence door-to-balloon times in clinical practice are much greater than those observed in randomized trials (12–14). Therefore, by combining fibrinolytic therapy with subsequent PCI in a pharmacoinvasive recanalization (15), the deficiencies of both

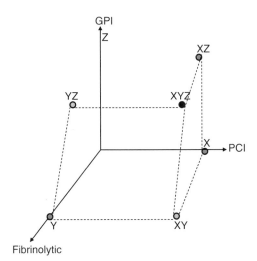

Figure 15.1 Various combinations of pharmacologic and reperfusion regimens in ST-elevation myocardial infarction using an X-Y-Z representation. X stands for PCI, Y for fibrinolytic, and Z for GP IIb/IIIa inhibitors. Their relative clinical utility are shown in green (safe and effective), yellow (limited clinical utility), and red (no proven role). Note that most studies combining fibrinolytic and GP IIb/IIIa inhibitors have studied reduced doses of the fibrinolytic agent, as represented by the lesser value along the Y-axis.

approaches can be minimized. The pharmacologic agents used for bridging the delay to PCI are essential in the success of this strategy.

The most widely studied and promising pharmacologic agents include fibrinolytics, glycoprotein (GP) IIb/IIIa inhibitors, and the combination of reduced-dose fibrinolytic + GP IIb/IIIa antagonist (Figure 15.1). Before reviewing the data for these various regimens, it is important to consider the key variable of "time," since the selection of treatments depends critically upon the anticipated timing of the PCI.

Time to reperfusion

The importance of time to restoration of myocardial blood flow simply cannot be overstated. As outlined in the recent guidelines for management of patients with STEMI (16), the choice between pharmacologic and mechanical strategies weighs heavily on two critical time variables: (1) time from symptom onset to presentation and (2) additional delay incurred by transfer to an expert PCI center (Figure 15.2).

The benefits of revascularization are dependent on establishing reperfusion early enough to salvage myocardium and preserve left ventricular ejection fraction (LVEF). This concept applies to both pharmacologic and interventional reperfusion (17–20). Newby *et al.* evaluated time to treatment onset in 39,833 patients receiving thrombolytic therapy for STEMI (17). Incrementally higher rates of inhospital mortality, 30-day mortality, and stroke were seen with each additional 2 h delay to treatment. Similarly, De Luca *et al.* evaluated 1,791 patients undergoing primary PCI for STEMI between 1994 and 2001 (19). After adjusting for age, diabetes, gender, and pervious revascularization, each 30-min delay was associated with an odds ratio (OR) of predischarge ejection fraction <30% of 1.09 (95% CI 1.023, 1.15; $P = 0.005$) and a relative risk (RR) of 1-year mortality of 1.08 (95% CI 1.008, 1.15; $P = 0.04$). This translated into a 7.5% risk of 1-year mortality for each 30-min delay (19). In comparing patients with symptom-to-balloon times of ≤2 h with >6 h, 1-year mortality was 4.4% and 9.7%, respectively ($P = 0.02$) (20).

While primary PCI is now the preferred method of treatment provided an experienced catheterization laboratory is available within 60–90 min (16), time delays are inherent to the system, particularly in community hospitals (20–23) and at night and over weekends (24). In fact, recent data from a U.S. national registry revealed that the median "door-to-balloon" time among patients who present to a community hospital and require transfer to a hospital with PCI facilities was 171–180 min (25,26). Analyses suggest that if primary PCI results in an incremental delay of >60 min beyond the time that fibrinolytic therapy could be initiated, patients may have better outcomes with fibrinolysis (27,28). Thus, several methods to combine the speed of pharmacologic reperfusion with primary PCI have been explored.

Routine PCI following fibrinolysis

Initial studies investigating early PCI after fibrinolysis failed to show any benefit and were associated with higher rates of bleeding, bypass graft surgery, and mortality (29–32). Michels *et al.* performed a meta-analysis or 16 trials evaluating PTCA after fibrinolysis (33). Mortality or nonfatal

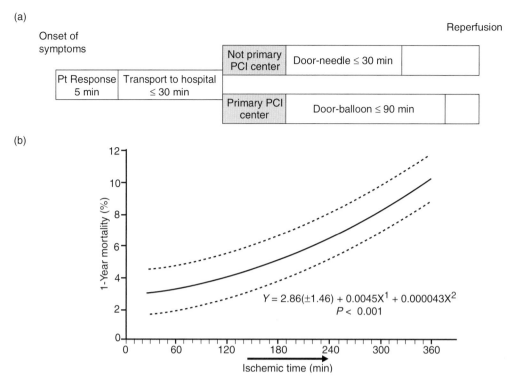

Figure 15.2 Time to reperfusion. (a) Represents step by step goal times to reperfusion as outlined by ACC/AHA guidelines. (b) Higher mortality levels are observed with longer time to reperfusion intervals. Dotted lines represent 95% confidence intervals. (*Source*: Reprinted from De Luca *et al*. (19).)

reinfarction at 6 weeks was not significantly different in any of the following groups: immediate vs no PTCA (OR 0.89, 95% CI 0.65, 1.21); early vs no PTCA (OR 1.06, 95% CI 0.89, 1.25); delayed vs no PTCA (OR 1.78, 95% CI 0.99, 3.19); immediate vs delayed PTCA (OR 1.61, 95% CI 0.91, 2.86). Similarly, no significant differences were observed in 1-year evaluations. Bleeding rates were not evaluated in this study. However, these early studies were performed (1985–1990) prior to the advent of advanced interventional tools and techniques, potent antiplatelet agents (GP IIb/IIIa inhibitors, thienopyridines), and reduced-dose heparin and fibrinolytic regimens. In the modern era, the strategy of fibrinolysis (for early reperfusion and myocardial salvage) followed by angioplasty with stenting may ensure reperfusion in cases of lytic failure as well as preventing reocclusion.

Following the disappointing early experience, more recent trials have reexplored routine PCI following fibrinolysis (Table 15.1). The Plasminogen-activator Angioplasty Compatibility Trial (PACT) trial (34) evaluated the efficacy of *half*-dose recombinant-tPA vs placebo immediately prior to angiography/PCI in 606 patients with STEMI. Although initial TIMI flow rates >2 were higher in patients receiving thrombolytics (61% vs 34%, $P < 0.001$), this did not improve LVEF at discharge, reocclusion rates, recurrent ischemia, stroke, emergency revascularization, major bleeding, or mortality. However, patients with initial TIMI 3 flow (vs TIMI grade <3) did have higher LVEF at 5–7 days (62.4% vs 57.9%, $P = 0.004$). This study is limited by a small sample size and infrequent use of stents (26%) and GP IIb/IIIa inhibitors (5%). This study confirms the importance of time to reperfusion, and shows that PCI can be safely performed soon after half-dose thrombolytic therapy.

In the present era, plain balloon angioplasty performed soon after thrombolysis did not alter reocclusion rates and was associated with higher complication rates (30,32,40). The invention of stents reduced restenosis and improved clinical outcomes (41,42). Therefore, the Grupo de Analisis

Table 15.1 Selected randomized trials of fibrinolytic therapy followed by PCI.

Trial name (N)	Experimental	Control	Main clinical endpoint	Major bleeding
Fibrinolytic + Immediate (<6 h) PCI				
PACT (34)	Half-dose tPA	Placebo	Reocclusion	12.9% vs 13.5%
(N = 606)	PCI: Immediate	PCI: Immediate	5.9% vs 3.7%	
SIAM-III (35)	Reteplase	Reteplase	Composite[a]	9.8% vs 7.4%
(N = 163)	Stent: Immediate	Stent: elective > 2 weeks	26% vs 51% (P = 0.001)	
GRACIA-2 (36)	Tenecteplase	No fibrinolytic	Composite[a]	2% vs 3%
(N = 212)	PCI: 3–12 h	PCI: Immediate	9% vs 12%	
CAPITAL-AMI (37)	Tenecteplase	Tenecteplase	Composite[a]	8.1% vs 7.1%
(N = 170)	Transfer for PCI: 3 h	Rescue PCI: ≥90 min	8.1% vs 21.4% (P = 0.02)	
ASSENT 4-PCI (38)	Tenecteplase	Control arm	Composite[a]	5.6% vs 4.4%
(N = 1,667)	PCI: ASAP after randomization	Primary PCI	19% vs 13% (P = 0.005)	
Fibrinolytic + Delayed (>6 h) PCI				
GRACIA-1 (39)	tPA	tPA	Composite[a]	1.6% vs 1.6%
(N = 500)	PCI: < 24 h	PCI: Ischemia-guided	9% vs 21% (P = 0.0008)	

ASAP, as soon as possible; h, hours; min, minutes; PCI, percutaneous coronary intervention; wks = weeks; P, NS for all comparisons unless otherwise stated.

[a]Composite endpoint—rates through 30 days of the following events: SIAM-III = death, reinfarction, target lesion revascularization, or ischemic events; GRACIA-1, GRACIA-2 = death, nonfatal reinfarction, or revascularization; CAPITAL-AMI = death, re-infarction, recurrent unstable ischemia, or stroke; ASSENT-4-PCI = 90 days death, heart failure, or shock.

de la Cardiopatia Isquemica Aguda (GRACIA)-1 trial (39) (conducted between March 2000 and November 2001) compared early (within 24 h) to ischemia-driven PCI in 500 patients treated with fibrinolysis. Rates of death, reinfarction, or revascularization at 1 year (the primary composite endpoint) was significantly reduced in the early PCI group (9% vs 21%, P = 0.0008). Additionally, length of stay (7.1 vs 10.5 days, P = 0.0001), revascularization during the index hospitalization (2% vs 12%, P < 0.0001) and by 1 year after discharge (4% vs 12%, P = 0.001) were significantly lower with the early strategy. Bleeding rates were similar in the early vs ischemia-driven intervention groups: any bleeding (2.4% vs 1.6%, P = 0.54) and major bleeding (1.6 vs 1.6, P = 0.73). In the invasive group, 80% received a stent and 32% received a GP IIb/IIIa inhibitor. Based on these and other similar results, reevaluation PCI following fibrinolysis, especially in the current era with improved devices and pharmacologic therapy was undertaken.

Subsequently, the GRACIA-2 study (43) randomized 212 patients to PCI within 3–12 h of thrombolysis vs primary PCI (<3 h). GP IIb/IIIa inhibitors were administered to 23% and 87% of patients in the pharmacoinvasive and primary PCI groups, respectively. The time from symptom onset to randomization was approximately 3.2 h in both groups. Although the pharmacoinvasive approach resulted in higher ST-segment resolution (at 6 h) (61% vs 43%, P = 0.03), infarct size was similar in both groups. The incidence of death, reinfarction, and ischemia-driven revascularization (the secondary composite endpoint) was lower in the pharmacoinvasive group but did not reach statistical significance (9% vs 12%). The incidence of major complications was not increased by a pharmacoinvasive strategy.

The Southwest German Interventional Study in Acute Myocardial Infarction (SIAM)-III investigators randomized patients treated with reteplase in hospitals without PCI availability to one of two strategies: transfer (<6 h to interventional center) for immediate PCI ($N = 82$) versus medical stabilization with elective stenting after 2 weeks (or sooner if ongoing ischemia; $N = 81$) (35). Time from thrombolysis to angiography in the immediate and conservative groups, respectively, was 3.5 h and 11.7 days ($P = 0.001$). Overall 9.8% and 16.0% ($P = 0.17$) of patients received abciximab in the two treatment groups respectively. The primary composite end point (ischemic events, death, reinfarction, or revascularization) after 287 days follow-up was reduced by 50% with immediate PCI (26% vs 51%, $P = 0.001$), driven mainly by a reduction in ischemic events (5% vs 28%, $P = 0.01$). At 2 weeks, LVEF was significantly higher in patients undergoing immediate PCI (57% vs 53%, $P = 0.037$). Also, LVEF improvement after 6 months reached statistical significance only in the immediate PCI group (57% → 62%, $P = 0.015$ vs 53% → 56%, $P = 0.082$).

In a recent Canadian study, the Combined Angioplasty and Pharmacological Intervention vs Thrombolysis Alone in Acute Myocardial Infarction (CAPITAL-AMI) investigators randomized 170 patients with STEMI to tenecteplase (TNK) followed by transfer for PCI (performed within 3 h of randomization) versus TNK alone (37). If indicated, rescue PCI was performed ≥90 min after initiation of therapy in the TNK alone group. Time from symptom onset to TNK administration was 120 min in both groups and symptom onset to first balloon inflation was 204 min in the PCI group. The composite of death, reinfarction, recurrent unstable ischemia, or stroke was lower in the PCI group during initial hospitalization (8.1% vs 21.4%; $P = 0.02$), at 3 months (9.3% vs 21.7%; $P = 0.03$), and at 6 months (primary endpoint 11.6% and 24.4%; $P = 0.04$). At all time points, a decrease in recurrent unstable ischemia (an end point which also included patients with re-infarction) was the driving force behind the superiority of the TNK-PCI strategy. The length of index hospitalization was also lower in the TNK-PCI group (5 vs 6 days; $P = 0.02$). Rates of major bleeding (8.1% vs 7.1%; $P > 0.9$) and intracranial hemorrhage (1.2% vs 1.2%; $P > 0.9$) were similar in the two groups (37). The above three small studies supported the emerging paradigm of early PCI (predominantly with stents) following fibrinolysis,

which was becoming more common in the United States and selected European countries.

The first trial adequately powered randomized clinical trial to assess clinical outcomes with PCI after fibrinolysis was the Assessment of the Safety and Efficacy of a New Thrombolytic Regiment (ASSENT)-4-PCI trial that compared PCI 1–3 h after full-dose TNK to primary PCI (38). The median time from randomization to first balloon was 115 vs 107 min ($P = 0.7$) in the fibrinolysis and PCI groups, respectively, and time from symptom onset to PCI was >4 h in both groups. The trial was terminated by the safety monitoring board after enrolling 1,667 of the 4,000 planned patients secondary to higher inhospital mortality in the TNK group (6% vs 3%; $P = 0.01$). The primary endpoint (90 days death, CHF, or shock) occurred more frequently in patients receiving fibrinolysis (19% vs 13%; $P = 0.0045$). Reinfarction rates (4.1% vs 1.9%; $P = 0.01$), abrupt vessel closure (1.9% vs 0.1%; $P < 0.001$), repeat TVR (4.4% vs 1.0%; $P < 0.001$); total inhospital stroke (1.8% vs 0.0%; $P < 0.0001$), intracranial hemorrhage (1.0% vs 0.0%; $P = 0.004$), and any bleeding (31.3% vs 23.4%; $P < 0.001$) were all significantly higher in patients receiving fibrinolytic therapy. Although TIMI 3 flow was higher in the fibrinolysis arm prior to PCI (43.0% vs 15.0%; $P < 0.001$), post-PCI TIMI 3 flow was higher in the primary PCI group (87.6% vs 88.7%; $P = 0.03$).

As was observed two decades ago, a strategy of routine early PCI following full-dose fibrinolytic in ASSENT-4 PCI resulted in worse clinical outcomes. There was a significantly higher rate of abrupt vessel closure in patients undergoing fibrinolysis followed by immediate PCI and more bleeding. In the absence of appropriate platelet inhibition (<10% of patients undergoing fibrinolysis received GP IIb/IIIa and 87% received clopidogrel/ticlopidine in this trial), fibrinolytic agents can be prothrombotic via platelet activation. It should be noted that in ASSENT-4 PCI, patients randomized in the ambulance had the lowest mortality and the highest pre-PCI TIMI 3 flow rates, once again emphasizing the benefits of earlier therapy.

Finally, a meta-analysis of 17 randomized controlled trials, Keeley *et al.* compared 42-day outcomes in patients undergoing pharmacoinvasive vs primary PCI (44). Here we report results from the subgroup of six trials (including ASSENT-4 PCI (38)) utilizing full-dose thrombolytic therapy prior to PCI. Event rates were higher in patients receiving fibrinolytics: death 6% vs 4% ($P = 0.042$), nonfatal reinfarction 4% vs 2% ($P = 0.006$), urgent TVR 5% vs 1% ($P < 0.0001$), major bleeding 7% vs 5% ($P = 0.17$), hemorrhagic stroke 1.0% vs 0.1% ($P = 0.0007$), and total stroke 1.6% vs 0.3% ($P = 0.0002$). These adverse outcomes were observed despite a higher initial TIMI 3 flow rate with a pharmacoinvasive approach (42% vs 15%; $P < 0.0001$). Results from this meta-analysis, ASSENT-4 PCI, and studies conducted in the 1980s support the existing guideline recommendations that elective PCI following fibrinolysis be limited to those high-risk patients who are at low bleeding risk and who experience recurrent ischemia (45). The Trial of Routine Angioplasty and Stenting after Fibrinolysis to Enhance Reperfusion in Acute Myocardial Infarction (Transfer AMI) (46) is underway evaluating full-dose TNK followed by PCI in patients with very long delays due to hospital transfer.

Glycoprotein IIb/IIIa inhibitors

Given that de novo plaque rupture as well as mechanical revascularization enhance platelet activation and aggregation (47), GP IIb/IIIa receptor antagonists that inhibit the final common pathway of platelet aggregation are logical candidates to utilize in a pharmacoinvasive approach. These agents bind fibrinogen and other proteins that bridge adjacent proteins. GP IIb/IIIa inhibition has been shown to prevent reocclusion of recanalized infarct arteries (48). Of the three commercially available GP IIb/IIIa inhibitors, most trials have been conducted with abciximab, a monoclonal antibody of the platelet GP IIb/IIIa receptor.

The addition of abciximab therapy to primary PCI has been shown to reduce mortality and cardiac complications (Table 15.2) (49–51). However, reducing the need for TVR accounts for most of the observed benefit. The ReoPro and Primary PTCA Organization and Randomized (RAPPORT) trial, one of the first trials of GP IIb/IIIa therapy in AMI, evaluated abciximab vs placebo therapy in 483 patients undergoing primary PCI (49). The primary end point (all-cause death,

reinfarction, any repeat TVR) was lower in patients treated with abciximab at 7 days (3.3% vs 9.9%, $P = 0.003$), 30 days (5.8% vs 11.2%, $P = 0.03$), and 180 days (11.6% vs 17.8%, $P = 0.048$). Separation of event curves was noted as early as day 1. Amid individual components of the composite end point, abciximab therapy significantly reduced the need for urgent TVR at all time points. Abciximab therapy reduced the need for "bail-out stenting" by 33%. Despite an increase in major bleeding (16.6% vs 9.5%, $P = 0.02$), abciximab therapy significantly reduced acute-phase ischemic events and was a favorable adjunct to primary PCI in this trial. Higher heparin doses (100 µ/kg vs the current standard of 60–70 µ/kg) used in the RAPPORT trial may account for the excess bleeding.

Zorman *et al.* randomized 163 patients undergoing primary PCI to immediate (prior to angiography), late (after initial angiography), or no abciximab (54). The incidence of initial TIMI ≥2 flow in the three groups, respectively, was 32%, 12%, and 18% ($P = 0.04$). Overall time from symptom onset to angioplasty was similar in the three groups and ranged from 297 to 374 min. Inhospital (0%, 7%, vs 10%, $P = 0.03$) and 6 months (0%, 9%, vs 14%, $P = 0.02$) mortality were significantly lower in the immediate and highest in the no abciximab groups. The incidence of bleeding (29%, 20%, vs 12%, $P = 0.10$) and thrombocytopenia (4%, 11%, vs 6%, $P = 0.10$) was similar in the three groups, respectively. Despite a small sample size, this study showed that early abciximab therapy can improve myocardial perfusion and clinical outcomes without increasing adverse events.

The Abciximab before Direct Angioplasty and Stenting in Myocardial Infarction Regarding Acute and Long-Term Follow-up (ADMIRAL) investigators randomized 300 patients with STEMI to abciximab (administered immediately after randomization—as early as in the mobile intensive care unit to as late as in the catheterization laboratory) vs placebo (50). All patients received the study medication prior to sheath placement and 92% received a stent. Initial TIMI 3 flow was higher in patients receiving abciximab (17% vs 5%; $P = 0.01$). Abciximab therapy reduced the composite, primary end point (death, reinfarction, or urgent TVR) at 30 (6.0% vs 14.6%; $P = 0.01$) and 180 days (7% vs 16%; $P = 0.02$). Minor bleeding

Table 15.2 Randomized trials of GP IIb/IIIa monotherapy in primary PCI.

Trial name (N)	30-day clinical composite[a]	Main safety outcome
Abciximab (ReoPro™)		
RAPPORT (49)	5.8% vs 11.2%	Major bleeds
(N = 483)	(P = 0.03)	16.6% vs 9.5%
		(P = 0.02)
Neumann et al. (52)	2.0% vs 9.2%	Transfusions
(N = 200)	(P = 0.03)	2.9% vs 6.0%
ISAR-2 (53)	5.0% vs 10.5%	Transfusions
(N = 401)	(P = 0.04)	3.5% vs 4.5%
Zorman et al. (54)	0% vs 7% vs 10%	Bleeding
(N = 163)	(P = 0.03)	29% vs 20% vs 12%
ADMIRAL (50)	6.0% vs 14.6%	Major bleeds
(N = 300)	(P = 0.01)	0.7% vs 0%
CADILLAC (51)	4.6% vs 7.0%	Major bleeds
(N = 2,082)	(P = 0.01)	0.6% vs 0.4%
Maioli et al. (55)	5.7% vs 8.6%	Bleeding
(N = 210)		8.6% vs 5.7%
Tirofiban (Aggrastat®)		
TIGER-PA (56)	6% vs 10%	Major bleeds
(N = 157)		2% vs 2%
SASTRE (57)	25% vs 43%	Any complication 11%
(N = 144)	(P < 0.001)	vs 11%
ON-TIME (58)	8.6% vs 4.4%	Major bleed
(N = 507)	(P = 0.06)	4.5% vs 3.2%
Eptifibatide (Integrilin™)		
INTAMI (59)	13.5% vs 6.1%	Severe bleed
(N = 106)		3.8% vs 4.1%
TITAN-TIMI 34 (60)	4.0% vs 2.8%	Major bleeding
(N = 343)		1.7% vs 3.5%

Values represent % patients with events in the GP IIb/IIIa inhibitor group vs comparator groups. In TIGER-PA, ON-TIME, and INTAMI, early vs late use of GP IIb/IIIa was compared, while all other trials were placebo-controlled.

P values are not significant unless otherwise specified.

[a]30-Day clinical composite endpoints as follows:

RAPPORT, ADMIRAL = death, reinfarction, urgent target vessel revascularization; Neumann, ISAR-2, INTAMI = death, reinfarction, or any target vessel revascularization; Zorman et al. = Inhospital mortality; CADILLAC = death, reinfarction, urgent repeat revascularization, or disabling stroke; Maioli et al. = Major adverse cardiac events; TIGER-PA = death, reinfarction, or rehospitalization; SASTRE = death, reinfarction, stroke, need for any revascularization, heart failure, new refractory ischemia, or severe ischemic-related hemodynamic instability; ON-TIME = death, reinfarction, stroke, or non-CABG related major bleeding;TITAN-TIMI 34 = 30 days death.

was significantly higher with abciximab therapy (12.1% vs 3.3%; P = 0.004). The ADMIRAL trial demonstrated that abciximab administration prior to primary PCI reduces acute ischemic events as well as end points related to coronary restenosis.

In a much larger trial, the The Controlled Abciximab and Device Investigators to Lower Late Angioplasty Complications (CADILLAC)

investigators randomized 2,082 patients with myocardial infarction and either ST-elevation or high-grade angiographic stenosis with an associated regional wall motion abnormality to one of four groups: PTCA alone, PTCA plus abciximab, stenting alone, or stenting plus abciximab (51). Abciximab therapy reduced 30-day composite end point (death, reinfarction, urgent repeat revascularization, or disabling stroke) by an absolute rate of 2.4% ($P = 0.01$). Rates of ischemic revascularization (2.5% vs 4.4%; $P = 0.02$), any revascularization (2.6% vs 4.7%; $P = 0.009$), and subacute thrombosis (0.4% vs 1.5%; $P = 0.01$) were also significantly reduced at 30 days. The incidence of moderate, severe, or intracranial hemorrhage was not significantly increased by abciximab therapy. Thrombocytopenia, however, occurred more often with abciximab therapy (4.5% vs 2.3%; $P = 0.008$). The ADMIRAL and CADILLAC trials confirmed the effectiveness of adjunctive GP IIb/IIIa inhibition in PCI without significant increases in bleeding complications.

A recent meta-analysis evaluated six randomized controlled trials (3,755 patients) of abciximab therapy in patients undergoing PCI for AMI (61). Outcomes were reported at 6 months (five trials) and 1 month (one trial). Abciximab therapy significantly reduced death (3.4% vs 4.9%; $P = 0.03$), target vessel revascularization (11.8% vs 14.4%; $P = 0.02$), and major cardiac events (17.0% vs 21.1%; $P = 0.001$). Major bleeding was increased in patients treated with higher doses of heparin: 100 U/kg (16.6% vs 9.5%, $P = 0.02$) vs 70 U/kg (4.3% vs 3.4%, $P = 0.28$) (abciximab vs control).

Another meta-analysis included eight randomized trials (3,949 patients) of abciximab as adjunctive therapy in primary angioplasty (62). The primary end points 30 days (2.4% vs 3.4%; $P = 0.047$; OR 0.68 [0.47–0.99]) and long-term mortality (4.4% vs 6.2%; $P = 0.01$; OR 0.69 [0.52–0.92]) were significantly reduced with abciximab therapy. Similarly, 30-day reinfarction (secondary endpoint) was lower with abciximab (1.0% vs 1.9%; $P = 0.03$). Abciximab did not portend a higher incidence of intracranial hemorrhage (0.06% vs 0.11%; $P = 0.96$) or bleeding complications (4.7% vs 4.1%; $P = 0.36$) (62). This meta-analysis demonstrates improved mortality (a "hard" end point) with abciximab therapy in addition to the decreased ischemic events seen in individual trials.

The previously mentioned Keeley meta-analysis also included a subgroup of nine studies (1,148 patients) utilizing GP IIb/IIIa antagonists vs placebo as adjuncts to PCI (up to 42 days follow-up) (44). Despite an improvement in initial TIMI 3 flow with GP IIb/IIIa inhibition (26% vs 15%; $P = 0.0001$), clinical end points were not significantly different between the two groups: death 3% vs 3% ($P = 0.94$), reinfarction 1% vs 1% ($P = 0.53$), urgent TVR 2% vs 2% ($P = 0.99$), major bleeding 7% vs 5% ($P = 0.30$), hemorrhagic stroke 0% vs 0.2% ($P = 0.68$), and total stroke 0% vs 0.4% ($P = 0.34$) (44). While GP IIb/IIIa inhibitors preceding PCI was not harmful with regards to any of the end points, it was not beneficial either in this analysis.

In a more recent meta-analysis, case specific data from three randomized trials were combined to evaluate GP IIb/IIIa inhibition in patients undergoing primary PCI and stenting (63). Patients were randomized to abciximab ($N = 550$) or placebo ($N = 551$) in all trials. Follow-up times for the three trials were 365 days in the ACE (64) trial and 1,095 days in the ISAR-2 (53), and ADMIRAL (50) studies. The cumulative hazard ratios were significantly lower with abciximab therapy: death or reinfarction (primary end point) 12.9% vs 19.0%, $P = 0.008$, NNT = 19; death 10.8% vs 14.3%, $P = 0.05$, NNT = 29; and reinfarction 2.3% vs 5.5%, $P = 0.01$, NNT = 31. The difference in major bleeding did not reach statistical significance between the abciximab (2.5%) and placebo (2.0%) groups ($P > 0.5$). When evaluating the primary end point in prespecified subgroups, abciximab afforded a significant benefit in diabetic patients (hazard rate (HR) 0.53; $P = 0.02$; NNT = 6) while reaching borderline significance in nondiabetics (HR 0.67; $P = 0.055$). This meta-analysis shows a 37% relative risk reduction in death or reinfarction with abciximab therapy and suggests that higher risk patients (e.g., patients with more comorbidities) may derive the most benefit.

Does timing of GP IIb/IIIa inhibition matter?

A prespecified subgroup analysis of the ADMIRAL trial demonstrated that earlier GP IIb/IIIa blockade (in the emergency department or ambulance) resulted in improved outcomes with respect to the primary clinical endpoint than therapy in the ICU or catheterization laboratory (50). A meta-analysis of 931 patients (six trials) aimed to compare administration of GP IIb/IIIa inhibitors prior to arrival in the catheterization laboratory vs immediately prior to PCI in patients with STEMI (65). Early treatment was associated with higher culprit vessel patency as indicated by TIMI 2 or 3 flow (41.7% vs 29.8%; NNT = 8; $P < 0.001$) and TIMI 3 flow (20.3% vs 12.2%; NNT = 12; $P < 0.0001$). Although there was a 28% reduction in mortality with early GP IIb/IIIa inhibition, the difference did not reach statistical significance. These results emphasize the need for larger randomized trials evaluating the impact early GP IIb/IIIa inhibition on clinical outcomes.

In a retrospective study of 446 patients undergoing primary PCI (66), early abciximab therapy (prior to transport to the catheterization laboratory) was compared to therapy in the catheterization laboratory. Of note, 70% of patients enrolled in this study were transferred from centers without PCI capabilities and 85% of patients received a stent. In the late group, abciximab therapy was delayed by 45 ± 15 min. A trend toward 6-month MACE-free survival (the primary end point) was observed with early abciximab administration (26.6% vs 36.4%, $P = 0.05$). Early treatment resulted in higher rates of TIMI 2–3 flow on initial angiography (35% vs 19%, $P < 0.001$). Additionally, the difference in major bleeding rates did not reach statistical significance between the two groups: 6.7% vs 5.8%, $P = 0.74$ (66).

Another recent meta-analysis (six trials) compared abciximab infusion prior to vs in the catheterization laboratory in 602 patients undergoing primary PCI (67). The initiation of abciximab therapy was a median of 50 and 5 min ($P < 0.001$) prior to visualization of the infarct related artery in the two groups. The composite of death, reinfarction, or TVR at 30-days was slightly lower in patients receiving early treatment (7.3% vs 9.7%; $P = 0.3$). The incidence of major bleeding was 3.5% in the early and 3.8% in the late treatment groups ($P = 0.8$). As with previous studies, initial TIMI 3 (20% vs 12%; $P = 0.01$) and TIMI 2/3 flow (42% vs 29%; $P = 0.001$) were significantly higher with early therapy. Similarly, post-PCI ST-resolution was seen in 59% and 41% ($P = 0.003$) of patients in the early and late groups, respectively (67).

In the Time to Integrilin Therapy in Acute Myocardial Infarction (TITAN) TIMI-34 trial, 343 patients undergoing primary PCI for STEMI were randomized to initiation of eptifibatide therapy in the emergency department vs in the catheterization laboratory (60). Earlier eptifibatide administration was associated with faster reperfusion as indicated

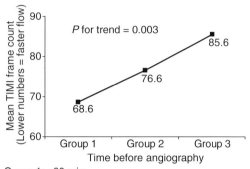

Figure 15.3 TIMI frame count and duration of GP IIb/IIIa inhibitor administration. Earlier administration of GP IIb/IIIa inhibitors before primary PCI results in faster coronary blood flow (lower TIMI frame counts) at the start of PCI. (*Source:* Reproduced from Gibson *et al.* (60) with permission.)

by lower pre-PCI corrected TIMI frame count (the primary end point: 77.5 vs 84.3; $P = 0.049$). In fact, there was a linear relationship between earlier GP IIb/IIIa inhibitor initiation and lower frame counts (Figure 15.3). Emergency department eptifibatide administration resulted in higher initial TIMI myocardial perfusion (24.3% vs 14.2%; $P = 0.03$) and global perfusion scores (42% vs 38%, $P = 0.008$). Although major (1.7% vs 3.5%) and major or minor (6.9% vs 7.8%) bleeding rates were lower with early therapy, the differences did not reach statistical significance. There was no difference in post-PCI angiographic results between the two groups. The incidence of clinical events (i.e., inhospital and 30-day death, reinfarction, abrupt vessel closure, new or worsening heart failure, rehospitalization for acute coronary syndrome) was low and was not statistically different between the two groups. Similar to previous studies, this trial shows faster reperfusion without increased bleeding with earlier GP IIb/IIIa inhibition. However, larger studies are needed to better assess the association of these findings with clinical outcomes.

More recently, Maioli and colleagues randomized 210 patients undergoing primary PCI for a first AMI to initiation of abciximab therapy in the emergency department vs catheterization laboratory after angiography (55). The study was conducted between 2003 and 2006. Initial TIMI 3 flow

(24% vs 10%; $P = 0.01$), the primary end point, and procedure times (11 ± 7 vs 15 ± 8; $P = 0.03$) were significantly improved with early therapy. The gain in LVEF at 1 month was also higher with early abciximab administration (8 ± 7% vs 6 ± 7%; $P = 0.02$). The incidence of adverse clinical outcomes did not significantly differ between the two groups: MACE 5.7% vs 8.6% ($P = 0.42$); 2.9% vs 5.7% ($P = 0.49$); reinfarction 1.9% vs 3.8% ($P = 0.68$); and bleeding complications 8.6% vs 5.7% ($P = 0.44$). In this small trial, early abciximab therapy did result in a significant improvement in LVEF while similar to previous studies; clinical outcomes were not significantly affected.

To date, studies demonstrate that early GP IIb/IIIa inhibition in patients undergoing PCI for STEMI results in early reperfusion and trends toward improved clinical outcomes. Based on small individual trials, the aforementioned meta-analyses, and results from larger studies conducted in other patient populations undergoing PCI (68), current STEMI guidelines support administering abciximab as soon as possible to patients undergoing primary PCI. However, given the lack of definitive large studies, use of abciximab as and adjunct to primary PCI has been assigned a class IIa indication. Since tirofiban and eptifibatide, compared to abciximab, have been less frequently studied in patients with STEMI, their use is assigned a class IIb recommendation (45). The optimal timing of GP IIb/IIIa blockade and efficacy in high risk vs lower risk subgroups still remains to be clarified with larger studies powered to evaluate clinical outcomes. The ongoing Facilitated Intervention with Enhanced Reperfusion Speed to Stop Events (FINESSE) trial (69) is evaluating early vs late abciximab therapy as well as the combination of half-dose reteplase plus abciximab in approximately 3,000 patients. This large randomized controlled trial should provide more definitive information regarding the clinical utility of early vs late GP IIb/IIIa inhibition in patients with STEMI undergoing primary PCI.

Combination reduced-dose fibrinolytic + GP IIb/IIIa inhibitor

The combination of half-dose fibrinolytics and GP IIb/IIIa inhibitors is another pharmacoinvasive strategy for restoring vessel patency. Two large randomized controlled trials (70,71) evaluating this pharmacoinvasive approach *without* subsequent PCI demonstrated similar mortality, more bleeding (especially in the elderly), but lower rates of recurrent ischemic complications with combination therapy compared to fibrinolytic monotherapy.

In a recent, nonrandomized study, 113 patients with STEMI who presented "after hours" (from 6 p.m. to 8 a.m. or on weekends) were treated with 20 mg of alteplase (single bolus) and standard dose abciximab while the catheterization laboratory was being prepared for PCI (72). The comparative group consisted of 95 patients who underwent primary PCI during "regular hours" (with 68% receiving abciximab). As expected, door-to-balloon times were higher in patients presenting "after hours" (72 vs 54 min; $P = 0.001$). Initial TIMI 3 flow was observed in 44.2% of patients receiving alteplase vs 1% of patients in the primary PCI arm ($P = 0.001$). The primary end point, postinterventional corrected TIMI frame count, was lower in the pharmacoinvasive group: 26 + 13 vs 30 + 19 ($P = 0.045$). These angiographic findings did not affect the mean improvement in LVEF at 1 month (8.3% vs 7.0%; $P = 0.26$). Pharmacoinvasive therapy was associated with a significantly higher 1-year MACE-free survival rates (89% vs 74%, $P = 0.02$). Although major bleeding was higher in patients receiving alteplase, this difference did not reach statistical significance (6.2% vs 3.0%, $P = 0.23$).

However, two small, randomized controlled trials of combination therapy preceding primary PCI (73,74), were disappointing (Table 15.3). For instance, the Bavarian Reperfusion Alternatives Evaluation (BRAVE) study investigators randomized 253 patients to abciximab plus half-dose reteplase or abciximab alone (74). In this study, conducted from 2001 to 2003, 186 patients presented to community hospitals and required transport to an interventional facility. The transport time ranged from 25 to 45 min and was similar in the two groups. Initial TIMI 3 flow was higher in patients receiving combination therapy (40% vs 18%; $P < 0.001$). The final infarct size as measured by nuclear scintigraphy at a median of 6.2 days (the primary end point) was 13.0% and 11.5% ($P = 0.81$) in the reteplase plus abciximab and abciximab alone groups respectively. The difference in the composite secondary end point of death, reinfarction, or

Table 15.3 Randomized trials of combination half-dose fibrinolytic + GP IIb/IIIa vs GP IIb/IIIa inhibitor monotherapy in primary PCI.

Trial name	Half-dose fibrinolytic	GP inhibitor	Main clinical outcome[a]	Bleeding
BRAVE (74) (N = 253)	Reteplase	Abciximab	Final infarct size 13% vs 11.5% (P = NS)	5.6% vs 1.6% (P = 0.16)
ADVANCE-MI (73) (N = 149)	Tenecteplase	Eptifibatide	Composite[b] 10.1% vs 2.6% (P = 0.09)	25% vs 10% (P = 0.02)

[a]Values represent % patients with events in the combination therapy group vs. GP IIb/IIIa monotherapy group.
[b]Death or new/worsening severe heart failure through 30 days.

stroke (6.4% vs 4.7%; P = 0.56) and major bleeding (5.6% vs 1.6%; P = 0.16) did not reach statistical significance in the two treatment groups. In this small study, improved coronary flow with combination therapy did not translate into better clinical outcomes.

After enrolling 148 patients, the Addressing the Value of Facilitated Angioplasty After Combination Therapy or Eptifibatide Monotherapy in Acute Myocardial Infarction (ADVANCE-MI) trial was prematurely terminated secondary to slow patient recruitment (73). Patients undergoing primary PCI within 4 h of hospital presentation were randomized to receive eptifibatide and either half-dose tenecteplase or placebo. The primary end point was death or severe CHF. Initial angiographic coronary flow was improved with combination therapy. Nonetheless, 30-day clinical end points were higher in the tenecteplase group: death 7% vs 0% (P = 0.03); severe CHF 7% vs 1% (P = 0.09); death or severe CHF 11% vs 1% (P = 0.02); death, reinfarction, or severe CHF 12% vs 3% (P = 0.03); major bleeding 23% vs 7% (P = 0.05). In this study, combination therapy resulted in higher adverse outcomes. However, given the small sample size and premature termination of this study, definitive conclusions should not be drawn from these results.

In their meta-analysis, Keeley et al. combined the data from these two studies combining half-dose fibrinolytics with GP IIb/IIIa inhibitors (399 patients) (44). Once again, higher initial TIMI 3 flow with combination therapy did not translate into improved clinical outcomes: death 4% vs 1% (P = 0.44), reinfarction 1% vs 1% (P = 0.98),

urgent TVR 3% vs 1% (endpoint from one study only; P = 0.17), hemorrhagic stroke 0.5% vs 0% (P = 0.76), and total stroke 0.5% vs 0% (P = 0.76). Moreover, the rate of major bleeding, was significantly higher in the combination group 12% vs 5% (P = 0.006) (44). Further data from adequately powered clinical studies such as the FINESSE trial (69) (see above) is awaited.

Another recent meta-analysis (75) evaluated 725 patients with STEMI (four trials) randomized to reduced-dose thrombolytics + GP IIb/IIIa inhibitors vs GP IIb/IIIa inhibitors alone prior to PCI (75). Although pre-PCI TIMI 3 flow was significantly higher with combination therapy (RR 2.18; 95% CI 1.7–2.81; P < 0.00001), no significant difference in specified clinical outcomes was observed: mortality (RR 1.47; 95% CI 0.52–4.14; P = 0.46); reinfarction (RR 0.96; 95% CI 0.23–4.02; P = 0.96); and post-PCI TIMI 3 flow (RR 0.99; 95% CI 0.86–1.14; P = 0.85). Major bleeding rates were higher in the pharmacoinvasive arm (RR 2.15; 95% CI 1.14–3.94; P = 0.01).

Discussion

In the current era, primary PCI is the preferred modality for treating patients with STEMI with a goal door-to-balloon time of <90 min (16). However, this modality is not available to all patients presenting with STEMI. In 1999, less than one in five United States hospitals and one in ten European hospitals had the capability to perform primary PCI. Even fewer hospitals are equipped to operate a 24-h catheterization laboratory (76). Given the importance of time to reperfusion (as previously outlined), a pharmacoinvasive approach is a logical strategy for patients with expected delays to PCI.

The current ACC/AHA STEMI guidelines provide an algorithm to help clinicians decide between primary PCI and fibrinolytic therapy (16). Primary PCI should be considered when:

- PCI laboratory is available with skilled operators and surgical backup
- Expected door-to-balloon time is <90 min
- High-risk patients (e.g., cardiogenic shock, Killip class III–IV)
- Patients have contraindications to thrombolytic therapy
- Patients present more than 3 h after symptoms onset
- Uncertainty exists in the diagnosis of STEMI. Fibrinolysis should be considered when:
- Primary PCI facility is not accessible
- Expected door-to-balloon time is >90 min
- Vascular access difficulties exist
- Patients present less than 3 h after symptoms onset.

Regarding pharmacoinvasive therapy, several questions still remain unanswered. For instance, larger trials powered to evaluate clinical outcomes are necessary to better understand the effects of various agents (e.g., GP IIb/IIIa inhibitors). We need to better define which pharmacoinvasive regimen is most ideal and which patients are good candidates for transfer to a PCI facility. Currently ongoing clinical trials (e.g., FINESSE trial) should help answer some of these questions.

References

1 Rogers WJ, Canto JG, Lambrew CT, *et al.* Temporal trends in the treatment of over 1.5 million patients with myocardial infarction in the US from 1990 through 1999: the National Registry of Myocardial Infarction 1, 2 and 3. *J Am Coll Cardiol.* December 2000;**36**(7):2056–2063.

2 Rosamond W, Flegal K, Friday G, *et al.* Heart disease and stroke statistics—2007 update: a report from the American Heart Association Statistics Committee and Stroke Statistics Subcommittee. *Circulation.* February 6, 2007;**115**(5):e69–e171.

3 Keeley EC, Boura JA, Grines CL. Primary angioplasty versus intravenous thrombolytic therapy for acute myocardial infarction: a quantitative review of 23 randomised trials. *Lancet.* January 4, 2003;**361**(9351):13–20.

4 Weaver WD, Simes RJ, Betriu A, *et al.* Comparison of primary coronary angioplasty and intravenous thrombolytic therapy for acute myocardial infarction: a quantitative review. *JAMA.* December 17, 1997;**278**(23):2093–2098.

5 Weaver WD, Cerqueira M, Hallstrom AP, *et al.* Prehospital-initiated vs hospital-initiated thrombolytic therapy. The Myocardial Infarction Triage and Intervention Trial. *JAMA.* September 8, 1993;**270**(10):1211–1216.

6 Fletcher AP, Alkjaersig N, Smyrniotis FE, Sherry S. The treatment of patients suffering from early myocardial infarction with massive and prolonged streptokinase therapy. *Trans Assoc Am Physicians.* 1958;**71**:287–296.

7 Boucek RJ, Murphy WP, Jr. Segmental perfusion of the coronary arteries with fibrinolysin in man following a myocardial infarction. *Am J Cardiol.* August 1960;**6**:525–533.

8 Gruntzig AR, Senning A, Siegenthaler WE. Nonoperative dilatation of coronary-artery stenosis: percutaneous transluminal coronary angioplasty. *N Engl J Med.* July 12, 1979;**301**(2):61–68.

9 Rentrop KP, Blanke H, Karsch KR, *et al.* Acute myocardial infarction: intracoronary application of nitroglycerin and streptokinase. *Clin Cardiol.* October 1979;**2**(5):354–363.

10 Antman EM. ST-elevation myocardial infarction: management. In: Zipes D, Libby P, Bonow R, Braunwald E, eds. *Braunwald's Heart Disease: A Textbook of Cardiovascular Medicine*, 7th ed. Philadelphia, PA: Elsevier Saunders; 2005:1167–1185.

11 Holmes DR, Lane G. Primary percutaneous coronary intervention in the management of acute myocardial infarction. In: Zipes D, Libby P, Bonow R, Braunwald E, eds. *Braunwald's Heart Disease: A Textbook of Cardiovascular Medicine*, 7th ed. Philadelphia, PA: Elsevier Saunders; 2005:1227–1242.

12 Zahn R, Schiele R, Schneider S, *et al.* Primary angioplasty versus intravenous thrombolysis in acute myocardial infarction: can we define subgroups of patients benefiting most from primary angioplasty? Results from the pooled data of the Maximal Individual Therapy in Acute Myocardial Infarction Registry and the Myocardial Infarction Registry. *J Am Coll Cardiol.* June 1, 2001;**37**(7):1827–1835.

13 The InTIME-II Investigators. Intravenous NPA for the treatment of infarcting myocardium early; InTIME-II, a double-blind comparison of single-bolus lanoteplase vs accelerated alteplase for the treatment of patients with acute myocardial infarction. *Eur Heart J.* December 2000;**21**(24):2005–2013.

14 Giugliano RP, Llevadot J, Wilcox RG, *et al.* Geographic variation in patient and hospital characteristics, management, and clinical outcomes in ST-elevation myocardial infarction treated with fibrinolysis. Results from InTIME-II. *Eur Heart J.* September 2001;**22**(18):1702–1715.

15 Dauerman HL, Sobel BE. Synergistic treatment of ST-segment elevation myocardial infarction with pharmacoinvasive recanalization. *J Am Coll Cardiol*. August 20, 2003;**42**(4):646–651.

16 Antman EM, Anbe DT, Armstrong PW, *et al*. ACC/AHA guidelines for the management of patients with ST-elevation myocardial infarction: a report of the American College of Cardiology/American Heart Association Task Force on Practice Guidelines (Committee to Revise the 1999 Guidelines on the Management of Patients With Acute Myocardial Infarction). *Circulation*. 2004;**110**(9):e82–e292.

17 Newby LK, Rutsch WR, Califf RM, *et al*. Time from symptom onset to treatment and outcomes after thrombolytic therapy. GUSTO-1 Investigators. *J Am Coll Cardiol*. June 1996;**27**(7):1646–1655.

18 Brodie BR, Stone GW, Morice MC, *et al*. Importance of time to reperfusion on outcomes with primary coronary angioplasty for acute myocardial infarction (results from the Stent Primary Angioplasty in Myocardial Infarction Trial). *Am J Cardiol*. November 15, 2001;**88**(10):1085–1090.

19 De Luca G, Suryapranata H, Ottervanger JP, Antman EM. Time delay to treatment and mortality in primary angioplasty for acute myocardial infarction: every minute of delay counts. *Circulation*. March 16, 2004; **109**(10):1223–1225.

20 De Luca G, Suryapranata H, Zijlstra F, *et al*. Symptom-onset-to-balloon time and mortality in patients with acute myocardial infarction treated by primary angioplasty. *J Am Coll Cardiol*. September 17, 2003;**42**(6): 991–997.

21 Rogers WJ, Canto JG, Barron HV, Boscarino JA, Shoultz DA, Every NR. Treatment and outcome of myocardial infarction in hospitals with and without invasive capability. Investigators in the National Registry of Myocardial Infarction. *J Am Coll Cardiol*. February 2000;**35**(2):371–379.

22 Krumholz HM, Chen J, Murillo JE, Cohen DJ, Radford MJ. Admission to hospitals with on-site cardiac catheterization facilities: impact on long-term costs and outcomes. *Circulation*. November 10, 1998;**98**(19): 2010–2016.

23 Llevadot J, Giugliano RP, Antman EM, *et al*. Availability of on-site catheterization and clinical outcomes in patients receiving fibrinolysis for ST-elevation myocardial infarction. *Eur Heart J*. November 2001;**22**(22): 2104–2115.

24 Magid DJ, Calonge BN, Rumsfeld JS, *et al*. Relation between hospital primary angioplasty volume and mortality for patients with acute MI treated with primary angioplasty vs thrombolytic therapy. *JAMA*. December 27, 2000;**284**(24):3131–3138.

25 Gibson CM. NRMI and current treatment patterns for ST-elevation myocardial infarction. *Am Heart J*. November 2004;**148**(5 Suppl):S29–S33.

26 Nallamothu BK, Bates ER, Herrin J, Wang Y, Bradley EH, Krumholz HM. Times to treatment in transfer patients undergoing primary percutaneous coronary intervention in the United States: National Registry of Myocardial Infarction (NRMI)-3/4 analysis. *Circulation*. February 15, 2005;**111**(6):761–767.

27 Nallamothu BK, Bates ER. Percutaneous coronary intervention versus fibrinolytic therapy in acute myocardial infarction: is timing (almost) everything? *Am J Cardiol*. October 1, 2003;**92**(7):824–826.

28 Pinto DS, Kirtane AJ, Nallamothu BK, *et al*. Hospital delays in reperfusion for ST-elevation myocardial infarction: implications when selecting a reperfusion strategy. *Circulation*. November 7, 2006;**114**(19): 2019–2025.

29 Topol EJ, Califf RM, George BS, *et al*. A randomized trial of immediate versus delayed elective angioplasty after intravenous tissue plasminogen activator in acute myocardial infarction. *N Engl J Med*. September 3, 1987;**317**(10):581–588.

30 The TIMI Study Group. Comparison of invasive and conservative strategies after treatment with intravenous tissue plasminogen activator in acute myocardial infarction. Results of the thrombolysis in myocardial infarction (TIMI) phase II trial. The TIMI Study Group. *N Engl J Med*. March 9, 1989;**320**(10):618–627.

31 The TIMI Research Group. Immediate vs delayed catheterization and angioplasty following thrombolytic therapy for acute myocardial infarction. TIMI II A results. The TIMI Research Group. *JAMA*. November 18, 1988;**260**(19):2849–2858.

32 Simoons ML, Arnold AE, Betriu A, *et al*. Thrombolysis with tissue plasminogen activator in acute myocardial infarction: no additional benefit from immediate percutaneous coronary angioplasty. *Lancet*. January 30, 1988;**1**(8579):197–203.

33 Michels KB, Yusuf S. Does PTCA in acute myocardial infarction affect mortality and reinfarction rates? A quantitative overview (meta-analysis) of the randomized clinical trials. *Circulation*. January 15, 1995;**91**(2): 476–485.

34 Ross AM, Coyne KS, Reiner JS, *et al*. A randomized trial comparing primary angioplasty with a strategy of short-acting thrombolysis and immediate planned rescue angioplasty in acute myocardial infarction: the PACT trial. PACT investigators. Plasminogen-activator Angioplasty Compatibility Trial. *J Am Coll Cardiol*. December 1999; **34**(7):1954–1962.

35 Scheller B, Hennen B, Hammer B, *et al*. Beneficial effects of immediate stenting after thrombolysis in acute myocardial infarction. *J Am Coll Cardiol*. August 20, 2003;**42**(4):634–641.

36 Fernandez Aviles F. GRACIA-2: PCI vs tenecteplase plus stenting in STEMI patients. Presented at the *Annual*

Meeting of the European Society of Cardiology. Vienna, Austria; 2003.

37 Le May MR, Wells GA, Labinaz M, *et al.* Combined angioplasty and pharmacological intervention versus thrombolysis alone in acute myocardial infarction (CAPITAL AMI study). *J Am Coll Cardiol.* August 2, 2005;**46**(3):417–424.

38 The ASSENT-4 PCI Investigators. Primary versus tenecteplase-facilitated percutaneous coronary intervention in patients with ST-segment elevation acute myocardial infarction (ASSENT-4 PCI): randomised trial. *Lancet.* February 18, 2006;**367**(9510):569–578.

39 Fernandez-Aviles F, Alonso JJ, Castro-Beiras A, *et al.* Routine invasive strategy within 24 hours of thrombolysis versus ischaemia-guided conservative approach for acute myocardial infarction with ST-segment elevation (GRACIA-1): a randomised controlled trial. *Lancet.* September 18, 2004;**364**(9439):1045–1053.

40 SWIFT trial of delayed elective intervention v conservative treatment after thrombolysis with anistreplase in acute myocardial infarction. SWIFT (Should We Intervene Following Thrombolysis?) Trial Study Group. *BMJ.* March 9, 1991;**302**(6776):555–560.

41 Alfonso F, Rodriguez P, Phillips P, *et al.* Clinical and angiographic implications of coronary stenting in thrombus-containing lesions. *J Am Coll Cardiol.* March 15, 1997;**29**(4):725–733.

42 Stone GW, Grines CL, Cox DA, *et al.* Comparison of angioplasty with stenting, with or without abciximab, in acute myocardial infarction. *N Engl J Med.* March 28, 2002;**346**(13):957–966.

43 Fernandez-Aviles F, Alonso JJ, Pena G, *et al.* Primary angioplasty vs. early routine post-fibrinolysis angioplasty for acute myocardial infarction with ST-segment elevation: the Gracia 2 non-inferiority, randomized, controlled trial. *Eur Heart J.* April 2007;**28**(8):949–960.

44 Keeley EC, Boura JA, Grines CL. Comparison of primary and facilitated percutaneous coronary interventions for ST-elevation myocardial infarction: quantitative review of randomised trials. *Lancet.* February 18, 2006;**367**(9510):579–588.

45 Smith SCJ, Feldman TE, Hirshfeld JWJ, *et al.* ACC/AHA/SCAI 2005 guideline update for percutaneous coronary intervention: a report of the American College of Cardiology/American Heart Association Task Force on Practice Guidelines (ACC/AHA/ACAI Writing Committee to Update the 2001 Guidelines for Percutaneous Coronary Intervention). American Heart Association Web Site. Available at http//www.americanheart.org. Accessed June 4, 2009.

46 Routine angioplasty and stenting after fibrinolysis for acute myocardial infarction. *Clinicaltrials.gov.* 2005. Available at http://www.clinicaltrials.gov/ct/gui/show/NCT00164190. Accessed June 4, 2009.

47 Ellis SG, Bates ER, Schaible T, Weisman HF, Pitt B, Topol EJ. Prospects for the use of antagonists to the platelet glycoprotein IIb/IIIa receptor to prevent post-angioplasty restenosis and thrombosis. *J Am Coll Cardiol.* May 1991;**17**(6 Suppl B):89B–95B.

48 Vivekananthan DP, Patel VB, Moliterno DJ. Glycoprotein IIb/IIIa antagonism and fibrinolytic therapy for acute myocardial infarction. *J Interv Cardiol.* April 2002;**15**(2):131–139.

49 Brener SJ, Barr LA, Burchenal JE, *et al.* Randomized, placebo-controlled trial of platelet glycoprotein IIb/IIIa blockade with primary angioplasty for acute myocardial infarction. ReoPro and Primary PTCA Organization and Randomized Trial (RAPPORT) Investigators. *Circulation.* August 25, 1998;**98**(8):734–741.

50 Montalescot G, Barragan P, Wittenberg O, *et al.* Platelet glycoprotein IIb/IIIa inhibition with coronary stenting for acute myocardial infarction. *N Engl J Med.* June 21, 2001;**344**(25):1895–1903.

51 Tcheng JE, Kandzari DE, Grines CL, *et al.* Benefits and risks of abciximab use in primary angioplasty for acute myocardial infarction: the Controlled Abciximab and Device Investigation to Lower Late Angioplasty Complications (CADILLAC) trial. *Circulation.* September 16, 2003;**108**(11):1316–1323.

52 Neumann FJ, Blasini R, Schmitt C, *et al.* Effect of glycoprotein IIb/IIIa receptor blockade on recovery of coronary flow and left ventricular function after the placement of coronary-artery stents in acute myocardial infarction. *Circulation.* December 15, 1998;**98**(24):2695–2701.

53 Neumann FJ, Kastrati A, Schmitt C, *et al.* Effect of glycoprotein IIb/IIIa receptor blockade with abciximab on clinical and angiographic restenosis rate after the placement of coronary stents following acute myocardial infarction. *J Am Coll Cardiol.* March 15, 2000;**35**(4):915–921.

54 Zorman S, Zorman D, Noc M. Effects of abciximab pretreatment in patients with acute myocardial infarction undergoing primary angioplasty. *Am J Cardiol.* September 1, 2002;**90**(5):533–536.

55 Maioli M, Bellandi F, Leoncini M, Toso A, Dabizzi RP. Randomized early versus late abciximab in acute myocardial infarction treated with primary coronary intervention (RELAx-AMI Trial). *J Am Coll Cardiol.* April 10, 2007;**49**(14):1517–1524.

56 Lee DP, Herity NA, Hiatt BL, *et al.* Adjunctive platelet glycoprotein IIb/IIIa receptor inhibition with tirofiban before primary angioplasty improves angiographic outcomes: results of the TIrofiban Given in the Emergency Room before Primary Angioplasty (TIGER-PA) pilot trial. *Circulation.* March 25, 2003;**107**(11):1497–1501.

57 Martinez-Rios MA, Rosas M, Gonzalez H, *et al.* Comparison of reperfusion regimens with or without tirofiban in ST-elevation acute myocardial infarction. *Am J Cardiol.* February 1, 2004;**93**(3):280–287.

58 van't Hof AW, Ernst N, de Boer MJ, *et al*. Facilitation of primary coronary angioplasty by early start of a glycoprotein 2b/3a inhibitor: results of the ongoing tirofiban in myocardial infarction evaluation (On-TIME) trial. *Eur Heart J*. May 2004;**25**(10):837–846.

59 Zeymer U, Zahn R, Schiele R, *et al*. Early eptifibatide improves TIMI 3 patency before primary percutaneous coronary intervention for acute ST elevation myocardial infarction: results of the randomized integrilin in acute myocardial infarction (INTAMI) pilot trial. *Eur Heart J*. October 2005;**26**(19):1971–1977.

60 Gibson CM, Kirtane AJ, Murphy SA, *et al*. Early initiation of eptifibatide in the emergency department before primary percutaneous coronary intervention for ST-segment elevation myocardial infarction: results of the Time to Integrilin Therapy in Acute Myocardial Infarction (TITAN)-TIMI 34 trial. *Am Heart J*. October 2006;**152**(4):668–675.

61 de Queiroz Fernandes Araujo JO, Veloso HH, Braga De Paiva JM, Filho MW, Vincenzo De Paola AA. Efficacy and safety of abciximab on acute myocardial infarction treated with percutaneous coronary interventions: a meta-analysis of randomized, controlled trials. *Am Heart J*. December 2004;**148**(6):937–943.

62 De Luca G, Suryapranata H, Stone GW, *et al*. Abciximab as adjunctive therapy to reperfusion in acute ST-segment elevation myocardial infarction: a meta-analysis of randomized trials. *JAMA*. April 13, 2005;**293**(14):1759–1765.

63 Montalescot G, Antoniucci D, Kastrati A, *et al*. Abciximab in primary coronary stenting of ST-elevation myocardial infarction: a European meta-analysis on individual patients' data with long-term follow-up. *Eur Heart J*. February 2007;**28**(4):443–449.

64 Antoniucci D, Rodriguez A, Hempel A, *et al*. A randomized trial comparing primary infarct artery stenting with or without abciximab in acute myocardial infarction. *J Am Coll Cardiol*. December 3, 2003;**42**(11):1879–1885.

65 Montalescot G, Borentain M, Payot L, Collet JP, Thomas D. Early vs late administration of glycoprotein IIb/IIIa inhibitors in primary percutaneous coronary intervention of acute ST-segment elevation myocardial infarction: a meta-analysis. *JAMA*. July 21, 2004;**292**(3):362–366.

66 Beeres SL, Oemrawsingh PV, Warda HM, *et al*. Early administration of abciximab in patients with acute myocardial infarction improves angiographic and clinical outcome after primary angioplasty. *Catheter Cardiovasc Interv*. August 2005;**65**(4):478-83.

67 Godicke J, Flather M, Noc M, *et al*. Early versus periprocedural administration of abciximab for primary angioplasty: a pooled analysis of 6 studies. *Am Heart J*. November 2005;**150**(5):1015.

68 Karvouni E, Katritsis DG, Ioannidis JP. Intravenous glycoprotein IIb/IIIa receptor antagonists reduce mortality after percutaneous coronary interventions. *J Am Coll Cardiol*. January 1, 2003;**41**(1):26–32.

69 Ellis SG, Armstrong P, Betriu A, *et al*. Facilitated percutaneous coronary intervention versus primary percutaneous coronary intervention: design and rationale of the Facilitated Intervention with Enhanced Reperfusion Speed to Stop Events (FINESSE) trial. *Am Heart J*. April 2004;**147**(4):E16.

70 Topol EJ. Reperfusion therapy for acute myocardial infarction with fibrinolytic therapy or combination reduced fibrinolytic therapy and platelet glycoprotein IIb/IIIa inhibition: the GUSTO V randomised trial. *Lancet*. June 16, 2001;**357**(9272):1905–1914.

71 Assessment of the Safety and Efficacy of a New Thrombolytic Regimen (ASSENT)-3 Investigators. Efficacy and safety of tenecteplase in combination with enoxaparin, abciximab, or unfractionated heparin: the ASSENT-3 randomised trial in acute myocardial infarction. *Lancet*. August 25, 2001;**358**(9282):605–613.

72 Maioli M, Gallopin M, Leoncini M, Bellandi F, Toso A, Dabizzi RP. Facilitated primary coronary intervention with abciximab and very low dose of alteplase during off-hours compared with direct primary intervention during regular hours. *Catheter Cardiovasc Interv*. August 2005;**65**(4):484–491.

73 Facilitated percutaneous coronary intervention for acute ST-segment elevation myocardial infarction: results from the prematurely terminated ADdressing the Value of facilitated ANgioplasty after Combination therapy or Eptifibatide monotherapy in acute Myocardial Infarction (ADVANCE MI) Investigators. *Am Heart J*. July 2005;**150**(1):116–122.

74 Kastrati A, Mehilli J, Schlotterbeck K, *et al*. Early administration of reteplase plus abciximab vs abciximab alone in patients with acute myocardial infarction referred for percutaneous coronary intervention: a randomized controlled trial. *JAMA*. February 25, 2004;**291**(8):947–954.

75 Sinno MC, Khanal S, Al-Mallah MH, Arida M, Weaver WD. The efficacy and safety of combination glycoprotein IIbIIIa inhibitors and reduced-dose thrombolytic therapy-facilitated percutaneous coronary intervention for ST-elevation myocardial infarction: a meta-analysis of randomized clinical trials. *Am Heart J*. April 2007;**153**(4):579–586.

76 Ryan TJ, Antman EM, Brooks NH, *et al*. 1999 update: ACC/AHA Guidelines for the Management of Patients With Acute Myocardial Infarction: Executive Summary and Recommendations: a report of the American College of Cardiology/American Heart Association Task Force on Practice Guidelines (Committee on Management of Acute Myocardial Infarction). *Circulation*. August 31, 1999;**100**(9):1016–1030.

CHAPTER 16

Streptokinase, alteplase, reteplase, or tenecteplase

Eric R. Bates

University of Michigan, Ann Arbor, MI, USA

Introduction

Acute thrombotic occlusion of a coronary artery usually results in ST-elevation myocardial infarction (STEMI), a major cause of cardiovascular morbidity and mortality. The goal of reperfusion therapy is to decrease STEMI complications by rapidly restoring complete and sustained infarct artery patency. When primary percutaneous coronary intervention is not immediately available, fibrinolytic therapy is recommended in patients with: (1) symptom onset within 12 h, (2) greater than 0.1 mV ST-segment elevation in at least two contiguous ECG leads or new left bundle branch block, and (3) low bleeding risk (1). By restoring infarct artery patency, fibrinolysis reduces infarct size, preserves left ventricular function, and decreases morbidity and mortality in patients with STEMI. This chapter will summarize information on the infusion (streptokinase and alteplase) and bolus (reteplase and tenecteplase) fibrinolytic agents. The characteristics of these drugs are shown in Table 16.1.

Streptokinase

Streptokinase is a single chain nonenzyme protein, which forms a 1:1 stoichiometric complex with

Pharmacology in the Catheterization Laboratory. Edited by Ron Waksman and Andrew E Ajani. © 2010 Blackwell Publishing, ISBN: 978-1-4051-5704-9.

plasminogen. The streptokinase–plasminogen activator complex then converts plasminogen to plasmin, which initiates fibrinolysis. The conventional intravenous dose is 1.5 million units over 60 min. Patency rates at 60 and 90 min are approximately 50% and 2–3 h patency rates are 70% (2).

The Gruppo Italiano per lo Studio della Streptochinasi nell'infarto Miocardico (GISSI)-1 (3) and International Study of Infarct Survival (ISIS)-2 (4) trials were the first properly powered trials to demonstrate the mortality advantage of intravenous fibrinolytic therapy. In the GISSI-1 trial, 11,712 patients were randomized to either intravenous streptokinase or control within 12 h of symptom onset. Only 21% of patients received anticoagulation therapy and only 14% received antiplatelet therapy. Mortality at 21 days was 10.7% in the streptokinase group vs 13% in the control group, an 18% risk reduction. The extent of the benefit was time-dependent, with relative reductions in inhospital mortality of 47% within 1 h of symptom onset, 23% within 3 h, and 21% within 6 h, but no benefit after 6 h. The benefit was maintained after hospital discharge up to 10 years, but there was no further mortality improvement (45.0% vs 46.9%) (5). The ISIS-2 trial randomized 17,187 patients within 24 h of the onset of symptoms of suspected MI to streptokinase, aspirin, both, or neither. Streptokinase alone reduced 5-week vascular mortality (9.2% vs 12%), a 23% risk reduction, and the combination of aspirin plus streptokinase additionally reduced

Table 16.1 Comparison of approved fibrinolytic agents.

Dose	Streptokinase 1.5 MU over 30–60 min	Alteplase Up to 100 mg in 90 min (based on weight)[a]	Reteplase 10 U over 2 min; repeat in 30 min	TNK-t-PA 30–50 mg (based on weight)[b]
Bolus administration	No	No	Yes	Yes
Antigenic	Yes	No	No	No
Allergic reactions (hypotension most common)	Yes	No	No	No
Systemic fibrinogen depletion	Marked	Mild	Moderate	Minimal
90-min patency rates (%)	~50%	~75%	~75%	~75%
TIMI grade 3 flow (%)	32%	54%	60%	63%
Cost per dose (3)	$613	$2,974	$2,750	$2,833 for 50 mg

Abbreviation: TIMI, Thrombolysis in Myocardial Infarction.

[a]Bolus 15 mg, infusion 0.75 mg/kg over 30 min (maximum 50 mg), then 0.5 mg/kg (maximum 35 mg) over the next 60 min to an overall maximum of 100 mg.

[b]30 mg for less than 60 kg; 35 mg for 60–69 kg; 40 mg for 70–79 kg; 45 mg for 80–89 kg; 50 mg for greater than or equal to 90 kg.

Source: Reprinted from Antman *et al*. (1).

mortality (8% vs 13.2%), a 39% risk reduction. Again, the benefit was maintained for 10 years, but did not change after 35 days (6).

Alteplase

Tissue plasminogen activator is a naturally occurring single-chain serine protease normally secreted by vascular endothelium. Native tissue plasminogen activator (t-PA) and alteplase (rt-PA) have a binding site for fibrin, which causes a great affinity for attaching to thrombus and preferentially lysing it, although systemic plasminogen activation occurs at clinical doses. The front-loaded or accelerated dosing recommendation is to give a bolus of 15 mg, followed by a 0.75 mg/kg infusion over 30 min (maximum 50 mg), and then a 0.5 mg/kg infusion over 60 min (maximum 35 mg). Ninety-minute patency rates are approximately 75% (Table 16.1).

The Anglo-Scandinavian Study of Early Thrombolysis (ASSET) (7,8) randomized 5,013 patients with less than 5 h of symptoms to alteplase or placebo. Although patients received intravenous heparin, aspirin was not given. At 1 month, mortality was reduced by 26% with alteplase (7.2% vs 9.8%). At 6 months, the rates were 10.4% with

alteplase and 13.1% with placebo. The effect was similar for anterior (15.6% vs 21.2%) and inferior (7.7% vs 12.8%) MI.

There have been two comparative trials of standard dose alteplase vs streptokinase. The GISSI-2 trial (9) tested a 3-h alteplase infusion and found no treatment advantage. The 12,490 patients from GISSI-2 were added to 8,401 recruited elsewhere to form the International Study (10), with no mortality difference between alteplase and streptokinase (8.9% vs 8.5%). Streptokinase was associated with fewer strokes and more allergic reactions and transfusions compared with alteplase.

In contrast, the Global Utilization of Streptokinase and Tissue Plasminogen Activator for Occluded Coronary Arteries trial (GUSTO)-I trial (11) tested the accelerated dose (two-thirds of the dose administered by 30 min instead of by 90 min) combined with intravenous heparin against streptokinase and found a significant mortality reduction (6.3% vs 7.3%) with alteplase. Also, there were significantly lower rates of heart failure, cardiogenic shock, sustained hypotension, asystole, atrioventricular block, atrial arrhythmias, and ventricular arrhythmias. There were two excess hemorrhagic strokes per 1,000 patients

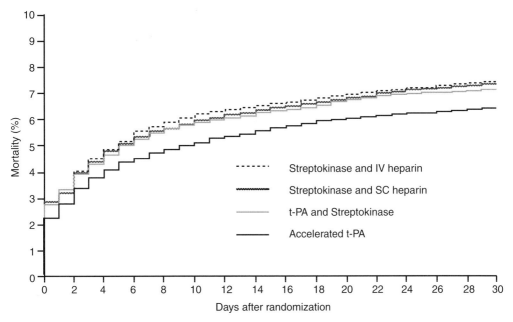

Figure 16.1 30-day mortality in the Global Utilization of Streptokinase and Tissue Plasminogen Activator for Occluded Coronary Arteries (GUSTO)-1 trial.

treated with alteplase, but the 30-day mortality or disabling stroke rate was lower with alteplase than streptokinase (6.9% vs 7.8%) (Figure 16.1). No real differences in bleeding were noted. At 1 year, the mortality advantage with alteplase was maintained (9.1% vs 10.1%) (12).

Reteplase

Reteplase (r-PA) is a mutant of alteplase in which the finger, kringle-1, and epidermal growth factor domains are removed. This results in decreased plasma clearance and less fibrin specificity. Reteplase is given as a double bolus of 10 units separated by 30 min, so it is easier to administer than alteplase and there may be fewer dosing errors. Patency rates are similar to alteplase (Table 16.1).

Reteplase was compared with streptokinase in the INJECT trial (13) where 6,010 patients with STEMI within 12 h of symptom onset were randomized. Thirty-five-day mortality with reteplase was at least equivalent to streptokinase (9.0% vs. 9.5%).

The GUSTO-III trial (14) was a superiority trial where 15,059 patients were randomized in a 2:1 ratio to reteplase or front-loaded alteplase. Mortality at 30 days was similar in both treatment

arms (7.47% vs 7.24%), as was the incidence of hemorrhagic stroke and major bleeding complications. Similar mortality rates were maintained for both treatment groups at 1-year follow-up (15).

The GUSTO-V trial randomized 16,588 patients to full-dose reteplase or half-dose reteplase (two boluses of 5 U) plus weight-adjusted abciximab (16). Thirty-day mortality rates were 5.9% for reteplase and 5.6% for combination therapy, fulfilling the criteria for noninferiority. Ischemic complications after STEMI were significantly reduced with combination therapy, but there were more moderate or severe nonintracranial bleeding complications (4.6% vs 2.3%). Intracranial hemorrhage rates were equal (0.6%), although the rate in patients above 75 years of age was almost twice as high with combination therapy (2.1% vs 1.1%).

Tenecteplase

Tenecteplase (TNK-t-PA) is also derived from alteplase. Mutations at three sites (T103, N117, KHRR296–299) increase plasma half-life, fibrin binding and specificity, and resistance to plasminogen activator inhibitor-1. Slower clearance allows convenient weight-adjusted single-bolus administration. Patency rates are similar to alteplase (Table 16.1).

In the ASSENT-2 trial (17), 16,949 patients were randomized to tenecteplase or front-loaded alteplase. Thirty-day mortality rates were equivalent (6.18% vs 6.15%) and remained so at 1-year follow-up (18). Intracranial hemorrhage rates were similar (0.93% vs 0.94%). Noncerebral bleeding complications and transfusions occurred less frequently with tenecteplase.

The effect of half-dose tenecteplase plus abciximab or full-dose tenecteplase with either unfractionated heparin or enoxaparin was studied in the ASSENT-3 trial (19). The primary end points were the composite of 30-day mortality, inhospital reinfarction, or refractory ischemia (primary efficacy end point), and the above plus inhospital intracranial hemorrhage or major bleeding (primary efficacy plus safety end point). Both enoxaparin and abciximab significantly reduced the risk for ischemic complications after treatment with tenecteplase, although 1-year mortality rates were similar across the three groups (20). Intracranial bleeding rates were also similar, but both major and minor bleeding complications were more frequent in the half-dose tenecteplase plus abciximab group. In the ExTRACT-TIMI 25 study (21), enoxaparin was associated with a significantly lower incidence of the composite endpoint of death, nonfatal reinfarction, or nonfatal intracranial hemorrhage compared with unfractionated heparin. Because LMWH offers several advantages over unfractionated heparin, including easier administration and no need for coagulation monitoring, the combination of tenecteplase and enoxaparin has emerged as the most attractive treatment strategy.

Complications

The major complication of fibrinolytic therapy is bleeding. The true incidence has been difficult to determine because of underreporting, the subjective nature of the events, different definitions for bleeding, and the variable use of invasive procedures. In GUSTO-I (11), the transfusion rate was 10%. Concomitant use of heparin increases bleeding risk, particularly when the aPTT exceeds 100 s (22). Many patients have conditions that increase the risk of serious bleeding and are absolute or relative contraindications for fibrinolytic therapy (Table 16.2) (1). Enoxaparin should be avoided in men with serum creatinine >2.0 mg/dL or in women with serum creatinine greater than 2.5 mg/dL, and in the morbidly obese. Bleeding rates are equivalent or higher compared with UFH (21).

When life-threatening bleeding occurs, heparin should be discontinued. Therapeutic interventions include protamine sulfate to normalize the aPTT, cryoprecipitate to increase fibrinogen levels, fresh frozen plasma to replace clotting factors, platelet transfusions if the bleeding time is prolonged, and packed red blood cells to restore hemoglobin mass. Protamine administration provides only partial reversal of the aPTT after enoxaparin. A computerized tomographic scan of the head should be performed to document suspected intracranial hemorrhage.

The most devastating complication of fibrinolytic therapy is intracerebral hemorrhage. The risk is 0.5–1%. At least half the patients die and severe disability occurs in an additional 25%. Increased risk is associated with age greater than 65 years, hypertension, and low bodyweight. More potent fibrinolytic agents increase risk. It is important to note, however, that fibrinolytic therapy decreases late, presumably thrombotic, stroke so there is no overall increase in stroke rates.

Streptokinase is antigenic. Because of antibody formation, retreatment should not be given after 4 days of the initial exposure to avoid neutralization of streptokinase activity. Moreover, mild allergic reactions (fever, rash, rigor, bronchospasm) occur in 5%, including anaphylactic shock in 0.2%, and release of bradykinin produces hypotension in 5–10%.

There does not appear to be any difference between agents in rates of recurrent ischemia (20%), reinfarction (4%), or bleeding.

Conclusion

Accelerated or front-loaded alteplase has proven to be as good as any fibrinolytic strategy tested to date in randomized clinical trials. Its superior ability to restore early normal blood flow to the infarct artery has been associated with lower mortality and morbidity rates than streptokinase.

Table 16.2 Contraindications and cautions for fibrinolytic use in STEMI.[a]

Absolute contraindications

- Any prior intracranial hemorrhage
- Known structural cerebral vascular lesion (e.g., AVM)
- Known malignant intracranial neoplasm (primary or metastatic)
- Ischemic stroke within 3 months EXCEPT acute ischemic stroke within 3 h
- Suspected aortic dissection
- Active bleeding or bleeding diathesis (excluding menses)
- Significant closed head or facial trauma within 3 months

Relative contraindications

- History of chronic severe poorly controlled hypertension
- Severe uncontrolled hypertension on presentation (SBP greater than 180 or DBP greater than 110 Hg)[b]
- History of prior ischemic stroke greater than 3 months, dementia, or known intracranial pathology not covered in contraindications
- Traumatic or prolonged (>10 min) CPR or major surgery (<3 weeks)
- Recent (within 2–4 weeks) internal bleeding
- Noncompressible vascular punctures
- For streptokinase/anistreplase: Prior exposure (especially within 5 days to 2 years) or prior allergic reaction to these agents
- Pregnancy
- Active peptic ulcer
- Current use of anticoagulants: the higher the INR, the higher the risk of bleeding

---

Abbreviations: AVN, arteriovenous malformation; INR, International Normalized Ratio; CPR, cardiopulmonary resuscitation; SBP, systolic blood pressure; DBP, diastolic blood pressure.

[a]Viewed as advisory for clinical decision-making and may not be all-inclusive or definitive.

[b]Could be an absolute contraindication in low-risk patients with myocardial infarction.

Source: Reprinted from Reference (1).

Bolus administration of reteplase or tenecteplase has not proven to be a more successful treatment strategy, but are more convenient to administer. Although primary PCI is considered to be the best reperfusion strategy, access is limited to those who live in proximity to hospitals with PCI capability: fibrinolytic therapy is more frequently utilized throughout the world. Moreover, delays in time-to-treatment decrease the benefits of primary PCI seen in randomized clinical trials and no differences in mortality rates between primary PCI and fibrinolytic therapy have been documented in registry reports (23).

Prehospital fibrinolytic therapy may be the best reperfusion strategy because the majority of patients can be treated within 2 h of symptom onset (23,24). Rescue PCI to improve early patency rates in patients with unsuccessful fibrinolytic therapy and clopidogrel, enoxaparin, and an early cardiac catheterization strategy with PCI to decrease reocclusion and reinfarction rates are other interventions that make fibrinolytic therapy competitive with a primary PCI strategy (25).

The major reductions in clinical events over the past two decades with improved reperfusion and adjunctive therapies have made it increasingly difficult to show incremental benefit with any new agent. The next major reduction in adverse events with STEMI will probably come from organizing better systems of care that allow more patients to receive reperfusion therapy with faster times-to-treatment.

References

1 Antman EM, Anbe DT, Armstrong PW, *et al.* ACC/AHA guidelines for the management of patients with ST-elevation myocardial infarction–executive summary: a report of the

American College of Cardiology/American Heart Association Task Force on Practice Guidelines (Writing Committee to Revise the 1999 Guidelines for the Management of Patients With Acute Myocardial Infarction). *Circulation*. 2004;**110**:588–636.

2 Granger CB, White H, Bates ER, *et al*. Patency profiles and left ventricular function after intravenous thrombolysis: a pooled analysis. *Am J Cardiol*. 1994;**74**:1220–1228.

3 Gruppo Italiano per lo Studio della Streptochinasi nell'infarto Miocardico (GISSI). Effectiveness of intravenous thrombolytic treatment in acute myocardial infarction. *Lancet*. 1986;**1**:397–401.

4 ISIS-2 (Second International Study of Infarct Survival) Collaborative Group. Randomised trial of intravenous streptokinase, oral aspirin, both, or neither among 17,187 cases of suspected acute myocardial infarction: ISIS-2. *Lancet*. 1988;**2**:349–360.

5 Franzosi MG, Santoro E, De Vita C, *et al*. Ten-year follow-up of the first megatrial testing thrombolytic therapy in patients with acute myocardial infarction; results of the Gruppo Italiano per lo studio della Sopravvivenza nell'infarto-1 study. The GISSI Investigators. *Circulation*. 1998;**98**:2659–2665.

6 Baigent C, Collins R, Appleby P, *et al*. ISIS-2: 10 year survival among patients with suspected acute myocardial infarction in randomized comparison of intravenous steptokinase, oral aspirin, both, or neither. *BMJ*. 1998;**316**:1337–1343.

7 Wilcox RG, von der Lippe G, Olsson CG, *et al*. Trial of tissue plasminogen activator for mortality reduction in acute myocardial infarction: the Anglo-Scandinavian Study of Early Thrombolysis (ASSET). *Lancet*. 1988; **2**:525–530.

8 Wilcox RG, von der Lippe G, Olsson CG, *et al*. Effects of alteplase in acute myocardial infarction: 6-month results from the ASSET study. *Lancet*. 190;**335**:1175–1178.

9 Gruppo Italiano per lo Studio Della Sopravvivenza nell'infarto Miocardico. GISSI-2: a factorial randomised trial of alteplase versus streptokinase and heparin versus no heparin among 12,490 patients with acute myocardial infarction. *Lancet*. 1990;**336**:65–71.

10 International Study Group. In-hospital mortality and clinical course of 20,891 patients with suspected acute myocardial infarction randomized between alteplase and streptokinase with or without heparin. *Lancet*. 1990;**336**:71–75.

11 The GUSTO Investigators: An international randomized trial comparing four thrombolytic strategies for acute myocardial infarction. *N Engl J Med*. 1993;**329**:673–682.

12 Califf RM, White HD, van de Werf F, *et al*. One-year results from the Global Utilization of Streptokinase and TPA for Occluded Coronary Arteries (GUSTO-1) trial. *Circulation*. 1996;**94**:1233–1238.

13 International Joint Efficacy Comparison of Thrombolytics. Randomised, double-blind comparison of reteplase double-bolus administration with streptokinase in acute myocardial infarction (INJECT): trial to investigate equivalence. *Lancet*. 1995;**346**:329–336.

14 The Global Use of Strategies to Open Occluded Coronary Arteries (GUSTO III) Investigators. A comparison of reteplase with alteplase for acute myocardial infarction. *N Engl J Med*. 1997;**337**:1118–1123.

15 Topol EJ, Ohman EM, Armstrong PW, *et al*. Survival outcomes 1 year after reperfusion therapy with either alteplase or reteplase for acute myocardial infarction: results from the Global Utilization of Streptokinase and t-PA for Occluded Coronary Arteries (GUSTO) III trial. *Circulation*. 2000;**102**:1761–1765.

16 The GUSTO-V Investigators. Reperfusion therapy for acute myocardial infarction with fibrinolytic therapy or combination reduced fibrinolytic therapy and platelet glycoprotein IIb/IIIa inhibition: the GUSTO V randomised trial. *Lancet*. 2001;**357**:1905–1914.

17 Assessment of the Safety and Efficacy of a New Thrombolytic Investigators. Single-bolus tenecteplase compared with front-loaded alteplase in acute myocardial infarction: the ASSENT-2 double-blind randomised trial. *Lancet*. 1999;**354**:716–722.

18 Sinnaeve P, Alexander J, Belmans A, *et al*. One-year follow-up of the ASSENT-2 trial: a double-blind, randomized comparison of single-bolus tenecteplase and front-loaded alteplase in 16,949 patients with ST-elevation acute myocardial infarction. *Am Heart J*. 2003;**146**:27–32.

19 The ASSENT-3 Investigators. Efficacy and safety of tenecteplase in combination with enoxaparin, abciximab, or unfractionated heparin: the ASSENT-3 randomised trial in acute myocardial infarction. *Lancet*. 2001; **358**:605–613.

20 Sinnaeve PR, Alexander JH, Bogaerts K, *et al*. Efficacy of tenecteplase in combination with enoxaparin, abciximab, or unfractionated heparin: one-year follow-up results of the Assessment of the Safety of a New Thrombolytic-3 (ASSENT-3) randomized trial in acute myocardial infarction. *Am Heart J*. 2004;**147**:993–998.

21 Antman EM, Morrow DA, McCabe CH, *et al*. Enoxaparin versus unfractionated heparin with fibrinolysis for ST-elevation myocardial infarction. *N Engl J Med*. 2006;**354**:1477–1488.

22 Granger CB, Hirsh J, Califf RM, *et al*. Activated partial thromboplastin time and outcome after thrombolytic therapy for acute myocardial infarction. Results from the GUSTO-I trial. *Circulation*. 1996;**93**:870–878.

23 Danchin N, Vaur L, Genes N, *et al*. Treatment of acute myocardial infarction by primary coronary angioplasty or intravenous thrombolysis in the "real world": one-year

results from a nationwide French survey. *Circulation.* 1999;**99**:2639–2644.

24 Steg PG, Bonnefoy E, Chabaud S, *et al.* Impact of time to treatment on mortality after prehospital fibrinolysis or primary angioplasty: data from the CAPTIM randomized clinical trial. *Circulation.* 2003;**108**:2851–2856.

25 Antman EM, Hand M, Armstrong PW, *et al.* 2007 focused update of the ACC/AHA 2004 Guidelines for the Management of Patients with ST-Elevation Myocardial Infarction: a report of the American College of Cardiology/American Heart Association Task Force on Practice Guidelines (Writing Group to Review New Evidence and Update the ACC/AHA 2004 Guidelines for the Management of Patients With ST-Elevation Myocardial Infarction). *J Am Coll Cardiol.* 2008;**51**:210–247.

CHAPTER 17

Intracoronary vs intravenous glycoprotein IIb/IIIa inhibitor use

Sanjiv Sharma[1,3], & Raj R. Makkar[2,3]

[1]Bakersfield Heart Hospital, Bakersfield, CA, USA
[2]Cedars-Sinai Medical Center, Los Angeles, CA, USA
[3]UCLA School of Medicine, Los Angeles, CA, USA

Introduction

The large-scale randomized controlled clinical studies documenting the safety and efficacy of the three clinically available glycoprotein IIb/III a inhibitors—Abciximab (ReoPro®), Eptifibatide (Integrilin®), and Tirofiban (Aggrastat®)—utilized intravenous administration of the drugs. Abciximab has been evaluated in comparative and randomized studies for intracoronary administration. Only case reports or unrandomized data exist for intracoronary use of Eptifibatide and Tirofiban. The data on intracoronary use of the glycoprotein IIb/IIIa (GP IIb/IIIa) inhibitors in the literature are reviewed.

Data from clinical studies

Abciximab

Abciximab reduces acute ischemic events by 35–56% at 30 days after percutaneous coronary intervention (PCI) (1–3), a benefit that persists long term with 22% reduction in mortality up to 3 years by combined analysis of EPIC, EPILOG, and EPISTENT trials (4). In acute myocardial infarction, abciximab opens the occluded artery, improves the success of stenting, reduces the rate of occlusion, and restores optimal flow for upto

Pharmacology in the Catheterization Laboratory. Edited by Ron Waksman and Andrew E Ajani. © 2010 Blackwell Publishing, ISBN: 978-1-4051-5704-9.

6 months, improving the left ventricular function and prognosis (ADMIRAL Study) (5).

In experimental animal studies, Mitchel *et al.* showed that intracoronary (IC) administration of abciximab leads to deposition of abciximab at the angioplasty site (6) and enhanced lysis of platelet-rich thrombi (7). Case reports have shown that IC abciximab dissolves intracoronary thrombus and resolves acute closure during PCI (8–13). Case series employing IC abciximab in the high-risk PCI, specifically in situations where there is anticipation of high embolic load from thrombus/plaque burden at the site of the culprit lesion, saphenous vein graft lesions, threatened abrupt closure, developing slow-flow/no reflow-phenomena with distal embolization (14) showed procedural success without any adverse side effects.

Retrospective studies have compared intracoronary (IC) to intravenous (IV) bolus abciximab administration in the setting of PCI. Wöhrle *et al.* retrospectively compared IC to IV abciximab bolus administration in patients with acute myocardial infarction (AMI) or unstable angina undergoing PCI (15). They found a 50% reduction of major adverse cardiac events (MACE) at 30 days in the IC group ($n = 294$) as compared with the IV group ($n = 109$) (10.2% vs 20.2% respectively, $P < 0.008$)—with significant reduction in all individual components of MACE (urgent revascularization, recurrent myocardial infarction, and death). The effect was most pronounced in patients with TIMI 0/1 flow, and not much different between the groups in patients with TIMI 2/3 flow. Kakkar *et al.* reported that the beneficial effects of IC ($n = 101$) over IV ($n = 72$) abciximab administration in coronary stenting persisted up to 6 months, when measured as a composite end point of death or myocardial infarction (5.9% vs 13.9 %, $P = 0.04$), without any increase in bleeding complications (16). Sharma *et al.* found that intragraft administration of abciximab combined with direct stenting prevents slow-flow and no-reflow phenomena in saphenous vein graft interventions (17).

Prospective randomized studies

Bellandi *et al.* prospectively randomized patients with AMI and occluded infarct-related artery undergoing primary PCI, to a strategy of IC bolus of abciximab through a dual lumen catheter after crossing the occlusion with a guidewire ($n = 22$), or the usual IV administration ($n = 23$) protocol (18). There was no difference in the short-term MACE. The corrected TIMI frame count (CTFC) and myocardial blush grade (MBG) were significantly better in the IC group. The final infarct size measured by serial perfusion technetium sestamibi SPECT scans (at 6 h, 7 and 30 days) was significantly smaller in the IC group, reflecting a greater degree of myocardial salvage. The ejection fraction improvement was greater in the IC group at the end of 1 month ($14.7 \pm 6.8\%$ vs $8 \pm 6.4\%$; $P = 0.013$).

Romagnoli *et al.* prospectively evaluated the coronary blood flow measured by the corrected TIMI frame count (CTFC) in the culprit vessel and nonculprit vessel of patients undergoing PCI for acute coronary syndromes who received IC bolus of abciximab ($n = 37$) (19). These patients were also compared to 37 matched controls who received only IV abciximab. The CTFC decreased significantly in the culprit vessel after IC abciximab from $48 + 37$ to $33 + 30$ ($p = 0.001$) while in the nonculprit, vessel it remained unchanged ($16 + 7$ pretreatment and $16 + 7$ post treatment, $p = 0.68$). The immediate post-IC bolus CTFC ($33 + 30$) was much lower than the CTFC after IV bolus ($49 + 48$) ($P = 0.001$), a benefit that persisted in the final CTFC as well IC group CTFC ($12 + 4$) vs IV group CTFC ($14 + 5$) ($P = 0.069$), with a trend toward lower posttreatment cardiac enzyme elevation in the IC group. This improvement in coronary angiographic flow occurred mostly in patients with angiographic evidence of thrombus and impaired antegrade coronary flow (TIMI 0 or 1).

In a prospective randomized trial of patients undergoing PCI, Osuna *et al.* compared the primary end point of major adverse cardiac events MACE (death, myocardial infarction, need for revascularization) and secondary end points of hemorrhagic complications and the troponin I level in patients randomized to receive IC abciximab ($n = 72$) or IV abciximab ($n = 65$) (20). They found no statistically significant difference between the MACE at 1 year; however, the level of myocardial injury marker troponin I was significantly decreased with IC abciximab as compared to IV administration. The likely difference between the study of Osuna *et al.* showing no difference in MACE and the retrospective studies by Wohrle and Kakkar *et al.* showing a benefit in short-term and medium-term MACE may relate to the a higher percentage of patients with TIMI 2–3 flow (about 90%) in the Osuna *et al.* study. Both the Osuna and Bellandi studies found that the level of myocardial injury (measured by different parameters) was decreased by IC administration of the drug.

Eptifibatide

In the ESPRIT trial, patients undergoing coronary stenting had a reduction of death, myocardial infarction, and urgent target vessel revascularization with the use of eptifibatide administered intravenously, a benefit that persisted long term (21,22).

A retrospective study of 59 patients with ST elevation myocardial infarction undergoing primary PCI who received IC eptifibatide (23) showed no adverse events. Normal TIMI 3 flow was achieved in 54% of patients. There were no deaths, reinfarctions, or urgent revascularizations. The same authors retrospectively analyzed data from 54 patients with unstable angina and non-ST elevation myocardial infarction undergoing PCI receiving IC eptifibatide (24). There was one myocardial infarction, though no deaths or urgent revascularizations. IC eptifibatide was shown to resolve no-reflow phenomenon in a case report of vein graft intervention (25). There are no studies comparing IC to IV administration of eptifibatide reported in the literature.

Tirofiban

In the RESTORE study, intravenous administration of tirofiban led to a reduction in the composite end points of death, MI, or refractory ischemia or repeat revascularization in patients undergoing PCI for acute coronary syndromes (26). There is one case report of treatment of no-reflow phenomenon after native coronary stenting with IC tirofiban (27). There is no comparative data on IC vs IV use of tirofiban in the literature.

Dose dependant effects of GP IIb/IIIa inhibitors and rationale for Intracoronary administration

IC bolus injection through the guiding catheter may achieve several fold higher concentration of the drug than with IV bolus. The ratio of IC to IV administered concentration of the drug at the lesion site may vary from 280:1 (minimal wash-out) and 1:1 (normal flow), depending upon the relation between inflow and washout from the residual perfusion and the size of the ischemic area (15). When coronary flow is significantly decreased, the IV administered drug may not reach the culprit lesion or the distal coronary bed until recanalization has been achieved, thereby limiting its beneficial effects.

The GP IIb/IIIa receptor is the final common pathway for platelet aggregation, with about 50,000–100,000 receptors on each platelet. One molecule of abciximab binds to a single GP IIb/IIIa receptor noncompetitively and firmly, causing steric hindrance. Eptifibatide and tirofiban bind competitively and reversibly to the RGD sequence of the GP IIb/IIIa receptor. There are several fold (>250) tirofiban and eptifibatide drug molecules per receptor (28). All agents exhibit dose-dependent inhibition of platelet function. Platelet inhibition starts at >50% receptor occupancy and is nearly complete at greater than 80% receptor occupancy.

GP IIb/IIIa inhibitors lead to a potent inhibition of platelet aggregation and thrombus formation at the site of the unstable or injured plaque. The drugs dissolve platelet-rich thrombi (dethrombosis) by competitive removal of fibrinogen (29), prevent platelet microembolization, improve microvascular perfusion, and suppress reperfusion injury and inflammation (30–32). In addition, abciximab binds to other integrin receptors (vitronectin and Mac-1), causing inhibition of the interaction between platelets and leukocytes, thus limiting the inflammatory response to PCI (4,31).

There is a dose–response in the effect of abciximab, eptifibatide, and tirofiban on fibrinolysis, platelet disaggregation, and other effects (29). High local doses of the drug allows diffusion of the drug inside the flow limiting thrombi, facilitating dethrombosis of thrombi at the culprit lesion and microemboli in distal microcirculation (4,15). These effects are likely beneficial in limiting distal embolization, microcirculatory dysfunction, reperfusion injury, local inflammation, and myocardial damage (30–32).

Dosage for intracoronary use

The dose of abciximab used in most studies was 0.25 mg/kg bolus through the guiding catheter (14,16–18). Some studies have employed a single dose of 5–20 mg abciximab (8,9,15). Some authors used an infusion catheter (8) or delivered the drug downstream to the occlusion through a dual lumen catheter (18). In the case series on IC eptifibatide, one or two boluses of 180 mcg/kg, were delivered through the guiding catheter (23,24). Eptifibatide is supplied in a vehicle that contains citric acid, with an acidic pH of 5.35 though no adverse events have been reported with IC administration (23). The pH of tirofiban is 5.5–6.5. There is only one case report where tirofiban 10 mcg/kg was administered through the guiding catheter (27). The dose of eptifibatide and tirofiban is adjusted in patients with renal insufficiency.

Summary of the data

A greater and more rapid platelet inhibition possibly ensues after IC administration of GP IIb/IIIa inhibitors. IC abciximab dissolves thrombus and resolves acute closure during PCI by causing platelet dethrombosis at the culprit lesion site. IC abciximab, eptifibatide, and tirofiban have been shown to treat and prevent slow-flow phenomenon in small studies or case reports, which signifies a benefit in treating distal embolization. The prevention of distal embolization, platelet plugging, associated microvascular dysfunction, and local inflammation reported with abciximab may account for the improvement in coronary flow and may make the process of reperfusion less damaging to the myocardium. This accounts for the decrease in myocardial damage seen after IC abciximab. These effects may translate into lower risk of major adverse cardiac events reported on short-term and long-term follow-up with IC abciximab. In most of these studies, the effects of IC abciximab are more pronounced when there is a decreased coronary flow and presence of thrombus. Data on IC eptifibatide are limited only to its safety of administration by IC route; efficacy data are not available. Tirofiban use by IC route has been reported in only one case report.

It may be reasonable to employ IC GP IIb/IIIa inhibitors in situations where there is presence of thrombus, or a high embolic load is anticipated or the coronary flow is diminished. This approach is safe, feasible, and possibly more effective, though larger randomized trials are required to validate the results of the pilot studies.

References

1 The EPIC Investigators. Use of monoclonal antibody directed against the platelet glycoprotein IIb/IIIa receptor in high-risk coronary angioplasty. *N Engl J Med.* 1994;**330**: 956–961.

2 The EPILOG Investigators. Platelet glycoprotein IIb/IIIa receptor blockade and low-dose heparin during percutaneous coronary revascularization. *N Engl J Med.* 1997;**336**:1689–1697.

3 Lincoff AM, Califf RM, Moliterno DJ, *et al.* Complimentary clinical benefits of coronary-artery stenting and blockade of platelet glycoprotein IIb/IIIa receptors. *N Engl J Med.* 1999;**341**:319–327.

4 Quinn MJ, Plow EF, Topol EJ. Platelet glycoprotein IIb/IIIa inhibitors. Recognition of a two edged sword? *Circulation.* 2002;**106**:379–385.

5 Montalescot G, Barragan P, Wittenberg O, *et al.* Platelet glycoprotein IIb/IIIa inhibition with coronary stenting for acute myocardial infarction. *N Engl J Med.* 2001;**344**:1895–1903.

6 Mitchel JF, Alberghini TV. Site specific thrombolysis with Reopro. *Circulation.* 1996;**94**:I 202.

7 Mitchel JF, Alberghini TV. Local delivery of Reopro: pharmacokinetics and effect on platelet deposition following balloon angioplasty. *Circulation.* 1996;**94**:I 202.

8 Bailey SR, O'Leary E, Chilton R. Angioscopic evaluation of site-specific administration of ReoPro. *Catheter Cardiovasc Diagn.* 1997;**42**:181–184.

9 Bartorelli AL, Trabattoni D, Galli S, Grancini L, Cozzi S, Ravagnani P. Successful dissolution of occlusive coronary thrombus with local administration of abciximab during PTCA. *Catheter Cardiovasc Interv.* 1999;**48**:211–213.

10 Sharma S, Bhambi B, Nyitray W, *et al.* Bivalirudin (Angiomax) use during intracoronary brachytherapy may predispose to acute closure. *J Cardiovasc Pharmacol Therap.* 2003;**8**:9–15.

11 Schlaifer JD, Horgan W, Malkowski MJ. Acute thrombotic occlusion of the left main coronary artery in a hypercoagulable patient treated with intracoronary abciximab. *Clin Cardiol.* 2001;**24**:788.

12 Thuraisingham S, Tan KH. Dissolution of thrombus formed during direct coronary angioplasty with a single 10 mg intracoronary bolus dose of abciximab. *Int J Clin Pract.* 1999;**53**:604–607.

13 Hang LC, Thye HK, Cheem TH. Instant dissolution of intracoronary thrombus by abciximab. *Int J Cardiol.* 2005;**104**:102–103.

14 Sharma S, Makkar R, Ladizabal J. Intracoronary administration of abciximab during percutaneous coronary interventions: should this be the routine and preferred approach? *J Cardiovac Pharmacol Ther.* 2006;**11**:136–141.

15 Wöhrle J, Grebe OC, Nusser T, *et al.* Reduction of major adverse cardiac events with intracoronary compared with intravenous bolus application of abciximab in patients with acute myocardial infarction or unstable angina undergoing coronary angioplasty. *Circulation.* 2003;**107**:1840–1843.

16 Kakkar AK, Moustapha A, Hanley HG, *et al.* Comparison of intracoronary vs. intravenous administration of abciximab in coronary stenting. *Catheter Cardiovasc Interv.* 2004;**61**:31–34.

17 Sharma S, Bhambi B, Nyitray W, *et al.* Intragraft administration of abciximab and verapamil combined with direct stenting prevents slow-flow during saphenous vein graft percutaneous coronary interventions. *Am J Cardiol.* 2002;**90**:154 H.

18 Bellandi F, Maioli M, Gallopin M, Toso A, Dabizzi RP. Increase of myocardial salvage and left ventricular function recovery with intracoronary abciximab downstream of the coronary occlusion in patients with acute myocardial infarction treated with primary coronary intervention. *Catheter Cardiovasc Interv.* 2004; **62**:186–192.

19 Romagnoli E, Burzotta F, Trani C, *et al.* Angiographic evaluation of the effect of intracoronary abciximab administration in patients undergoing urgent PCI. *Int J Cardiol.* 2005;**105**:250–255.

20 Galache Osuna JG, Sanchez-Rubio J, Calvo I, *et al.* Does intracoronary abciximab improve the outcome of

percutaneous coronary interventions? A randomized controlled trial. *Rev Esp Cardiol.* 2006;**59**:567–574.

21 ESPRIT investigators. Novel dosing regimen of eptifibatide in planned coronary stent implantation (ESPRIT): a randomised, placebo-controlled trial. *Lancet.* 2000;**356**:2037–2044.

22 O'Shea JC, Buller CE, Cantor WJ, *et al.* Long-term efficacy of platelet glycoprotein IIb/IIIa integrin blockade with eptifibatide in coronary stent intervention. *JAMA.* 2002;**287**:618–621.

23 Pinto DS, Kirtane AJ, Ruocco NA, *et al.* Administration of intracoronary eptifibatide during ST-elevation myocardial infarction. *Am J Cardiol.* 2005;**96**:1494–1497.

24 Deibele AJ, Kirtane AJ, Pinto DE, *et al.* Intracoronary bolus administration of eptifibatide during percutaneous coronary stenting for non ST elevation myocardial infarction and unstable angina. *J Thromb Thrombolysis.* 2006;**22**:47–50.

25 Iancu AC, Lazar A. Successful management of the no-reflow syndrome after venous graft stenting. *J Invasive Cardiol.* 2005;**17**:E50–E51.

26 The RESTORE Investigators. Effects of platelet glycoprotein IIb/IIIa blockade with tirofiban on adverse cardiac events in patients with unstable angina or acute myocardial infarction undergoing coronary angioplasty. *Circulation.* 1997;**96**:1445–1453.

27 Yang TY, Chang ST, Chung CM, *et al.* Restoration of normal coronary flow with tirofiban by intracoronary administration for no-reflow phenomenon after stent deployment. *Int Heart J.* 2005;**46**:139–145.

28 Schror K, Weber AA. Comparative pharmacology of GP IIb/IIIa antagonists. *J Thromb Thrombolysis.* 2003;**15**:71–80.

29 Moser M, Bertram U, Peter K, *et al.* Abciximab, eptifibatide, and tirofiban exhibit dose-dependent potencies to dissolve platelet aggregates. *J Cardiovac Pharmacol.* 2003;**41**:586–592.

30 Prati F, Kwiatkowski P, Caroselli C, *et al.* Use of abciximab prevents microcirculatory impairment in patients treated with coronary angioplasty for unstable angina: Results of a prospective randomized study. *Catheter Cardiovasc Interv.* 2005;**66**:165–169.

31 Lincoff AM, Kereiakes DJ, Mascelli MA, *et al.* Abciximab suppresses the rise in levels of circulating inflammatory markers after percutaneous coronary revascularization. *Circulation.* 2001;**104**:163–167.

32 Aymong ED, Curtis MJ, Youssef M, *et al.* Abciximab attenuates coronary microvascular endothelial dysfunction after coronary stenting. *Circulation.* 2002;**105**:2981–2985.

CHAPTER 18

Upstream vs procedural use of glycoprotein IIb/IIIa inhibitors in acute coronary syndromes

Ralph Wessel[1] & John A. Ambrose[1,2]

[1]UCSF Fresno, Fresno, CA, USA
[2]University of California, San Francisco, CA, USA

Role of platelets in pathogenesis of acute coronary syndrome

Platelets play a key role in the pathogenesis of acute coronary syndromes. Platelet thrombus forms as a result of fibrous cap disruption or erosion, and percutaneous coronary intervention itself may initiate or potentiate this process. Exposure of Von Willebrand's factor and collagen in the subendothelial matrix initiates platelet adhesion to the vessel wall and leads to activation of the platelet, resulting in the activation of the glycoprotein IIb/IIIa (GP IIb/IIIa) receptor. This receptor, which is abundantly represented on the surface of the platelet when activated, binds either fibrinogen or Von Willebrand's factor linking one platelet to another. The aggregated platelets form a "white thrombus." The platelet-rich thrombus ordinarily is nonocclusive and if clinically symptomatic, may be the immediate cause of non-ST-elevation myocardial infarction (NSTEMI) or unstable angina. The platelet-rich thrombus can also embolize into the distal coronary arterial bed, which may potentiate myocardial ischemia or infarction. The activation of the GP IIb/IIIa receptor is the single final pathway leading to platelet aggregation and platelet-rich thrombus formation. Inhibition of the GP IIb/IIIa receptor is a logical and effective strategy in the

Pharmacology in the Catheterization Laboratory. Edited by Ron Waksman and Andrew E Ajani. © 2010 Blackwell Publishing, ISBN: 978-1-4051-5704-9.

management of acute coronary syndromes and during percutaneous coronary interventions.

Glycoprotein IIb/IIIa inhibitors

Four GP IIb/IIIa inhibitors have been developed and studied for use in the management of acute coronary syndromes and during percutaneous coronary interventions. Three of these agents are available for clinical use in North America. These are abciximab (ReoPro), eptifibatide (Integrelin), and tirofiban (Aggrastat). Lamifiban is available outside of North America.

The first agent developed was abciximab. It is the most extensively studied GP IIb/IIIa inhibitor. As a monoclonal antibody fragment, it is a large molecule made up of a portion of mouse-derived Fab fragment linked to a human immunoglobulin G Fab moiety. Due to its high-affinity binding to the GP IIb/IIIa receptor, it has a low dissociation constant. It has a prolonged antiplatelet effect after cessation of its infusion, which persists up to 2 weeks after discontinuation of treatment. Abciximab is avidly bound to the GP IIb/IIIa receptor, leaving little free abciximab circulating in the plasma, which allows for rapid reversal of its antiplatelet effect with platelet transfusions that increase the pool of circulating platelets and their available unbound GP IIb/IIIa receptors.

Eptifibatide, tirofiban, and lamifiban are small-molecule, synthetic, GP IIb/IIIa inhibitors with low affinity but high specificity for the GP IIb/IIIa receptor. They are competitive inhibitors with rapid reversibility that results in large amounts of the drug circulating in the plasma at steady state. Due to the large quantities of unbound drug, platelet transfusion is not effective in reversing antiplatelet effects. These agents are eliminated with first-order kinetics and have a short duration of platelet inhibition of only a few hours after discontinuation of their infusion as long as kidney function is normal.

There are significant cost differences between abciximab and the small-molecule inhibitors with a course of abciximab being approximately 3–4 times the cost of the small-molecule agents for their recommended infusion strategies and cost-effectiveness for quality-adjusted life-year added (1).

As eptifibatide and tirofiban are excreted by the kidneys, they require dosing adjustments in patients with renal insufficiency. Dosing guideline for use of GP IIb/IIIa inhibitors are shown in Table 18.1.

Guidelines for therapy of acute coronary syndrome: Early invasive verse conservative selective invasive approach and use of glycoprotein IIb/IIIa inhibitors

Prior to availability of GP IIb/IIIa inhibitors and intracoronary stents, a routine early invasive strategy for the management non-ST-elevation acute coronary syndromes compared to an conservative selective invasive approach appeared not to be beneficial and possible harmful as suggested in the Veterans Affair Non-Q Wave Infarction Strategies In-Hospital (VANQWISH) trial (2). With the introduction of GP IIb/IIIa inhibitors and intracoronary stents, the balance shifted to demonstrate the superiority of an early invasive strategy in most randomized clinical trials.

The FRagmin and Fast Revascularization during Instability in Coronary artery disease (FRISC II) study (3) randomized acute coronary syndrome patients to a (delayed) routine invasive strategy within the first 7 days or a noninvasive strategy and either to dalteparin, a low-molecular-weight heparin (LMWH), or placebo. There was a significant decrease in the composite end point of

Table 18.1 Dosing guidelines for GP IIb/IIIa inhibitors.

In Acute Coronary Syndromes:
- Eptifibatide (Integrilin)
- Bolus of 180 µg/kg followed by 2 µg/kg/min IV infusion for up to 72 h
- Tirofiban (Aggrastat)
- Bolus of 0.4 µg/kg/min (given over 30 min) followed by a 0.1 µg/kg/min IV
- Infusion for up to 72 h

During PCI:
- Abciximab (Reopro)
- Bolus of 0.25 mg/kg followed by a 0.125 µg/kg/min IV infusion for 12 h
- Eptifibatide (Integrilin)
- Double bolus of 180 mg/kg (10 min apart) followed by 2 µg/kg/min IV infusion
- Infusion for 18–24 h
- Tirofiban (Aggrastat)
- Bolus of 10 µg/kg followed by 0.15 µg/kg/min IV infusion for 24 h

With Renal Insufficiency:
- Eptifibatide (Integrilin)
- If CrCl <50 mL/min reduce continuous IV infusion to 1 µg/kg/min
- Contraindicated in patients on renal dialysis
- Tirofiban (Aggrastat)
- Decrease bolus and infusion dose to 50% if CrCl <30 mL/min
- Abciximab (Reopro)
- No dose adjustment needed. Not dependent on renal excretion

death or myocardial infarction in patients with signs of ischemia on ECG or elevated biochemical markers of myocardial damage with the routine invasive strategy. Early revascularization was associated with a nonstatistically significant higher risk of early death and myocardial infarction because of procedure-related events which were offset by a lower risk of spontaneous events after revascularization.

The Treat angina with Aggrastat and determine Cost of Therapy with Invasive or Conservative Strategy—Thrombolysis In Myocardial Infarction 18 (TACTICS-TIMI 18) trial (4) in which more than 90% of the early invasive patients were treated with a GP IIb/IIIa inhibitor (tirofiban) and more than 80% had intracoronary stents deployed revealed a significant benefit of the early invasive approach. The primary composite end point of death, nonfatal MI, and rehospitalization for ACS at 6 months was significantly reduced from 19.4% with the conservative strategy to 15.9% with the early invasive strategy ($p = 0.025$). The benefit of an early invasive strategy in reducing the primary composite end point at 6 months was only seen in patients with an elevated troponin T with 14.8% in the invasive strategy and 24.3% in the conservative strategy having a primary composite event ($p \leq 0.001$). There was no significant benefit in patients without troponin T elevation. Of the patients randomized to the invasive strategy, 97% underwent cardiac catheterization, out of which 41% proceeded to undergo percutaneous coronary intervention, 20% underwent coronary artery bypass grafting, while 39% received optimal medical therapy alone. The median time after randomization with the invasive strategy to catheterization was 22 h; to percutaneous coronary revascularization was 25 h; and to coronary artery bypass grafting was 89 h. In the conservative group, as a result of spontaneous or provoked recurrent ischemia, 51% underwent cardiac catheterization, 24% had percutaneous coronary intervention, and 13% had coronary artery bypass grafting. Tirofiban was administered in 94% of the patients in the invasive strategy and 59% in the conservative strategy for a duration of 48 and 50 h, respectively. The routine use of upstream GP IIb/IIIa in this trial may have eliminated the excess risk of an early acute MI (within 7 days) of an invasive strategy seen in FRISC II and other trials that did not routinely use upstream GP IIb/IIIa inhibition.

As a result of the FRISC II, TACTICS-TIMI 18, and other smaller studies, the ACC/AHA practice guidelines update for management of patients with unstable angina and non-ST-segment elevation myocardial infarction—2002 (5) gave its strongest recommendation of Class I (Level of Evidence: A) for an early invasive strategy in patients with UA/NSTE-MI and a high-risk indicator, including an elevated troponin (T or I) level (Table 18.2).

Additional contemporary randomized trials [Treatment of Refractory Unstable angina in Geographically isolated areas without Cardiac Surgery (TRUCS), Value of First Day Angiography/Angioplasty In Evolving Non-ST Segment Elevation Myocardial Infarction: An

Table 18.2 Selection of initial treatment strategy: invasive vs conservative strategy.

Preferred strategy	Patient characteristics
Invasive	Recurrent angina or ischemia at rest or with low-level activities despite intensive medical therapy
	Elevated cardiac biomarkers (TnT or TnI)
	New or presumable new ST-segment depression
	Signs or symptoms of HF or new or worsening mitral regurgitation
	High-risk findings from noninvasive testing
	Hemodynamic instability
	Sustained ventricular tachycardia
	PCI with 6 months
	Prior CABG
	High-risk score (e.g., TIMI, GRACE)
	Reduced left ventricular function (LVEF less than 40%)
Conservative	Low-risk score (e.g., TIMI, GRACE)
	Patient or physician preference in the absence of high-risk features

Abbreviations: CABG, coronary artery bypass graft surgery; GRACE, Global Registry of Acute Coronary Events; HF, heart failure; LVEF, left ventricular ejection fraction; PCI, percutaneous coronary intervention; TIMI, Thrombolysis in Myocardial Infarction; TnI, troponin I; TnT, troponin T.

Open Multicenter Randomized Trial (VINO), Randomized Intervention Trail of unstable Angina 3 trial (RITA-3), and Invasive vs Conservative Treatment in Unstable Coronary Syndromes (ICTUS)] (6–9) along with FRISC-II (3) and TACTICS-TIMI 18 (4) were reviewed in a meta-analysis by Bavry *et al.* (10) and confirmed the benefit of an early invasive strategy in the management of non-ST-segment elevation acute coronary syndromes with improvement in long-term survival and reduction of late myocardial infarction and rehospitalization for unstable angina.

It is of note that the most recently reported large randomized study (ICTUS) found no benefit for the routine invasive vs the selectively invasive approach (9). Furthermore, the ICTUS investigators (9) reported an increase in myocardial infarction with the early invasive strategy. We believe there are other possible causes for the increase in acute myocardial infarction seen in the invasive arm of this trial other than the obvious reason that early invasive strategy is detrimental. In this trial, this increase may be explained by the liberal definition of myocardial infarction, which was an elevation of the CK-MB above the upper limit of normal. The small elevations in CK-MB seen in the early invasive group may have been a function of the natural course of the delayed appearance of the CK-MB seen when percutaneous coronary intervention was performed soon after admission of a myocardial infarction (median of 20 h). The absence of a Clinical Events Committee (to adjudicate end points) in this trial, in our opinion, makes it difficult to interpret the significance of these small CK-MB bumps after percutaneous coronary intervention in patients presenting with chest pain and brought rapidly to the catheterization laboratory.

At 1 year, there was a high rate of revascularization in both groups in ICTUS: 79% in the invasive group (78% PCI, 22% CABG) and 54% in the conservative group (74% PCI, 26% CABG). This high rate of revascularization in the selectively invasive arm may have also diluted the benefit of an early invasive strategy as found in other trials with a lower rate of revascularization in the selectively invasive arm. Nevertheless, the incidence of spontaneous myocardial infarction in the follow-up of ICTUS demonstrated a trend toward reduction with the early invasive strategy. There was a significant reduction in rehospitalization due to angina at the 1-year follow-up with the early invasive strategy, although mortality was not different between the two strategies. In spite of these trial results, we do not believe that the results negate the proven benefit of the early invasive strategy as previously reported.

With regard to the optimal timing of the early invasive strategy, the meta-analysis of Bavry (10) revealed no incremental benefit in case of a very early invasive strategy (median time to angiography of 9.3 h) compared to a later early invasive strategy (median time to angiography of 39.4 h). In an analysis of data from the Can Rapid risk stratification of Unstable angina patients Suppress ADverse outcomes with Early Implementation of the ACC/AHA guidelines (CRUSADE) National Quality Initiative (11), patients presenting with non-ST-

segment acute coronary syndromes on weekends had a longer time to angiography (median of 46.3 h) compared to patients presenting on weekdays (median of 23.4 h). This delay was not associated with increased inhospital adverse events, including death (weekend 4.4% vs weekday 4.1%, $p = 0.23$), recurrent MI (2.9% vs 3.0%, $p = 0.36$), or their combination (6.6% vs 6.6%, $p = 0.86$).

A strategy of delaying the invasive evaluation to provide an extended period of antithrombotic treatment for "cooling-off" the culprit plaque (plaque passivation) was evaluated in the Intracoronary Stenting with Antithrombotic Regimen Cooling-Off (ISAR-COOL) trial (12). Patients with non-ST-segment elevation acute coronary syndromes were randomly assigned to antithrombotic pretreatment with ASA, clopidogrel, tirofiban, and heparin either for 72–120 h or <6 h. Median time to catheterization was 2.4 h in the early intervention group and 86 h in the cooling-off group. The primary end point, combined death and nonfatal myocardial infarction within 30 days, was reached in 11.6% of patients in the cooling-off group compared with only 5.9% in the early intervention group ($p = 0.04$). Therefore, from analysis of all of the above data, the optimal time to proceed to cardiac catheterization appears to be within 48 h of presentation. There may be no need to proceed to cardiac catheterization in an emergent manner unless the patient is clinically or hemodynamically unstable in spite of medical therapy. These data also support the use of upstream GP IIb/IIIa inhibitor therapy in these patients.

Use of GP IIb/IIIa inhibitors during PCI for non-ST-elevation acute coronary syndromes

The benefit of routine use of GP IIb/IIIa inhibitors with percutaneous intervention has been documented in numerous trials, several of which were exclusively or largely composed of patients with non-ST-elevation acute coronary syndromes (5). The efficacy of the routine usage of GP IIb/IIIa inhibitors in patients with an acute coronary syndrome prior to percutaneous intervention or in patients who were not routinely scheduled for an invasive strategy with early coronary revascularization as warranted is less clearly established.

A meta-analysis by Boersma (13) of multiple large (>1,000 patients) randomized trials evaluating the benefit of routine GP IIb/IIIa on the cardiac outcomes of patients with non-ST-elevation acute coronary syndromes without recommendation of early (<48 h) coronary revascularization revealed a reduction in the occurrence of death or myocardial infarction with the use of a GP IIb/IIIa inhibitor. The benefit was statistically significant only in patients with an elevated troponin T or I level. The benefit was greatest in patients who underwent percutaneous coronary intervention or coronary artery bypass grafting within 5 days after randomization with a 31% risk reduction of death or myocardial infarction at 30 days. Major bleeding was increased with the use of GP IIb/IIIa inhibitors compared to placebo (2.5% vs 1.4%, $p < 0.0001$). There was no difference in intracranial hemorrhage or total stroke. Only the small-molecule GP IIb/IIIa inhibitors demonstrated a benefit. The large-molecule GP IIb/IIIa inhibitor, abciximab, as used in Global use of Strategies to Opened Occluded Coronary Arteries—IV—Acute Coronary Syndromes (GUSTO IV-ACS) (14), did not reveal any benefit and had a trend toward adverse cardiac outcomes.

As a result of the above studies, the 2002 ACC/AHA practice guidelines update for management of unstable angina and non-ST-elevation myocardial infarction (5) gave its strongest recommendation of Class I (Level of Evidence: A) for the administration of a platelet GP IIb/IIIa antagonist, in addition to ASA and heparin, to patients in whom catheterization and PCI are planned. The GP IIb/IIIa antagonist may also be administered just prior to PCI. A less strong recommendation of Class IIa (Level of Evidence: A) for the administration of eptifibatide or tirofiban, in addition to ASA and LMWH or UFH, to patients with continuing ischemia, an elevated troponin or with other high-risk features in whom an invasive management strategy is not planned. However, it is our opinion that the later recommendation for the use of GP IIb/IIIa inhibitors for medical passivation of the plaque when PCI or CABG is not contemplated is rarely warranted.

The recently revised ACC/AHA 2007 guidelines for the management of unstable angina/non-ST-elevation myocardial infarction (15) have a Class I recommendation for UA/NSTEMI patients in whom an initial invasive strategy is selected. Antiplatelet therapy in addition to aspirin should be initiated before diagnostic angiography (upstream) with either clopidogrel or an intravenous GP IIb/IIIa inhibition. (Level of Evidence: A). Abciximab as the choice for upstream GP IIb/IIIa therapy is indicated only if there is no appreciable delay to perform angiography and PCI is likely to be performed. Otherwise, IV eptifibatide or tirofiban is the preferred choice of GP IIb/IIIa inhibitor. (Level of Evidence: B) A Class I recommendation was also given for UA/NSTEMI patients in whom an initial conservative strategy is selected, if recurrent symptoms/ischemia, heart failure, or serious arrhythmias subsequently appear. Then diagnostic angiography should be performed. Either an intravenous GP IIb/IIIa inhibiter (eptifibatide or tirofiban; Level of Evidence A) or clopidogrel (Level of Evidence: A) should be added to ASA and anticoagulant therapy before diagnostic angiography (upstream) (Level of Evidence: C).

Upstream versus deferred use of GP IIb/IIIa inhibitors in non-ST-elevation acute coronary syndromes

The timing of initiation of GP IIb/IIIa inhibitor therapy is an unsettled issue. This could be, in part, responsible for a failure of adherence to the above guideline recommendation for the early administration of a GP IIb/IIIa antagonist in non-ST-elevation myocardial infarctions. The National Registry of Myocardial Infarction (NRMI) 4 database (16) of 60,770 NSTE MI patients who were eligible for early GP IIb/IIIa inhibitor therapy presenting from July 2000 to July 2001 revealed that only 15,379 patients (25%) received such therapy within 24 h of admission. The CRUSADE National Quality Improvement Initiative (17) revealed of patients presenting between March 31, 2000 and December 31, 2002 that only 39.9% of males and 30.5% of females who were troponin positive received a GP IIb/IIIa inhibitor within 24 h of admission. The more recent data are not more promising. Of 31,665 patients entered into the CURSADE database (16) from July 1, 2005 to June 30, 2006, only 46% of eligible patient received a GP IIb/IIIa inhibitor within 24 h of admission.

An observational study of the above mentioned patients in the NRMI 4 database (16) demonstrated that patients treated with early GP IIb/IIIa inhibitor therapy vs patients who were not treated had a lower unadjusted inhospital mortality (3.3% vs 9.6%, $p < 0.0001$) and it remained significantly lower after adjustment for patient risk, treatment propensity, and hospital characteristics (adjusted odds ratio = 0.88; 95% confidence interval, 0.79–0.97). The magnitude of mortality benefit was remarkably consistent with those estimated from a meta-analysis of the major GP IIb/IIIa inhibitor trials by Kong (18) with a 30-day mortality risk reduction with treatment of 0.87 (95% CI, 0.74–1.02). However, major bleeding was slightly increased from 9.5% without the early use of a GP IIb/IIIa inhibitor to 10.0% with the early use of a GP IIb/IIIa inhibitor ($p = 0.038$). There was no significant increased risk of blood transfusion (8.5% vs 8.7%) or hemorrhagic stroke (0.1% vs 0.1%) associated with GP IIb/IIIa inhibition. The benefits of early GP IIb/IIIa therapy persisted after excluding those who had PCI or cardiac catheterization.

The EVEREST Trial (19) was a randomized comparison of upstream tirofiban vs downstream (at the time of PCI) high bolus dose (HBD) tirofiban or abciximab on tissue-level perfusion and troponin release in high-risk acute coronary syndromes treated with percutaneous coronary interventions. The primary end point of better tissue-level perfusion and attenuated myocardial damage was significantly improved with upstream therapy. All patients had elevated preprocedural troponin I levels without significant difference in peak pre-PCI levels between the groups. The results of the EVEREST trial (20) are shown in Table 18.3. The TIMI myocardial perfusion grade 0/1 was significantly less frequent with upstream tirofiban compared with HBD tirofiban and abciximab before PCI and after PCI. Upstream tirofiban was associated with a significant higher intracoronary myocardial contrast echocardiography score index. Postprocedural troponin I elevation was significantly less frequent with upstream tirofiban. The troponin I levels after PCI were also significantly lower with upstream tirofiban. The time to PCI for upstream tirofiban was 30.4 ± 13.6 h, HBD tirofiban was 26.0 ± 12.4 h, and abciximab was 26.1 ± 18.7 h ($p = $ NS). Preprocedural clopidogrel

Table 18.3 Results of EVERST trial.

	Upstream Tirofiban	HBD Tirofiban	Abciximab	P
TMPG 0/1[a]				
Before PCI	28.1%	66.7%	71%	.0009[b]
After PCI	6.2%	20%	35.5%	.0015[b]
MCESI[c]	0.87 ± 0.19	0.77 ± 0.32	0.71 ± 0.35	<.05[b]
Normal Tissue-level Perfusion by MCE (% of patients)	96.2%	75%	72.4%	.04[b]
Post-Procedural cTnI Elevation	9.4%	30%	38.7%	.018[b]
cTnI Level post-PCI	3.8 ± 4.1	7.2 ± 12	9 ± 13.8	.015
	3.8 ± 4.1			.0002
Bleeding[d]				
Major	0%	0%	3.2%	NS
Minor	15.6%	13.3%	15.6%	NS

[a]TIMI Myocardial Perfusion Grade (% of patients).

[b]P value for Upstream tirofiban vs (HBD tirofiban and abciximab).

[c]Myocardial Contrast Echocardiography Score Index.

[d]Major bleeding—Fall of Hgb ≥2.0 mmol/L and need for transfusion of ≥2 U of blood, corrective groin surgery, or both, or as bleeding that resulted in documented intracranial, GI, or retroperitoneal hemorrhage.

Minor bleeding—Fall of Hgb ≤2.0 mmol/L without the need for a transfusion.

was given, with a loading dose of 300 mg, respectively, to 78%, 77%, and 68% of patients in each group. There was no difference in major or minor bleeding between the treatment groups. This was the first randomized study comparing upstream vs downstream GP IIb/IIIa inhibitor therapy in the setting of an early invasive strategy for NSTE MI. The improved tissue-level perfusion and attenuated myocardial damage observed with upstream GP IIb/IIIa inhibitor therapy used in conjunction with an early invasive strategy for NSTE MI confirm and expand previous experimental data and coupled with the clinical finding from the TACTICS-TIMI 18 trial strongly suggest that upstream therapy will lead to more favorable outcomes.

A cost-effective analysis of upstream vs in-catheterization laboratory initiation of GP IIb/IIIa inhibitor therapy using decision analysis methodology found that upstream use of the cheaper small-molecule inhibitors was more cost-effective compared to the use of the more expensive abciximab when the patients had a moderate- to high-risk TIMI risk score (1). The strategy of upstream use of a small molecule GP IIb/IIIa inhibitor was superior to selective use, and economically acceptable, with a cost-effectiveness ratio of $18,000 per year of life gained.

The most recent trial to address this issue of upstream GP IIb/IIIa use was Acute Catheterization and Urgent Intervention Triage Strategy trial (ACUITY) (21). ACUITY evaluated heparin plus GP IIb/IIIa inhibition compared with the direct thrombin inhibitor bivalirudin with or without GP IIb/IIIa inhibition among patients with an acute coronary syndrome. A separate analysis of the timing of GP IIb/IIIa inhibitors, either upstream or delayed administration just prior to PCI, was also conducted by the ACUITY investigators in the ACUITY Timing Trial (22). In the ACUITY Timing Trial angiography was performed an average of 6.2 h after randomization and cardiac enzymes (troponin or CKMB) were elevated at baseline in 57% of the patients. This is in contrast to the median time to catheterization of 21 h of patients reported in the CRUSADE registry. Also, in the main ACUITY trial, a 26% (95% CI, 0.67–1.05) risk reduction of death, MI, or unplanned revascularization was found in the patients whose angiography was performed between 3 and 19.7 h after

randomization with use of heparin and GP IIb/IIIa inhibitor compared to bivalirudin alone. Only a 4% (95% CI, 0.39–1.22) risk reduction was found in patient whose angiography was performed in <3 h in the ACUITY trial, which suggests that the benefit of GP IIb/IIIa is seen primarily with an early but not immediate invasive approach.

The primary outcome of the ACUITY Timing trial was assessment of noninferiority of deferred GP IIb/IIIa inhibitor use compared with upstream administration for the prevention of composite ischemic events. The triple composite ischemic end point of death, MI, and unplanned revascularization for ischemia at 30 days revealed a nonsignificant trend in favor of upstream GP IIb/IIIa inhibition (7.1% in the upstream group compared with 7.9% in the delayed group). The criterion for the primary outcome of noninferiority of deferred therapy was not met. Furthermore, there was no difference in mortality (1.3% for upstream vs 1.5% for delayed) or MI (4.9% vs 5.0%) but unplanned revascularization for ischemia was lower in the upstream group (2.1% vs 2.8%, $p = 0.03$). In the cohort of patients who received PCI, the composite ischemic end point was significantly lower in the upstream therapy group vs the delayed therapy group (8.0% vs 9.5%). However, major bleeding was significant lower in the delayed group (4.9% vs 6.1%, $p = 0.009$). There was no difference when using the TIMI major bleeding criteria (1.9% vs 1.5%, $p = 0.20$) but TIMI minor bleeding was lower in the delayed group (5.4% vs 7.2%, $p < 0.001$). The final conclusions of the ACUITY Timing trial were that among patients with moderate- and high-risk ACS undergoing an invasive strategy, deferring the routine upstream use of GP IIb/IIIa inhibitors for selective administration in the cardiac catheterization laboratory only to patients undergoing percutaneous coronary intervention resulted in a numerical increase in composite ischemia that, while not statistically significant, did not meet the criterion for noninferiority. This finding was offset by a significant reduction in major bleeding with the delayed strategy.

Conclusions

1 Platelet activation and aggregation plays a key role in the pathogenesis of acute coronary syndromes.

2 GP IIb/IIIa inhibitors block the final common pathway leading to platelet aggregation and thrombus formation in the acute coronary syndrome.

3 An early invasive strategy with revascularization predominately by percutaneous coronary intervention and coronary artery bypass grafting as warranted is the preferred strategy for management of acute coronary syndromes particularly with an elevated troponin level.

4 In the patient with an acute coronary syndrome who stabilizes on admission, there is no apparent necessity to proceed immediately to angiography. Angiography should be performed within 72 h (preferably within 48 h) of presentation.

5 Upstream GP IIb/IIIa inhibition with a small molecule inhibitor (eptifibatide or tirofiban) along with aspirin and heparin (UFH or LMWH) should be considered, unless contraindicated, in patients with an acute coronary syndrome and the following:

   a. Elevated troponin (T or I) levels.

   b. Not proceeding immediately to angiography.

   c. Thienopyridine (clopidogrel or ticlopidine) therapy has not been started prior to angiography.

6 Abciximab or a small-molecule GP IIb/IIIa inhibitor should be considered in acute coronary syndrome patients undergoing percutaneous coronary intervention in the absence of upstream GP IIb/IIIa inhibitor therapy or thienopyridine therapy started with an appropriate loading dose prior to PCI. Even in patients loaded with clopidogrel prior to intervention the use of abciximab has recently been shown in Intracoronary Stenting and Antithrombotic Regimen: Rapid Early Action for Coronary Treatment 2 trial (ISAR-REACT-2) to improve outcome following PCI in patients with a baseline elevated troponin (23).

7 The benefit of upstream GP IIb/IIIa inhibitor therapy with a reduction in death, nonfatal MI, rehospitalization for recurrent acute coronary syndrome, or unplanned revascularization is partially but not fully offset by a significant increase in bleeding, which is predominately TIMI minor bleeding at the vascular assess site.

8 Finally, concerning the upstream use of GP IIb/IIIa inhibitors vs delayed (at the time of PCI) or no GP IIb/IIIa inhibition, one must always weigh the potential benefits vs the risk of bleeding in a given patient. Thus, there is no substitute for sound clinical judgment in the evaluation and management of these patients.

References

1 Glasser R, Glick HA, Herman HC, Kimmel SE. The role of risk stratification in the decision to provide upstream versus selective glycoprotein IIb/IIIa inhibiters for acute coronary syndromes: a cost-effectiveness analysis. *J Am Coll Cardiol.* 2005;**47**:529–537.

2 Boden WE, O'Rourke RA, Crawford MH, *et al.* Outcomes in patients with acute non-Q wave myocardial infarction randomly assigned to an invasive as compared with a conservative management strategy. *N Engl J Med.* 1998;**338**:1785–1792. Erratum, *N Engl J Med.* 1998;**339**:1091.

3 FRagmin and Fast Revascularization during Instability in Coronary Artery Disease (FRISC II) Investigations. Invasive compared with non-invasive treatment in unstable coronary artery disease: the FRISC II invasive randomized trial. *Lancet.* 1999;**354**:708–715.

4 Cannon CP, Weintraub WS, Dermopoulos LA, *et al.* Comparison of early invasive and conservative strategies in patients with unstable coronary syndromes treated the glycoprotein IIb/IIIa inhibitor Tirotibam. *N Engl J Med.* 2001;**344**:1879–1887.

5 Braunwald E, Autman JM, Beasley JF, *et al.* ACC/AHA 2002 Guideline update for the management of patients with unstable angina and non-ST segment elevation myocardial infarction: a report of the American College of Cardiology/American Heart Association Task Force on Practice Guidelines (Committee on the Management of Patients with the Unstable Angina) 2002. Available at www.acc.org/qualityand science/clinical/guidelines/unstable/incorporated/UA_incorporated.pdf. Accessed July 1, 2007.

6 Michalis LK, Stroumbis CS, Pappas K, *et al.* Treatment of refractory unstable angina in geographically isolated areas without cardiac surgery. Invasive versus conservative strategy (TRUCS Study). *Eur Heart J.* 2000;**20**:1954–1959.

7 Spacek R, Widimsky P, Straka Z, *et al.* Valve of first day coronary angiography/angioplasty in evolving non-ST segment elevation myocardial infarction: a open multicenter randomized trial. The VINO Study. *Eur Heart J.* 2002;**23**:230–238.

8 Fox KA, Poole-Wilson PA, Henderson RA, *et al.* Interventional versus conservative treatment for patients with unstable angina or non-ST elevation myocardial infarction: the British Heart Foundation RITA 3 randomized trial. Randomized Intervention Trial of Unstable Angina. *Lancet.* 2002;**360**:743–751.

9 de Winter RJ, Windhausen F, Cornel JH, *et al*. Early invasive versus selectively invasive management for acute coronary syndromes. *N Engl J Med*. 2005;**353**: 1095–1014.

10 Bavry AA, Kumbhani DJ, Rassi AN, *et al*. Benefit of early invasive therapy in acute coronary syndromes: a meta-analysis of contemporary randomized clinical trials. *J Am Coll Cardiol*. 2006;**48**:1319–1325.

11 Ryan JW, Peterson ED, Chen AY, *et al*. Optimal timing of intervention in non-ST-segment elevation acute coronary syndromes: in sight from the CRUSADE (Can Rapid risk stratification of Unstable angina patients Suppress Adverse outcomes with Early implementation of the ACC/AHA guidelines) registry. *Circulation*. 2005;**112**:3049–3057.

12 Neumann F-J, Kastrati A, Pogatsa-Murray G, *et al*. Evaluation at prolonged antithrombotic pretreatment ("Cooling-Off" strategy) before intervention in patients with unstable coronary syndromes. A randomized controlled trial. *JAMA*. 2003;**290**:1593–1599.

13 Boersma E, Harrington RA, Moliterno DJ, *et al*. Platelet glycoprotein IIb/IIIa inhibitors in acute coronary syndromes: a meta-analysis of all major randomized clinical trials. *Lancet*. 2002;**359**:189–198.

14 The GUSTO IV—ACS Investigators. Effect of glycoprotein IIb/IIIa receptor blocker abciximab on outcome in patients with acute coronary syndromes without early coronary revascularization: the GUSTO IV-ACS randomized trial. *Lancet*. 2001;**357**:1915–1924.

15 Anderson KL, Adams CP, Autman EM, *et al*. ACC/AHA 2007 guidelines for the management of patients with unstable angina/non-ST-elevation myocardial infarction. *J Am Coll Cardiol*. 2007;**50**:e1–e157.

16 Peterson ED, Pollack CV, Roe MT, *et al*. Early use of glycoprotein IIb/IIIa inhibitors in non-ST-elevation acute myocondrial infarction: observations from the National Registry of Myocardial Infarction 4. *J Am Coll Cardiol*. 2003;**42**:45–53.

17 Blomkaln AL, Chen AY, Hochman JS, *et al*. Gender disparities in the diagnosis and treatment of non-ST-segment elevation acute coronary syndromes: large-scale observations from the CRUSADE National Quality Improvement Initiative. *J Am Coll Cardiol*. 2005;**45**:832–837.

18 Kong DF, Califf RM, Miller DP, *et al*. Clinical outcomes of therapeutic agents that block the platelet glycoprotein IIb/IIIa integrin in ischemic heart disease. *Circulation*. 1998;**98**:2829–2835.

19 Bolognese L, Falsini G, Liistro F, *et al*. Randomized comparison of upstream tirofiban versus downstream high bolus dose tirofiban or ab ciximab on tissue-level perfusion and troponin release in high-risk acute coronary interventions: the EVEREST trial. *J Am Card Cardiol*. 2006;**47**: 522–528.

20 CRUSADE data. Available at www.crusadeqi.com.

21 Stone GW, McLaurin BT, Cox DA, *et al*. Bivalirudin for patients with acute coronary syndromes. *N Engl J Med*. 2006;**355**:2203–2216.

22 Stone GW, Bertrand ME, Moses JW, *et al*. Routine upstream initiation vs. deferred selective use of glycoprotein IIb/IIIa inhibitors in acute coronary syndromes: the ACUITY timing trial. *JAMA*. 2007;**297**:591–602.

23 Kastrati A, Mehilli J, Neumann FJ, *et al*. Abciximab in patients with acute coronary syndromes undergoing percutaneous coronary intervention after clopidogrel pretreatment: the ISAR-REACT 2 randomized trial. *JAMA*. 2006;**295**:1531–1538.

CHAPTER 19

High-dose tirofiban

Bart Dawson, Debabrata Mukherjee, &
David J. Moliterno
University of Kentucky, Lexington, KY, USA

Glycoprotein (GP) IIb/IIIa inhibitors reduce a composite of cardiovascular ischemic events (death, myocardial infarction [MI], and urgent target vessel revascularization [TVR]) after percutaneous coronary intervention (PCI) (1). The degree of pharmacologically-induced platelet inhibition during PCI has been shown to be an independent predictor of major adverse cardiovascular events (MACE) after PCI (2). Early dose-finding studies of tirofiban showed >85% platelet inhibition *ex vivo* by light transmission aggregometry in response to a 0.4 µg/kg/min bolus over 30 min plus a 0.15 µg/kg/min infusion (3). Subsequent randomized controlled trials have shown a reduction in ischemic events utilizing this dose of tirofiban in patients with acute coronary syndromes (ACS) undergoing PCI (4,5).

Despite a large body of evidence demonstrating improved outcomes with the use of GP IIb/IIIa inhibitors in ACS patients undergoing PCI (5–7), head-to-head data among the three available agents abciximab, tirofiban, and eptifibatide are lacking. The only such completed trial to date is TARGET (Do Tirofiban And Reo Pro Give Similar Efficacy Outcome Trial) (8). In the TARGET trial, the 30-day composite end point of death, MI, and urgent TVR was reduced with abciximab compared

to tirofiban. The lower incidence of the combined end point was reflected in large part by the reduction in periprocedural MI in the first 12–24 h after PCI in the abciximab cohort. Kabbani *et al.* subsequently demonstrated that inhibition of platelet function within 60 min of PCI is greater with abciximab than with tirofiban given at the dose used in the TARGET trial (9). On the other hand, the extent of platelet inhibition >2 h after PCI is similar between the two agents (10). This finding of suboptimal early platelet inhibition with a 10 µg/kg bolus dose of tirofiban vs abciximab at the time of PCI likely contributed to the greater incidence of periprocedural events observed in the tirofiban arm.

These observations have led to more recent mechanistic studies of the antiplatelet effects and safety of a higher bolus dose of tirofiban in patients undergoing PCI. Schneider *et al.* performed further dose-finding studies, which demonstrated that a 25 µg/kg bolus plus a 0.15 µg/kg/min-infusion of tirofiban produces >90% platelet inhibition by light transmission aggregometry from 15–60 min after the onset of treatment in patients with ACS (11). Furthermore, Ernst *et al.* have demonstrated that in patients with ST-segment elevation myocardial infarction (STEMI), the degree of platelet aggregation inhibition at the time of PCI is highly variable among individuals, and that a higher bolus dose tirofiban protocol was the only regimen that produced a mean periprocedural level of platelet aggregation inhibition >80% (12). Similar effects on the angiographic outcome and left ventricular

Pharmacology in the Catheterization Laboratory. Edited by Ron Waksman and Andrew E Ajani. © 2010 Blackwell Publishing, ISBN: 978-1-4051-5704-9.

function recovery in STEMI have been observed between high-dose bolus tirofiban and abciximab (12,13). Most recently, Mardikar *et al.* conducted the MR PCI study to determine the degree of platelet aggregation inhibition achieved by high-dose bolus tirofiban with and without clopidogrel compared to standard dose eptifibatide with and without clopidogrel in patients undergoing elective high-risk PCI (14). Inhibition of platelet aggregation was significantly higher with high-dose tirofiban compared to eptifibatide at 10 min and 6–8 h independent of the addition of clopidogrel. Differences in clinical outcomes between these regimens were not noted but the study was not powered to assess differences in outcome.

Based on these platelet function data, several small studies have been performed to compare clinical endpoints when higher-dose bolus tirofiban is compared to abciximab in patients undergoing PCI (Table 19.1). Danzi *et al.* showed that the higher-dose bolus of tirofiban was safe and not associated with an increased risk of major bleeding or access site complications in comparison with abciximab (15). Gunasekara and coworkers demonstrated no difference in 6-month MACE rates between the higher-dose bolus of tirofiban and abciximab in patients undergoing PCI for STEMI, NSTEMI, or unstable angina pectoris (16). Bolognese *et al.* found that in patients undergoing high-risk PCI, a high-dose bolus tirofiban regimen is an effective strategy in ACS (17). Valgimigli and colleagues demonstrated that in patients with STEMI, a strategy of high-dose bolus tirofiban-supported sirolimus-eluting stenting reduced the cumulative incidence of MACE when compared to abciximab-supported bare metal stenting (18). The TENACITY (Tirofiban Evaluation of Novel Dosing vs Abciximab with Clopidogrel and Inhibition of Thrombin) trial was designed to prospectively compare clinical outcomes between high-dose bolus tirofiban and abciximab in over 8,000 patients undergoing PCI, but was terminated prematurely for financial reasons (19).

Recently, a pooled analysis from these five clinical trials was performed to assess clinical outcomes and bleeding risk between high-dose bolus tirofiban and abciximab (20). The primary end point in this meta-analysis was the composite of death, MI, and urgent TVR at 30 days. Major and minor bleeding and the incidence of thrombocytopenia were also assessed. A total of 1,392 patients (689 tirofiban, 703 abciximab) were included. The incidence of the combined ischemic end point at 30 days was 6.1% with tirofiban and 7.3% with abciximab ($p = 0.46$). Also, no differences were found in the individual primary end points of death, MI, TVR, major or minor bleeding, or thrombocytopenia between the two groups, though the small sample precluded any statistically meaningful assessments.

Limited data suggests a substantial cost savings by using high-dose bolus tirofiban vs abciximab in patients undergoing PCI. Gunasekara *et al.* demonstrated similar clinical end points using high-dose bolus tirofiban with a substantial pharmaceutical cost savings ($332 for high-dose bolus tirofiban vs $1350 for abciximab) (16). Valgimigli *et al.* showed that at current European market prices, a high-dose bolus tirofiban regimen would offset the additional cost of a drug-eluting stent when compared to abciximab ($742 for tirofiban vs $2,432 for abciximab in pharmaceutical costs) (18).

Based on the available data, in patients undergoing PCI, use of high-dose bolus tirofiban (25 μg/kg bolus plus a 0.15 μg/kg/min infusion) appears to result in similar outcomes with a comparable safety profile to standard dose abciximab though definitive data are lacking. Tirofiban could substantially reduce the pharmaceutical cost of PCI relative to abciximab. A large randomized trial comparing the two strategies would more accurately assess their equivalence, countering the short follow-up and lack of statistical power in the current literature.

References

1 Topol EJ, Byzova TV, Plow EF. Platelet GPIIb-IIIa blockers. *Lancet.* 1999;**353**:227–231.

2 Steinhubl SR, Talley JD, Braden GA, *et al.* Point-of-care measured platelet inhibition correlates with a reduced risk of an adverse cardiac event after percutaneous coronary intervention: results of the GOLD (AU-Assessing Ultegra) multicenter study. *Circulation.* 2001;**103**:2572–2578.

3 Kereiakes DJ, Kleiman NS, Ambrose J, *et al.* Randomized, double-blind, placebo-controlled dose-ranging study of tirofiban (MK-383) platelet IIb/IIIa blockade in high risk patients undergoing coronary angioplasty. *J Am Coll Cardiol.* 1996;**27**:536–542.

Table 19.1 Characteristics and outcomes of high-dose tirofiban trials.

	Danzi et al. (15)	Gunasekara et al. (16)	Bolognese et al. (17)	Valgimigli et al. (18)	Moliterno et al. (19)
Patient population	PCI for AMI, UAP, stable angina (20% AMI) (n = 554)	PCI for STEMI, NSTEMI, UA, stable angina (80% STEMI/NSTEMI (n = 219)	PCI for Tn-I + ACS (n = 93)	PCI for STEMI (n = 175)	Intermediate- to high-risk PCI (NSTEMI, STEMI, UAP PCI) (n = 373)
Treatment arms	HDB tirofiban + infusion vs standard dose abciximab	HDB tirofiban + infusion vs standard dose abciximab	Upstream standard dose tirofiban vs HDB tirofiban at PCI vs abciximab at PCI	HDB tirofiban + infusion with sirolimus-eluting stent vs standard dose abciximab with bare metal stenting	HDB tirofiban + heparin or bivalrudin vs abciximab + heparin or bivalrudin
Additional medications	ASA, ticlopidine (32%), UFH	ASA, clopidogrel (36% tirofiban vs 24% abciximab), UFH	ASA, clopidogrel or ticlopidine, UFH	ASA, clopidogrel, UFH	ASA, Clopidogrel
Primary end points	Major bleeding + access site complications	Major/minor TIMI bleeding, access site complications, Tn-I rise, thrombocytopenia	Difference in TMPG before PCI	Freedom from death, nonfatal MI, stroke, binary restenosis at 8 months	30-day composite death, MI, urgent TVR
Secondary end points	Combined death, Q/non-Q MI, CABG, emergent TVR at 30 days	Combined death, Q/non-Q MI, CABG, stroke, emergent TVR at 30 days and 6 months	TIMI grade flow, cTFC, TMPG before and after PCI, MCE score and Tn-I release after PCI	Freedom from MACE (death, reinfarction, stroke, TVR), TIMI major and minor bleeding, thrombocytopenia at 30 days and 8 months	6-month death, MI, any TVR, 1-year mortality, major bleeding
Major results	Major bleeding 0 vs 1.4% (p = 0.14), no difference in access site complications, MACE 6.4 vs 5.4% (p = 0.77)	Major bleeding 7.3 vs 3% (p = 0.118), minor bleeding 24 vs 15.5% (p = 0.118), thrombocytopenia 0.9 vs 2% (p = 0.556), 30-day MACE 14.5 vs 9% (p = 0.200), 6-month MACE 23 vs 20% (p = 0.711)	No difference in overall TMPG before PCI, MCE score, or post-PCI Tn-I release between HDB tirofiban and abciximab	No differences in 30-day MACE, 8-month MACE 18 vs 32% (p = 0.04), driven by reduction in TVR in tirofiban group, no difference in major/minor bleeding, or severe thrombocytopenia	No difference in 30-day composite or major bleeding between HDB tirofiban and abciximab

ACS, acute coronary syndrome; AMI, acute myocardial infarction; ASA, aspirin; CABG, coronary artery bypass graft surgery; cTFC, corrected TIMI frame count; HDB, high-dose bolus; MACE, major adverse cardiovascular events; MCE, myocardial contrast echo; NSTEMI, non-ST-segment elevation myocardial infarction; PCI, percutaneous coronary intervention; STEMI, ST elevation myocardial infarction; TIMI, thrombolysis in myocardial infarction; TMPG, TIMI myocardial perfusion grade; TVR, target vessel revascularization; UAP, unstable angina pectoris; UFH, unfractionated heparin.

4 The RESTORE Investigators. Effects of platelet glycoprotein IIb/IIIa blockade with tirofiban on adverse cardiac events in patients with unstable angina or acute myocardial infarction undergoing coronary angioplasty. The RESTORE Investigators. Randomized Efficacy Study of Tirofiban for Outcomes and REstenosis. *Circulation.* 1997;**96**:1445–1453.

5 PRISM-PLUS Study Investigators. Inhibition of the platelet glycoprotein IIb/IIIa receptor with tirofiban in unstable angina and non-Q-wave myocardial infarction. Platelet Receptor Inhibition in Ischemic Syndrome Management in Patients Limited by Unstable Signs and Symptoms (PRISM-PLUS) Study Investigators. *N Engl J Med.* 1998;**338**:1488–1497.

6 The EPIC Investigators. Use of a monoclonal antibody directed against the platelet glycoprotein IIb/IIIa receptor in high-risk coronary angioplasty. The EPIC Investigation. *N Engl J Med.* 1994;**330**:956–961.

7 The PURSUIT Trial Investigators. Inhibition of platelet glycoprotein IIb/IIIa with eptifibatide in patients with acute coronary syndromes. The PURSUIT Trial Investigators. Platelet glycoprotein IIb/IIIa in unstable angina: receptor suppression using integrilin therapy. *N Engl J Med.* 1998;**339**:436–443.

8 Topol EJ, Moliterno DJ, Herrmann HC, *et al.* Comparison of two platelet glycoprotein IIb/IIIa inhibitors, tirofiban and abciximab, for the prevention of ischemic events with percutaneous coronary revascularization. *N Engl J Med.* 2001;**344**:1888–1894.

9 Kabbani SS, Aggarwal A, Terrien EF, DiBattiste PM, Sobel BE, Schneider DJ. Suboptimal early inhibition of platelets by treatment with tirofiban and implications for coronary interventions. *Am J Cardiol.* 2002;**89**:647–650.

10 Neumann FJ, Hochholzer W, Pogatsa-Murray G, Schomig A, Gawaz M. Antiplatelet effects of abciximab, tirofiban and eptifibatide in patients undergoing coronary stenting. *J Am Coll Cardiol.* 2001;**37**:1323–1328.

11 Schneider DJ, Herrmann HC, Lakkis N, *et al.* Enhanced early inhibition of platelet aggregation with an increased bolus of tirofiban. *Am J Cardiol.* 2002;**90**:1421–1423.

12 Ernst NM, Suryapranata H, Miedema K, *et al.* Achieved platelet aggregation inhibition after different antiplatelet regimens during percutaneous coronary intervention for ST-segment elevation myocardial infarction. *J Am Coll Cardiol.* 2004;**44**:1187–1193.

13 Danzi GB, Sesana M, Capuano C, Mauri L, Berra Centurini P, Baglini R. Comparison in patients having primary coronary angioplasty of abciximab versus tirofiban on recovery of left ventricular function. *Am J Cardiol.* 2004;**94**:35–39.

14 Mardikar HM, Hiremath MS, Moliterno DJ, *et al.* Optimal platelet inhibition in patients undergoing PCI: data from the Multicenter Registry of High-Risk Percutaneous Coronary Intervention and Adequate Platelet Inhibition (MR PCI) study. *Am Heart J.* August 2007;**154**(2): 344.e1–344.e5.

15 Danzi GB, Capuano C, Sesana M, Baglini R. Safety of a high bolus dose of tirofiban in patients undergoing coronary stent placement. *Catheter Cardiovasc Interv.* 2004;**61**:179–184.

16 Gunasekara AP, Walters DL, Aroney CN. Comparison of abciximab with "high-dose" tirofiban in patients undergoing percutaneous coronary intervention. *Int J Cardiol.* 2006;**109**:16–20.

17 Bolognese L, Falsini G, Liistro F, *et al.* Randomized comparison of upstream tirofiban versus downstream high bolus dose tirofiban or abciximab on tissue-level perfusion and troponin release in high-risk acute coronary syndromes treated with percutaneous coronary interventions: the EVEREST trial. *J Am Coll Cardiol.* 2006;**47**:522–528.

18 Valgimigli M, Percoco G, Malagutti P, *et al.* Tirofiban and sirolimus-eluting stent vs abciximab and bare-metal stent for acute myocardial infarction: a randomized trial. *JAMA.* 2005;**293**:2109–2117.

19 Moliterno DJ. *Do Tirofiban and Reo Pro Give Similar Efficacy Outcome Trial.* Presented at Transcatheter Cardiovascular Therapeutics (TCT), Washington DC, November 2005.

20 Dawson C, Mukherjee D, Valgimigli M, *et al.* Meta-analysis of high-dose single-bolus tirofiban versus abciximab in patients undergoing PCI. American Heart Association Scientific Sessions 2006 (poster presentation). November 12–15, 2006; Chicago, IL.

CHAPTER 20

Oral anticoagulation issues in percutaneous coronary intervention

Scott Martin[1], Allen Jeremias[1], & Luis Gruberg[2]

[1]Stony Brook School of Medicine, Stony Brook, NY, USA
[2]Stony Brook University Medical Center, Stony Brook, NY, USA

Introduction

Anticoagulant therapies have been an essential part of the treatment of acute and chronic coronary artery disease since the late 1970s, when it was recognized that intracoronary thrombosis was a key mechanism in the pathophysiology of acute myocardial infarction (1). In particular, intravenous anticoagulation with unfractionated heparin or low-molecular-weight heparins has been standard practice during percutaneous coronary intervention (PCI) to prevent thrombosis since the first series of balloon angioplasties reported by Gruntzig (2). Oral anticoagulation with warfarin or related compounds that inhibit the production of vitamin K-dependent coagulation factors (factors VII, IX, X, II) has had a more limited role in the treatment of coronary artery disease in the PCI era, largely due to the hemorrhagic side-effects of anticoagulation and the development of potent antiplatelet regimens. In this chapter, we review the use of oral anticoagulation in coronary artery disease in current PCI practice. This includes historical data from the angioplasty era; the early stent years (prior to the use of the thienopyridine derivatives ticlopidine and clopidogrel), when oral anticoagulation was commonly used as part of an

aggressive antithrombotic treatment to prevent stent thrombosis, and limited contemporary data. We also discuss the issues in pharmacotherapy during and after PCI in patients who require oral anticoagulation for other thrombotic indications, such as prosthetic heart valves, atrial fibrillation, or venous thromboembolic disease.

Oral anticoagulation and balloon angioplasty

While intravenous anticoagulation is the standard practice during balloon angioplasty procedures, oral anticoagulation is rarely used. Three studies have been conducted to evaluate the role of oral anticoagulation during and after balloon angioplasty. The first two studies, both conducted in the early years of angioplasty, concluded that oral anticoagulants were not more effective than aspirin alone after angioplasty. However, it is important to note that these studies focused mainly on the prevention of restenosis. Thornton and colleagues (3) randomized 248 patients after successful percutaneous transluminal coronary balloon angioplasty (PTCA) to either aspirin or coumarin, with a goal INR of 2.0–2.5. Coumarin was used regularly in only 74% of the patients, and an adequate prothrombin time was achieved in only 35% of them. Patients were followed by stress testing and angiography 3–6 months after angioplasty. Although the rates of clinical events were not reported, the rate of recurrent stenosis was not significantly different

Pharmacology in the Catheterization Laboratory. Edited by Ron Waksman and Andrew E Ajani. © 2010 Blackwell Publishing, ISBN: 978-1-4051-5704-9.

between the two groups. The second study, by Urban and colleagues (4) included 110 patients, comparing treatment with aspirin to warfarin with goal INR >2.5. No information on the level of anticoagulation achieved was reported. Clinical, stress testing, and angiographic data were obtained at 5 months and showed no significant difference between the aspirin and warfarin groups. The third study of oral anticoagulation and balloon angioplasty by ten Berg and colleagues (5) was larger and included pretreatment with oral anticoagulation prior to balloon angioplasty. A total of 1,058 patients were randomized prior to PTCA to aspirin or coumarin with a goal INR of 2.1–4.8. Treatment began prior to PTCA and continued for 6 months afterward. In contrast to the earlier studies, these authors found a significant benefit to coumarin administration in decreasing the composite primary end point of death, myocardial infarction, target lesion revascularization, or stroke at 30 days, from 6.4% in the aspirin group to 3.4% in the oral anticoagulation group and from 20.3% to 14.3% at 1 year ($p < 0.05$) (Figures 20.1 and 20.2). Provisional stenting was done in 35% of patients, and there was no difference between the two groups (5). However, there was also a small but significant increase in the incidences of major (2.2% vs 0.2%) and minor (4.0% vs 0.4%) bleeding complications in the coumarin group. In a follow-up study (6), the authors found that 82% of patients in the oral anticoagulant group had achieved the target INR, and that those patients who achieved the target

level of anticoagulation had a 61% reduction in the relative risk of reaching the primary end point compared to patients treated with aspirin.

These conflicting results between the three trials may be largely due to differences in anticoagulation levels. While the two trials showing anticoagulation therapy to be ineffective achieved only low rates of adequate anticoagulation (3,4) or did not report on anticoagulation levels, ten Berg and colleagues found beneficial effects of long-term anticoagulation with 82% of patients achieving adequate anticoagulation levels (6). Based on this data, it appears likely plausible that adequate oral anticoagulation reduces the risk of major adverse cardiovascular events over aspirin alone after PCI. In support of this theory, trials of oral anticoagulation in post-myocardial infarction patients treated conservatively have shown a similar dichotomy, with trials of inadequate anticoagulation levels such as CARS and CHAMP (7,8) showing no benefit, while trials with a substantial numbers of patients achieving adequate anticoagulation levels, such as WARIS-2 and ASPECT-2 (9,10), demonstrating a significant decrease in major adverse cardiovascular events over aspirin alone. A meta-analysis of trials using high-intensity treatment with oral anticoagulants in post-myocardial infarction patients (INR 2.8–4.8) (11) confirmed a significant reduction in recurrent myocardial infarction, thromboembolic events, and mortality, but at the cost of a significant sixfold increase in the incidence of major bleeding.

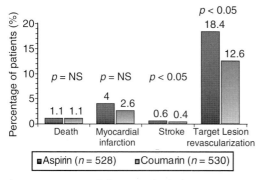

Figure 20.1 One-year follow-up individual primary end points. Patients randomized to the aspirin group (black bar) vs those treated with coumarin (gray bar). (*Source*: Data abstracted from ten Berg *et al.* (5).)

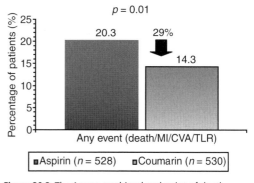

Figure 20.2 The 1-year combined end point of death, myocardial infarction (MI), target lesion revascularization (TLR), or stroke (CVA) in patients randomized to aspirin (black bar) vs those treated with coumarin (gray bar). (*Source*: Data abstracted from ten Berg *et al.* (5).)

Oral anticoagulation and coronary stenting

As most stents are made of stainless steel, they are a nidus for thrombus formation. Stent thrombosis can occur within the first 24 h (acute), within the first month after stent placement (subacute) or after 30 days (late stent thrombosis). In early clinical trials of coronary stents, there were very high rates of subacute stent thrombosis, ranging from 16% in the Palmaz-Schatz study (12) to 24% in the Wallstent Study (13), mostly occurring within the first 2 weeks after stent placement. The antithrombotic regimens used in these studies included aspirin, dipyridamole, heparin, and low-molecular-weight dextran. The high rates of stent thrombosis led to the adoption of more aggressive antiplatelet and anticoagulant regimen including the above agents followed by oral warfarin for weeks to months. Subsequent trials (14,15) using this aggressive antithrombotic treatment reduced the risk of acute and subacute stent thrombosis to approximately 3.5%. Unfortunately, this aggressive pharmacological regimen also doubled the hospital length-of-stay (from 3 to 6 days) and increased the rate of hemorrhagic and vascular complications to 7–13% compared to 3–4% with plain balloon angioplasty alone. Stenting also resulted in significantly higher costs at 1 year, largely due to longer initial hospital stay and higher rates of vascular complications (16). Although early clinical data suggested that stents were effective in reversing coronary occlusions and reducing restenosis, few physicians used them routinely mainly because of fear of the aforementioned complications. In the study by ten Berg *et al.*, 188 patients were concomitantly treated with stents in the aspirin group and 181 patients in the coumarin group. Interestingly, the late outcome was identical in the two groups and there was no longer a benefit from the administration of coumarin, with a 12.4% and 13.0% 1-year event rate, respectively (5).

Improvements in stenting techniques, including high-pressure stent deployment and dual antiplatelet therapy with aspirin and the thienopyridine ticlopidine (and later clopidogrel), dramatically reduced the incidence of stent thrombosis. The landmark Stent Anticoagulation Restenosis Study (STARS) (17) effectively ended the era of oral anticoagulation after stenting by showing that a regimen of aspirin and ticlopidine was superior to aspirin and warfarin at preventing stent thrombosis (0.5% vs 2.7%). This result was then confirmed by several other randomized trials. The Intracoronary Stenting and Antithrombotic Regimen (ISAR) Trial (18) showed that aspirin and ticlopidine decreased stent thrombosis compared to aspirin and intense anticoagulation with the warfarin-like compound phenprocoumon with goal INR of 3.5–4.5. The reduction in risk with aspirin and ticlopidine was solely attributable to patients at high risk for adverse cardiac events; for example, patients who underwent stenting for acute myocardial infarction had a 3.3% risk of stent thrombosis with aspirin and ticlopidine vs 2.1% with aspirin and oral anticoagulation. The Full Anticoagulation vs Aspirin and Ticlopidine (FANTASTIC) study (19) showed significant decreases in major adverse cardiovascular events, bleeding complications, and length of hospital stay with aspirin and ticlopidine vs aspirin and oral anticoagulant with goal INR 2.5–3.0. The Multicenter Aspirin and Ticlopidine Trial after Intracoronary Stenting (MATTIS) (20) also compared aspirin and ticlopidine with aspirin and oral anticoagulant with goal INR 2.5–3.0 and found a significant decrease in 30-day major adverse cardiovascular events (11% vs 5.6%) with the antiplatelet regimen.

With the benefits of dual antiplatelet therapy using aspirin and ticlopidine or clopidogrel well established, few if any cardiologists routinely treat post-PCI patients with oral anticoagulation to prevent stent thrombosis. The usefulness of adding warfarin to dual antiplatelet therapy (e.g., in a patient with recurrent stent thrombosis on dual antiplatelet therapy) has not been established. The only published data on this topic is a retrospective analysis from Mattichak and colleagues (21), who found that patients discharged on dual antiplatelet therapy plus warfarin had no significant difference in major adverse cardiovascular events, but a trend toward increased reinfarction at 6 and 12 month follow-up. Additionally, warfarin-treated patients had a significantly higher risk of bleeding and need for blood transfusion (21% vs 0%). While adding warfarin to dual antiplatelet therapy may be reasonable in the highest risk patients, no data supports this strategy.

Chronic oral anticoagulation

We frequently encounter patients presenting for cardiac catheterization who are chronically anticoagulated for indications such as mechanical heart valves, venous thromboembolism, atrial fibrillation, or left ventricular thrombus. While there are case series reporting the relative safety of cardiac catheterization and PCI in patients anticoagulated with warfarin (22), oral anticoagulation is routinely withheld prior to cardiac catheterization for elective cases to decrease the INR to <1.8 in order to minimize the risk of vascular access complications. Patients at particularly high thrombotic risk can be treated with unfractionated heparin, or more commonly subcutaneous low-molecular-weight heparin, while oral anticoagulation is withheld.

The effect of adding aspirin and a thienopyridine (ticlopidine or clopidogrel) to chronic warfarin therapy in patients undergoing PCI has not been well studied. Small series published on this topic have shown significant rates of hemorrhage with the combination of dual antiplatelet plus oral anticoagulant therapy ("triple therapy"). Orford and colleagues (23) performed a retrospective study of 65 patients requiring triple therapy and found a 9.2% incidence of bleeding events, with 3.1% having major bleeding episodes. Buresly and colleagues (24) conducted a database cohort study of elderly Canadians that showed that the addition of warfarin or a thienopyridine derivative to aspirin is associated with at least a twofold increase in bleeding risk among elderly patients. None of these patients sustained intracranial hemorrhage during exposure to the dual antiplatelet combination. On the other hand, there was a tendency toward an increased risk in intracranial bleeding in the aspirin plus warfarin combination compared with aspirin alone (11.1% vs 6.4%, $p = 0.14$). Of note, there were only a small number of patients in the cohort treated with triple therapy and they did not have significantly more bleeding events than the other groups.

Most recently, Khurram and colleagues published a retrospective cohort study of 107 patients on chronic oral anticoagulation who underwent PCI (25). These patients were subsequently treated with triple therapy of aspirin, clopidogrel, and warfarin and were compared to 107 randomly selected

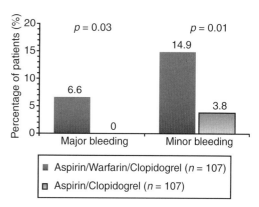

Figure 20.3 Major bleeding and minor bleeding complications in patients randomized to triple therapy (black bar) vs those treated with dual antiplatelet therapy (gray bar). (*Source*: Data abstracted from Khurram *et al.* (25).)

patients who were treated with dual antiplatelet therapy after PCI. Following stenting, patients on triple therapy had more incidences of major and minor bleeding compared to patients on dual antiplatelet therapy (Figure 20.3). After adjusting for confounding variables using multivariate analysis, triple therapy was found to be an independent predictor of bleeding (hazard ratio = 5.44; $p = 0.001$). Among patients on triple therapy, clopidogrel was discontinued prematurely in 8%, while coumadin was stopped in 6% due to bleeding complications.

Oral anticoagulation and drug-eluting stents

In the current era of widespread use of drug-eluting stents, which require prolonged dual antiplatelet therapy with aspirin and clopidogrel, rational strategies need to be employed to prevent stent thrombosis. A recent report by Iakovou and colleagues showed that the use of drug-eluting stents in the general population was associated with higher rates of late stent thrombosis than those reported in clinical trials (26). Furthermore, stent thrombosis was associated with 45% mortality and nonfatal myocardial infarction rates. According to this study, before time or "premature" discontinuation of antiplatelet therapy was the strongest predictor of stent thrombosis in patients treated with drug-eluting stents. Although it is estimated that 5% of patients undergoing percutaneous coronary intervention require long-term anticoagulation because of an underlying chronic medical condition, continuing treatment with triple therapy increases the risk of bleeding. In most patients, triple antithrombotic therapy seems justified for a short period of time and currently there is no data on the effectiveness and/or safety of triple therapy in patients treated with drug-eluting stents.

Several strategies can be employed to minimize the bleeding risk associated with triple therapy. In some patients, temporarily withholding oral anticoagulation may be an option, particularly in patients who have had bleeding complications on oral anticoagulation therapy alone. Only in those patients at a very high risk for thromboembolic events (patients with mechanical prosthetic heart valves or atrial fibrillation with multiple risk factors) will the risk of thromboembolism while withholding oral anticoagulation exceed the risk of major bleeding on triple therapy. Arab and colleagues (27) published an algorithm for patients receiving long-term anticoagulation undergoing PCI and recommend this approach for patients with low to moderate thromboembolic risk with a high risk of bleeding. If it is deemed imprudent to withhold oral anticoagulation for 3 to 6 months (or more) of dual antiplatelet therapy recommended after drug-eluting stent placement, bare metal stent should be used with a briefer withdrawal of oral anticoagulation as an option. Another option, which has not been explored in any trials to date, is to substitute low-molecular-weight heparin for oral anticoagulation during the period of dual antiplatelet treatment. The combination of aspirin, a thienopyridine, and low-molecular-weight heparin should be adequate to prevent thromboembolism and may theoretically cause fewer bleeding complications than the combination of aspirin, a thienopyridine, and warfarin. However, like triple therapy with oral anticoagulation, low-molecular-weight heparin-based triple therapy has been shown to cause more bleeding complications than dual antiplatelet treatment alone (28). One strategy that should be avoided is early discontinuation of aspirin or thienopyridine (e.g., treating with warfarin plus aspirin and prematurely stopping clopidogrel following stent implantation). Multiple aforementioned trials

have shown the beneficial effects of dual antiplatelet therapy over the aspirin/warfarin combination. However, lowering the aspirin dose to <100 mg daily may reduce bleeding complications while continuing to prevent stent thrombosis. Finally, patients at a high risk for thromboembolic events and high risk for bleeding should consider delaying any nonemergent PCI if their risk factors can be modified and abide to a conservative line of treatment. Otherwise they face a risk of bleeding and/or thrombosis that may be prohibitive.

Oral direct thrombin inhibitors

The oral direct thrombin inhibitor ximelagatran held great promise as a potential replacement for warfarin in a variety of indications, including anticoagulation post–myocardial infarction and also in the setting of PCI. The use of ximelagatran does not require INR monitoring. The phase II Efficacy and Safety of the Oral Direct Thrombin Inhibitor Ximelagatran in Patients with Recent Myocardial Damage (ESTEEM) trial (29) evaluated ximelagatran in combination with aspirin as long-term therapy in a predominantly noninterventional, post–myocardial infarction setting and showed encouraging results. This study showed a 24% reduction in the primary end point of death, myocardial infarction, and severe recurrent ischemia in the ximelagatran group vs placebo. Major bleeding was infrequent in both groups and was not significantly increased with ximelagatran. Unfortunately, ximelagatran was subsequently withdrawn from the market by its manufacturer in 2006 due to safety concerns including several deaths from liver failure in clinical trials. No other oral direct thrombin inhibitors are currently available.

Summary

Although oral antithrombotic agents had a role in the early days of percutaneous coronary intervention, its current role has become more limited with the advent of new, powerful, and highly selective antiplatelet agents. The use of oral anticoagulants has also been curtailed mainly by the need for frequent blood tests to assess coagulation status and by high rates of bleeding complications seen with these agents. At the present time, only a minority of patients require combined antiplatelet and antithrombotic therapy following PCI, and they should be maintained on this combination for the shortest possible period to avoid serious bleeding complications.

References

1 DeWood MA, Spores J, Notske R, *et al.* Prevalence of total coronary occlusion during the early hours of transmural myocardial infarction. *N Engl J Med.* 1980;**303**:897–902.

2 Gruntzig AR, Senning A, Siegenthaler WE. Nonoperative dilatation of coronary-artery stenosis: percutaneous transluminal coronary angioplasty. *N Engl J Med.* 1979;**301**:61–68.

3 Thornton MA, Gruentzig AR, Hollman J, *et al.* coumarins and aspirin in prevention of recurrence after transluminal coronary angioplasty: a randomized study. *Circulation.* 1984;**69**:721–727.

4 Urban P, Buller N, Fox K, *et al.* Lack of effect of warfarin on the restenosis rate or on clinical outcome after balloon coronary angioplasty. *Br Heart J.* 1988;**60**:485–488.

5 ten Berg JM, Kelder JL, Sutturp MJ, *et al.* Effect of coumarins started before coronary angioplasty on acute complications and long term follow-up. *Circulation.* 2000;**102**:386–391.

6 ten Berg JM, Hutten BA, Kelder JL, *et al.* Oral anticoagulant therapy during and after coronary angioplasty: the intensity and duration of anticoagulation are essential to reduce thrombotic complications. *Circulation.* 2001;**103**:2042–2047.

7 Coumadin Aspirin Reinfarction Study (CARS) Investigators. Randomised double-blind trial of fixed low-dose warfarin with aspirin after myocardial infarction. *Lancet.* 1997;**350**:389–396.

8 Fiore LD, Ezekowitz MD, Brophy MT, *et al.* Department of Veterans Affairs cooperative studies program clinical trial comparing combined warfarin and aspirin with aspirin alone in survivors of acute myocardial infarction: primary results of the CHAMP study. *Circulation.* 2002;**105**:557–563.

9 Hurlen M, Abdelnoor M, Smith P, *et al.* Warfarin, aspirin, or both after myocardial infarction. *N Engl J Med.* 2002;**347**:969–974.

10 van Es RF, Jonker JJ, Verheugt Fw, *et al.* Aspirin and coumadin after acute coronary syndromes (the ASPECT-2 study): a randomised controlled trial. *Lancet.* 2002;**360**(9327):109–113.

11 Anand SS, Yusuf S. Oral anticoagulant therapy in patients with coronary artery disease: a meta-analysis. *JAMA.* 1999;**282**:2058–2067.

12 Schatz RA, Baim DS, Leon M, *et al.* Clinical experience with the Palmaz-Schatz coronary stent: initial results of a multicenter study. *Circulation.* 1991;**83**:148–161.

13 Serruys PW, Strauss BH, Beatt KJ, *et al.* Angiographic follow-up after placement of a self-expanding coronary-artery stent. *N Engl J Med.* 1991;**324**:13–17.

14 Fischman DL, Leon BM, Baim DS, *et al.* A randomized comparison of coronary-stent placement and balloon angioplasty in the treatment of coronary artery disease. *N Engl J Med.* 1994;**331**:496–501.

15 Serruys PW, de Jaegere P, Kiemeneij F, *et al.* A comparison of balloon-expandable-stent implantation with balloon angioplasty in patients with coronary artery disease. *N Engl J Med.* 1994;**331**:489–95.

16 Cohen DJ, Krumholz HM, Sukin CA, *et al.* In-hospital and one-year economic outcomes after coronary stenting or balloon angioplasty: results from a randomized clinical trial: Stent Restenosis Study Investigators. *Circulation.* 1995;**92**:2480–2487.

17 Leon MB, Baim DS, Popma JJ, *et al.* A clinical trial comparing three antithrombotic-drug regimens after coronary artery stenting. *N Engl J Med.* 1998;**339**: 1665–1671.

18 Schomig A, Neumann F-J, Kastrati A, *et al.* A randomized comparison of antiplatelet and anticoagulant therapy after the placement of coronary-artery stents. *N Engl J Med.* 1996;**334**:1084–1089.

19 Bertrand ME, Legrand V, Boland J, *et al.* Randomized multicenter comparison of conventional anticoagulation versus antiplatelet therapy in unplanned and elective coronary stenting. *Circulation.* 1998;**98**:1597–1603.

20 Urban P, Macaya C, Rupprecht HJ, *et al.* Randomized evaluation of anticoagulation versus antiplatelet therapy after coronary stent placement in high-risk patients. *Circulation.* 1998;**98**:2126–2132.

21 Mattichak SJ, Reed PS, Gallagher MS, *et al.* Evaluation of the safety of warfarin in combination with antiplatelet therapy for patients treated with coronary stents for acute myocardial infarction. *J Interventional Cardiol.* 2005;**18**:163–166.

22 Kahn JK, Kodali U, Savas V, Gordon R. Effects of chronic warfarin therapy on complications of coronary angioplasty during acute myocardial infarction. *Am J Cardiol.* 1995;**75**:724.

23 Orford JL, Fasseas P, Melby S, *et al.* Safety and efficacy of aspirin, clopidogrel, and warfarin after coronary stent placement in patients with an indication for anticoagulation. *Am Heart J.* 2004;**147**:463–467.

24 Buresly K, Eisenberg MJ, Zhang X, Pilote L. Bleeding complications associated with combinations of aspirin, thienopyridine derivatives, and warfarin in elderly patients following acute myocardial infarction. *Arch Intern Med.* 2005;**165**:784–789.

25 Khurram Z, Chou E, Minutello R, *et al.* Combination therapy with aspirin, clopidogrel and warfarin following coronary stenting is associated with a significant risk of bleeding. *J Invasive Cardiol.* 2006;**18**:162–164.

26 Iakovou I, Schmidt T, Bonizzoni E, *et al.* Incidence, predictors, and outcome of thrombosis after successful implantation of drug-eluting stents. *JAMA.* 2005; **293**:2126–2130.

27 Arab D, Lewis B, Cho L, *et al.* Review: antiplatelet therapy in anticoagulated patients requiring coronary intervention. *J Invasive Cardiol.* 2005;**17**:549–554.

28 Batchelor WB, Mahaffey KW, Berger PB, *et al.* A randomized, placebo-controlled trial of enoxaparin after high-risk coronary stenting: the ATLAST trial. *J Am Coll Cardiol.* 2001;**38**:1608–1613.

29 Wallentin L, Wilcox RG, Weaver WD, *et al.* Oral ximelagatran for secondary prophylaxis after myocardial infarction: the ESTEEM randomised controlled trial. *Lancet.* 2003;**362**:789–797.

PART IV

IV

Elective PCI miscellaneous

CHAPTER 21

Agents to optimize access of radial artery approach

Tift Mann
Wake Heart Associates, Raleigh, NC, USA

The benefits of the transradial approach for percutaneous coronary intervention have been well documented in the past several years (1–10). Technological advances in the field of interventional cardiology as well as extensive experience with the transradial technique have resulted in primary success rates that now approach that of femoral procedures (11). Pharmacologic agents are an integral part of these improved success rates, and the purpose of the present chapter is to review these agents.

Prevention of radial artery vasospasm

The radial artery is a muscular vessel with a rich supply of alpha-1 adrenoreceptors (12). Smooth muscles cells within the vessel wall contract in response to stimulation of these adrenoreceptors, resulting in a significant reduction in lumen diameter. The radial artery has been classified as a type III vessel, reflecting the high rates of spasm found with this vessel as compared to others (13). Circulating catecholamines and mechanical stimulation result in significant vasospasm, which can prevent arterial access and interfere with catheter manipulation causing significant patient arm discomfort. Thus,

Pharmacology in the Catheterization Laboratory. Edited by Ron Waksman and Andrew E Ajani. © 2010 Blackwell Publishing, ISBN: 978-1-4051-5704-9.

prevention of vasospasm pharmacologically is mandatory for successful transradial procedures.

Sedation

Control of patient anxiety throughout the procedure will minimize circulating catecholamines. However, oversedation may limit postprocedure ambulation, one of the important advantages of the transradial approach. Patients at our center generally do not receive preprocedure medications, but diphenhydramine 25 mg IV is administered upon arrival in the catheterization laboratory. Midazolam 0.5–1 mg IV increments are administered as needed.

Analgesia

Local anesthesia is provided with subcutaneous lidocaine. We generally give only small amounts (1–2 cc) so as not to interfere with palpation of the radial pulse. Fentanyl in 25 mg increments is administered intravenously to control any other patient discomfort during the procedure.

Spasmolytics

One of the major advances in transradial catheterization has been the use of an intra-arterial cocktail to prevent vasospasm. Radial artery spasm can be objectively quantified using an automatic pullback device (14). Without the use of the spasmolytic cocktail, vasospasm will cause arm pain in a significant number of patients (15,16). He and Yang demonstrated rapid, prolonged relaxation of radial artery segments taken from patients undergoing coronary bypass surgery in vitro after a combination of verapamil plus nitroglycerin (17,18). Subsequent studies in patients have confirmed that this combination substantially reduces the incidence of vasospasm in patients undergoing transradial procedures and is more effective than other agents (15,16). Most experienced operators now administer verapamil 2.5–5 mg plus nitroglycerin 100–200 mcg diluted in 10 cc of saline directly into the radial artery through the side arm of the arterial sheath prior to catheter insertion. This solution may cause burning and is thus administered incrementally with further dilution using blood withdrawn from the side arm of the arterial sheath. Vasodilatation occurs immediately as seen using radial artery intravascular ultrasound (Figure 21.1) (19). In this study, radial artery area increased 44% after the administration of verapamil plus sublingual nitroglycerin with only a moderate reduction in mean arterial pressure and no significant change in heart rate (Figure 21.2) (19).

As previously mentioned, mechanical stimulation may evoke radial artery spasm. This particularly may occur after initial unsuccessful attempts to cannulate the vessel. In a recent study, the local subcutaneous administration of 400 mcg nitroglycerin resulted in a rapid return of pulse and facilitated cannulation (20). The use of hydrophilic coated arterial sheath also reduced patient arm discomfort (21,22). Presumably, the increased lubricity of the sheath resulted in less mechanically induced vasospasm.

Magnesium sulfate has been evaluated as a spasmolytic agent with potential additional advantages of analgesia and absent hemodynamic changes (23,24). Magnesium sulfate, administered as a 150 mg intra-arterial bolus over 1 min, resulted in a 36% increase in radial artery diameter with a reduced hemodynamic effect compared to verapamil (23). A major disadvantage to the use of this drug at our hospital is that individual doses must be mixed in the pharmacy increasing cost. Phentolamine 2.5 mg administered intravenously has been used by some physicians as a radial vasodilator (25).

Prevention of radial artery occlusion

Anticoagulants

Anticoagulation with unfractionated heparin even during diagnostic procedures is necessary to prevent procedural-related radial artery occlusion (26,27). We routinely administer 5,000 units of unfractionated heparin intravenously for diagnostic procedures, and additional heparin is administered as required for interventional procedures. Regardless of the anticoagulation administered, including group IIb/IIIa glycoprotein inhibitors and/or thrombolytic agents, the arterial sheath is removed at the conclusion of the procedure and a hemostasis device applied. The ease of selective radial artery compression for effective hemostasis is the reason why access site complications are virtually eliminated with the transradial approach (11).

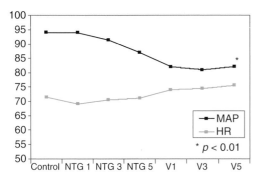

Figure 21.1 Hemodynamic effects of drug administration. MAP (mean arterial pressure, mmHg). HR (beats per minute). NTG (nitroglycerin; numbers indicate minutes after sublingual administration). V (verapamil; numbers indicate minutes after intra-arterial administration). *$p < .01$ as compared to control value.

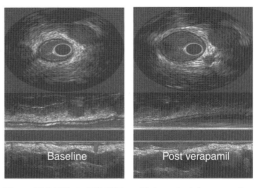

Figure 21.2 Effect of SL NTG and intra-arterial verapamil on the radial artery IVUS. Cross-sectional view above and serial pullback mode below.

The use of bivalirudin during ad hoc transradial interventions is a specialized situation since this drug is not packaged for diagnostic procedures. Thus, in order to protect against radial artery occlusion, we administer a reduced heparin dose for the diagnostic portion of the procedure (28). The balance of the 5,000-unit total heparin dose is then administered at the conclusion of the diagnostic procedure if an intervention is not performed. On the other hand, standard bivalirudin dosage is given should an interventional procedure be necessary. In this study, administration of the standard bivalirudin dosage after 1,000–2,500 units heparin did not cause bleeding complications, and dividing the heparin dose for a diagnostic procedure did not increase the incidence of radial artery occlusion (28).

With adequate anticoagulation, control of radial artery spasm, avoidance of oversized catheters, and expeditious removal of the hemostasis device, the incidence of radial occlusion is low (3,4,20,21). Although undesirable, radial artery occlusion is usually a benign, asymptomatic complication. A significant percentage of these cases will recanalize, and with the dual blood supply to the hand, hand ischemia due to a transradial procedure is rare.

References

1 Kiemeneij F, Laarman GJ, Slagboom T, van der Wieken R. Outpatient coronary stent implantation. *J Am Coll Cardiol.* 1997;**29**:323–327.

2 Kiemeneij F, Laarman GJ, Odekerken D, Slagboom T, van der Wieken R. A randomized comparison of percutaneous transluminal coronary angioplasty of the radial, brachial and femoral approaches: the ACCESS study. *J Am Coll Cardiol.* 1997;**29**:1269–1275.

3 Mann T, Cubeddu G, Bowen J, *et al.* Stenting in acute coronary syndromes: a comparison of radial versus femoral access sites. *J Am Coll Cardiol.* 1998;**32**:572–576.

4 Mann T, Cowper PA, Peterson ED, *et al.* Transradial coronary stenting: comparison with femoral access closed with an arterial suture device. *Catheter Cardiovasc Interv.* 2000;**49**:150–156.

5 Hildick-Smith DJ, Walsh JT, Lowe, MD, Shaprio LM, Petch MC. Transradial coronary angiography in patients with contraindications to the femoral approach: an analysis of 500 cases. *Catheter Cardiovasc Interv.* 2004; **61**:60–66.

6 Hildick-Smith DJ, Lowe MD, Walsh JT, *et al.* Coronary angiography from the radial artery—experience, complications and limitations. *Int J Cardiol.* 1998;**64**:231–239.

7 Louvard Y, Lefevre T, Allain A, Morice M. Coronary angiography through the radial or the femoral approach: the CARAFE study. *Catheter Cardiovasc Interv.* 2001;**52**:181–187.

8 Lotan C, Hasin Y, Mosseri M, *et al.* Transradial approach for coronary angiography and angioplasty. *Am J Cardiol.* 1995;**76**:164–167.

9 Cooper CJ, El-Shiekh RA, Cohen DJ, Blaesing L, Burket MW, Basu A. Effect of transradial access on quality of life and cost of cardiac catheterization: a randomized comparison. *Am Heart J.* 1999;**138**:430–436.

10 Saito S, Tanaka S, Hiroe Y, *et al.* Comparative study on transradial approach vs. transfemoral approach in primary stent implantation for patients with acute myocardial infarction: results of the test for myocardial infarction by prospective unicenter randomization for access sites (TEMPURA) trial. *Catheter Cardiovasc Interv.* 2003;**59**:26–33.

11 Agostoni P, Biondi-Zoccai G, Benedictis M, *et al.* Radial versus femoral approach for percutaneous diagnostic and interventional procedures. *J Am Coll Cardiol.* 2004;**44**:349–356.

12 He G-W, Yang C-Q. Characteristics of adrenoreceptors in the human radial artery; clinical implications. *J Thorac Cardiovasc Surg.* 1998;**115**:1136–1141.

13 He G-W, Yang C-Q. Comparison among arterial grafts and coronary artery: an attempt at functional classification. *J Thorac Cardiovasc Surg.* 1995;**109**:707–715.

14 Kiemeneij F, Vajifdar B, Eccleshall S, Laarman G, Slagboom T, van der Wieken R. Measurement of radial artery spasm using an automatic pullback device. *Catheter Cardiovasc Interv.* 2001;**54**:437–441.

15 Kiemeneij F, Vajifdar B, Eccleshall S, Laarman G, Slagboom T, van der Wieken R. Evaluation of a spasmolytic cocktail to prevent radial artery spasm during coronary procedures. *Catheter Cardiovasc Interv.* 2003;**58**:261–284.

16 Varenne O, Jegou A, Cohen R, *et al.* Prevention of arterial spasm during percutaneous coronary interventions through radial artery: the SPASM study. *Catheter Cardiovasc Interv.* 2006;**68**:231–235.

17 He G-W, Yang C-Q. Use of verapamil and nitroglycerine solution for preparation of radial artery for coronary bypass grafting. *Ann Thorac Surg.* 1996;**61**:610–614.

18 He G-W, Yang C-Q. Verapamil plus nitroglycerine solution maximally preserves endothelial function of the radial artery: comparison with papaverine solution. *J Thorac Cardiovasc Surg.* 1998;**115**:1321–1327.

19 Edmundson A, Mann T. Nonocclusive radial artery injury resulting from transradial coronary interventions: radial artery IVUS. *J Invas Cardiol.* 2005;**17**:528–531.

20 Pancholy S, Coppola J, Patel T. Subcutaneous administration of nitroglycerin to facilitate radial artery cannulation. *Catheter Cardiovasc Interv.* 2006;**68**:389–391.

21 Saito S, Tanaka S, Hiroe Y, *et al.* Usefulness of hydrophilic coating on arterial sheath introducer in transradial coronary intervention. *Catheter Cardiovasc Interv.* 2002;**56**:328–332.

22 Kiemeneij F, Fraser D, Slagboom T, Laarman G, van der Wieken R. Hydrophilic coating aids radial sheath withdrawal and reduces patient discomfort following transradial coronary intervention: a randomized double-blind comparison of coated and uncoated sheaths. *Catheter Cardiovasc Interv.* 2003;**59**:161–164.

23 Byrne J, Spence M, Haegeli L, *et al.* Magnesium sulphate during transradial cardiac catheterization: a new use for an old drug? *J Invasive Cardiol.* 2008;**20**:539–542.

24 Zellner C, Boyle A, Yeghiazarians Y. Magnesium sulfate for transradial cardiac catheterization: teaching an old dog new tricks. *Invasive Cardiol.* 2008;**20**:543–544.

25 Ruiz-Salmerón R, Mora R, Masotti M, Betriu A. Assessment of the efficacy of phentolamine to prevent radial artery spasm during cardiac catheterization procedures: a randomized study comparing phentolamine vs. verapamil. *Catheter Cardiovasc Interv.* 2005;**66**:192–198.

26 Stella PR, Kiemeneij F, Laarman G, Odekerken D, Slagboom T, van der Wieken R. Incidence and outcome of radial artery occlusion following transradial artery coronary angioplasty. *Cathet Cardiovasc Diagn.* 1997;**40**:156–158.

27 Spaulding C, Lefevre T, Funck F, *et al.* Left radial approach for coronary angiography: results of a prospective study. *Cathet Cardiovasc Diagn.* 1996;**39**:365–370.

28 Venkatesh K, Mann T. Transitioning from heparin to bivalirudin in patients undergoing ad hoc transradial interventional procedures: a pilot study. *J Invas Cardiol.* 2006;**18**:120–124.

PART V

High-risk PCI

CHAPTER 22

Diabetes mellitus

Joseph Lindsay
Washington Hospital Center, Washington, DC, USA

Overview of the problem

Diabetes mellitus confers a dramatically increased risk of death and myocardial infarction in comparison to patients without that disorder (1,2). Because its prevalence in the general population is steadily increasing, individuals with this disorder will inevitably constitute a growing proportion of patients presenting for cardiac catheterization (3). In as much as outcomes of percutaneous coronary intervention (PCI) in this group are inferior to nondiabetic patients, it is particularly appropriate to examine diabetes in some detail in connection with therapy in the cardiac catheterization laboratory.

Nearly all diabetes encountered in the catheterization laboratory is type 2. Glucose dysregulation is triggered not by an inadequate insulin production as in type 1 diabetes but by resistance to insulin activity at the tissue level. Hyperglycemia appears only after the pancreatic islet cells become unable to match with increased insulin production the tissue resistance in glucose disposal pathways into skeletal muscle and adipose tissue. Further, insulin-mediated reduction in hepatic production of glucose is blunted by insulin resistance (4). Importantly, it seems likely that damage to the vascular wall begins with the onset of insulin resistance, well before the appearance of hyperglycemia (5). Insulin resistance, adiposity, or associated dyslipidemia may each play a role in the premature coronary disease associated with the metabolic syndrome (6).

Pathogenetic mechanisms for diabetic vascular disease
Hyperglycemia/insulin resistance

It is increasingly recognized that the insulin-resistant/hyperglycemic state sets in motion complex metabolic pathways, resulting in oxidative stress in endothelial cells, vascular smooth muscle cells, leukocytes, and platelets (4,6,7). Oxygen free radicals promote a prothrombotic, proapoptotic, and proinflammatory state, thereby advancing the atherothrombotic process.

In contrast, insulin is protective of the vasculature. It produces vasodilatation through the nitric oxide-cyclic GMP pathway as well as anti-inflammatory effects on mononuclear leukocytes and endothelial cells (4,7). If, as in the case in insulin-resistant states such as the metabolic syndrome or type-2 diabetes, insulin receptors in the various cells do not respond normally to insulin, the beneficial effects of the hormone are blunted or lost (5–8).

It is important also to recall that a dysfunctional endothelium produced by the oxidative stress not only produces a diminished amount of NO but also increased amounts of vasoconstrictor prostanoids and endothelin. These may further promote

Pharmacology in the Catheterization Laboratory. Edited by Ron Waksman and Andrew E Ajani. © 2010 Blackwell Publishing, ISBN: 978-1-4051-5704-9.

inflammation and stimulate smooth muscle cell contraction and growth (4,7).

Moreover, diabetic vasculopathy appears to promote plaque rupture. Increased smooth muscle cell apoptosis in plaques leaves fewer such cells, and the elaboration of inflammatory cytokines diminishes smooth muscle cell synthesis of collagen and increases production of matrix metalloproteinase (4).

Altered platelet function and coagulation factors

The intracellular glucose concentration in platelets mirrors the extracellular environment. Consequently, hyperglycemia results in increased intracellular production of superoxide anions, resulting in decreased platelet-derived NO. These and other intracellular mechanisms increase the likelihood of platelet aggregation and adhesion. Coupled with these platelet-related events are increases in coagulation factors and reductions in endogenous anticoagulants. Further, increased production of plasminogen activator inhibitor-1 reduces the fibrinolytic process. All these processes contribute to a prothrombotic state (4).

Thus, through complex mechanisms, insulin and hyperglycemia have opposing effects. The former is anti-inflammatory and antithrombotic and the latter is proinflammatory and prothrombotic (7,8).

Free fatty acid liberation

Excess liberation of free fatty acids from adipose tissue and reduction of their uptake by skeletal muscle in insulin-resistant patients result in increased circulating levels. Free fatty acids are an additional disturbance to endothelial function because of their association with an increase in oxygen free radicals (4). Moreover, the liver responds to the increase in circulating free fatty acids by increasing production of triglyceride-rich lipoproteins, resulting in hypertriglyceridemia. A reduction in HDL-cholesterol (HDL-C) and an increase in small, dense LDL-cholesterol (LDL-C) ensue. The changes in HDL-C and in the nature of LDL-C result in a greater atherogenic potential as well as endothelial dysfunction (4).

Diabetes and outcomes of percutaneous coronary intervention

Reviews comparing catheter-based treatment of coronary stenoses in diabetic patients with those without the disorder indicate that procedural success and inhospital complication rates are similar whether the comparison is made in the balloon angioplasty era (9) or subsequent to the introduction of stenting (10). Intermediate and late outcomes, however, have been inferior to those in nondiabetic patients with regard to late mortality and rate of myocardial infarction (10,11).

Comparisons of late outcomes of coronary bypass surgery (CABG) and PCI have generally reflected comparable late mortality and myocardial infarction rates in nondiabetic patients but a survival advantage for CABG in diabetic patients with multivessel coronary disease (12,13). Uncertainty continues, however, since in both trials PCI was performed prior to the stent era and without GP IIb/IIIa blocking agents. Since the procedure now includes routine use of stents including drug-eluting stents, this topic remains controversial (14–18). Now in its follow-up phase, the BARI 2-D trial (19) addresses the role of revascularization by either catheter-based or operative techniques in patients with closely managed diabetes.

In addition to the more rapid progression of atherosclerosis inherent in the diabetic process, a substantially increased rate of restenosis in these patients with its attendant need for additional revascularization no doubt plays a role in the increased risk of late death and myocardial infarction. The addition of stenting reduced the rate of restenosis in diabetic patients just as it did in the overall PCI population (20,21). Although use of drug-eluting stents has reduced the frequency of restenosis in diabetic patients to less than 10%, the need for additional revascularization is still more frequent than that in nondiabetic patients (22,23).

It is important also to recall that diabetes mellitus is an independent predictor of procedure-associated nephropathy. This complication predicts adverse late outcomes (24), therefore its prevention by attention to hydration and by reduction of the contrast agent load to the least amount required are imperative. Moreover, consideration should be given to the use of whatever measures are currently employed in the laboratory to protect against this dangerous complication. This topic is discussed further in the chapter devoted to this topic.

Potential therapeutic strategies for improving outcomes in diabetic patients

Since it is late outcomes that are inferior in diabetic patients, the success of catheterization laboratory strategies will have to be gauged by the degree to which they are improved. Adverse late outcomes can plausibly be attributed to both progression of coronary atherothrombosis and to the higher rate of restenosis attendant on the diabetic state. Thus, the interventional cardiologist must attempt to reduce the restenosis rate and apply the latest secondary prevention strategies for this population. Secondary prevention recommendations for diabetic vascular disease are beyond the scope of this review. The reader is referred to the very recent review of the topic (25).

Antithrombotic therapy

In view of the prothrombotic state associated with diabetes, it is surprising that the recently published ACC/AHA guidelines for percutaneous intervention do not recommend any adjustments in antithrombotic therapy specifically for diabetic patients (26). As with nondiabetic patients, periprocedural administration of antithrombin agents (i.e., heparin, low-molecular-weight heparin, or bivalirudin) together with dual antiplatelet therapy (aspirin and clopidogrel or ticlopidine) is recommended.

Glycoprotein IIb/IIIa receptor blockers

In the light of the known platelet abnormalities associated with diabetes (27), a special role for inhibitors of platelet GP IIb/IIIa receptors was anticipated (28). Early trials of these agents conducted in patients with and without diabetes demonstrated improved survival for acute coronary syndromes in both groups (29,30). The pertinence of such therapy to contemporary coronary

intervention has been questioned on the grounds that the randomized trials supporting such a special role were conducted before the routine use of stents and dual antiplatelet therapy.

The first major randomized trial specifically for diabetic patients with *stable* coronary disease supports the position that current PCI strategies obviate the role of GP IIb/IIIa blocking agents (30). The ISAR-SWEET investigators found that outcomes of PCI are not improved by GP IIb/IIIa blocking drugs when a 600 mg clopidogrel loading dose is employed. It is, however, important to recognize that this study does not address patients with *unstable* coronary syndromes for whom the ACC/AHA guidelines continue to call for IIb/IIIa inhibitor for all patients undergoing PCI when clopidogrel is not being administered and indicate that it is *reasonable* to administer such agents if clopidogrel is being given.

There is suggestive evidence (30,31) that these agents reduce the rate of target vessel revascularization (TVR) in diabetic patients. It has been proposed that IIb/IIIa inhibitors reduce the amount of mural thrombus at the site of arterial injury from the PCI and the subsequent contribution of that thrombus to the formation of the pseudo-intimal proliferation that produces restenosis. A subsequent study employing intracoronary ultrasound did not support this hypothesis (32).

Insulin-sparing diabetic agents

The advent of insulin-sparing drugs for the care of diabetic patients (19), particularly the thiazolidinedione (TZD) class of antidiabetic agents, has generated great interest. These agents are agonists of the peroxisome proliferator-activated receptor-γ (PPAR-γ). They reduce insulin resistance and thereby improve glucose control and spare insulin production. In addition, they may beneficially modify dyslipidemia, the procoagulant state, intravascular inflammation, and blood pressure. They offer at least theoretical benefits for insulin-resistant patients even those without overt hyperglycemia. The effects of these agents have resulted in improved cardiovascular outcomes in experimental animals and in preliminary clinical trials (33).

The impact of TZD's on restenosis has been inconsistent, but a recent meta-analysis (34) identified a small beneficial effect on TVR in both diabetic and nondiabetic patients. On the other hand, a meta-analysis of TZD trials not limited to those in which PCI was performed sounds a discouraging note. Data from this analysis suggest that these agents may produce an adverse effect on survival (35). The ongoing BARI-2D trial should provide clearer insight into the effects of these promising agents (19).

Glycemic control

Regulation of the blood glucose/insulin balance, an intervention directed at the heart of the pathogenetic process, may offer the greatest promise for improving the results of PCI in diabetic patients. Indeed, Corpus *et al.* (36) found that adequate glycemic control, as evidenced by hemoglobin A1C levels ≤7% at the time of the PCI, is associated with need for TVR equal to that of patients without diabetes while those with less good glycemic control had much higher rates. Consistent with these findings are those of Robertson (37) who demonstrated an association between a preprocedural glucose level of 200 mg/dL or more and an increased frequency of a rise in CKMB and serum creatinine following PCI. Both of these are markers of late adverse outcomes (24). The deleterious effects of poor glycemic control on the vascular wall over time can reasonably be invoked to account for these two observations.

Not readily explicable by poor chronic glycemic control are observations indicating that "stress hyperglycemia" in diabetic patients as well as in those in whom the diagnosis was unknown is a more powerful predictor of both early and late mortality than the patient's usual blood sugar level or chronic glycemic control as reflected by hemoglobin A1c levels (8,38,39). Zarich and Nesto (8) summarize the putative mechanisms by which acute hyperglycemia produces a deleterious effect and insulin, a beneficial one.

It is plausible that the association of "stress hyperglycemia" and adverse outcomes is an epiphenomenon relating to the severity of illness and has no causative relationship, however against this possibility are recent observations indicating that acute intensive insulin therapy aimed at restoring near normal blood glucose levels reduces the risk of mortality and other complications in patients with acute myocardial infarction (8), other severe illness (40), and with coronary bypass surgery (41). Thus, it can be posited that acute hyperglycemia, independent of chronic glycemic control, results in significant vascular and tissue injury and thereby an adverse outcome and further that aggressive therapy to restore normal blood sugar can reverse its deleterious effects.

We observed an additional consequence of acute hyperglycemia during a preliminary investigation of restenosis in diabetic patients. We found in a cohort of stable diabetic patients (unlikely to have "stress hyperglycemia" from severe illness) undergoing PCI that preprocedure glucose level had a greater effect on nine-month TVR rate than chronic glycemic control as evidenced by hemoglobin A1c level (42). Thus, it seems possible that the metabolic state at the time of the vascular injury imposed by the procedure had effects prolonged enough to affect the process of restenosis.

The reasonable person might ask for the experimental underpinnings of the hypothesis that acute hyperglycemia is an important metabolic factor in diabetic vascular disease. Gresele *et al.* (43) demonstrated in 12 diabetic patients studied with glucose clamping that during hyperglycemia there was greater platelet activation than during euglycemia. Esposito *et al.* (44) found increased circulating inflammatory cytokines during controlled hyperglycemia in subjects with impaired glucose tolerance. Moreover, Kawano *et al.* (45) found that abnormal endothelial function appeared during the hyperglycemic phase of an oral glucose tolerance test in diabetics subjects as well as those with impaired or with normal glucose tolerance. Finally, taking advantage of technology to measure blood sugar continuously, Monnier *et al.* (46) demonstrated that metabolic evidence of oxidative stress was more closely associated with wide swings in glucose levels than with chronic glycemic control as measured by hemoglobin A1c.

Thus, there is experimental and clinical evidence that intensive control of blood glucose levels at the time of vascular injury (as in PCI) offers an opportunity for improving the outcomes of PCI. Clinical application of this strategy in the cardiac catheterization laboratory waits additional testing.

References

1 Bonow RO, Gheorghiade M. The diabetes epidemic: a national and global crisis. *Am J Med.* 2004;**116**:2–10.

2 Berry C, Tardif J-C, Bourassa MG. Coronary heart disease in patients with diabetes. Part I Recent advances in prevention and noninvasive management. *J Am Coll Cardiol.* 2007;**49**:631–642.

3 Fox CS, Coady S, Sorlie PD, *et al.* Increasing cardiovascular disease burden due to diabetes mellitus. *Circulation.* 2007;**115**:1544–1550.

4 Creager MA, Luscher TF, Cosentino F, Beckman JA. Diabetes and vascular disease: pathophysiology, clinical consequences, and medical therapy: Part I. *Circulation.* 2003;**108**:1527–1532.

5 Prior JO, Quinones MJ, Hernandez-Pampaloni M, *et al.* Coronary circulatory dysfunction in insulin resistance, impaired glucose tolerance, and type 2 diabetes mellitus. *Circulation.* 2005;**111**:2291–2298.

6 Wilson PWF, D'Agostino RB, Parise H, Sullivan L, Meigs JB. Metabolic syndrome as a precursor of cardiovascular disease and type 2 diabetes mellitus. *Circulation.* 2005;**112**:3066–3072.

7 Dandona P, Chaudhuri A, Ghanim H, Mohanty P. Effect of hyperglycemia and insulin in acute coronary syndromes. *Am J Cardiol.* 2007;**99**(suppl):12H–18H.

8 Zarich SW, Nesto RW. Implications and treatment of acute hyperglycemia in the setting of acute myocardial infarction. *Circulation.* 2007;**115**:e436–e439.

9 Stein B, Weintraub WS, Gebhart SSP, *et al.* Influence of diabetes mellitus on early and late outcomes after percutaneous transluminal coronary angioplasty. *Circulation.* 1995;**91**:979–989.

10 Mathew V, Gersh BJ, Williams BA, *et al.* Outcomes in patients with diabetes mellitus undergoing percutaneous coronary intervention in the current era. *Circulation.* 2004;**109**:476–480.

11 Wilson SR, Vakili BA, Sherman W, Sanborn TA, Brown D. Effect of diabetes on long-term mortality following contemporary percutaneous coronary intervention. *Diabetes Care.* 2004;**27**:1137–1142.

12 The BARI Investigators. The final 10-year follow-up results from the BARI randomized trial. *J Am Coll Cardiol.* 2007;**49**:1600–1606.

13 King SB, III, Kosinski AS, Guyton RA, Lembo NJ, Weintraub WS, for the Emory Angioplasty vs Surgery Trial (EAST) Investigators. Eight-year mortality in the Emory Angioplasty Versus Surgery Trial (EAST). *J Am Coll Cardiol.* 2000;**35**:1116–1121.

14 King SB, III. Surgery is preferred for the diabetic with multivessel disease. *Circulation.* 2005;**112**:1500–1507, 1514.

15 Dangas G, Moses JW. Debate on revascularization strategy for diabetic patients with multivessel coronary artery disease. *Circulation.* 2005;**112**:1507–1515.

16 Flaherty JD, Davidson CJ. Diabetes and coronary revascularization. *JAMA.* 2005;**293**:1501–1508.

17 Berry C, Tardif J-C, Bourassa MG. Coronary heart disease in patients with diabetes. Part II: recent advances in coronary revascularization. *J Am Coll Cardiol.* 2007;**49**:643–656.

18 Briguori C, Condorelli G, Airoldi F, *et al.* Comparison of coronary drug-eluting stents versus coronary artery bypass grafting in patients with diabetes mellitus. *Am J Cardiol.* 2007;**99**:779–784.

19 Sobel BE, Frye R, Detre KM. Burgeoning dilemmas in the management of diabetes and cardiovascular disease. Rationale for the Bypass Angioplasty Revascularization Investigation 2 Diabetes (BARI 2D) trial. *Circulation.* 2003;**107**:636–642.

20 Elezi S, Kastrati A, Pache J, *et al.* Diabetes mellitus and the clinical and angiographic outcome after coronary stent placement. *J Am Coll Cardiol.* 1998;**32**:1866–1873.

21 Cutlip DE, Chauhan MS, Baim DS, *et al.* Clinical restenosis after coronary stenting: perspectives from multicenter trials. *J Am Coll Cardiol.* 2002;**40**:2082–2089.

22 Moussa I, Leon MB, Baim DS, *et al.* Impact of sirolimus-coated stents in diabetic patients. *Circulation.* 2004;**109**:2273–2278.

23 Sabaté M, Jiménez-Quevedo P, Angiolillo DJ, *et al.* Randomized comparison of sirolimus-eluting stent versus standard stent for percutaneous coronary revascularization in diabetic patients. The diabetes and sirolimus-eluting stent (DIABETES) trial. *Circulation.* 2005;**112**:2175–2183.

24 Lindsay J, Canos DA, Apple S, Pinnow E, Aggrey G, Pichard AD. Causes of acute renal dysfunction after percutaneous coronary intervention and comparison of late mortality rates with post procedure rise of creatine kinase-MB versus rise of serum creatinine. *Am J Cardiol.* 2004;**94**:786–789.

25 Berry C, Tardif J-C, Bourassa MG. Coronary disease in patients with diabetes. Part I: recent advances in prevention and noninvasive measures. *J Am Coll Cardiol.* 2007;**49**:631–642.

26 Smith SC, Jr, Feldman TE, Hirshfeld JW, Jr, *et al.* ACC/AHA/SCAI: guideline update for percutaneous coronary intervention—summary article. *Circulation.* 2006;**113**:156–175.

27 Colwell JA, Nesto RW. The platelet in diabetes. *Diabetes Care.* 2003;**26**:2181–2188.

28 Lincoff AM. Important triad in cardiovascular medicine. Diabetes, coronary intervention, and platelet glycoprotein IIb/IIIa receptor blockade. *Circulation.* 2003;**107**:1556–1559.

29 Roffi M, Chew DP, Mukherjee D, *et al.* Platelet glycoprotein IIb/IIIa inhibitors reduce mortality in diabetic patients with non-ST-segment-elevation acute coronary syndromes. *Circulation.* 2001;**104**:2767–2771.

30 Marso SP, Lincoff AM, Ellis SG, *et al.* Optimizing the percutaneous interventional outcomes for patients with diabetes mellitus. *Circulation.* 1999;**100**:2477–2484.

31 Mehilli J, Kastrati A, Schühlen H, *et al.* Randomized clinical trial of abciximab in diabetic patients undergoing elective percutaneous coronary interventions after treatment with a high loading dose of clopidogrel. *Circulation.* 2004;**110**:3627–3635.

32 Chaves AJ, Sousa AGMR, Mattos LA, *et al.* Volumetric analysis of in-stent intimal hyperplasia in diabetic patients treated with and without Abciximab. *Circulation.* 2004;**109**:861–866.

33 Hsueh WA, Bruemmer D. Peroxisome proliferator-activated receptor: implications for cardiovascular disease. *Hypertension.* 2004;**43**(part 2):2987–2305.

34 Riche DM, Valderrama R, Henyan NN. Thiazolidinediones and risk of repeat target vessel revascularization following percutaneous coronary intervention. *Diabetes Care.* 2007;**30**:384–388.

35 Nissen SE, Woloski K. Effect of rosiglitazone on the risk of myocardial infarction and death from cardiovascular causes. *N Engl J Med.* 2007;**356**:2457–2471.

36 Corpus RA, George PB, House JA, *et al.* Optimal glycemic control is associated with a lower rate of target vessel revascularization in treated type II diabetic patients undergoing elective percutaneous coronary intervention. *J Am Coll Cardiol.* 2004;**43**:8–14.

37 Robertson BJ, Gascho JA, Gabbay RA, McNulty PH. Usefulness of hyperglycemia in predicting renal and myocardial injury in patients with diabetes mellitus undergoing percutaneous coronary intervention. *Am J Cardiol.* 2004;**94**:1027–1029.

38 Ceriello A. Acute hyperglycemia: a "new" risk factor during acute myocardial infarction. *Eur Heart J.* 2005;**26**:328–331.

39 Timmer JR, Ottervanger JP, Bilo HJG, *et al.* Prognostic value of admission glucose and glycosylated haemoglobin levels in acute coronary syndromes. *Q J Med.* 2006;**99**:237–243.

40 Van den Berghe G, Wouters P, Weekers F, *et al.* Intensive insulin therapy in critically patients. *N Engl J Med.* 2001;**345**:1359–1367.

41 Lazar HL, Chipkin SR, Fitzgerald CA, Bao Y, Cabral H, Apstein CS. Tight glycemic control in diabetic coronary artery bypass graft patients improves perioperative outcomes and decreases recurrent ischemic events. *Circulation.* 2004;**109**:1497–1502.

42 Lindsay J, Sharma AK, Canos D, *et al.* Preprocedure hyperglycemia is more strongly associated with restenosis in diabetic patients after percutaneous coronary intervention than is hemoglobin A1C. *Cardiovasc Revasc Med.* 2007;**8**:15–20.

43 Gresele P, Guglielmini G, De Angelis M, *et al.* Acute, short-term hyperglycemia enhances shear-stress-induced platelet activation in patients with type II diabetes mellitus. *J Am Coll Cardiol.* 2003;**41**:1013–1020.

44 Esposito K, Nappo F, Marfella R, *et al.* Inflammatory cytokine concentrations are acutely increased by hyperglycemia in humans. *Circulation.* 2002;**106**:2067–2072.

45 Kawano H, Motoyama T, Hirashima O, *et al.* Hyperglycemia rapidly suppresses flow-mediated-endothelium dependent vasodilatation of the brachial artery. *J Am Coll Cardiol.* 1999;**34**:146–154.

46 Monnier L, Mas E, Ginet C, *et al.* Activation of oxidative stress by acute glucose fluctuations compared with sustained chronic hyperglycemia in patients with type 2 diabetes. *JAMA.* 2006;**295**:1681–1687.

CHAPTER 23

Cardiogenic shock

Pantelis Diamantouros[1] & E. Magnus Ohman[2]
[1]University of Western Ontario, London, ON, Canada
[2]Duke University Medical Center, Durham, NC, USA

In this chapter, we will be reviewing the diagnosis, etiology, risk factors, and prognosis of cardiogenic shock. The evidence for the mainstays of treatment of cardiogenic shock will also be discussed. The complimentary pharmacologic management of shock including the use of inotropic agents and anticoagulation for devices will be reviewed in the following chapters.

Pathophysiology

Definition and diagnosis

Cardiogenic shock is defined as a state of inadequate tissue perfusion due to severe impairment of ventricular function in the setting of adequate intravascular volume. The criteria required for the diagnosis of cardiogenic shock used in the SHOCK trial (Should we emergently revascularize Occluded Coronaries for cardiogenic shocK (1)) entail

- a systolic blood pressure <90 mmHg or supported to >90 mmHg;
- heart rate > 60/min;
- not responsive to fluid administration;
- secondary to cardiac dysfunction;

- associated with signs of hypoperfusion (oliguria <30 mL/h, altered mental state, cold extremities); and
- cardiac index <2.2 L/min/m² and pulmonary capillary wedge pressure >15 mmHg.

Cardiogenic shock often develops within 48 h after initial presentation but can develop considerably later, sometimes as late as 2 weeks after infarction (2). Patients presenting in cardiogenic shock comprise 15% of cases with 85% of patients developing cardiogenic shock after admission.

Etiology

Although acute myocardial infarction (AMI), resulting in left ventricular dysfunction, is the most common cause of cardiogenic shock (3), other etiologies in the setting of AMI include ventricular septal rupture, ventricular free-wall rupture, and acute mitral regurgitation which together account for 12% of cases (4–6). Right ventricular dysfunction accounts for around 3% of cases (7). As well, cardiogenic shock can also occur in the setting of a non-ST elevation acute coronary syndrome complicating about 2.5% of such cases (8–10). Most patients with AMI complicated by shock have severe coronary disease with 16% of those who underwent coronary angiography having left main disease and 53% of those having triple vessel disease (11). Worse coronary artery disease is associated with more severe MR (12).

Some of the other noncoronary causes of cardiogenic shock include severe valvular heart

Pharmacology in the Catheterization Laboratory. Edited by Ron Waksman and Andrew E Ajani. © 2010 Blackwell Publishing, ISBN: 978-1-4051-5704-9.

disease, myocarditis, and hypertrophic obstructive cardiomyopathy.

Mechanism

Most patients develop shock because of extensive myocardial necrosis or ischemia, resulting in reduced stroke volume and arterial pressure. What then follows is a series of neurohormonal responses that include activation of the renin–angiotensin system and the sympathetic nervous system due to the perceived reduction in effective circulating volume and pressure (Figure 23.1). These responses cause vasoconstriction and salt and water retention, which lead to diminished coronary artery perfusion, thereby, triggering a downward spiral of further myocardial ischemia and necrosis, which further lowers arterial pressure, resulting in lactic acidosis, organ failure, and ultimately death (13). In addition, excessive nitric oxide synthase production in the setting of AMI and shock results in high levels of nitric oxide that cause inappropriate vasodilation, leading to further systemic and coronary hypoperfusion and depression of the myocardium (14,15).

Clinical information

Risk of developing cardiogenic shock

Due to the increased mortality associated with cardiogenic shock, identification of high-risk subgroups of patients presenting with acute coronary syndromes likely to develop shock is important for timely diagnosis and rapid treatment of this high-risk group. Certain clinical and demographic variables have been found to strongly correlate with the development of cardiogenic shock. Age is the variable with the strongest association with an increased risk of 47% for developing shock with every 10-year increase in age. Along with age, systolic blood pressure, heart rate, and Killip class provide more than 85% of the predictive information needed (16).

Prognosis

Despite significant advances in the treatment of AMI over the last 25 years, the proportion of AMI cases complicated by cardiogenic shock has remained unchanged at 5–10% (17–19). Shock

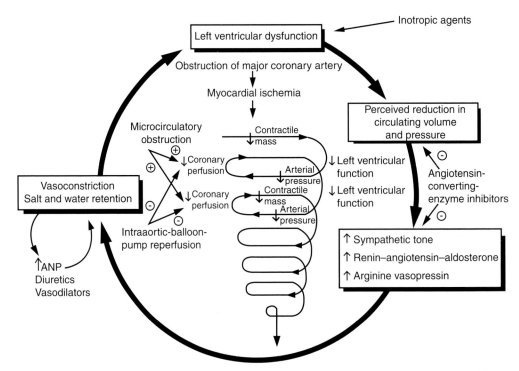

Figure 23.1 The downward spiral of cardiogenic shock. (*Source: J Intensive Care Med.* 2005;**20**:188–198; adapted from *N Engl J Med.* 1994;**330**:1724–1730.)

continues to be the leading cause of death in patients presenting with acute myocardial infarction (20–22) with mortality rates as high as 80% historically. Lower rates of inhospital mortality have been noted more recently ranging from 56% to 74% (9,18,19,21,23) and may reflect early revascularization strategies and increased use of IABC. Contemporary data from the SHOCK trial shows 1-year survival rates for the early revascularization group of 46.7% compared to 33.6% for the initial medical stabilization group (24). Long-term (6-year) data report survival rates of 32.8% and 19.6% in patients managed with an early revascularization strategy compared to initial medical stabilization, respectively (25).

The timing of the development of cardiogenic shock relative to presentation appears to have an effect on prognosis as well. Patients with early shock development (within 48 h) appear to have significantly lower mortality rates than those with later shock development (26). However, patients that present in cardiogenic shock appear to have a higher inhospital mortality rate of 75% and tend to die more rapidly (27).

Patients presenting with ST-elevation myocardial infarction (STEMI) complicated by shock have similar mortality rates to those presenting with non-STEMI complicated by shock (10).

Predictors of mortality

Once cardiogenic shock has developed, there are some risk factors that may identify patients at higher risk for mortality. Analysis from the GUSTO-I database identified increasing age as a predictor of mortality with an odds ratio of 1.49 for each 10-year increase in age (28). In an analysis of the SHOCK registry, cardiac power, defined as the product of simultaneously measured cardiac output and mean arterial pressure, was found to be the strongest hemodynamic predictor of mortality (29). Echocardiographically, the only independent predictors of outcome were left ventricular ejection fraction and severity of mitral regurgitation (30).

Management strategy

The management of cardiogenic shock will be discussed in the context of AMI since this is the most common etiology. The goal in any patient presenting with cardiogenic shock is efficient stabilization and transfer for revascularization to the cardiac catheterization laboratory, surgical suite, or to another facility with these capabilities. Therapies for cardiogenic shock can be thought of in the context of initial stabilizing measures, left ventricular support, and counteraction of MI expansion.

Initial stabilization

Initial stabilization and resuscitation involves the administration of intravenous fluids to exclude the possibility of hypovolemia unless the patient is in obvious pulmonary edema. An empiric volume challenge of isotonic saline can be administered. Further boluses can be administered under the guidance of hemodynamic measures from the right heart catheter. In cases of right ventricular shock, preload is critical and, therefore, fluid support and avoidance of nitrates are indicated.

Patients with pulmonary edema may require therapy with diuretics, morphine, and supplemental oxygen. Endotracheal intubation and mechanical ventilation are often indicated for airway support and ventilation. Sedation and muscle paralysis improves procedural safety and decreases oxygen demand. In selected patients, a trial of noninvasive positive pressure ventilation may be attempted. The use of mechanical ventilation may increase the likelihood of successful weaning from IABC support. In a small study (28 patients), a significantly larger proportion of ventilated patients were weaned from IABC (90% vs 44%) and discharged from the hospital (80% vs 28%) (31).

Sustained brady- and tachy-dysrhythmias should be treated appropriately as per ACLS (Advances Cardiac Life Support) protocols in order to maximize cardiac output. Metabolic derangements that may predispose to dysrhythmias should be identified and corrected. As well, normalization of glucose levels with an insulin infusion is a class I recommendation in patients with STEMI and cardiogenic shock whether or not they have a diagnosis of diabetes mellitus (32).

Drugs that have a negative inotropic effect should be avoided in cardiogenic shock. Included in this group are beta blockers, calcium channel antagonists and antiarrhythmic agents with negative inotropic or vasodilating effects such as procainmide, bretylium, and quindine (32). Amiodarone is the antiarrhythmic agent of choice if one is required although it does have some beta-blocking properties.

Insertion of a Swan-Ganz catheter and an intra-arterial blood pressure monitoring catheter are recommended. Repeated hemodynamic determination will help to help evaluate the response to therapeutic interventions (13,32,33). In addition, hemodynamic data may be used to help in the detection and quantification of intracardiac shunting from ventricular septal rupture in AMI.

Counteracting extension of myocardial infarction
Pharmacologic therapies
Aspirin

Aspirin at a dose of 160–325 mg is recommended for all patients with cardiogenic shock complicating AMI (32). Even though aspirin has not been studied in this specific setting, it significantly reduces mortality from AMI. If unable to be taken orally, alternative routes include administration via a nasogastric tube, via rectal suppository, or crushed for absorption through the buccal mucosa.

Clopidogrel

Clopidogrel at a loading dose of 300–600 mg is recommended for all patients with cardiogenic shock complicating AMI who have had stenting of the infarct-related artery (IRA) (34). Given the need for emergency surgery in a large proportion of these patients, it is reasonable to defer the administration of clopidogrel therapy until the revascularization strategy has been determined. If the patient is unable to take medication orally, the clopidogrel can be crushed and given via a nasogastric tube. Loading strategies and other considerations regarding clopidogrel therapy will be discussed in more detail in Chapter 6.

Heparin

Intravenous unfractionated heparin (bolus 60 U/kg, maximum 4,000 U IV bolus; initial infusion of 12 U/kg/h, maximum 1,000 U/h) is recommended for patients with AMI complicated by cardiogenic shock. These patients are in a low-flow state with high fibrinogen concentrations and, therefore, are at risk for left ventricular and deep venous thrombosis. Even though heparin has not been specifically evaluated in cardiogenic shock, it reduces mortality in AMI (32). The use of heparin as an adjunct to mechanical devices used in cardiogenic shock will be discussed further in Chapter 1.

Glycoprotein IIb/IIIa inhibitors

Platelet glycoprotein (GP) IIb/IIIa blockade has been studied extensively in the setting of AMI but the data for its use in AMI complicated by cardiogenic shock comes mostly from nonrandomized studies. The benefit of IIb/IIIa blockade in this setting appears to be its ability to help prevent the no-reflow phenomenon. Although the exact mechanism is unclear, it is postulated that the no-reflow phenomenon is caused by abnormalities at the level of the microvasculature (35). IIb/IIIa blockade prevents platelet and neutrophil adhesion and helps mitigate against the no re-flow phenomenon by reducing microthrombus formation and relief of microvasculature obstruction (36,37). A more detailed review of the no-reflow phenomenon and its medical management can be found in Chapter 28.

In a study by Giri *et al.*, abciximab was shown to improve 30-day outcomes (composite event rate of death, reinfarction, and target vessel revascularization) of primary PCI with and without stenting in AMI complicated by cardiogenic shock (31% vs 63%, $p = 0.002$) (38). In a later study by Antoniucci *et al.* where all patients with AMI and cardiogenic shock underwent stenting, the use of abciximab significantly reduced 1-month mortality (18% vs 42%, $p < 0.020$) (39). In a multivariate analysis, abciximab was the only variable independently related to 1-month mortality (OR 0.36%, $p = 0.021$, 95% confidence intervals 0.15–0.86) (39). High procedural success rates and improved outcomes in AMI complicated by cardiogenic shock were also observed with abciximab use in the nonrandomized REO-SHOCK trial (40). Furthermore, a retrospective observational review from 1988 to 2003 by Huang *et al.* demonstrated that stent use with IIb/IIIa blockade using abciximab and antiplatelet therapy was significantly associated with survival in AMI complicated by cardiogenic shock (adjusted $p = 0.007$) (41). These findings were supported by a prospective review by

Chan *et al.* who showed that stenting and abciximab use in AMI complicated by CS was superior to stent only, PTCA plus abciximab, and PTCA alone with mortality rates at 2.5 years of follow-up of 33%, 43%, 61%, and 68%, respectively (log-rank $p = 0.028$) (42).

The only available randomized data for the use of IIb/IIIa blockade in AMI complicated by cardiogenic shock comes from a post hoc analysis of the PURSUIT trial (9). This demonstrated that patients with unstable angina and NSTEMI complicated by shock treated with eptifibatide had significantly reduced 30-day mortality rates (52.7% vs 77.2%, $p = 0.001$).

In a meta-analysis of randomized clinical trials evaluating the use of abciximab vs placebo in primary percutaneous coronary intervention, treatment with abciximab significantly reduced the 30-day composite end point of death, reinfarction, or ischemic or urgent target vessel revascularization (OR = 0.54; 95% CI, 0.40–0.72) (43). The clinical benefit of reduction of early adverse ischemic events seen with abciximab use was maintained at 6-month follow-up (OR = 0.80; 95% CI, 0.67–0.97).

Therefore, it is recommended that patients with cardiogenic shock undergoing PCI receive abciximab with eptifibatide being a viable alternative, in the absence of contraindications. The recommended dosing regimens are as follows:

Abciximab—0.25 mg/kg IV bolus then a 12 h infusion at 10 mg/min.

Eptifibatide—180 mg/kg bolus followed by a second 180 mg/kg bolus with an infusion at 2 mg/kg/min started after the first bolus for 18 h. Infusion decreased to 1 mg/kg/min if impaired renal function present.

Fibrinolysis

Due to the significant amount of evidence in their favor, PPCI and CABG are the preferred methods for reperfusion in AMI complicated by cardiogenic shock. In canine models, Prewitt *et al.* have shown that coronary clot lysis is dependent on perfusion pressure and coronary blood flow (44). In the setting of AMI complicated by cardiogenic shock, these parameters are impaired and this may account for the benefit of mechanical vs pharmacologic reperfusion seen in the SHOCK trial. However,

fibrinolytic therapy may be indicated if delays are anticipated. It may also be administered to patients who are not candidates for early revascularization with no contraindications (32). Tenecteplase is as effective as alteplase and, due to its ease of administration and less noncerebral bleeding and need for transfusion, it has become the most commonly used fibrinolytic agent.

If thrombolysis is chosen as the revascularization strategy, Prewitt *et al.* have shown that in canine models with states of moderate hypotension, IABC enhanced the rate of rTPA (recombinant tissue plasminogen activator)–induced coronary thrombolysis in canines (45).

As well, in humans, the TACTICS trial assessed the benefit of adding 48 h of IABC therapy to fibrinolysis in patients with AMI complicated by sustained hypotension, possible cardiogenic shock, or possible heart failure. Only 57 patients were randomized and the trial was stopped early due to poor enrollment but, when analyzed, the data showed that patients with Killip class III or IV heart failure showed a trend toward greater benefit from having early IABC added to their fibrinolytic therapy (6-month mortality 39% vs 80%, $p = 0.05$) (46).

Mechanical reperfusion strategies
SHOCK trial

Nonrandomized studies have suggested that mechanical reperfusion of occluded coronary arteries by PCI or CABG may improve survival in AMI patients with cardiogenic shock. The SHOCK trial confirmed this approach and was a multicenter, prospective, randomized study, which enrolled 302 patients. At 30 days, overall mortality did not significantly differ between the revascularization and medical therapy groups (46.7% and 56.0%, respectively, $p = 0.11$). However, at 6 months, mortality was significantly lower in the revascularization group (50.3% vs 63.1%, $p = 0.027$) (1). The 12-month mortality remained significantly lower for the emergency revascularization group (PCI or CABG) compared to the medical stabilization group (53.3% vs 66.4%, $p < 0.03$) (see Figure 23.2) (24). Prespecified subgroup analysis showed an even greater benefit of early revascularization in patients less than 75 years of age. The benefit of early revascularization is long-lasting

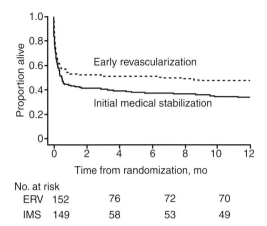

Figure 23.2 SHOCK trial Kaplan–Meier survival curve 1-year postrandomization. Log-rank test $p = 0.04$. (*Source*: Hochman et al. (25).)

and resulted in a 13.2% absolute and a 67% relative improvement in 6-year survival compared with initial medical stabilization (25). However, in patients older than 75 years, there was no treatment benefit seen. Similar results were seen in the SMASH (Swiss Multicenter trial of Angioplasty for Shock) trial although the results in this 55-patient study did not reach statistical significance (47).

Patients presenting to a nonacute care facility in cardiogenic shock should be transferred to a tertiary care facility with PCI and CABG capabilities. Analysis of the SHOCK trial and registry demonstrates the same relative benefit between transferred and directly admitted patients (48). IABP placement before transport will help stabilize the patient, if skilled personnel are available.

Given the large treatment effect (13 lives saved per 100 patients treated), emergency revascularization is recommended for patients under the age of 75 years. Interventions should be performed as soon as possible with a goal of revascularization occurring within 18 h of the development of shock.

Emergency revascularization in the elderly

For patients over the age of 75 years, results from the SHOCK trial are not conclusive since there were only 56 such patients enrolled. Data from the larger, nonrandomized SHOCK registry where

patients over the age of 75 years were clinically selected to receive emergency revascularization reveal a marked survival benefit in these patients even after covariate adjustment and exclusion of early deaths (49). Furthermore, in a closer analysis of the SHOCK trial data for patients over the age of 75, Dzavik et al. concluded that the survival benefit of early revascularization is applicable to patients over the age of 75 years as well (50). The lack of apparent benefit from early revascularization may be due to differences in important baseline characteristics, specifically LV function, and play of chance arising from such a small sample size. Other registries investigating elderly patients with AMI complicated by CS report a decline in hospital mortality over time that corresponds with a more aggressive early revascularization strategy (51). As well, a strategy of routine early revascularization is highly feasible and results in lower hospital mortality rates (44–56%) in a real-world selection of elderly shock patients than those reported for the elderly in the SHOCK trial (81%) (52–54).

Coronary artery bypass grafting

CABG is the preferred mode of revascularization for left main or triple vessel disease to achieve complete revascularization preferably within 6 h of the development of shock (55,56). In the SHOCK trial, 30-day outcome was similar between the PCI and CABG groups despite more severe coronary disease and more diabetes in the CABG group (57). Surgical revascularization should be considered in shock patients with severe mitral insufficiency or multivessel disease not amenable to complete percutaneous revascularization (58). For moderate three-vessel disease, the SHOCK trial recommends PCI of the IRA followed by delayed CABG for those who stabilize (15,23). Other strategies include PTCA of the IRA and IABC as a bridge to emergency CABG.

Left ventricular and blood pressure support
Tilarginine

Generation of excess nitric oxide during AMI complicated by cardiogenic shock is believed to contribute to inappropriate vasodilation and contribute to the high mortality seen in cardiogenic shock. One of the more novel approaches to the treatment of cardiogenic shock under investigation recently is the inhibition of nitric oxide synthase (NOS) using tilarginine (L-N^{G}-monomehtylarginine [L-NMMA]). This is a nonselective NOS inhibitor that was studied in the TRIUMPH trial (59). This randomized, double-blind, placebo-controlled trial had a primary outcome of all-cause mortality. The trial was terminated early after enrollment of 398 out of a planned 658 patients based on a prespecified futility analysis. Although there was a significant increase in the systolic blood pressure of the group treated with tilarginine, there was no difference in 30-day (48% vs 42%, risk ratio 1.14; 95% CI 0.92–1.41; $p = 0.24$) or 6-month (58% vs 59%, risk ratio 1.04; 95% CI 0.79–1.36; $p = 0.80$) all-cause mortality between the tilarginine and placebo groups, respectively (59). Therefore, although it held much promise and significantly raised blood pressure in cardiogenic shock patients, tilarginine has no effect on mortality in this high-risk group at the dose (1 mg/kg bolus and 1 mg/kg/h for 5 h) studied in the TRIUMPH trial (see Figure 23.3). That fact that NOS inhibition by tilarginine raised blood pressure further supports the theory of excess nitric oxide production playing a role in the pathophysiology of cardiogenic shock.

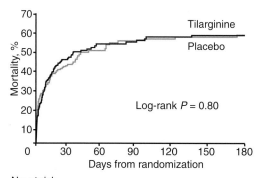

Figure 23.3 Kaplan–Meier mortality over 6 months of follow-up in the TRIUMPH trial. (*Source*: *JAMA*. March 26, 2007.)

Intra-aortic balloon counterpulsation (IABC)

An intra-aortic balloon pump is usually inserted through the femoral artery and placed in the descending thoracic aorta distal to the left subclavian artery. The balloon is inflated during cardiac diastole to augment diastolic blood pressure and thereby increase the coronary artery perfusion pressure and myocardial oxygen supply. It is deflated during the isovolumetric phase of left ventricular contraction and this decreases systemic afterload, aortic impedance, and myocardial oxygen consumption. The net effect is a favorable shift in the myocardial oxygen supply/demand ratio with a small increase in systemic perfusion (60).

The appropriate sized balloon is one that when placed just distal to the left subclavian artery does not obstruct the renal arteries. After appropriate placement and preparation, the balloon is filled and the pump's ratio is set to 1:1 for cardiac assist in the acute setting and is then weaned as deemed appropriate by the clinical situation usually 24–48 h after reperfusion. Careful surveillance for complications is required during IABC.

Anticoagulation is required for the prevention of thromboembolic complications (see Chapter 33 for more details).

The use of IABC alone in many patients reverses end organ hypoperfusion and stabilizes patients but often does not allow for weaning of the device and does not alter mortality because coronary flow has not been reestablished with reperfusion therapy (61,62). However, although there is no randomized clinical data, when IABC is used in conjunction with reperfusion therapy, outcomes appear to be improved (46,63–65). If IABC is to be used, there is registry data that supports its insertion before intervention in the catheterization laboratory. In a report by Brodie *et al.*, IABC was a significant independent predictor of freedom from catheterization laboratory events (ventricular fibrillation, cardiopulmonary arrest, prolonged hypotension) in patients with cardiogenic shock (14.5% vs 35.1%, $p = 0.009$) (66). If a strategy of pharmacologic reperfusion has been chosen, the administration of thrombolytic therapy should not be delayed once the diagnosis of AMI has been made. Insertion of an IABC catheter via a femoral artery should be carefully undertaken by experienced operators in order to avoid any bleeding complications.

Table 23.1 ACC/AHA recommendations for cardiogenic shock.

Class I

1 Intra-aortic balloon counterpulsation is recommended for STEMI patients when cardiogenic shock is not quickly reversed with pharmacological therapy. The IABP is a stabilizing measure for angiography and prompt revascularization. *(Level of Evidence: B)*

2 Intra-arterial monitoring is recommended for the management of STEMI patients with cardiogenic shock. *(Level of Evidence: C)*

3 Early revascularization, either PCI or CABG, is recommended for patients less than 75 years old with ST elevation or LBBB who develop shock within 36 h of MI and who are suitable for revascularization that can be performed within 18 h of shock unless further support is futile because of the patient's wishes or contraindications or unsuitability for further invasive care. *(Level of Evidence: A)*

4 Fibrinolytic therapy should be administered to STEMI patients with cardiogenic shock who are unsuitable for further invasive care and do not have contraindications to fibrinolysis. *(Level of Evidence: B)*

5 Echocardiography should be used to evaluate mechanical complications unless these are assessed by invasive measures. *(Level of Evidence: C)*

Class IIa

1 Pulmonary artery catheter monitoring can be useful for the management of STEMI patients with cardiogenic shock. *(Level of Evidence: C)*

2 Early revascularization, either PCI or CABG, is reasonable for selected patients 75 years or older with ST elevation or LBBB who develop shock within 36 h of MI and who are suitable for revascularization that can be performed within 18 h of shock. Patients with good prior functional status who agree to invasive care may be selected for such an invasive strategy. *(Level of Evidence: B)*

Source: Adapted from Antman *et al.* (32).

Guidelines published by the ACC/AHA in 2004 gave a class I recommendation for the use of IABC as a stabilizing measure in AMI in patients with cardiogenic shock not quickly reversed pharmacologically or with acute MR or ventricular septal defect (see Table 23.1) (32).

Left ventricular assist device (LVAD)

A percutaneous left ventricular assist device (LVAD) was compared to IABC in a small randomized trial. Although hemodynamic and metabolic parameters were reversed more effectively by the LVAD, complications (severe bleeding and limb ischemia) were more common and there was no difference in mortality (67). Therefore, pending any newer, the use of percutaneous LVADs is not recommended in cardiogenic shock unless in the setting of a randomized trial.

References

1 Hochman JS, Sleeper LA, Webb JG, *et al.* Early revascularization in acute myocardial infarction complicated by cardiogenic shock. SHOCK Investigators. Should we emergently revascularize occluded coronaries for cardiogenic shock. *N Engl J Med.* August 26, 1999;**341**(9):625–634.

2 Lindholm MG, Kober L, Boesgaard S, Torp-Pedersen C, Aldershvile J. Cardiogenic shock complicating acute myocardial infarction; prognostic impact of early and late shock development. *Eur Heart J.* February 2003;**24**(3):258–265.

3 Menon V, White H, LeJemtel T, Webb JG, Sleeper LA, Hochman JS. The clinical profile of patients with suspected cardiogenic shock due to predominant left ventricular failure: a report from the SHOCK Trial Registry. SHould we emergently revascularize Occluded Coronaries in cardiogenic shocK? *J Am Coll Cardiol.* September 2000;**36**(3 Suppl A):1071–1076.

4 Thompson CR, Buller CE, Sleeper LA, *et al.* Cardiogenic shock due to acute severe mitral regurgitation complicating acute myocardial infarction: a report from the SHOCK Trial Registry. SHould we use emergently revascularize Occluded Coronaries in cardiogenic shocK? *J Am Coll Cardiol.* September 2000;**36**(3 Suppl A): 1104–1109.

5 Menon V, Webb JG, Hillis LD, *et al.* Outcome and profile of ventricular septal rupture with cardiogenic shock after myocardial infarction: a report from the SHOCK Trial Registry. SHould we emergently revascularize Occluded Coronaries in cardiogenic shocK? *J Am Coll Cardiol.* September 2000;**36**(3 Suppl A):1110–1116.

6 Slater J, Brown RJ, Antonelli TA, *et al.* Cardiogenic shock due to cardiac free-wall rupture or tamponade after acute myocardial infarction: a report from the SHOCK Trial Registry. Should we emergently revascularize occluded coronaries for cardiogenic shock? *J Am Coll Cardiol.* September 2000;**36**(3 Suppl A):1117–1122.

7 Jacobs AK, Leopold JA, Bates E, *et al.* Cardiogenic shock caused by right ventricular infarction: a report from the SHOCK registry. *J Am Coll Cardiol.* April 16, 2003;**41**(8):1273–1279.

8 Jacobs AK, French JK, Col J, *et al.* Cardiogenic shock with non-ST-segment elevation myocardial infarction: a report from the SHOCK Trial Registry. SHould we emergently revascularize Occluded coronaries for Cardiogenic shocK? *J Am Coll Cardiol.* September 2000;**36**(3 Suppl A):1091–1096.

9 Hasdai D, Harrington RA, Hochman JS, *et al.* Platelet glycoprotein IIb/IIIa blockade and outcome of cardiogenic shock complicating acute coronary syndromes without persistent ST-segment elevation. *J Am Coll Cardiol.* September 2000;**36**(3):685–692.

10 Holmes DR, Jr, Berger PB, Hochman JS, *et al.* Cardiogenic shock in patients with acute ischemic syndromes with and without ST-segment elevation. *Circulation.* November 16, 1999;**100**(20):2067–2073.

11 Wong SC, Sanborn T, Sleeper LA, *et al.* Angiographic findings and clinical correlates in patients with cardiogenic shock complicating acute myocardial infarction: a report from the SHOCK Trial Registry. SHould we emergently revascularize Occluded Coronaries for cardiogenic shocK? *J Am Coll Cardiol.* September 2000;**36**(3 Suppl A):1077–1083.

12 Berkowitz MJ, Picard MH, Harkness S, Sanborn TA, Hochman JS, Slater JN. Echocardiographic and angiographic correlations in patients with cardiogenic shock secondary to acute myocardial infarction. *Am J Cardiol.* October 15, 2006;**98**(8):1004–1008.

13 Califf RM, Bengtson JR. Cardiogenic shock. *N Engl J Med.* June 16, 1994;**330**(24):1724–1730.

14 Akiyama K, Kimura A, Suzuki H, *et al.* Production of oxidative products of nitric oxide in infarcted human heart. *J Am Coll Cardiol.* August 1998;**32**(2):373–379.

15 Hochman JS. Cardiogenic shock complicating acute myocardial infarction: expanding the paradigm. *Circulation.* June 24, 2003;**107**(24):2998–3002.

16 Hasdai D, Califf RM, Thompson TD, *et al.* Predictors of cardiogenic shock after thrombolytic therapy for acute myocardial infarction. *J Am Coll Cardiol.* January 2000;**35**(1):136–143.

17 Hasdai D, Topol EJ, Califf RM, Berger PB, Holmes DR, Jr. Cardiogenic shock complicating acute coronary syndromes. *Lancet.* August 26, 2000;**356**(9231):749–756.

18 Goldberg RJ, Gore JM, Thompson CA, Gurwitz JH. Recent magnitude of and temporal trends (1994–1997) in the incidence and hospital death rates of cardiogenic shock complicating acute myocardial infarction: the second national registry of myocardial infarction. *Am Heart J.* January 2001;**141**(1):65–72.

19 Holmes DR, Jr, Bates ER, Kleiman NS, *et al.* Contemporary reperfusion therapy for cardiogenic shock: the GUSTO-I trial experience. The GUSTO-I Investigators. Global utilization of streptokinase and tissue plasminogen activator for occluded coronary arteries. *J Am Coll Cardiol.* September 1995;**26**(3):668–674.

20 Goldberg RJ, Gore JM, Alpert JS, *et al.* Cardiogenic shock after acute myocardial infarction. Incidence and mortality from a community-wide perspective, 1975 to 1988. *N Engl J Med.* October 17, 1991;**325**(16):1117–1122.

21 Goldberg RJ, Samad NA, Yarzebski J, Gurwitz J, Bigelow C, Gore JM. Temporal trends in cardiogenic shock complicating acute myocardial infarction. *N Engl J Med.* April 15, 1999;**340**(15):1162–1168.

22 Zeymer U, Vogt A, Zahn R, *et al.* Predictors of in-hospital mortality in 1333 patients with acute myocardial infarction complicated by cardiogenic shock treated with primary percutaneous coronary intervention (PCI); Results of the primary PCI registry of the Arbeitsgemeinschaft Leitende Kardiologische Krankenhausarzte (ALKK). *Eur Heart J.* February 2004;**25**(4):322–328.

23 Hochman JS, Boland J, Sleeper LA, *et al.* Current spectrum of cardiogenic shock and effect of early revascularization on mortality. Results of an International Registry. SHOCK Registry Investigators. *Circulation.* February 1, 1995;**91**(3):873–881.

24 Hochman JS, Sleeper LA, White HD, *et al.* One-year survival following early revascularization for cardiogenic shock. *JAMA.* January 10, 2001;**285**(2):190–192.

25 Hochman JS, Sleeper LA, Webb JG, *et al.* Early revascularization and long-term survival in cardiogenic shock complicating acute myocardial infarction. *JAMA.* June 7, 2006;**295**(21):2511–2515.

26 Webb JG, Sleeper LA, Buller CE, *et al.* Implications of the timing of onset of cardiogenic shock after acute myocardial infarction: a report from the SHOCK Trial Registry. SHould we emergently revascularize Occluded Coronaries for cardiogenic shocK? *J Am Coll Cardiol.* September 2000;**36**(3 Suppl A):1084–1090.

27 Jeger RV, Harkness SM, Ramanathan K, *et al.* Emergency revascularization in patients with cardiogenic shock on admission: a report from the SHOCK trial and registry. *Eur Heart J.* March 2006;**27**(6):664–670.

28 Hasdai D, Holmes DR, Jr, Califf RM, *et al.* Cardiogenic shock complicating acute myocardial infarction: predictors of death. GUSTO Investigators. Global utilization of streptokinase and tissue-plasminogen activator for occluded coronary arteries. *Am Heart J.* July 1999;**138**(1 Pt 1):21–31.

29 Fincke R, Hochman JS, Lowe AM, *et al.* Cardiac power is the strongest hemodynamic correlate of mortality in cardiogenic shock: a report from the SHOCK trial registry. *J Am Coll Cardiol.* July 21, 2004;**44**(2):340–348.

30 Picard MH, Davidoff R, Sleeper LA, *et al.* Echocardiographic predictors of survival and response to early revascularization in cardiogenic shock. *Circulation.* January 21, 2003;**107**(2):279–284.

31 Kontoyannis DA, Nanas JN, Kontoyannis SA, Stamatelopoulos SF, Moulopoulos SD. Mechanical ventilation in conjunction with the intra-aortic balloon pump improves the outcome of patients in profound cardiogenic shock. *Intensive Care Med.* August 1999;**25**(8):835–838.

32 Antman EM, Anbe DT, Armstrong PW, *et al.* ACC/AHA guidelines for the management of patients with ST-elevation myocardial infarction: a report of the American College of Cardiology/American Heart Association Task Force on Practice Guidelines (Committee to Revise the 1999 Guidelines for the Management of Patients with Acute Myocardial Infarction). *Circulation.* August 31, 2004;**110**(9):e82–e292.

33 Mueller HS, Chatterjee K, Davis KB, *et al.* ACC expert consensus document. Present use of bedside right heart catheterization in patients with cardiac disease. American College of Cardiology. *J Am Coll Cardiol.* September 1998;**32**(3):840–864.

34 Smith SC, Jr, Feldman TE, Hirshfeld JW, Jr, *et al.* ACC/AHA/SCAI 2005 guideline update for percutaneous coronary intervention: a report of the American College of Cardiology/American Heart Association Task Force on Practice Guidelines (ACC/AHA/SCAI Writing Committee to Update 2001 Guidelines for Percutaneous Coronary Intervention). *Circulation.* February 21, 2006;**113**(7):e166–e286.

35 Rezkalla SH, Kloner RA. No-reflow phenomenon. *Circulation.* February 5, 2002;**105**(5):656–662.

36 Topol EJ, Yadav JS. Recognition of the importance of embolization in atherosclerotic vascular disease. *Circulation.* February 8, 2000;**101**(5):570–580.

37 Williams MS, Coller BS, Vaananen HJ, Scudder LE, Sharma SK, Marmur JD. Activation of platelets in platelet-rich plasma by rotablation is speed-dependent and can be inhibited by abciximab (c7E3 Fab; ReoPro). *Circulation.* August 25, 1998;**98**(8):742–748.

38 Giri S, Mitchel J, Azar RR, *et al.* Results of primary percutaneous transluminal coronary angioplasty plus abciximab with or without stenting for acute myocardial infarction complicated by cardiogenic shock. *Am J Cardiol.* January 15, 2002;**89**(2):126–131.

39 Antoniucci D, Valenti R, Migliorini A, *et al.* Abciximab therapy improves survival in patients with acute myocardial infarction complicated by early cardiogenic shock undergoing coronary artery stent implantation. *Am J Cardiol.* August 15, 2002;**90**(4):353–357.

40 Zeymer U, Tebbe U, Weber M, *et al.* Prospective evaluation of early abciximab and primary percutaneous intervention for patients with ST elevation myocardial infarction complicated by cardiogenic shock: results of the REO-SHOCK trial. *J Invasive Cardiol.* July 2003;**15**(7):385–389.

41 Huang R, Sacks J, Thai H, *et al.* Impact of stents and abciximab on survival from cardiogenic shock treated with percutaneous coronary intervention. *Catheter Cardiovasc Interv.* May 2005;**65**(1):25–33.

42 Chan AW, Chew DP, Bhatt DL, Moliterno DJ, Topol EJ, Ellis SG. Long-term mortality benefit with the combination of stents and abciximab for cardiogenic shock complicating acute myocardial infarction. *Am J Cardiol.* January 15, 2002;**89**(2):132–136.

43 Kandzari DE, Hasselblad V, Tcheng JE, *et al.* Improved clinical outcomes with abciximab therapy in acute myocardial infarction: a systematic overview of randomized clinical trials. *Am Heart J.* March 2004;**147**(3):457–462.

44 Prewitt RM, Gu S, Schick U, Ducas J. Effect of a mechanical vs a pharmacologic increase in aortic pressure on coronary blood flow and thrombolysis induced by IV administration of a thrombolytic agent. *Chest.* February 1997;**111**(2):449–453.

45 Prewitt RM, Gu S, Schick U, Ducas J. Intraaortic balloon counterpulsation enhances coronary thrombolysis induced by intravenous administration of a thrombolytic agent. *J Am Coll Cardiol.* March 1, 1994;**23**(3):794–798.

46 Ohman EM, Nanas J, Stomel RJ, *et al.* Thrombolysis and counterpulsation to improve survival in myocardial infarction complicated by hypotension and suspected cardiogenic shock or heart failure: results of the TACTICS Trial. *J Thromb Thrombolysis.* February 2005;**19**(1):33–39.

47 Urban P, Stauffer JC, Bleed D, *et al.* A randomized evaluation of early revascularization to treat shock complicating acute myocardial infarction. The (Swiss) Multicenter Trial of Angioplasty for Shock-(S)MASH. *Eur Heart J.* July 1999;**20**(14):1030–1038.

48 Jeger RV, Tseng CH, Hochman JS, Bates ER. Interhospital transfer for early revascularization in patients with ST-elevation myocardial infarction complicated by cardiogenic shock—a report from the SHould we revascularize Occluded Coronaries for cardiogenic shocK? (SHOCK) trial and registry. *Am Heart J.* October 2006;**152**(4):686–692.

49 Dzavik V, Sleeper LA, Cocke TP, *et al.* Early revascularization is associated with improved survival in elderly patients with acute myocardial infarction complicated by cardiogenic shock: a report from the SHOCK Trial Registry. *Eur Heart J.* May 2003;**24**(9):828–837.

50 Dzavik V, Sleeper LA, Picard MH, *et al.* Outcome of patients aged >or= 75 years in the SHould we emergently revascularize Occluded Coronaries in cardiogenic shocK (SHOCK) trial: do elderly patients with acute myocardial infarction complicated by cardiogenic shock respond differently to emergent revascularization? *Am Heart J.* June 2005;**149**(6):1128–1134.

51 Dauerman HL, Goldberg RJ, Malinski M, Yarzebski J, Lessard D, Gore JM. Outcomes and early revascularization for patients > or = 65 years of age with cardiogenic shock. *Am J Cardiol.* April 1, 2001;**87**(7):844–848.

52 Migliorini A, Moschi G, Valenti R, *et al.* Routine percutaneous coronary intervention in elderly patients with cardiogenic shock complicating acute myocardial infarction. *Am Heart J.* November 2006;**152**(5):903–908.

53 Dauerman HL, Ryan TJ, Jr, Piper WD, *et al.* Outcomes of percutaneous coronary intervention among elderly patients in cardiogenic shock: a multicenter, decade-long experience. *J Invasive Cardiol.* July 2003;**15**(7):380–384.

54 Prasad A, Lennon RJ, Rihal CS, Berger PB, Holmes DR, Jr. Outcomes of elderly patients with cardiogenic shock treated with early percutaneous revascularization. *Am Heart J.* June 2004;**147**(6):1066–1070.

55 Allen BS, Rosenkranz E, Buckberg GD, *et al.* Studies on prolonged acute regional ischemia. VI. Myocardial infarction with left ventricular power failure: a medical/surgical emergency requiring urgent revascularization with maximal protection of remote muscle. *J Thorac Cardiovasc Surgery.* November 1989;**98**(5 Pt 1):691–702; discussion 3.

56 Allen BS, Buckberg GD, Fontan FM, *et al.* Superiority of controlled surgical reperfusion versus percutaneous transluminal coronary angioplasty in acute coronary occlusion. *J Thorac Cardiovasc Surg.* May 1993;**105**(5):864–879; discussion 79–84.

57 White HD, Assmann SF, Sanborn TA, *et al.* Comparison of percutaneous coronary intervention and coronary artery bypass grafting after acute myocardial infarction complicated by cardiogenic shock: results from the Should We Emergently Revascularize Occluded Coronaries for Cardiogenic Shock (SHOCK) trial. *Circulation.* September 27, 2005;**112**(13):1992–2001.

58 Webb JG, Lowe AM, Sanborn TA, *et al.* Percutaneous coronary intervention for cardiogenic shock in the SHOCK trial. *J Am Coll Cardiol.* October 15, 2003; **42**(8):1380–1386.

59 The TRIUMPH Investigators. Effect of tilarginine acetate in patients with acute myocardial infarction and cardiogenic shock: the TRIUMPH randomized controlled trial. *JAMA.* 2007;**297**:1657–1666.

60 Nanas JN, Moulopoulos SD. Counterpulsation: historical background, technical improvements, hemodynamic and metabolic effects. *Cardiology.* 1994;**84**(3):156–167.

61 Scheidt S, Wilner G, Mueller H, *et al.* Intra-aortic balloon counterpulsation in cardiogenic shock. Report of a co-operative clinical trial. *N Engl J Med.* May 10, 1973;**288**(19):979–984.

62 Goldberger M, Tabak SW, Shah PK. Clinical experience with intra-aortic balloon counterpulsation in 112 consecutive patients. *Am Heart J.* March 1986;**111**(3):497–502.

63 Anderson RD, Ohman EM, Holmes DR, Jr, *et al.* Use of intraaortic balloon counterpulsation in patients presenting with cardiogenic shock: observations from the GUSTO-I Study. Global Utilization of Streptokinase and TPA for Occluded Coronary Arteries. *J Am Coll Cardiol.* September 1997;**30**(3):708–715.

64 Barron HV, Every NR, Parsons LS, *et al.* The use of intra-aortic balloon counterpulsation in patients with cardiogenic shock complicating acute myocardial infarction: data from the National Registry of Myocardial Infarction 2. *Am Heart J.* June 2001;**141**(6):933–939.

65 Sanborn TA, Sleeper LA, Bates ER, *et al.* Impact of thrombolysis, intra-aortic balloon pump counterpulsation, and their combination in cardiogenic shock complicating acute myocardial infarction: a report from the SHOCK Trial Registry. SHould we emergently revascularize Occluded Coronaries for cardiogenic shocK? *J Am Coll Cardiol.* September 2000; **36**(3 Suppl A):1123–1129.

66 Brodie BR, Stuckey TD, Hansen C, Muncy D. Intra-aortic balloon counterpulsation before primary percutaneous transluminal coronary angioplasty reduces catheterization laboratory events in high-risk patients with acute myocardial infarction. *Am J Cardiol.* July 1, 1999;**84**(1):18–23.

67 Thiele H, Sick P, Boudriot E, *et al.* Randomized comparison of intra-aortic balloon support with a percutaneous left ventricular assist device in patients with revascularized acute myocardial infarction complicated by cardiogenic shock. *Eur Heart J.* July 2005; **26**(13):1276–1283.

CHAPTER 24

High-risk coronary intervention and renal dysfunction

Geoffrey Lee, Ronen Gurvitch, & Andrew E. Ajani
The Royal Melbourne Hospital, Melbourne, Victoria, Australia

Background

A potential complication of coronary intervention is contrast medium-induced nephropathy (CIN), leading to transient or permeant renal dysfunction. CIN is defined as an increase in serum creatinine of 0.5 mg/dL or a 25% or greater relative increase from baseline within 72 h of iodinated contrast medium infusion (1–4).

Pathogenesis

The exact mechanism of CIN has not been established although several causes have been described. These include increased adenosine-, endothelin-, and free radical-induced vasoconstriction and reduced nitric oxide- and prostaglandin-induced vasodilatation. The final common pathway, however, is thought to be an ischemic injury to the outer renal medulla, although contrast agents can also have direct toxic effects on renal tubular cells (5).

The true incidence of CIN is unknown, but in the general unselected population, it is said to in the order of 2%. However, this risk can be as high as 20–30% (1–4) in patients with risk factors.

These risk factors include underlying chronic renal impairment, diabetes mellitus, congestive heart failure, and older age. Apart from patient factors, higher contrast volume load is also an important factor. CIN is usually transient with serum creatinine levels peaking at 3 days and returning back to normal after 10 days. It is not a benign condition and has been linked to increase morbidity, increased length of stay, and also increased costs of hospital stay (6). Renal failure after contrast administration requiring inhospital dialysis is associated with poor outcome including 36% inhospital mortality and 19% 2-year survival (5,7).

Risk-prediction models for the risk factors of CIN have been looked at in the setting of percutaneous coronary interventions (8). Independent risk factors include: hypotension (if systolic blood pressure <80 mm Hg for at least 1 h requiring inotropic support), use of intra-aortic balloon pump, congestive heart failure (if class III/IV by New York Heart Association classification or history of pulmonary edema), age (>75 years), anemia (if hematocrit >39% for men and >36% for women), diabetes mellitus, contrast media volume (incremental risk per 100 mL contrast agent used), and estimated glomerular filtration. Preprocedural creatinine >3 mg/dL and preexisting renal impairment were all shown to be important determinates for the development of CIN.

The decision to proceed to high-risk coronary intervention is based on a balanced risk benefit evaluation by the clinician. Unfortunately, in

Pharmacology in the Catheterization Laboratory. Edited by Ron Waksman and Andrew E Ajani. © 2010 Blackwell Publishing, ISBN: 978-1-4051-5704-9.

the acute situation, often there is no alternative strategy and coronary intervention must proceed with the caveat that nephrotoxicity from contrast media may occur. It is therefore mandatory to adopt prophylactic protocols to prevent radio contrast nephropathy and rationalize adjunctive coronary medications that may also be nephrotoxic.

Preventive strategies

There have been many strategies described in the literature to prevent CIN in general radiological imaging procedures and also during coronary angiography. These include intervention such as prehydration, use of nonionic low-osmolal contrast agents, oral and intravenous N-acetylcysteine (NAC), and prehydration, dopamine and fenoldopam infusion, vasodilation using intravenous theophylline, and the use of pre- and post-procedural hemodialysis. To date, there is no firm evidence to support any of these strategies in large randomized controlled trials.

Contrast media

Contrast media is divided into high, low and iso-osmolar depending on their relative osmolality to plasma. The introduction of low osmolar contrast media has lead to a decrease incidence of CIN and this decreased risk seems to be more pronounced in those with higher preprocedural serum creatinine (1–4).

Apart from the type of contrast media, the volume of contrast media is also an independent risk factor for the development of CIN. It has been suggested to limit the total contrast volume to 3 mL/kg, by limiting the number angiographic views taken and reduce the number of test injections during interventional wire and device placement (9). Although studies have shown mixed results of these studies, there is a general acceptance to use the smallest possible amount of a nonionic, low-osmolal contrast agent, and to avoid repeated contrast administration within a short period of time.

Prehydration

Correction of hypovolemia is important before percutaneous coronary intervention and the administration of contrast media. It is generally recommended that fluid hydration be employed is a simple and effective means to reduce CIN. However, there are no conclusive large prospective trials that randomize patients to pre- or no hydration to prevent CIN.

There are many trials looking at different intravenous hydration protocols to prevent CIN, however, there is no fluid hydration protocol that seems to be superior over another (10–13). Stevens et al. studied patients with preexisting renal insufficiency undergoing percutaneous coronary intervention, and randomized them to fluid hydration, IV hydration plus frusemide, hydration plus IV frusemide plus dopamine, IV hydration plus IV frusemide plus dopamine plus mannitol, and found no differences in outcomes between all groups (12).

Despite the lack of conclusive evidence, intravenous hydration with 0.9% isotonic saline in the periprocedural period can be used to try and prevent CIN. Care must be taken in the acute infarct setting where patients may be in heart failure and fluid overloaded.

N-acetylcysteine

The data on the efficacy of NAC to prevent CIN have been mixed. There are several prospective, randomized trials that have shown administration of NAC and IV hydration to reduce the incidence of CIN in high-risk patients with preexisting renal impairment. The reason for this disparity in reported efficacy is thought to be due to a heterogeneity between these studies in their hydration protocols, dosage, of NAC used, different volumes and types of contrast media used, and also different procedures performed (14).

Despite the mixed results of trials, NAC is often given to those with the highest risk (i.e., those with elevated serum creatinine) in part because of its favorable side effect profile, low cost, and ease of administration. There are different NAC protocols but a typical dosing regimen would be NAC at a dose of 600 mg bid for 24 h before and after the procedure along with IV fluid hydration.

Rationalization of cardiac medications

In the setting of the high-risk acute coronary intervention, worsening cardiac and vascular function may lead to a decreased cardiac output a reduction of the circulating blood volume and a decrease in the intrarenal perfusion pressure. Maintenance of the glomerular filtration rate is maintained by the activation of the renin–angiotensin–aldosterone system. In particular, there is an increase effect of angiotensin II, leading to a preferential increase in resistance at the efferent postglomerular arteriole.

Medications that blunt renal vascular autoregulation such as angiotensin-converting enzyme inhibitors (ACE inhibitors), angiotensin II receptor blockers (A2RB), and nonsteroidal anti-inflammatory drugs need to be rationalized in this setting. Likewise, potential direct nephrotoxic agents such as gentamicin should be ceased prior to the procedure.

ACE inhibitors and A2RB

Both ACE inhibitors and A2RB drugs affect the renin–angiotensin–aldosterone system. One of the major effects of ACE inhibitors is to inhibit the conversion of angiotensin I to the vasoconstrictor angiotensin II while A2RB blocks the binding receptor of angiotensin II. Long-term suppression of the renin–angiotensin system with ACE inhibitors and angiotensin-2 receptor blockers has been shown to be of benefit in a variety of settings including in acute myocardial infarcts, systolic heart failure, hypertension, and in the diabetic population.

However, during high-risk coronary intervention, which often occurs in the milieu of cardiogenic shock, hypotension, hypovolemia, and the use of high-contrast media volumes concomitant ACE inhibition or A2RB inhibition can increase the risk of contrast-induced nephropathy. In this setting, these drugs should be ceased before the procedure if patients are already taking these medications or started/restarted for long-term benefit when renal function has stabilized in the postprocedure period.

Nonsteroidal anti-inflammatory drugs

Nonsteroidal anti-inflammatory drugs (NSAIDs) in the form of selective and nonselective cyclooxygenase inhibitors are a commonly used class of medications for the treatment of pain. The predominate action of NSAIDs is to inhibit cyclooxygenase, an enzyme responsible for the production of important biological mediators called prostanoids (including prostaglandins (PG), prostacyclin, and thromboxane).

NSAID medications are well known to potentially cause acute renal failure in the general population. A recent nested case-control study by Huerta *et al.* (15) found that the incidence rate of nonfatal acute renal failure was 1.1 cases/10,000 person-years and that users of NSAIDs had a threefold greater risk of developing first ever ARF than nonusers (15).

NSAID-induced acute renal failure is caused by two distinct mechanisms. First, its hemodynamic effects on renal perfusion mediated by inhibition of prostaglandin synthesis. Inhibition of renal prostaglandin production impairs the normal compensatory renal vasodilatory response induced by activation of the renin–angiotensin–aldosterone system. Second, NSAIDs can lead to acute renal failure by causing an acute interstitial nephritis. Recent evidence suggests that selective COX-2 inhibitors have the same nephrotoxic risk as nonselective COX inhibitors (16).

Because of the additive risk of renal impairment, NSAIDs should be avoided during the index admission for high-risk coronary intervention. More recently, both cyclooxygenase 2 selective (COX-2 inhibitors) and nonselective NSAIDs have captured the attention of the popular press due to the increased cardiovascular risk signal generated from these medications, in particular the selective COX-2 inhibitor. As such, they should be used with caution in those with either preexisting cardiovascular disease or in those with cardiovascular risk factors (17).

Metformin

Preexisting biguanide metformin (dimethylbiguanide) use is likely in the diabetic patient undergoing high-risk coronary intervention. Metformin for treatment of noninsulin-dependant diabetes has been shown to reduce microvascular events and also reduce cardiovascular events in the obese population (18). Metformin has 90% renal excretion in the first 24 h of oral administration. However, in the setting of renal insufficiency (glomerular filtration rate <70 mL/min, or serum creatinine >1.6 mg/dL [140 μmol/L]), there is retention of these biguanides in the tissues and a potential to develop lactic acidosis (19).

Lactic acidosis as a complication of metformin use is rare and has a reported incidence of one to five cases per 100,000 (20). There has been no evidence of lactic acidosis being precipitated by the use of contrast media in the setting of normal renal function. All the reported cases in the literature have been in the setting of preexisting renal impairment and tissue hypoxia such as in the setting of acute myocardial infarction.

Recent recommendations have been suggested to discontinue metformin when tissue hypoxia is suspected and to withdraw for 3 days after contrast medium-containing iodine has been given, and start treatment with metformin only after renal function has been checked (21).

Summary

Contrast-induced nephropathy in the setting of high-risk coronary intervention is a serious complication that can lead to increased morbidity. Those at greatest risk are those with preprocedural creatinine >3 mg/dL and preexisting renal impairment. Those with normal renal function and without recognized risk factors for CIN do not need measurement of creatinine or preventative strategies. Although evidence on the best strategy to prevent this complication is mixed, there are a few general measures that can be undertaken to potentially reduce the risk and can be summarized as follows:

- Use smallest possible amount of a nonionic, low-osmolal or iso-osmolal contrast agent, and avoid repeated contrast administration within a short period of time.
- Periprocedural intravenous hydration to avoid hypovolemia.
- Consideration of the use of NAC in the periprocedural period.
- Cessation of nephrotoxic medications such as gentamicin and NSAIDS (both selective and nonselective COX inhibitors).
- Temporary cessation of ACE inhibitors and A2RB inhibitors if patient is at high risk of contrast-induced nephropathy (until renal function stabilizes).
- Cessation of metformin in the setting of preexisting renal impairment, tissue hypoxia, or possible CIN. Withdraw metformin for 3 days after exposure to iodinated contrast media and restart treatment only after renal function has stabilized.

References

1 Murphy SW, Barrett BJ, Parfrey PS. Contrast nephropathy. *J Am Soc Nephrol.* 2000;**11**:177–182.

2 Fishbane S, Durham JH, Marzo K, Rudnick M. N-Acetylcysteine in the prevention of radio contrast-induced nephropathy. *J Am Soc Nephrol.* 2004;**15**: 251–260.

3 Gleeson TG, Bulugahapitiya S. Contrast-induced nephropathy. *AJR Am JRoentgenol.* 2004;**183**:1673–1689.

4 Maeder M, Klein M, Fehr T, Rickli H. Contrast nephropathy: review focusing on prevention. *J Am Coll Cardiol.* 2004;**44**:1763–1771.

5 Persson PB, Hansell P, Liss P. Pathophysiology of contrast medium induced nephropathy. *Kidney Int.* 2005;**68**:14–22.

6 McCullough PA, Wolyn R, Rocher LL, Levin RN, O'Neill WW. Acute renal failure after coronary intervention: incidence, risk factors, and relationship to mortality. *Am J Med.* 1997;**103**:368–375.

7 Gruberg L, Mehran R, Dangas G, *et al.* Acute renal failure requiring dialysis after percutaneous coronary interventions. *Cathet Cardiovasc Interv.* 2001;**52**:409–416.

8 Mehran R, Aymong ED, Nikolsky E, *et al.* A simple risk score for prediction of contrast-induced nephropathy after percutaneous coronary intervention: development and initial validation. *J Am Coll Cardiol.* 2004;**44**:1393–1399.

9 Baim DS, Grossman W. *Grossmans's Cardiac Catheterization, Angiography, and Intervention,* 6th Edition. © 2000 by Lippincott Williams & Wilkins Pg 59.

10 Taylor AJ, Hotchkiss D, Morse RW, McCabe J. PREPARED: Preparation for Angiography in Renal Dysfunction: a randomized trial of inpatient vs outpatient hydration protocols for cardiac catheterization in mild-to-moderate renal dysfunction. *Chest.* 1998;**114**:1570–1574.

11 Solomon R, Werner C, Mann D, D'Elia J, Silva P. Effects of saline, mannitol, and furosemide to prevent acute decreases in renal function induced by radio contrast agents. *N Engl J Med.* 1994;**331**:1416–1420.

12 Stevens MA, McCullough PA, Tobin KJ, *et al.* A prospective randomized trial of prevention measures in patients at high risk for contrast nephropathy: results of the P.R.I.N.C.E. Study: Prevention of Radio contrast Induced Nephropathy Clinical Evaluation. *J Am Coll Cardiol.* 1999;**33**:403–411.

13 Mueller C, Buerkle G, Buettner HJ, *et al.* Prevention of contrast media-associated nephropathy: randomized comparison of 2 hydration regimens in 1620 patients

undergoing coronary angioplasty. *Arch Intern Med.* 2002;**162**:329–336.

14 Tepel M, Aspelin P, Lameire N. Contrast-induced nephropathy: a clinical and evidence-based approach. *Circulation.* 2006;**113**;1799–1806.

15 Huerta C, Castellsague J, Varas-Lorenzo C, García Rodríguez LA. Nonsteroidal anti-inflammatory drugs and risk of ARF in the general population. *Am J Kidney Dis.* March 2005;**45**(3):531–539.

16 Gambaro G, Perazella MA. Adverse renal effects of anti-inflammatory agents: evaluation of selective and non-selective cyclo-oxygenase inhibitors. *J Intern Med.* June 2003;**253**(6):643–652. Review.

17 Graham DJ, Campen D, Hui R, *et al*. Risk of acute myocardial infarction and sudden death in patients treated with cyclo-oxygenase 2 selective and non-selective non-steroidal anti inflammatory drugs: nested case control study. *Lancet.* 2005;**365**:475–478.

18 UK Prospective Diabetes Study Group. Effect of intensive blood glucose control with metformin on complications in overweight patients with type 2 diabetes (UKPDS 34). *Lancet* 1998;**352**:854–865.

19 Thomsen HS, Morcos SK, ESUR Contrast Media Safety Committee. Contrast media and metformin: guidelines to diminish the risk of lactic acidosis in non-insulin-dependent diabetics after administration of contrast media. *Eur Radiol.* 1999;**9**:738–740.

20 Brown JB, Pedula, MS, Barzilay J, Herson MK, Latare P. Lactic acidosis rates in type 2 diabetes. *Diabetes Care.* 1998;**21**:1659–1663.

21 Jones GC, Macklin JP, Alexander WD. Contraindications to the use of metformin. *BMJ.* 2003;**326**:4–5.

CHAPTER 25

Renal-protective agents

Giancarlo Marenzi & Antonio L. Bartorelli
University of Milan, Milan, Italy

Contrast-induced nephropathy (CIN) following the administration of contrast media is a common and potentially serious clinical problem, particularly in patients with chronic kidney disease. This complication of radiographic and cardiologic procedures has an adverse effect on prognosis and adds to health care cost. Multiple pharmacologic approaches have been devised to mitigate the risk of CIN in patients with preexisting renal disease (1). The mechanism by which contrast agents cause nephrotoxicity is poorly understood but probably includes a reduction in renal perfusion, resulting in vasoconstriction and regional hypoxia, as well as direct tubular toxicity (2). Accordingly, a number of studies have targeted renal vasoconstriction and hypoxia-induced oxidative stress and evaluated the role of pharmacologic adjunct therapies designed to inhibit them. However, with the exception of volume expansion and antioxidant agents, few of these adjunctive therapies have shown any clear and consistent benefit (Table 25.1).

Fluid administration

Hydration remains the cornerstone for the prevention of CIN, although few studies have addressed this issue directly, and there have been no

Table 25.1 Pharmacologic strategies evaluated for contrast-induced nephropathy risk reduction.

Positive results (potentially beneficial)
Hydration (isotonic saline, sodium bicarbonate)
Theophylline/aminophylline
NAC
Ascorbic acid
Statins
Prostaglandin E_1
Trimezatidine
Captopril

Neutral results (no consistent effect)
Fenoldopam
Dopamine
Calcium channel blockers
Amlodipine
Felodipine
Nifedipine
Nitrendipine
Atrial natriuretic peptide
L-Arginine

Negative results (potentially detrimental)
Furosemide
Mannitol
Endothelin receptor antagonist

NAC = *N*-acetylcysteine.

randomized controlled trial comparing a strategy of volume expansion with no volume expansion (Figure 25.1). Hydration results in plasma volume expansion with concomitant suppression of the renin-angiotensin-aldosteron system, downregulation

Pharmacology in the Catheterization Laboratory. Edited by Ron Waksman and Andrew E Ajani. © 2010 Blackwell Publishing, ISBN: 978-1-4051-5704-9.

195

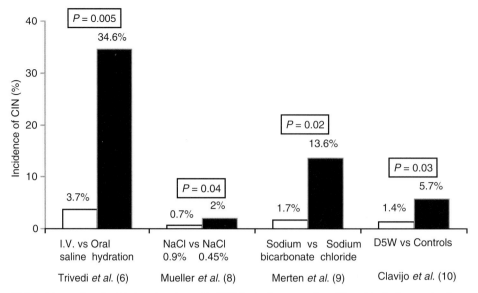

Figure 25.1 Incidence of contrast-induced nephropathy (CIN) in studies comparing different hydration protocols. NaCl, sodium chloride; D5W, 5% dextrose; I.V., intravenous.

of the tubuloglomerular feedback, dilution of the contrast media—and thus prevention of renal cortical vasoconstriction—and avoidance of tubular obstruction (3). Multiple trials have addressed type, amount, duration, and route of volume repletion to prevent CIN (4–7). However, many of these aspects remain undefined. Trivedi *et al.* (6) found that oral hydration alone appeared to be inferior to intravenous hydration with respect to the development of CIN. By comparing patients treated with hydration and mannitol and hydration and furosemide, Solomon *et al.* (4) demonstrated that intravenous infusion of 0.45% saline (1 mL/kg/h), starting 4–6 h before contrast medium administration, and continued for 24 h afterward, reduced the risk of CIN in patients with mild renal insufficiency undergoing cardiac angiography. More recent evidence suggests that hydration with isotonic saline is superior to half-isotonic saline, likely because of the enhanced ability of isotonic fluids to expand intravascular volume (8). The advantage of isotonic hydration is certainly demonstrated in patients with normal renal function and with a low risk of CIN, but these results on the superiority of isotonic vs half-isotonic hydration cannot be transferred conclusively to patients with moderate and severe chronic renal failure. Recently, Merten *et al.* (9) demonstrated that hydration with sodium

bicarbonate (154 mEq/L of sodium bicarbonate in dextrose and water at a rate of 3 mL/kg/h per 1 h before CM exposure, followed by 1 mL/kg/h during, and for 6 h after the procedure) is more effective than hydration with sodium chloride and may provide additional renoprotection by alkalinizing renal tubular fluid and thereby minimizing tubular damage. Finally, Clavijo *et al.* (10) have most recently reported a retrospective analysis showing that a rapid intra-arterial infusion of dextrose 5% (1 L administered though the femoral artery sheath as a bolus >5 min immediately before angiography), was well tolerated and effective against CIN in patients with a creatinine clearance <60 mL/min.

Although a clearly emerging concept is that volume expansion is critical in the prevention of CIN, the prognostic impact of hydration is still controversial, and we have no definite information on the possible advantage of this strategy on CIN-associated cardiovascular complications and mortality rate in high-risk population. We also lack data from controlled clinical trials that define the most effective hydration period, infusion rate, or hydration volume. Additional studies are also required to investigate the role of hydration in patients with congestive heart failure and renal insufficiency, a population that has always been poorly represented in previous studies, and in which vigorous hydration before percutaneous cardiovascular interventions is logistically difficult and poorly tolerated.

Vasodilators

Due to the potential role of hemodynamic effects induced by contrast agents, numerous vasodilators drugs have been tested for prevention of acute reduction in renal function. The possible role of endothelin-induced renal vasoconstriction has led to the evaluation of a nonselective endothelin receptor antagonist in a multicenter, double-blind randomized trial of high-risk patients undergoing coronary angiography (11). Compared with those randomized to placebo, a significantly higher percentage of patients who received active therapy developed CIN (56% vs 29%; $p = 0.002$). However, this study evaluated a mixed endothelin A and B receptor antagonist, and this disappointing result may tentatively be explained by endothelin B receptor inhibition, which favors vasoconstriction. To date, it is not known whether selective endothelin A blockade may be beneficial in preventing CIN.

Atrial natriuretic peptide has been considered as prophylaxis in high-risk patients, since its administration has been associated with beneficial effects in animal models of CIN. However, no benefit was observed with the intravenous administration of this agent in a large multicenter, prospective, double-blind, placebo-controlled randomized trial (12).

Calcium channel blockers, such as verapamil, diltiazem, and amlodipine, have been found to attenuate the renal vasoconstrictor response to radiocontrast media and to inhibit CIN in rats. A randomized placebo-controlled study of 35 patients with renal insufficiency has shown that oral nitrendipine (20 mg/day for 3 days) is effective for preventing the decrease in glomerular filtration rate (13). In contrast, other studies with nitrendipine, felodipine, and amlodipine did not confirm the beneficial effects of calcium antagonists for prevention of CIN. However, it must be emphasized that only dihydropyridine calcium channel blockers have been clinically tested so far. These agents have a more potent peripheral vasodilating effect than verapamil or diltiazem. Therefore, a possible

protective renal effect from calcium channel inhibition, which leads to lower renal perfusion pressure, may be offset by the hypotensive effect caused by these drugs. Currently, the use of calcium channel blockers to prevent CIN is not recommended.

Prostaglandin E_1 (PGE) has vasodilatory effects and may be promising as a prophylactic agent against CIN. A recent randomized, placebo-controlled pilot study suggests that prophylactic administration of iloprost, a prostacyclin (PGI_2) analogue, at a dose of 1 ng/kg/min, in patients with chronic renal failure undergoing a coronary procedure, is safe and may effectively prevent CIN (14). Nevertheless, further studies are needed to confirm the effectiveness of this agent. Contrast media stimulate the intra-renal secretion of adenosine, which binds to the renal adenosine receptor and acts as a potent vasoconstrictor, primarily in the efferent arterioles, reducing renal blood flow. As this vasoconstrictive response can be blunted with theophylline in experimental animals, multiple investigators have evaluated the adenosine antagonists (aminophylline and theophylline) as a potential means of reducing the risk of CIN in human subjects. However, these studies have been limited by a small sample size, variation in timing and dosage of drug administration, and variation in the definition of CIN. A meta-analysis of seven trials including 480 patients suggest that theophylline may be helpful (15), and further studies are needed to definitively determine its efficacy, safety, and utility. In particular, the potential benefits of theophylline must be weighed against the potential for serious adverse effects including gastrointestinal, neurological, and cardiovascular effects (16).

Although theoretically justified, studies testing the effectiveness of low (<2 µg/kg/min) doses of dopamine have shown negative or neutral results (17,18). The failure of dopamine may be due to hypovolemia and tachyarrhythmia induced by its diuretic and proarrhythmogenic effects, both leading to reduced cardiac output and reduced effective circulating arterial volume. In contrast to dopamine, fenoldopam is a selective dopamine-1 receptor agonist with systemic and renal arteriolar vasodilatory properties that does not stimulate dopamine-2 or adrenergic receptors, even when administered in higher doses. Fenoldopam significantly increases renal blood flow and decreases renal vascular resistance, without altering glomerular filtration rate (19). Following preliminary studies showing a benefit in reducing CIN, a more recent prospective, randomized trial (CONTRAST), evaluating fenoldopam in 315 patients at risk for developing CIN undergoing diagnostic and/or interventional cardiology procedures, has shown negative results (20).

Theoretically, L-arginine might be renoprotective because it is a substrate for nitric oxide synthesis. However, a single infusion of L-arginine (300 mg/kg) immediately before coronary angiography did not prevent CIN in patients with mild-to-moderate renal failure included in a randomized, placebo controlled trial (21).

The role of angiotensin-converting enzyme inhibitors for the prevention of CIN is still controversial. Preliminary studies suggest that abnormalities of renal perfusion, possibly mediated by the renin angiotensin system, are responsible for the development of CIN, and administration of captopril may offer protection against its development, particularly in diabetic patients (22).

Antioxidants

In recent years, in an attempt to prevent CIN, many clinical studies have been conducted with the use of antioxidant compounds. N-Acetylcysteine (NAC), the most widely studied of all prophylaxis strategies, has direct vasodilating effects on kidneys vessels, contributing to improved renal hemodynamics. It may also attenuate endothelial dysfunction, and, more notably, it is able to scavenge oxygen-free radicals, thus preventing direct oxidative tissue damage occurring in patients receiving contrast. Tepel et al. (23) first reported that NAC (600 mg orally twice daily) plus hydration before and after contrast administration offers good protection against CIN in patients with renal insufficiency undergoing computed tomography with a constant dose (75 mL) of contrast (2% vs 21%; $p = 0.01$). This finding was supported by some, but not all, subsequent clinical trials investigating the efficacy of NAC in preventing CIN, both in patients with preexisting renal insufficiency and in those with normal renal function (24–27).

Several meta-analysis studies have been published on this topic to date (Table 25.2) (28–38). By combining the data from available prospective controlled clinical trials that used NAC, they recorded an overall significant relative risk reduction in chronic renal failure patients given NAC (39). Nine have presented pooled risk estimates suggesting benefit. However, as the literature currently available is greatly heterogeneous, the benefit of oral NAC among all individuals with renal insufficiency cannot be clearly demonstrated (31). Differences in contrast media type and volumes, definitions of CIN, patient selection, interventions, applied hydration regimens, NAC dose (cumulative dosage varied between 1,500 and 6,000 mg), and route of administration (intravenous vs oral), as well as the timing of the procedure (urgent vs elective) may have contributed to the heterogeneity observed in the pooled analysis. Some recent studies utilizing a greater dose of NAC seem to support the hypothesis of a dose-dependent protective effect of NAC (Figure 25.2) (40–42). Moreover, a very recent randomized trial demonstrated an improved preventive effect against CIN when two different antioxidant strategies, such as NAC and bicarbonate, were combined (43). This seems to confirm the relevant pathogenetic role of oxidative stress in CIN development.

Additional evidence of the effectiveness of an antioxidant strategy comes from the recent observation by Spargias et al. (44) who investigated the impact of ascorbic acid in a randomized, double-blind, placebo-controlled trial including 231 patients with a serum creatinine concentration ≥1.2 mg/dL who underwent coronary angiography and/or intervention. Ascorbic acid (3 g at least 2 h before the procedure and 2 g in the night and the morning after the procedure) or placebo were administered orally. CIN occurred in 9% in the ascorbic acid group and in 20% in the placebo group ($p = 0.02$). The antioxidant ascorbic acid has been shown to attenuate renal damage caused by a variety of insults, such as postischemic stress, cis-platin, aminoglycosides, and potassium bromate in animals. When added to NAC, however, ascorbic acid did not show any improvement as compared to NAC alone (43). Thus, the possible benefits of ascorbic acid deserve further studies.

It has been suggested that statins may reduce CIN because they have beneficial effects on endothelial

Table 25.2 Meta-analyses of studies on the prophylactic use of *N*-acetylcysteine to prevent contrast-induced nephropathy.

Source	Procedure	Type of study	Number of trials	Number of patients	Heterogeneity (p value)	Pooled estimate (95% CI)	Author conclusions
Birk et al. (28)	CT or angiography	A	7	805	Present (p = 0.02)	RR 0.44 (0.22–0.88)	Beneficial
Isenbarger et al. (29)	CT or angiography	A	7	805	Present (p = 0.01)	OR 0.37 (0.16–0.84)	Beneficial
Alonso et al. (30)	CT or angiography	A, B	8	805	Not reported	RR 0.41 (0.22–0.79)	Beneficial
Kshirsager et al. (31)	CT or angiography	A, B	16	1,538	Present (p < 0.001)	Not reported	Inconclusive
Pannu et al. (32)	CT or angiography	A, B, D	15	1,776	Present (p = 0.02)	RR 0.65 (0.43–1.00)	Inconclusive
Guru and Fremes (33)	CT or angiography	A, C	11	1,213	Present (p = 0.01)	OR 0.46 (0.32–0.66)	Beneficial
Bagshaw and Ghail(34)	Angiography	A	14	1,261	Present (p = 0.03)	OR 0.54 (0.32–0.91)	Inconclusive
Misra et al. (35)	Angiography	A	5	643	Present (p = 0.05)	RR 0.30 (0.11–0.82)	Beneficial
Nallamothu et al. (36)	CT or angiography	A, D	20	2,195	Present (p = 0.01)	RR 0.73 (0.52–1.0)	Inconclusive
Liu et al. (37)	CT or angiography	A, B	9	1,028	Present (p = 0.03)	RR 0.43 (0.24–0.75)	Beneficial
Duong et al. (38)	CT or angiography	A, C	14	1,584	Present (p = 0.01)	RR 0.57 (0.37–0.84)	Beneficial

A = randomized controlled trials (articles), B = randomized controlled trials (abstracts), C = not randomized trials (articles), D = unpublished; CT = computed tomography; RR = relative risk; OR = odd ratio; CI = confidence intervals.

Source: Modified from Bagshaw SM et al. *Arch Intern Med.* 2006;**166**:161–166.

Elective PCI (Data from Briguori *et al.* (41))

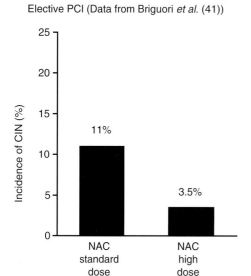

Primary PCI (Data from Marenzi *et al.* (42))

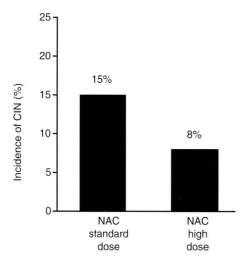

Figure 25.2 Dose-dependent protective effect of *N*-acetylcysteine (NAC) against contrast-induced nephropathy (CIN). PCI: percutaneous coronary intervention.

function and reduce oxidative stress. A retrospective review of 1,002 patients with renal insufficiency undergoing coronary angiography suggested that the risk of CIN was lower in patients in whom a statin was initiated just before the procedure (45). The results of a large PCI registry study including 29,409 patients also confirmed this conclusion (46). Nevertheless, to date, there is not enough evidence to support the use of statins in patients undergoing radiologic procedures in whom these drugs are not otherwise indicated.

Trimezatidine has been initially described as a cellular anti-ischemic agent. Previous studies, however, demonstrated that trimezatidine exerts potent antioxidant activity in myocardial, renal, and hepatic ischemia–reperfusion injury. In a recent randomized, controlled trial, trimezatidine (20 mg t.i.d orally for 72 h starting 48 h before the procedure) in addition to standard intravenous saline hydration was compared with hydration alone in 82 patients with mild chronic renal insufficiency undergoing elective coronary procedures (47). The incidence of CIN was significantly lower in patients receiving trimezatidine (2.5% vs 16.6%; $p < 0.05$). The potential usefulness of this drug in the prevention of CIN, particularly in higher risk patients, should be investigated in larger prospective clinical studies.

Conclusions

Current evidence indicates that hydration remains the cornerstone prophylactic strategy of CIN. Patients at risk of this complication should receive adequate intravenous volume expansion with isotonic saline for at least 6 h before the procedure and for 6–24 h afterward. Although no adjunctive pharmacologic treatment has been proved conclusively to reduce the risk for CIN, consideration could be given to prophylactic treatment with any of the agents that have shown promising results, specifically sodium bicarbonate, NAC, theophilline, ascorbic acid, and prostaglandin E_1.

References

1 Briguori C, Marenzi G. Pharmacologic prophylaxis. *Kidney Intern* 2006;**69**:S30–S38.

2 Tumlin J, Stacul F, Adam A, *et al.* Pathophysiology of contrast-induced nephropathy. *Am J Cardiol.* 2006;**98**: 14K–20K.

3 Erley CM. Does hydration prevent radiocontrast-induced acute renal failure? *Nephrol Dial Transplant.* 1999;**14**: 1064–1066.

4 Solomon R, Werner C, Mann D, D'Elia J, Silva P. Effects of saline, mannitol, and furosemide on acute decreases in renal function induced by radiocontrast agents. *N Engl J Med.* 1994;**331**:1416–1420.

5 Taylor AJ, Hotchkis D, Morse RW, McCabe J. PREPARED: preparation for angiography in renal dysfunction. A randomized trial of inpatient vs outpatient hydration protocols for cardiac catheterization in mild to moderate renal dysfunction. *Chest*. 1998;**114**:1570–1574.

6 Trivedi HS, Moore H, Nasr S, *et al.* A randomized prospective trial to assess the role of saline hydration on the development of contrast nephropathy. *Nephron Clin Pract*. 2003;**93**:C29–C34.

7 Stevens MA, McCullough PA, Tobin KJ, *et al.* A prospective randomized trial of prevention measures in patients at high risk for contrast nephropathy: results of the PRINCE study. *J Am Coll Cardiol*. 1999;**33**:403–411.

8 Mueller C, Buerkle G, Buettner HJ, *et al.* Prevention of contrast media-associated nephropathy: randomized comparison of 2 hydration regimens in 1620 patients undergoing coronary angioplasty. *Arch Intern Med*. 2002;**162**:329–336.

9 Merten GJ, Burgess WP, Gray LV, *et al.* Prevention of contrast-induced nephropathy with sodium bicarbonate. A randomized controlled trial. *JAMA*. 2004;**291**: 2328–2334.

10 Clavijo LC, Pinto TL, Kuchulakanti PK, *et al.* Effect of a rapid intra-arterial infusion of dextrose 5% prior to coronary angiography on frequency of contrast-induced nephropathy in high-risk patients. *Am J Cardiol*. 2006;**97**:981–983.

11 Wang, A, Holcslaw, T, Bashore, TM, *et al.* Exacerbation of radiocontrast nephrotoxicity by endothelin receptor antagonism. *Kidney Int*. 2000;**57**:1675–1680.

12 Kurnik, BR, Allgren, RL, Genter, FC, *et al.* Prospective study of atrial natriuretic peptide for the prevention of radiocontrast-induced nephropathy. *Am J Kidney Dis*. 1998;**31**:674–680.

13 Neumayer HH, Junge W, Kufner A, Wenning A. Prevention of radiocontrast-media-induced nephrotoxicity by the calcium channel blocker nitrendipine: a prospective randomized clinical trial. *Nephrol Dial Transplant*. 1989;**4**:1030–1036.

14 Spargias K, Adreanides E, Giamouzis G, *et al.* Iloprost for prevention of contrast-mediated nephropathy in high-risk patients undergoing a coronary procedure. Results of a nonrandomized pilot study. *Eur J Clin Pharmacol*. 2006;**62**:589–595.

15 Ix JH, McCulloch CE, Chertow GM. Theophylline for the prevention of radiocontrast nephropathy: a meta-analysis. *Nephrol Dial Transplant*. 2004;**19**:2747–2753.

16 Cooling DS. Theophylline toxicity. *J Emerg Med*. 1993; **11**:415–425.

17 Abizaid A, Clark CE, Mintz GS, *et al.* Effects of dopamine and aminophylline on contrast-induced acute renal failure after coronary angioplasty in patients with preexisting renal insufficiency. *Am J Cardiol*. 1999;**83**:260–263.

18 Gare M, Haviv YS, Ben-Yehuda A, *et al.* The renal effect of low-dose dopamine in high-risk patients undergoing coronary angiography. *J Am Coll Cardiol*. 1999;**34**:1682–1688.

19 Mathur V, Swan S, Lambrecht L, *et al.* The effects of fenoldopam, a selective dopamine receptor agonist, on systemic and renal hemodynamic in normotensive subjects. *Crit Care Med*. 1999;**27**:1832–1837.

20 Stone GW, McCullough PA, Tumlin JA, *et al.* Fenoldopam mesylate for the prevention of contrast-induced nephrotoxicity. *JAMA*. 2003;**290**:2284–2291.

21 Miller HI, Dascalu A, Rassin TA, *et al.* Effects of an acute dose of L-arginine during coronary angiography in patients with chronic renal failure: a randomized, parallel, double-blind clinical trial. *Am J Nephrol*. 2003;**23**:91–95.

22 Gupta RK, Kapoor A, Tewari S, Sinha N, Sharma RK. Captopril for prevention of contrast-induced nephropathy in diabetic patients: a randomized study. Indian Heart J. 1999;**51**:521–526.

23 Tepel M, Van der Giet M, Schwarzfeld C, Laufer U, Liermann D, Zidek W. Prevention of radiographic-contrast-agent-induced reductions in renal function by acetylcysteine. *N Engl J Med*. 2000;**343**:180–184.

24 Diaz-Sandoval LJ, Kosowsky BD, Losordo DW. Acetylcysteine to prevent angiography-related renal tissue injury (the APART trial). *Am J Cardiol*. 2002; **89**:356–358.

25 Shyu KG, Cheng JJ, Kuan P. Acetylcysteine protects against acute renal damage in patients with abnormal renal function undergoing a coronary procedure. *J Am Coll Cardiol*. 2002;**40**:1383–1388.

26 Kay J, Chow WH, Chan TM, *et al.* Acetylcysteine for prevention of acute deterioration of renal function following elective coronary angiography and intervention: a randomized controlled trial. *JAMA*. 2003;**289**:553–558.

27 Briguori C, Manganelli F, Scarpato P, *et al.* Acetylcysteine and contrast-agent associated nephrotoxicity. *J Am Coll Cardiol*. 2002;**40**:298–303.

28 Birck R, Krzossok S, Markowetz F, *et al.* Acetylcysteine for prevention of contrast nephropathy. *Lancet*. 2003; **362**:598–603.

29 Isenbarger D, Kent S, O'Malley P. Meta-analysis of randomized clinical trials on the usefulness of acetylcysteine for prevention of contrast nephropathy. *Am J Cardiol*. 2003;**92**:1454–1458.

30 Alonso A, Lau J, Jaber BL, *et al.* Prevention of radiocontrast nephropathy with N-acetylcysteine in patients with chronic kidney disease: a meta-analysis of randomized, controlled trials. *Am J Kidney Dis*. 2004;**43**:1–9.

31 Kshirsagar A, Poole C, Mottl A, *et al.* N-acetylcysteine for the prevention of radiocontrast induced nephropathy: a meta-analysis of prospective controlled trials. *J Am Soc Nephrol*. 2004;**15**:761–769.

32 Pannu N, Manns B, Lee H, Tonelli M. Systematic review of the impact of N-acetylcysteine on contrast nephropathy. *Kidney Int*. 2004;**65**:1366–1374.

33 Guru V, Fremes S. The role of N-acetylcysteine in preventing radiographic contrast-induced nephropathy. *Clin Nephrol*. 2004;**62**:77–83.

34 Bagshaw S, Ghali WA. Acetylcysteine for prevention of contrast-induced nephropathy: a systematic review and meta-analysis. *BMC Med*. 2004;**2**:38.

35 Misra D, Leibowitz K, Gowda R, Shapiro M, Khan I. Role of N-acetylcysteine in prevention of contrast-induced nephropathy after cardiovascular procedures: a meta-analysis. *Clin Cardiol*. 2004;**27**:607–610.

36 Nallamothu BK, Shojania KG, Saint S, *et al.* Is acetylcysteine effective in preventing contrast-related nephropathy? A meta-analysis. *Am J Med*. 2004;**117**:938–947.

37 Liu R, Nair D, Ix J, Moore D, Bent S. N-acetylcysteine for prevention of contrast-induced nephropathy: a systematic review and meta-analysis. *J Gen Intern Med*. 2005; **20**:193–200.

38 Duong M, MacKenzie T, Malenka D. N-acetylcysteine prophylaxis significantly reduces the risk of radiocontrast-induced nephropathy. *Catheter Cardiovasc Interv*. 2005; **64**:471–479.

39 Tepel M, Aspelin P, Lameire N. Contrast-induced nephropathy: a clinical and evidence-based approach. *Circulation*. 2006;**113**:1799–1806.

40 Baker CSR, Wragg A, Kumar S, *et al.* A rapid protocol for the prevention of contrast-induced renal dysfunction: the RAPPID study. *J Am Coll Cardiol*. 2003;**41**:2114–2118.

41 Briguori C, Colombo A, Violante A, *et al.* Standard vs double dose of N-acetylcysteine to prevent contrast agent associated nephrotoxicity. *Eur Heart J*. 2004;**25**:206–211.

42 Marenzi G, Assanelli E, Marana I, *et al.* N-acetylcysteine and contrast-induced nephropathy in primary angioplasty. *N Engl J Med*. 2006;**354**:2773–2782.

43 Briguori C, Airoldi F, D'Andrea D, *et al.* Renal insufficiency following contrast adminstration trial (REMEDIAL). A randomized comparison of 3 preventive strategies. *Circulation*. 2007;**115**:1211–1217.

44 Spargias K, Alexopoulos E, Kyrzopoulos S, *et al.* Ascorbic acid prevents contrast-mediated nephropathy in patients with renal dysfunction undergoing coronary angiography or intervention. *Circulation*. 2004;**110**:2837–2842.

45 Attallah N, Yassine L, Musial J, Yee J, Fisher K. The potential role of statins in contrast nephropathy. *Clin Nephrol*. 2004;62:273–278.

46 Khanal S, Attallah N, Smith DE, *et al.* Statin therapy reduces contrast-induced nephropathy: an analysis of contemporary percutaneous interventions. *Am J Med*. 2005;118:843–849.

47 Onbasili AO, Yeniceriglu Y, Agaoglu P, *et al.* Trimetazidine in the prevention of contrast-induced nephropathy after coronary procedures. *Heart*. 2007;93:654–655.

CHAPTER 26

Radiocontrast-induced nephropathy

Giancarlo Marenzi & Antonio L. Bartorelli
University of Milan, Milan, Italy

Contrast-induced nephropathy (CIN) is a common and potentially serious complication that can follow the administration of iodinated contrast agents to patients who are at risk of acute renal injury. With the ever-expanding number and growing complexity of diagnostic and interventional procedures requiring the use of contrast media, and with more elderly patients with comorbidities undergoing radiological procedures, CIN is becoming increasingly important in the modern medical practice. Indeed, approximately 11% of the cases of hospital-acquired renal failure can be attributed to its occurrence (1).

Although there is no universally accepted definition, CIN refers to development of acute renal impairment following intravascular administration of radiocontrast in the absence of other identifiable causes of renal failure. The most commonly used definition in clinical trials is an absolute increase in serum creatinine of 0.5 mg/dL (44 μmol/L), or a relative 25% increase from the baseline value, assessed 48–72 h after the systemic administration of contrast agents.

Based on these definitions, the overall incidence of CIN in the general population is estimated to be lower than 3%, but it can rise up to 50% or more in patients with multiple risk factors. However, the reported frequencies probably underrepresent the magnitude of the problem, because serum creatinine is not measured routinely following percutaneous coronary interventions (PCI) or after contrast exposure in radiological procedures.

Pathophysiology of CIN

The exact mechanism of the development of CIN has not been completely elucidated and is still under investigation. However, there is increasing evidence that it is caused by a combination of direct toxic effects on tubular epithelial cells and renal ischemia (2). Direct toxic effects in the proximal convoluted tubular cells and in the inner cortex of the kidneys, including epithelial cell vacuolization, interstitial inflammation, and cellular necrosis, have been demonstrated following exposure to a variety of iodinated contrast agents. Studies in animals have suggested that oxidant-mediated injury, due to enhanced production of oxygen-free radicals and lipid peroxidation of biological membranes, might be implicated as a cause of CIN. The ability to accommodate oxidant injury decreases with age, and is thought to contribute to the increased risk of CIN among older patients. Moreover, increased oxidative stress is present in patients with chronic renal failure and diabetes (3,4). Apoptosis, resulting from cellular injury, has also been considered to have a role.

As regards ischemic injury, several studies have documented immediate vasoconstriction and reduction in renal blood flow occurring after

Pharmacology in the Catheterization Laboratory. Edited by Ron Waksman and Andrew E Ajani. © 2010 Blackwell Publishing, ISBN: 978-1-4051-5704-9.

contrast medium administration. Subsequent studies have shown that the changes in renal plasma flow are not uniform and that contrast media appear to exert regional effects within the kidney, with increases in blood flow to the renal cortex and simultaneous flow reduction to the outer medulla. The deeper portion of the outer medulla of the kidney is particularly susceptible to ischemic injury, since this area is maintained at the verge of hypoxia, with pO_2 levels often as low as 20 mmHg; in contrast, perfusion is high for the cortex. In addition to the low oxygen tension, the metabolic activity of the outer medulla is high, and the relative high oxygen requirements due to salt reabsorption account for this vulnerability (5).

Two possible mechanisms by which medullary hypoxia and ischemia may occur in response to contrast agent's exposure have been proposed. First, contrast agents may cause renal vasoconstriction, and both increased activity of several intrarenal mediators (adenosin, vasopressin, angiotensin II, dopamine-1, and endothelin) and decreased activity of renal vasodilators (nitric oxide and prostaglandins) have been implicated as causative factors (2,5). Second, contrast media may decrease renal blood flow indirectly by causing erythrocyte aggregation. Iso-osmolar dimeric contrast media have been reported to cause more red blood cell aggregation, cessation of flow in the renal microcirculation, and greater reduction of renal blood flow than low-osmolar monomeric contrast media, probably due to their increased viscosity (6). A diminished transit time of the higher viscosity dimeric contrast agent in the tubule may lead to a decrease of both glomerular filtration rate and renal blood flow by compression of peritubular vessels. Moreover, the diminished tubular transit time of the nonionic dimers may result in an increased time for solute transport and increased oxygen utilization. Experimental studies on the role of osmolality *per se* in the pathogenesis of CIN have provided conflicting data. Although clinical trials indicate a lower incidence of CIN when using low-osmolality compared with high-osmolality contrast agents, the advantage of using iso-osmolality rather than low-osmolality compounds is still uncertain.

In brief, the nephrotoxic effects of iodinated contrast media may occur primarily through direct citotoxicity and renal medullary ischemia, and factors other than osmolality (such as viscosity and hydrophilicity) may contribute substantially to their toxic effect.

Risk factors and risk stratification

Identification of patients at increased risk for the development of CIN is of major importance; whether or not a patient develops clinically significant acute renal failure depends very much on the presence and combination of certain risk factors. A large body of data indicates that the risk of CIN is related to patient characteristics, clinical setting, and other modifiable factors (Table 26.1) (7). Evidence provided from clinical studies indicates that renal impairment has a strong and consistent association with CIN development. The higher the baseline creatinine value, the greater is the risk of CIN. However, baseline creatinine is not reliable enough for identification of patients with increased risk. This is because the creatinine concentration in the blood is affected by a number of factors other than creatinine filtration, including diet, age, gender, and muscle mass. Thus, the serum creatinine concentration may remain within the normal range, despite a substantial decrease in glomerular filtration rate. To evaluate renal function reliably, assessment of creatinine clearance, based on the Cockgroft-Gault formula (8) or calculation of estimated glomerular filtration rate by the Modification of Diet in Renal Disease (MDRD) equation (9), has been recommended (Table 26.2). Several studies have shown that an estimated glomerular filtration rate of 60 mL/min/1.73 m^2 is a reliable cutoff point for identifying patients at high risk for the development of CIN. The clinical evidence also supports an association between the severity of renal dysfunction below this threshold and the risk of CIN (Figure 26.1) (10). The presence of diabetes mellitus may significantly increase the risk in patients with pre-existing renal dysfunction. Studies have shown that these patients have a fourfold higher rate of CIN as compared to those without diabetes or renal impairment. However, it is not clear whether the risk of CIN is significantly increased in patients with diabetes who do not have renal impairment. The duration of diabetes and the presence of diabetic complications have also been reported to increase the risk of CIN (11). Additional

Table 26.1 Risk factors for contrast-induced nephropathy.

Patient related

Chronic kidney disease (stage III or greater)

Diabetes mellitus (type 1 or type 2)

Volume depletion

Older age

Congestive heart failure
(or left ventricular ejection fraction <40%)

Hypertension

Anemia and blood loss

Hypoalbuminemia (<35 g/L)

Nephrotoxic drug use
(NSAIDs, cyclosporine, aminoglycosides)

Diuretics

ACE inhibitors

Hypotension or preprocedural hemodynamic instability

Urgent procedure (acute myocardial infarction)

Intra-aortic balloon pump use

Renal transplant

Not patient related

Contrast properties

High osmolar contrast

Ionic contrast

Contrast viscosity

Contrast volume

Intra-arterial administration

Abbreviations: NSAIDs, nonsteroidal anti-inflammatory drugs; ACE, angiotensin-converting enzyme.

Table 26.2 Cockgroft-Gault formula, and modification of diet in renal disease equation.

Cockgroft-Gault formula for estimation of creatinine clearance (CrCl) from serum creatinine:

$$CrCl\ (mL/min) = \frac{(140 - age\ in\ years) \times body\ weight\ in\ kg}{72 \times serum\ creatinine\ in\ mg/dL}$$

The resulting value must be multiplied by 0.85 for women.

Modification of Diet in Renal Disease equation for estimation of glomerular filtration rate (eGFR) from serum creatinine:

$$eGFR\ (mL/min/1.73\ m^2) = (186.3 \times [serum\ creatinine^{-1.154}] \times [age^{-203}])$$

Calculated values are multiplied by 0.742 for women and by 1.21 for African Americans.

risk factors include older age (most likely in relation to the decline in renal function with aging), congestive heart failure, reduced effective arterial volume (as in case of dehydration, nephrosis, and cirrhosis), type and volume of contrast agents, anemia and procedure-related blood loss, concurrent use of potentially nephrotoxic drugs such as diuretics, aminoglycosides, as well as drugs impairing the renovascular autoregulation such as nonsteroidal anti-inflammatory drugs (10,12). Although hypovolemia and decreased effective circulating volume are well-recognized risk factors for CIN, their direct effect have never been assessed in clinical trials, and indirect evidence comes from studies showing the benefit of intravenous hydration and the deleterious effect of diuretics.

Apart from the known unfavorable association of diabetes and renal insufficiency, the presence of two or more risk factors is additive, possibly by a variety of interacting mechanisms, and the likelihood of CIN rises sharply as the number of risk factors

increases (12). This was first evidenced in a study of renal angiography by Cochran *et al.* (13), who found a 50% risk of CIN in patients with five risk factors. Evidence of a synergistic effect comes also from another study in which CIN occurred in 1.2% of the patients without risk factors, 11.2% with one risk factor, and in >20% of the patients with two or more risk factors (14). Information derived from multiple large-scale studies has led to the development of multivariate prediction scoring schemes for patients undergoing PCI. Application of these risk scores showed that patients with multiple risk factors have a very high, if not certain, expectation for CIN development after contrast exposure. Bartholomew *et al.* (15) identified (in over 20,000 patients) eight variables associated with CIN that were incorporated in a risk score (creatinine clearance <60 mL/min, use of intra-aortic balloon pump, urgent coronary procedure, diabetes, congestive heart failure, hypertension, peripheral vascular disease, and contrast volume). A significant increase of CIN rate after PCI was found for each increment in the risk score. It is noteworthy that no patient with a risk score of <1 developed CIN, whereas 26% of those with the highest score (>9) developed CIN. Mehran *et al.* (12) identified (in more than 8,000 patients) three additional factors that were associated with increased risk: age >75 years, the presence of hypotension, and anemia. The occurrence of CIN was found to increase progressively from 7.5% for patients with a low (0–5) risk score, up to 57.3% for those with a high (>16) risk score (Figure 26.2). Finally, five independent

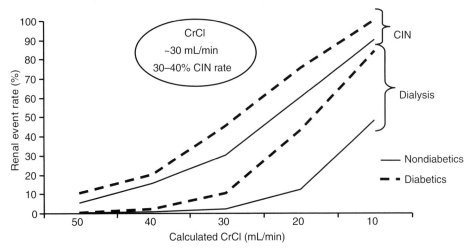

Figure 26.1 Validated risk of contrast-induced nephropathy (CIN) and acute renal failure requiring dialysis after diagnostic angiography and *ad hoc* angioplasty in nondiabetic and diabetic patients. A mean contrast dose of 250 mL and a mean age of 65 years is assumed. CrCl = creatinine clearance. (Modified from McCullough PA, Sandeberg KR. Epidemiology of contrast-induced nephropathy. *Rev Cardiovasc Med*. 2003;**4** (Suppl 5):S3–S9.)

Risk factors	Integer score
• Hypotension	5
• Intra-aortic balloon pump	5
• Heart failure (NYHA III–IV)	5
• Age >75 years	4
• Anemia	3
• Diabetes	3
• Contrast volume	1 for each 100 mL
• Serum creatinine >1.5 mg/dL or	4
• eGFR <60 mL/min/1.73 m^2	2 (40–60); 4 (20–40); 6 (<20)

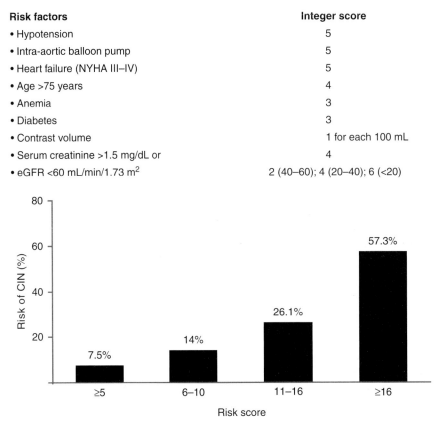

Figure 26.2 Risk prediction scheme for the development of contrast-induced nephropathy (CIN). eGFR = estimated glomerular filtration rate (modified from Mehran R, *et al.* (12)).

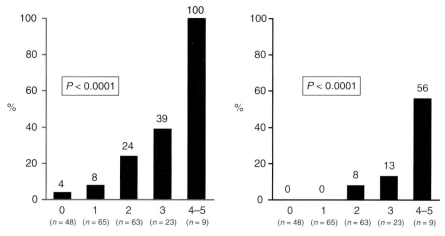

Figure 26.3 Incidence of contrast-induced nephropathy (left panel) and of in-hospital death (right panel) after primary angioplasty, according to the risk score (modified from Marenzi *et al.* (16)).

predictors of CIN were identified in the setting of acute myocardial infarction treated with primary angioplasty: (1) age >75 years, (2) anterior infarction location, (3) time-to-reperfusion >6 h, (4) contrast agent volume >300 mL, and (5) use of an intra-aortic balloon pump (16). These variables were included as risk indicators for CIN in a risk scoring system. The incidence of CIN, as well as the in-hospital mortality rate, revealed a significant gradation as the risk score increased in the study population (Figure 26.3). Notably, all patients with four or five risk factors developed CIN. It should be emphasized, however, that all these scores have been evaluated retrospectively, and none has been prospectively validated in different populations. Thus, current recommendation for the clinical use of risk scoring based on these data cannot be made.

Clinical presentation and prognostic implications of CIN

The clinical course of CIN is usually characterized by spontaneous recovery of renal function. The serum creatinine level begins to rise within 24 h after administration of a contrast medium in 80% of patients in whom CIN develops, typically peaking on the second or third day (16,17). Serum creatinine usually returns to baseline value within 7–10 days. Although the clinical relevance of CIN may not be immediately evident, given the subclinical course and the high frequency of recovery of renal function, some degree of residual renal impairment has been reported in as many as 30% of those affected and up to 7% of patients may require temporary dialysis or progress to end-stage renal failure (18). Serious clinical consequences, including death, may occur in patients developing CIN. Patients with CIN were observed to have several noncardiac in-hospital complications, including hematoma formation, pseudoaneurysms, stroke, coma, adult respiratory distress syndrome, pulmonary embolism, and gastrointestinal hemorrhage (19). Patients who develop CIN after PCI have a 15-fold higher rate of major adverse cardiac events during hospitalization than patients without this complication. They also have a sixfold increase in myocardial infarction and an 11-fold increase in coronary vessel reocclusion (15). Although few patients with CIN require dialysis (<1%), they have a more complicated clinical outcome than those who do not require renal replacement therapy, including a significantly higher rate of non-Q-wave myocardial infarction (46% vs 15%), pulmonary edema (65% vs 3%), and gastrointestinal bleeding (16% vs 1%). Moreover, they have a 15-fold longer stay in the Intensive Care Unit, and a five-fold longer hospital stay (20). In contemporary studies, CIN requiring dialysis developed in 3.1% of patients with underlying renal impairment and in

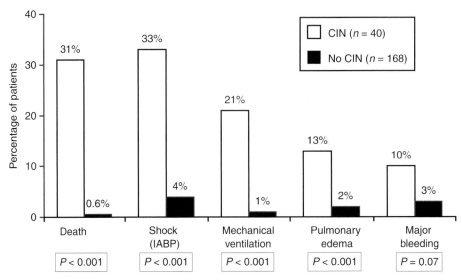

Figure 26.4 In-hospital complications of patients who developed contrast-induced nephropathy (CIN) following primary angioplasty and of those who did not in the study by Marenzi *et al.* (16) IABP = intra-aortic balloon pump.

3% of patients undergoing primary PCI for acute myocardial infarction (16,21). Patients undergoing primary PCI are a particularly high-risk group. In one series of patients with primary angioplasty, major in-hospital complications, including acute pulmonary edema, respiratory failure, cardiogenic shock, and the need for a pacemaker, were significantly more common in patients developing CIN (Figure 26.4) (16).

It has been recognized that the development of CIN is linked to an increased risk of in-hospital and long-term mortality, probably as a result of the morbidities described. Several studies have reported an increased mortality rate in patients developing CIN. In a large retrospective study, including more than 16,000 patients undergoing procedures requiring contrast medium, the risk of death during hospitalization was 34% in patients who developed CIN, compared with 7% in matched controls who received contrast medium but did not developed CIN (22). The high risk of in-hospital death associated with CIN has also been noted in a retrospective analysis of 7,586 patients (19). The hospital mortality rate was 22% in the patients developing CIN, compared with only 1.4% in patients who did not have this complication. In this study, the increased risk of death persisted over time, with significantly higher mortality rates at 1 year (12.1%) and at 5 years (44.6%), compared

with rates of 3.7% and 14.5%, respectively, in patients who did not develop CIN. Other studies confirmed this observation, with in-hospital mortality rates ranging from 7.1% to 14.9%, and with 1-year mortality rates from 30% to 37%, depending on the patient's baseline risk profile (10,23). In the latter two studies, in-hospital and 1-year mortality rates were significantly higher (up to 54%) for patients who developed CIN and required dialysis after the procedure.

In patients undergoing primary PCI for myocardial infarction, a higher mortality rate was also documented in patients developing CIN, compared with those without CIN (31% vs 0.6%; $p = 0.0001$) (16).

Conclusion

There is increasing evidence that CIN represents an important clinical problem with an adverse effect on short- and long-term prognosis, particularly in high-risk patients undergoing PCI. The continuously growing number of diagnostic and therapeutic procedures that require contrast agents highlights the importance of identifying patients at risk of CIN, on the basis of their history, as well as of the presence of renal dysfunction and other contributing factors, in order to develop and implement appropriate prophylactic strategies.

References

1 Nash K, Hafeez A, Hou S. Hospital-acquired renal insufficiency. *Am J Kidney Dis.* 2002;**39**:930–936.

2 Persson PB, Tepel M. Contrast medium-induced nephropathy: the pathophysiology. *Kidney Int.* 2006;**69** (Suppl 100):S8–S10.

3 Massy ZA, Nguyen-Khoa T. Oxidative stress and chronic renal failure: markers and management. *J Nephrol.* 2002;**15**:336–341.

4 Scott JA, King GL. Oxidative stress and antioxidant treatment in diabetes. *Ann N Y Acad Sci.* 2004;**1031**:204–213.

5 Tumlin J, Stacul F, Adam A, *et al.* Pathophysiology of contrast-induced nephropathy. *Am J Cardiol.* 2006; **98**(suppl):14K–20K.

6 Schrader R. Contrast material-induced renal failure: an overview. *J Interven Cardiol.* 2005;**18**:417–423.

7 McCullough PA, Adam A, Becker CR, *et al.* Risk prediction of contrast-induced nephropathy. *Am J Cardiol.* 2006; **98**(suppl):27K–36K.

8 Cockcroft DW, Gault MH. Prediction of creatinine clearance from serum creatinine. *Nephron.* 1976;**16**:31–41.

9 Levey AS, Bosch JP, Lewis JB, Greene T, Rogers N, Roth D. A more accurate method to estimate glomerular filtration rate from serum creatinine: a new prediction equation. Modification of Diet in Renal Disease Study Group. *Ann Intern Med.* 1999;**130**:461–470.

10 McCullough PA, Wolyn R, Rocher LL, Levin RN, O'Neill WW. Acute renal failure after coronary intervention: incidence, risk factors and relationship to mortality. *Am J Med.* 1997;**103**:368–375.

11 Kamdar A, Weidmann P, Makoff DL, Massry SG. Acute renal failure following intravenous use of radioghraphic contrast dyes in patients with diabetes mellitus. *Diabetes.* 1977;**26**:643–649.

12 Mehran R, Aymong ED, Nikolsky E, *et al.* A simple risk score for prediction of contrast-induced nephropathy after percutaneous coronary intervention. *J Am Coll Cardiol.* 2004;**44**:1393–1399.

13 Cochran ST, Wong WS, Roe DJ. Predicting angiography-induced acute renal function impairment: clinical risk model. *Am J Roentgenol.* 1983;**141**:1027–1033.

14 Rich MW, Crecelius CA. Incidence, risk factors and clinical course of acute renal insufficiency after cardiac catheterization in patients 70 years of age or older. A prospective study. *Arch Intern Med.* 1990;**150**:1237–1242.

15 Bartholomew BA, Harjai KJ, Dukkipati S, *et al.* Impact of nephropathy after percutaneous coronary intervention and a method for risk stratification. *Am J Cardiol.* 2004;**93**:1515–1519.

16 Marenzi G, Lauri G, Assanelli E, *et al.* Contrast-induced nephropathy in patients undergoing primary angioplasty for acute myocardial infarction. *J Am Coll Cardiol.* 2004;**44**:1780–1785.

17 Barrett BJ, Parfrey PS. Preventing nephropathy induced by contrast medium. *N Engl J Med.* 2006;**354**:379–386.

18 Gruber L. Clinical features and prognostic implications of contrast-induced nephropathy. In: Bartorelli AL, Marenzi G, eds. *Contrast-induced Nephropathy.* London, England: Taylor & Francis; 2006:35–45.

19 Rihal CS, Textor SC, Grill DE, *et al.* Incidence and prognostic importance of acute renal failure after percutaneous coronary intervention. *Circulation.* 2002;**105**:2259–2264.

20 Gruber L, Mehran R, Dangas G, *et al.* Acute renal failure requiring dialysis after percutaneous coronary interventions. *Catheter Cardiovasc Interv.* 2001;**52**:409–416.

21 Nicolsky E, Mehran R, Turcot D, *et al.* Impact of chronic kidney disease on prognosis of patients with diabetes mellitus treated with percutaneous coronary intervention. *Am J Cardiol.* 2004;**94**:300–305.

22 Levy EM, Viscoli CM, Horwitz RI. The effect of acute renal failure on mortality: a cohort analysis. *JAMA.* 1996;**275**:1489–1494.

23 Gruberg L, Mintz GS, Mehran R, *et al.* The prognostic implications of further renal function deterioration within 48 hours of interventional coronary procedures in patients with pre-existent chronic renal insufficiency. *J Am Coll Cardiol.* 2000;**36**:1542–1548.

CHAPTER 27

Ideal contrast agent

Luis Gruberg
Stony Brook University Medical Center, Stony Brook, NY, USA

Introduction

The Nephrology Panel of the Committee on Adverse Reactions officially adopted the term "toxic nephropathy" in the 1950s to describe any adverse functional or structural change in the kidney due to the effect of a chemical or biological product that is inhaled, injected, or absorbed, or that yields toxic metabolites with an identifiable effect on the kidneys (1). Injectable and absorbable contrast media for the use in radiology, all which contain iodine as an essential component, has been and continues to be one of the main causes of hospital-acquired renal failure. The incidence of serious events with contrast agents was a strong deterrent to the use of contrast material in the early days of radiography following several reports of nephrotoxicity, contrast-induced nephropathy (CIN), and severe adverse reactions (2–5). Although numerous preventative methods has been explored to avoid renal contrast damage, radiocontrast-induced nephropathy continues to be a concern in patients with preexisting renal insufficiency who undergo contrast-enhanced radiographic examinations (6–8).

Definition

A rise in serum creatinine ≥25% from baseline or an absolute increase of >0.5 mg/dL from baseline

Pharmacology in the Catheterization Laboratory. Edited by Ron Waksman and Andrew E Ajani. © 2010 Blackwell Publishing, ISBN: 978-1-4051-5704-9.

are the two most common definitions of CIN available in the literature. This rise occurs within the first 24 h in the majority of patients, peaking on the third to fifth day after the procedure, and is coupled with a reduction in creatinine clearance. Unfortunately, serum creatinine measurement is an insensitive method to monitor renal function, as >50% reduction in glomerular filtration rate may occur before any increase is observed. A more accurate way to assess the renal function is to calculate the creatinine clearance by applying the Cockcroft-Gault formula or by calculating the glomerular filtration rate using the Modification of Diet in Renal Disease (MDRD) formula (9).

Implications

In patients with normal renal function, the incidence of CIN is relatively rare (1%), but its frequency increases in patients with abnormal renal function, and all the more in diabetic patients with preexisting renal insufficiency. The complications and prognosis of patients who develop CIN are significantly different when compared to those patients who do not. An early study by McCullough and colleagues of over 1,800 continuous patients undergoing coronary intervention revealed that acute renal failure requiring dialysis was associated with high rates of inhospital mortality (35.7%) and poor 2-year survival (18.8%) (10). A recent report by Rihal *et al.* (11), supporting McCullough's work, examined the prognostic implications of CIN after percutaneous coronary intervention. In this retrospective analysis of 7,586 patients who underwent percutaneous coronary intervention, 254 developed acute renal insufficiency (3.3%). Patients who developed CIN were at a significantly higher risk of death, both inhospital and in the long term. Among patients with normal renal function or moderate renal insufficiency (serum creatinine ≤2.0 mg/dL), the risk of developing renal insufficiency was significantly higher in diabetic patients compared to nondiabetic patients (4.5% vs 1.9%, $p < 0.001$). We also examined the prognostic importance of deterioration of renal function after percutaneous coronary intervention (12). In a consecutive series of 439 patients with chronic renal insufficiency (serum creatinine ≥1.8 mg/dL) who underwent coronary intervention, 37% developed CIN. Patients who developed CIN had significantly higher inhospital mortality rates compared to patients whose renal function was preserved (14.9% vs 4.9%; $p = 0.001$). A total of 31 of these patients required inhospital dialysis. The inhospital mortality of patients requiring dialysis was 22.6% and their cumulative 1-year mortality was 45.2%. In patients who developed CIN, the overall 1-year mortality rate was 35.4% compared to 19.4% in patients who did not develop CIN ($p = 0.001$). Recently Nash *et al.* (13) prospectively evaluated 4,622 consecutive patients for the development of hospital-acquired renal insufficiency. Diagnostic cardiac catheterization and coronary angioplasty caused renal insufficiency in 49% of patients who developed hospital acquired renal insufficiency after undergoing a study with radiocontrast material. Whether the development of CIN is just a marker of a severe comorbid state or directly contributes to the poor outcome of these patients has not been fully elucidated. Since the prognosis for patients who develop CIN following coronary angiography with or without intervention is significantly worse, prevention is a key issue needed to protect these patients.

Contrast media

Volume

One of the most important factors predicting CIN is the volume of contrast delivered to the patient (14,15). Cigarroa *et al.* devised an empiric formula for calculating the maximal amount of contrast material that can be administered safely: 5 mL of contrast/kg body weight (maximum, 300 mL)/serum creatinine (mg/dL) (16). An increase in serum creatinine ≥1.0 mg/dL was seen in 21% of patients who received an excess of contrast material, compared to only 2% of patients who received less than the calculated amount. In the Blue Cross Blue Shield of Michigan Cardiovascular Consortium (BMC2) Trial, Freeman *et al.* (17) explored the role of a weight- and creatinine-adjusted maximum radiographic contrast dose (MRCD) in patients developing contrast nephropathy who required dialysis. The MRCD was calculated as: MRCD = 5 mL × body weight (kg)/serum creatinine (mg/dL) and was the strongest independent predictor of contrast nephropathy that required dialysis. Inhospital mortality and CIN that required hemodialysis were both significantly higher in patients who exceeded the MRCD compared to patients who did not ($p < 0.001$). Results from the Michigan experience underscore the clinical implications and potential toxicity of large volumes of radiocontrast agents. In a multiple regression analysis of 1,869 consecutive patients who underwent coronary intervention by McCullough *et al.*, no patient who received less than 100 mL of contrast developed contrast nephropathy (10). Thus, every effort should be made to limit the amount of contrast media in patients with impaired baseline renal function.

Type of contrast media

Direct toxicity to the tubular cells of the kidneys and renal medullary ischemia are believed to be the main causes of contrast-induced renal function deterioration, as was reported more than 50 years ago. Tri-iodinated benzoic acid derivatives are water-soluble, ionic monomeric compounds that have an osmolality up to eight times greater than that of human plasma (>1,500 mOsm/kg, high-osmolar contrast media, HOCM) (Table 27.1). Newer low-osmolar contrast media (LOCM) agents have lower osmolality, but still more than double of that of plasma (>900 mOsm/kg) and are considered to be less nephrotoxic compared to HOCM. Iodixanol is the only nonionic agent that is iso-osmolar to blood (IOCM) that has been extensively studied (Table 27.1). Previous studies have shown that LOCM are less nephrotoxic when

Table 27.1 Type and ionicity of contrast media.

High-osmolality (HOCM) [1,500–2,000 mOsm/kg]	Low-osmolality (LOCM) [600–1,000 mOsm/kg]		Iso-osmolality (IOCM) [280–290 mOsm/kg]
	Ionic dimer	Nonionic	Nonionic dimer
Diatrizoate	Ioxaglate	Iohexanol	Iodixanol
Metrizoate		Iopamidol	Iotrolan
Ioxithalamate		Iopentol	
Iothalamate		Iopromide	
		Iomeprol	
		Iobitridol	
		Ioversol	

compared to HOCM. A meta-analysis of over 25 trials by Barrett *et al.* (18) showed that the use of LOCM caused a statistically detectable smaller decline in renal function compared to HOCM. Close examination of the results from these studies revealed a fairly consistent, albeit small, difference favoring LOCM. Esplugas *et al.* (19) compared several types of contrast media and concluded that in order to prevent CIN, minimal doses of either LOCM or IOCM should be used along with intravenous hydration and the use of HOCM should be avoided. Additionally, the use of either ionic LOCM (ioxaglate) or nonionic IOCM (iodixanol) was recommended in patients undergoing percutaneous coronary intervention because of antithrombotic advantages over nonionic LOCM. Grines *et al.* (20) compared LOCM ionic vs nonionic contrast media in 211 randomized patients with acute coronary syndrome undergoing percutaneous coronary intervention. Patients were additionally followed for 1 month for clinical events. Ionic contrast media was less likely to decrease blood flow during the procedure (8.1% vs 17.8%, $p < 0.04$) and was associated with fewer recurrent ischemic events requiring repeat catheterizations (3.0% vs 11%, $p < 0.02$). After 1 month, patients receiving ionic contrast media reported fewer symptoms of angina (8.5% vs 20.0%, $p < 0.04$), angina at rest (1.4% vs 11.8%, $p < 0.01$), and had a reduced need for subsequent bypass surgery (0% vs 5.9%, $p < 0.04$). Furthermore, LOCM causes less discomfort and fewer cardiovascular adverse effects than HOCM; however, the higher cost of LOCM has been a limiting factor for their universal use.

Contrarily to the Michigan experience by Grines *et al.*, several other trials have reported that nonionic contrast media is associated with less adverse effects than ionic contrast media (21,22). A study by Schrader *et al.* (21) prospectively randomized 2,000 patients undergoing percutaneous coronary intervention in a double-blind fashion to either the nonionic LOCM iomeprol in 1,001 patients or the LOCM ionic ioxaglate in 999 patients. The results of the study showed that there were no statistically significant differences between the two groups regarding abrupt vessel closure, emergency bypass surgery, myocardial infarction, or cardiac death. The only significant difference was that the patients receiving nonionic (iomeprol) contrast media had increased incidence of coronary artery dissection (30.2% vs 25.0%, $p = 0.01$) and elastic recoil (4.6% vs 2.8%, $p = 0.04$), two phenomena not related to the contrast media. In the COURT trial, a multicenter, prospective, double-blinded trial, Davidson *et al.* (22) randomized 856 patients undergoing percutaneous coronary intervention to either the isosmolar nonionic contrast agent (iodixanol, $n = 405$) or the low osmolar ionic contrast agent ioxaglate ($n = 410$). Patients receiving the nonionic contrast agent (iodixanol) experienced a 45% reduction in inhospital major adverse clinical events (5.4% vs 9.5%, $p = 0.027$), with a reduction in abrupt vessel closure and nonfatal myocardial infarction. This study was performed with contemporary coronary intervention techniques, including stents and GP IIb/IIIa inhibitors. The NEPHRIC study is a randomized, double-blind, multicenter, prospective study that assessed the

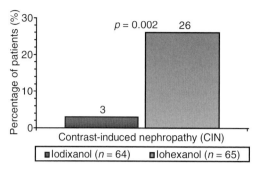

Figure 27.1 The incidence of contrast-induced nephropathy in patients undergoing angiography in the NEPHRIC Study with either iodixanol (light gray bar) or Iohexol (black bar). (*Source*: Data abstracted from Aspelin *et al.* (23).)

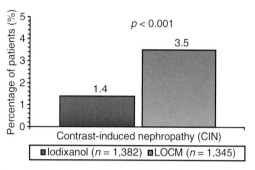

Figure 27.2 Incidence of contrast-induced nephropathy in all patients who received either iodixanol (light gray bar) or low-osmolality contrast agents (LOCM) (black bar). (*Source*: Data abstracted from McCullough *et al.* (24).)

incidence of CIN in high-risk patients with diabetes (type I or II) and serum creatinine 1.5–3.5 mg/dL undergoing coronary or aortofemoral angiography (23). This study compared 64 patients who received iodixanol (IOCM) and 65 patients that received iohexol (LOCM). Patients in the iohexol arm of the study experienced a significant increase in peak serum creatinine within 3 days (0.55 vs 0.13 mg/dL; $p = 0.001$). Contrast nephropathy occurred in 3% (2/64) of the iodixanol group compared to 26% (17/65) of the iohexol group ($p = 0.002$) (Figure 27.1). After 7 days, the mean change in serum creatinine was significantly greater in the iohexol group (0.24 mg/dL) compared to the iodixanol group (0.07 mg/dL) ($p = 0.003$). Despite differences in baseline clinical characteristics and in the procedure itself between the two groups, the investigators concluded that in high-risk patients, the chance of developing CIN is significantly less with iodixanol compared to iohexol (23). A recent meta-analysis by McCullough and colleagues pooled data from 2,727 patients from control-led, randomized studies that compared serum creatinine changes after the administration of iodixanol (IOCM) vs all types of LOCM in a large patient population (24). Although the population examined was heterogeneous with respect to risk factors, the incidence of CIN and serial measure-ments of serum creatinine levels, data are available on a total of 1,382 patients treated with iodixanol and 1,340 patients treated with LOCM. The inci-dence of CIN was significantly lower in patients who received iodixanol, particularly in the subgroup of patients with preexisting chronic

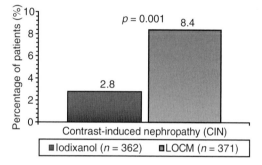

Figure 27.3 Incidence of contrast-induced nephropathy in patients with chronic kidney disease who received either iodixanol (light gray bar) or low-osmolality contrast agents (LOCM) (black bar). (*Source*: Data abstracted from McCullough *et al.* (24).)

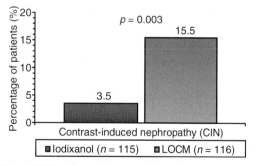

Figure 27.4 Incidence of contrast-induced nephropathy in patients with chronic kidney and diabetes mellitus disease who received either iodixanol (light gray bar) or low-osmolality contrast agents (LOCM) (black bar). (*Source*: Data abstracted from McCullough *et al.* (24).)

kidney disease or chronic kidney disease and dia-betes (Figures 27.2–27.4). Interestingly, diabetes alone was not associated with a higher incidence of CIN in this study. Therefore, the results of this meta-analysis of pooled data indicate that the use of the IOCM iodixanol is associated with a significantly lower rate of CIN, especially in patients with chronic kidney disease with and without diabetes. Similar conclusions were drawn by the CIN Consensus Working Panel that recommended that in patients with chronic kidney disease (estimated glomerular filtration rate <60 mL/min per 1.73 m^2), IOCM should be used (25).

Alternative contrast materials

Gadolinium and CO_2

Other contrast agents that are being used as alternatives to iodinated compounds in interventional radiology are carbon dioxide and the gadolinium compounds (26–28). Recent publications have shown that gadolinium can be used as an alternative or in combination with iodine-based compounds in patients with chronic renal insufficiency. However, further research is needed to determine if these compounds can be implemented in coronary intervention. Yet, other studies have reported cases of acute renal failure after the use of gadolinium-based contrast agents and even a higher rate of CIN in chronic kidney disease patients undergoing percutaneous coronary interventions (29,30). In view of these reports, the use of gadolinium-based contrast media to avoid CIN in chronic kidney disease patients cannot be recommended at this time. The use of CO_2 has also been proposed as an alternative to guide vascular interventions, especially in patients with chronic renal disease undergoing endovascular renal artery intervention. It must be remembered that CO_2 is not approved for angiography and cannot be used above the diaphragm (25,31).

Summary

The plethora of literature and medical research on the ideal contrast material indicates the concern among physicians regarding CIN and its dire consequences in patients undergoing percutaneous coronary interventions. Various prospective, randomized, controlled studies have shown that the type of contrast agent used has an important role on the potential etiology of CIN and now routine use of either ionic or nonionic low osmolar contrast is implemented in contrast-based procedures. Currently, the best strategy for prevention of CIN is risk recognition (chronic kidney disease and diabetes), limiting the volume of contrast medium utilized (less than 100 mL where possible), using an IOCM or LOCM and allowing 2 weeks between staged procedures. Assessment of the number of risk factors present in each patient prior to contrast administration affords the clinician the opportunity to utilize one, if not several, protective mechanisms in order to decrease the chances of CIN.

References

1 Schreiner GE. Nephrotoxicity and diagnostic agents. *JAMA*. 1966;**196**:413–415.

2 Pendergrass EP, Chamberlin GW, Godfrey EW, Burdick ED. A survey of deaths and unfavorable sequelae following administration of contrast media. *Am J Roentgen*. 1942;**48**:741–762.

3 Miller GM, Wylie EJ, Hinman F Jr. Renal complications from aortography. *Surgery*. 1954;**35**:885–896.

4 Idbohrn H. Tolerance to contrast media in renal angiography. *Acta Radiol*. 1956;**45**:141.

5 McAfee JG. A survey of complications of abdominal aortography. *Radiology*. 1957;**68**:825–838.

6 Gruberg L, Mehran M, Dangas G, et al. Acute renal failure requiring dialysis after percutaneous coronary interventions. *Catheter Cardiovasc Interv*. 2001;**52**:409–416.

7 Gruberg L, Dangas G, Mehran R, et al. Clinical outcome following percutaneous interventions in patients with chronic renal failure. *Catheter Cardiovasc Interv*. 2002;**55**:66–72.

8 Gruberg L, Weissman NJ, Waksman R, et al. Comparison of outcomes of percutaneous coronary revascularization with stents in patients with and without mild chronic renal failure. *Am J Cardiol*. 2002;**89**:54–57.

9 National Kidney Foundation. Clinical practice guidelines for chronic kidney disease: evaluation, classification and stratification. *Am J Kidney Dis*. 2002;**2**(suppl 1):S46–S75.

10 McCullough PA, Wolyn R, Rocher LL, Levin RN, O'Neill WW. Acute renal failure after coronary intervention: incidence, risk factors, and relationship to mortality. *Am J Med*. 1997;**103**:368–375.

11 Rihal CS, Textor SC, Grill DE, et al. Incidence and prognostic importance of acute renal failure after percutaneous coronary intervention. *Circulation*. 2002;**105**:2259–2264.

12 Gruberg L, Mintz GS, Mehran R, et al. The prognostic implications of further renal function deterioration within 48 h of interventional coronary procedures in patients with pre-existing chronic renal insufficiency. *J Am Coll Cardiol*. 2000;**36**:1542–1548.

13 Nash K, Hafeez A, Hou S. Hospital-acquired renal insufficiency. *Am J Kidney Dis.* 2002;**39**:930–936.

14 Mueller C, Buerkle G, Buettner HJ, *et al.* Prevention of contrast media-associated nephropathy: randomized comparison of 2 hydration regimens in 1620 patients undergoing coronary angioplasty. *Arch Intern Med.* 2002;**162**:329–336.

15 Trivedi HS, Moore H, Nasr S, *et al.* A randomized prospective trial to assess the role of saline hydration on the development of contrast nephrotoxicity. *Nephron.* 2003;**93**:C29–C34.

16 Cigarroa RG, Lange RA, Williams RH, Hillis LD. Dosing of contrast material to prevent contrast nephropathy in patients with renal disease. *Am J Med.* 1989;**86**:649–652.

17 Freeman RV, O'Donell M, Share D, *et al.* Nephropathy requiring dialysis after percutaneous coronary intervention and the critical role of an adjusted contrast dose. *Am J Cardiol.* 2002;**90**:1068–1073.

18 Barrett BJ, Carlisle EJ. Metaanalysis of the relative nephrotoxicity of high- and low-osmolality iodinated contrast media. *Radiology.* 1993;**188**:171–178.

19 Esplugas E, Cequier A, Gomez-Hospital JA. Comparative tolerability of contrast media used for coronary interventions. *Drug Saf.* 2002;**25**(15):1079–1098.

20 Grines CL, Schreiber TL, Savas V, *et al.* A randomized trial of low osmolar ionic versus nonionic contrast media in patients with myocardial infarction or unstable angina undergoing percutaneous transluminal coronary angioplasty. *J Am Coll Cardiol.* 1996;**27**:1381–1386.

21 Schrader R, Esch I, Ensslen R, *et al.* A randomized trial comparing the impact of a nonionic (iomeprol) versus an ionic (ioxaglate) low osmolar contrast medium on abrupt vessel closure and ischemic complications after coronary angioplasty. *J Am Coll Cardiol.* 1999; **33**:395–402.

22 Davidson CJ, Laskey WK, Hermiller JB, *et al.* Randomized trial of contrast media utilization in high-risk PTCA, the COURT trial. *Circulation.* 2000;**101**:2172–2177.

23 Aspelin P, Aubry P, Fransson SG, *et al.* Nephrotoxic effects in high-risk patients undergoing angiography. *N Engl J Med.* 2003;**348**:491–499.

24 McCullough PA, Bertrand ME, Brinker JA, Stacul F. A meta-analysis of the renal safety of isosmolar iodixanol compared with low-osmolar contrast media. *J Am Coll Cardiol.* 2006;**48**:692–699.

25 Davidson C, Stacul F, McCullough PA, *et al.*, on behalf of the CIN consensus working panel. Contrast medium use. *Am J Cardiol.* 2006;**98**(suppl):42K–58K.

26 Sterner G, Nyman U, Valdes T. Low risk of contrast-medium-induced nephropathy with modern angiographic technique. *J Intern Med.* 2001;**250**:429–434.

27 Spinosa DJ, Kaufmann JA, Hartwell GD. Gadolinium chelates in angiography and interventional radiology: a useful alternative to iodinated contrast media for angiography. *Radiology.* 2002;**223**:319–325.

28 Rieger J, Sitter T, Toepfer M. Gadolinium as an alternative contrast agent for diagnostic and interventional angiographic procedures in patients with impaired renal function. *Nephrol Dial Transplant.* May 2002; **17**:824–828.

29 Thomsen HS. Gadolinium-based contrast media may be nephrotoxic even at approved doses. *Eur Radiol.* 2004;**14**:1654–1656.

30 Briguori C, Colombo A, Airoldi F, *et al.* Gadolinium-based contrast agents and nephrotoxicity in patients undergoing coronary artery procedures. *Catheter Cardiovasc Interv.* 2006;**67**:175–180.

31 Kessel DO, Robertson I, Patel JV, *et al.* Carbon-dioxide-guided vascular interventions: technique and pitfalls. *Cardiovasc Intervent Radiol.* 2002;**25**:476–483.

VI

PART VI

PCI complications

CHAPTER 28

The no reflow phenomenon: Etiology, prophylaxis, and treatment

Tim A. Fischell

Michigan State University, Kalamazoo, MI, USA

Introduction

Slow or no reflow is a serious problem that complicates approximately 2–3% of native vessel percutaneous coronary artery interventions (PCIs) and 15–25% of percutaneous transluminal coronary angioplasty (PTCA) and stent cases in degenerated saphenous vein bypass grafts (1–4). This complication may be increased in patients treated with atherectomy and/or stents, in PCI for ST-elevation myocardial infarction (STEMI) (5–7), and in patients who undergo coronary intervention after non-Q wave myocardial infarction (MI). The risk of slow or no-reflow is significantly higher during PCI in degenerated saphenous vein grafts than in native vessels (3,4).

Slow or no-reflow are defined, respectively, as the impairment, or loss, of antegrade blood flow after PCI in the absence of a residual obstructive lesion in the conductance (epicardial) vessel. This complication may lead to as much as a 10-fold increase in the incidence of both inhospital death and/or acute myocardial infarction (1–4). Fortunately, there are a growing number of strategies to prevent and/or reverse this morbid complication.

Etiology

The etiology of no-reflow or slow flow after angioplasty of native vessels and degenerated vein grafts is likely twofold. There is evidence that in many cases, there is a mechanical component of small vessel obstruction from distal embolization of the friable plaque debris and/or thrombus from the dilated lesion site (8,9). In both native and vein graft lesions, plaque components, including organized thrombus and cholesterol crystals, have been documented to embolize downstream (Figure 28.1). There appears to be a higher risk of no reflow and distal embolization in degenerated vein grafts due to the soft and friable nature of these lesions (8–14).

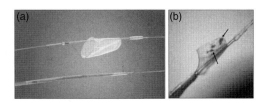

Figure 28.1 Filterwire™ device for distal embolic protection. (a) The Filterwire™ system (Boston Scientific, Natick, MA) is shown in its predeployed state (lower panel) and after filter deployment (upper panel). (b) Embolic debris is observed in the filter section after the stent-based intervention in a degenerated saphenous vein graft. Arrows highlight the embolic debris captured in the filter.

Pharmacology in the Catheterization Laboratory. Edited by Ron Waksman and Andrew E Ajani. © 2010 Blackwell Publishing, ISBN: 978-1-4051-5704-9.

Although mechanical (embolic) obstruction of the distal microvascular bed clearly plays a role in slow/no reflow, evidence suggests that intense microvascular vasoconstriction, leading to increased distal microvascular resistance may play a dominant role in the majority of cases (15–20). There are several studies that clearly demonstrate that there is a high concentration of potent, soluble vasoconstricting substances released to the distal microcirculatory bed from the effluent released from the target site during PCI (18–20).

Additional microvascular vasoconstriction may be triggered by embolization of thrombotic and atheromatous debris into the distal vascular bed, causing local activation of platelets, with release of platelet-derived vasoconstrictors such as thromboxane A2 and serotonin (20). The consistent and often dramatic responses to vasodilating agents such as verapamil, diltiazem, nicardipine, nitroprusside, and adenosine also support the hypothesis that microvascular spasm plays a major etiologic role in this syndrome (21–30). The remainder of this review will highlight the currently available, and newer, investigational approaches to treat and/or prevent no reflow during PCI.

Pharmacologic approaches to reverse and/or prevent no reflow

Historically, intracoronary (IC) nitroglycerin was used as a mainstay in the treatment of no reflow. Although nitroglycerin is a potent vasodilator of the epicardial coronary artery (17), it has weak effects as a microvascular/arteriolar vasodilator. In one series comparing the calcium channel blocker, verapamil, to nitroglycerin for the treatment of no reflow, the patients treated with nitroglycerin had no significant improvement in flow, and an increase in adverse clinical outcomes (2). Although intracoronary nitroglycerin can be recommended as the agent of choice for the reversal of large (epicardial) coronary artery spasm, it should not be considered as an appropriate treatment for the treatment of no reflow.

Adenosine is one of the most potent arteriolar vasodilating agents available to reverse no reflow in degenerated saphenous vein grafts. Since IC adenosine has a very short duration of action (half-life ~15–20 s) (31), repeated boluses (10–20,

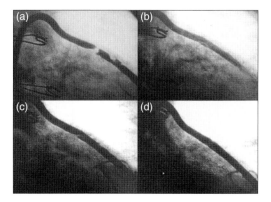

Figure 28.2 Angiographic example of rapid injection of intracoronary adenosine for reversal of no-reflow following saphenous vein graft intervention. In Panel a, an ulcerated and partially thrombotic lesion is seen in the midportion of the vein graft to the LAD. Panel b, shows balloon angioplasty, there is some improvement in the lesion morphology but TIMI I flow as depicted by lack of filling the vein graft at 60 frames following contrast injection. Panel c demonstrates reversal to TIMI III flow following intracoronary adenosine boluses, with complete filling at frame count 20. Panel d shows final result following stent placement.

12–24 µg/boluses) are needed to reverse no reflow. Because of its short half-life, adenosine is not an agent of choice for the prevention of no reflow. In two series (22,23), repeated and rapid bolus administration of IC adenosine via a guiding catheter, ideally using small (3 mL) syringes, has been highly effective in reversing no reflow (Figure 28.2). In both series, no reflow was reversed to TIMI 3 flow in 90–95% of patients within 3–5 min of onset. Although IC adenosine can theoretically cause A–V block when administered in the right or dominant left circumflex arteries, this effect is very rare and is short lived due to the short half-life of the drug.

Intracoronary nitroprusside may also be effective in the treatment of no reflow (29,30). Nicorandil, an ATP-sensitive potassium channel opener, has been shown to decrease the risk of no-reflow during rotational atherectomy compared to verapamil (28), and to help to preserve microvascular integrity and myocardial viability in patients with anterior wall myocardial infarction (32). These agents may work via their action as in enhancing NO release or availability at the arteriolar level. These drugs may be administered via an intracoronary route via the distal lumen of a balloon catheter or an infusion catheter, or through injection through the guiding catheter. Although a number of laboratories have used successfully used nitroprusside and nicorandil there are relatively few published reports to allow us to evaluate the efficacy of these drugs compared to other agents.

Calcium channel blockers to reverse no-reflow

Calcium channel blockers appear to have a substantial beneficial effect in reversing and preventing no reflow. Verapamil, diltiazem, and nicardipine have all been used successfully to reverse and/or prevent no reflow (2,21,25–27,33–35).

Intracoronary administration of verapamil (100–900 μg total dose given in 100 μg boluses) has been demonstrated to improve antegrade blood flow in patients with no reflow (2,3). This therapy has been reported to be effective in 67–89% of the cases (1–3). In the largest reported series (2), 81% of patients were reversed to TIMI 3 flow. Thus, verapamil appears to have reasonable efficacy. However, there are still occasional and morbid failures of this agent. In addition, the use of intracoronary verapamil may carry a risk of potentially serious adverse effects including prolonged heart block (~3–5%) and a potential for negative myocardial inotropic responses.

Intracoronary diltiazem may also be effective in reversing no reflow (21). In the series reported by Mooney et al., no reflow was significantly improved in 23/24 patients (95%). In this study, IC diltiazem was administered in 0.5–2.5 mg boluses, up to a total dose of 0.5–8.5 mg. The drug was well tolerated and only 1 of the 24 patients in this series suffered a non-Q wave MI. One study has also suggested the potential to reduce the risk of no-reflow with the preadministration of IC diltiazem prior to directional atherectomy (34).

Nicardipine may be the most potent calcium channel blocker for the reversal and/or prophylaxis for no reflow (25–27,35,36). In one comparative study, Doppler wire measurements were used to compare the magnitude and duration of arteriolar vasodilatation with verapamil, diltiazem, and nicardipine (36). Nicardipine had substantially greater maximal arteriolar vasodilating effects than either verapamil or diltiazem (36). In addition,

the duration of this effect with nicardipine (mean 4–5 min coronary blood flow >2 times basal flow) was significantly longer than the other two calcium channel blockers. The risk of heart block and negative inotropic effects should also be very small with this dihydropyridine calcium channel blocker.

This agent has been shown to be very effective in reversing no reflow. Huang et al. have recently reported great success using intracoronary nicardipine to reverse no-reflow complicating both native vessel and saphenous vein graft interventions (26). In this study of 72 patients, no-reflow was reversed to normal flow in 98.6% of cases (26).

"Pharmacologic" distal protection during SVG intervention

Verapamil, diltiazem, nicorandil, and nicardipine have all been shown to have efficacy in the prevention of no reflow events in high risk PCI (25,32–35). In the VAPOR trial, Michaels et al. demonstrated the feasibility of using prophylactic, intracoronary verapamil to prevent no reflow during SVG intervention (33).

Because of its duration of action and potency (37–39), IC nicardipine may be the agent of choice for the prophylaxis of no-reflow. Fischell et al. (25,35) have studied the use of intragraft nicardipine as a means to prevent no-reflow during SVG stenting (25,35). In a case study, this pharmacologic approach to prevent no-reflow was used successfully in two patients who required triple SVG intervention (25). In a second, larger series, prophylactic nicardipine was used, without adjunctive distal (mechanical) protection, as a method to minimize the incidence of no reflow in saphenous vein graft interventions (35). In this consecutive series of 83 elective "real-world" SVG interventions, there was a low, 4.4% 30-day MACE and 4.4% incidence of CPK MB elevation greater than three times the upper limit of normal, using prophylactic intragraft nicardipine (35). These results compare favorably with data from mechanical distal protection trials, such as the SAFER Trial (PercusurgeTM) (40), the PRIDE Trial (41), and the FIRE trial (Filterwire) (42).

Unlike mechanical distal protection, which may not be anatomically feasible in the 25–30% of lesions, "pharmacologic" distal protection with

Table 28.1 Pharmacologic management of no reflow.

Drug	Route/dose	Prevention no reflow y/n/unknown	Reversal no reflow y(%effective)/n	Approximate duration of action
Diltiazem	IC/0.5–10 mg; 0.5–1 mg/bolus	Unknown	Yes (>90%)	2–3 min
Verapamil	IC/100–900 µg; 100 µg/bolus	Yes	Yes (67–87%)	2–3 min
Nicardipine	IC/50–500 µg; 50–200 µg/bolus	Yes	Yes (>98.6%)	3–5 min
Nitroprusside	IC/50–500 µg; 50–200 µg/bolus	Unknown	Yes (>90%)	uncertain
Adenosine	IC/10–20 boluses; 12–24 µg/bolus	No	Yes (90–95%)	10–30 s
Nitroglycerin	IC/100–300 µg	No	No	2–5 min
Nicorandil	IC/100–400 µg	With rotational atherectomy	Uncertain	uncertain

nicardipine or verapamil can be used in all SVG interventions. In some cases, there may also be trauma and possible initiation of no reflow by the passage and manipulation of the distal protection device across a severe stenosis.

Finally, the pharmacologic distal protection using nicardipine provides a time-efficient and cost-effective intervention, compared to the routine use of distal (mechanical) protection devices. This may translate to a >90% cost reduction using this pharmacologic approach as an alternative to mechanical distal or proximal protection (35). We currently recommend administration of 200–300 µg of IC nicardipine to be given just prior to the vein graft manipulation, with repeated doses every 4–5 min as needed. Pharmacologic prophylaxis may also be used adjunctively with mechanical distal protection in high-risk interventions, when it is anatomically feasible.

Antiplatelet agents to prevent no-reflow

Finally, the antiplatelet GP IIb/IIIa blockers may play a small, and somewhat provocative, role in the prevention of no reflow in saphenous vein graft interventions, and in acute MI. These drugs have been evaluated in randomized trials, including the EPIC, EPILOG, and EPISTENT studies (43,44). In the substudy examining interventions in "degenerated" vein grafts from the EPIC and EPILOG studies, the bolus plus infusion of abciximab was associated with a significant reduction in clinically apparent distal embolization (2% abciximab vs 18% in placebo group,

$p = 0.017$) (43). At this time, we have relatively little data regarding the use of the other IIb/IIIa inhibitors in this setting.

A summary of the vasodilating agents that may be used in the management of no reflow is provided in Table 28.1.

Devices for the prevention of no reflow

There are a number of devices that are either approved or under investigation for the treatment of intracoronary thrombus and/or the prevention of no reflow during coronary interventions (45–53).

The Angiojet Rheolytic™ Thrombectomy System (Possis Medial, Inc., Minneapolis, MN) is a novel device that uses high-velocity saline jets to create a "localized Bernoulli effect," to allow the mechanical removal of organized thrombus (45,46). This FDA approved device is capable of efficient thrombus removal. Limitations of this technology may include capital costs, hemolysis, and difficulty in advancing the device through the obstructing lesion. There may also be issues regarding the Angiojet's effectiveness in the removal of atheroembolic debris during the treatment of degenerated saphenous vein grafts (SVGs). The use of this device in a randomized clinical trial in patients presenting with ST elevation MI failed to demonstrate and benefit over conventional treatment. Thrombectomy with this device did not improve flow, reduce the incidence of no-reflow, nor improve clinical outcomes when used adjunctively in the setting of acute MI PCI in native vessels (50).

Other thrombectomy catheters are also available and allow a somewhat simpler means for thrombus debulking/aspiration. Although these devices, like the Angiojet, are capable of mechanical debulking of thrombus, the role of this approach to prevent no-reflow in native vessels or SVGs in controversial (47,50).

The PercuSurge system consists of a 0.014" wire with a balloon near the distal end (GuardWire™). The wire can be passed through the thrombotic lesion and advanced to the distal vessel. The balloon is inflated and the PTCI is performed over this GuardWire™. Following the intervention, an aspiration catheter is advanced over this wire and is used to suction out loose thrombotic or athero-embolic debris that was released into the closed space created by the balloon occlusion. This device has been used successfully in pilot series in SVGs (51). In this pilot, particulate debris was retrieved in 21/23 cases. Non-Q wave MI occurred in 11% of cases, but only one case had CPK elevation of greater than three times the upper limit of normal. The average particle size retrieved was 204 × 83 μm. The advantage of this system is the potential to physically remove most of the debris released during intervention. In the SAFER study, this device was been shown to be efficacious in reducing the risk of no reflow and myonecrosis when used adjunctively, during PCI of diseased saphenous vein bypass grafts (40). In this trial, the risk of embolization with myocardial infarction was reduced from 14.7% in the control group to 8.6% in the PercuSurge group (40). This device is FDA-approved. One significant disadvantage with this system is the need to work quickly, with multiple exchanges, while there is ischemia induced by the distal balloon occlusion.

The PRIDE trial looked at results with three different mechanical distal protection systems. In that study, the incidence of MI after elective SVG intervention was higher than the MI rate in patients treated with prophylactic nicardipine (35). The MI rates were 11.9% for Filterwire™, 11.3% for Guardwire™, and 7.6% for TriActiv™. In the Filterwire™ subgroup, there was a 7.1% incidence of >8 fold CPK MB increase compared to 0/68 (0%) cases in nicardipine "pharmacologic" prophylaxis study (35).

Another device-related approach to this problem utilizes the concept of a distal expandable and retractable filter (41,42,49). The Filterwire™, manufactured by Boston Scientific (Natick, MA), is the most widely used FDA approved, device of this type. The filter has the potential advantage of allowing distal blood flow while collecting the larger embolic debris. These devices can play an important role in the prevention of no reflow in high-risk saphenous vein graft interventions, when the anatomy is suitable (41,42,49). One of the disadvantages of these filters is the inability to stop the downstream effects of soluble vasoconstrictors that may provoke no reflow (18–20).

Conclusions

In summary, no/slow reflow is a relatively common and morbid complication of percutaneous coronary intervention. This complication is most frequent in the setting of thrombus-laden lesions, PCI in acute MI, and during the treatment of degenerated saphenous vein bypass grafts. The use of atherectomy and stenting may also increase the incidence of this complication.

If no reflow does occur, there are a number of pharmacologic options that appear to be effective in reversing the vast majority of these events in a short period of time. Intracoronary nicardipine with or without repeated boluses of IC adenosine may be the most effective treatment to reverse no reflow after vein graft interventions. Intracoronary verapamil, diltiazem, nitroprusside, and nicorandil also appear to be effective agents. Nitroglycerin is a potent epicardial coronary artery vasodilator, but should not be used as an agent to prevent or reverse the microvascular vasoconstriction that causes no-reflow.

In terms of preventing no-reflow, there is little convincing evidence that clot "debulking" reduces the risk of no-reflow in SVG or native coronary artery lesions. Proximal and distal embolic protection systems do have a role in high-risk lesions. Prophylactic intragraft administration of nicardipine, followed by direct stenting appears to be a safe simple, and cost-effective alternative, or adjunct, to mechanical distal protection for elective SVG interventions. Comparisons of device and pharmacologic or combination treatments should be evaluated in future clinical trials.

References

1 Abbo KM, Dooris M, Glazier S, *et al.* Features and outcome of no-reflow after percutaneous coronary intervention. *Am J Cardiol.* 1995;**75**:778–782.

2 Kaplan BM, Benzuly KH, Kinn JW, *et al.* Treatment of no-reflow in degenerated saphenous vein graft interventions: comparison of intracornary verapamil and nitroglycerin. *Cathet Cardiovasc Diag.* 1996;**39**:113–118.

3 Piana RN, Paik GY, Moscucci M, *et al.* Incidence and treatment of "no-reflow" after percutaneous coronary intervention. *Circulation.* 1994;**89**:2514–2518.

4 Eeckhout E, Kern MJ. The coronary no-reflow phenomenon: a review of mechanisms and therapies. *Eur Heart J.* 2001;**22**(9):729–739.

5 De Lemos JA, Antman EM, Giugliano RP, *et al.* ST-segment resolution and infarct related artery patency and flow after thrombolytic therapy. Thrombolysis in Myocardial Infarction (TIMI) 14 investigators. *Am J Cardiol.* 2000;**85**:299–304.

6 Feld H, Lichstein E, Schachter J, Shani J. Early and late angiographic findings of the "no-reflow" phenomenon following direct angioplasty as primary treatment for acute myocardial infarction. *Am Heart J.* 1992;**123**:782–784.

7 Morishima I, Sone T, Okumura K, *et al.* Angiographic no-reflow phenomenon as a predictor of adverse long-term outcome in patients treated with percutaneous transluminal coronary angioplasty for first acute myocardial infarction. *J Am Coll Cardiol.* 2000;**36**:1202.

8 Kalan JM, Robers WC. Morphologic changes in saphenous veins used as coronary arterial bypass conduits for longer than one year: necropsy analysis of 53 patients, 123 saphenous veins and 1865 five millimeter segments of veins. *Am Heart J.* 1990;**119**:1164–1184.

9 Saber RS, Edwards WD, Bailey KR, McGovern TW, Schwartz RS, Holmes DR, Jr. Coronary embolization after balloon angioplasty or thrombolytic therapy: an autopsy study of 32 cases. *J Am Coll Cardiol.* 1993;**22**:1283–1288.

10 White CJ, Ramee SR, Collins TJ, Mesa JE, Jain A. Percutaneous angioscopy of saphenous vein coronary bypass grafts. *J Am Coll Cardiol.* 1993;**21**:1181–1185.

11 de Feyter P, Serruys P, van den Brand M, Meester H, Beatt K, Suryapranata H. Percutaneous transluminal angioplasty of totally occluded bypass graft: a challenge that should be resisted. *Am J Cardiol.* 1989;**64**:88–90.

12 Kahn KJ, Rutherford BD, McConahay DR, *et al.* Initial and long-term outcome of 83 patients after balloon angioplasty of totally occluded bypass grafts. *J Am Coll Cardiol.* 1994;**23**:1038–1042.

13 Henriques JP, Zijlstra F, Ottevanger JP, *et al.* Incidence and clinical significance of distal embolization during primary angioplasty for acute myocardial infarction. *Eur Heart J.* 2002;**23**:1112–1117.

14 Kotani J, Mintz GS, Pregowski J, *et al.* Volumetric intravascular ultrasound evidence that distal embolization during acute infarct intervention contributes to inadequate myocardial perfusion grade. *Am J Cardiol.* 2003;**92**:728–732.

15 Wilson RF, Laxson DD, Lesser JR, White CW. Intense microvascular constriction after angioplasty of acute thrombotic coronary arterial lesions. *Lancet.* 1989;**I**: 807–811.

16 Kloner RA, Ganote CE, Jennings, RB. The "no-reflow" phenomenon after temporary coronary occlusion in the dog. *J Clin Invest.* 1974;**54**:1496–1508.

17 Fischell TA, Derby G, Tse TM, Stadius ML. Coronary artery vasoconstriction routinely occurs following percutaneous transluminal coronary angioplasty: a quantitative arteriographic analysis. *Circulation.* 1988; **78**(6):1323–1334.

18 Leineweber K, Bose D, Vogelsang M, *et al.* Intense vasoconstriction in response to aspirate from stented saphenous vein aortocoronary bypass grafts. *J Am Coll Cardiol.* 2006;**47**:981–986.

19 Salloum J, Tharpe C, Vaughn D, Zhao DX. Release and elimination of soluble vasoactive factors during percutaneous coronary intervention of saphenous vein grafts: analysis using the PercuSurge GuardWire distal protection device. *J Invasive Cardiol.* 2005;**17**(11):575–579.

20 Paik GY, Caputo RP, Nunez BD, *et al.* Thrombus contains soluble factor which decrease blood flow in swine coronary arteries through a nitrous oxide-dependent pathway. *J Am Coll Cardiol.* 1994;**23**:64A.

21 Weyrens FJ, Mooney J, Lesser J, Mooney MR. Intracoronary diltiazem for microvascular spasm after interventional therapy. *Am J Cardiol.* 1995;**75**:849–850.

22 Fischell TA, Carter AJ, Foster MT, *et al.* Reversal of "no reflow" during vein graft stenting using high velocity boluses of intracoronary adenosine. *Cathet Cardiovasc Diagn.* 1998;**45**:360–365.

23 Sdringola A, Assali A, Ghani M, *et al.* Adenosine use during aortocoronary vein graft interventions reverses but does not prevent the slow-no reflow phenomenon. *Catheter Cardiovasc Interv.* 2000;**50**:156.

24 Fischell TA, Lauer MA. Prevention and management of "no-reflow" during coronary interventions. In: Nissen S, Popma J, Kern M, eds. *Cardiac Catheterization and Interventional Self-Assessment Program (CathSap II).* Bethesda, Maryland: American College of Cardiology Foundation; 2001:255–258.

25 Haller S, Ashraf K, Fischell TA. Intragraft nicardipine prophylaxis to prevent no reflow in triple-vessel,

saphenous vein graft intervention. *J Invasive Cardiol.* 2005;**17**(6):334–337.

26 Huang RI, Patel P, Walinsky P, *et al.* Efficacy of intracoronary nicardipine in the treatment of no-reflow during percutaneous coronary intervention. *Catheter Cardiovasc Interv.* 2006;**68**:671–676.

27 Fischell TA, Mashwari A. Current applications for nicardipine in invasive and interventional cardiology. *J Invasive Cardiol.* 2004;**16**(8):428–432.

28 Tsubokawa A, Ueda K, Sakamoto H, *et al.* Effect of intracoronary nicorandil administration on prevention no-reflow/slow flow phenomenon during rotational atherectomy. *Circ J.* 2002;**66**:1119–1123.

29 Wang HJ, Lo PH, Lin JJ, *et al.* Treatment of slow/no-reflow phenomenon with intracoronary nitroprusside injection in primary coronary intervention for acute myocardial infarction. *Catheter Cardiovasc Interv.* 2004;**63**:171–176.

30 Hillegass WB, Dean NA, Liao L, *et al.* Treatment of no-reflow and impaired flow with the nitric oxide donor nitroprusside following percutaneous coronary interventions: initial human clinical experience. *J Invasive Cardiol.* 2001;**37**:1335–1343.

31 Wilson RF, Wyche K, Christensen BV, Zimmer S, Laxson DD. Effects of adenosine on human coronary arterial circulation. *Circulation.* 1990;**82**:1595–1605.

32 Ito H, Taniyama Y, Iwakura K, *et al.* Intravenous nicorandil can preserve microvascular integrity and myocardial viability in patients with reperfused anterior wall myocardial infarction. *J Invasive Cardiol.* 1999;**33**:654–660.

33 Michaels AD, Appleby M, Otten MH, *et al.* Pretreatment with intragraft verapamil prior to percutaneous coronary intervention of saphenous vein graft lesions: results of the randomized, controlled vasodilator prevention on no-reflow (VAPOR) trial. *J Invasive Cardiol.* 2002; **14**(6):299–302.

34 Jalinours F, Mooney JA, Mooney MR. Pretreatment with intracoronary diltiazem reduces non-Q wave myocardial infarction following directional atherectomy. *J Invasive Cardiol.* 1997;**9**:270–273.

35 Fischell TA, Subraya RG, Ashraf K, Carter AJ, Perry B, Haller SD. "Pharmacologic" Distal protection using prophylactic, intragraft nicardipine to prevent no-reflow and non-Q was MI during SVG interventions. *J Invasive Cardiol.* 2007;**19**(2):58–62.

36 Fugit MD, Rubal BJ, Donovan DJ. Effects of intracoronary nicardipine, diliazem and verapamil on coronary blood flow. *J Invasive Cardiol.* 2000;**12**(2):80–85.

37 Whiting RL, Dow RJ, Graham DJ, Mroszczak EJ. An overview of the pharmacology and pharmacokinetics of nicardipine. *Angiology.* 1990;**41**(11 Pt 2):987–991.

38 Lambert CR, Pepine CJ. Effects of intravenous and intracoronary nicardipine. *Am J Cardiol.* 1989;**64**(15): 8H–15H.

39 Singh BN, Josephson MA. Clinical pharmacology, pharmacokinetics, and hemodynamic effects of nicardipine. *Am Heart J.* 1990;**119**(2 Pt 2):427–434.

40 Baim DS, Wahr D, Gorge B, *et al.* Randomized trial of a distal protection device during percutaneous intervention of saphenous vein aorto-coronary bypass grafts. *Circulation.* 2002;**105**:1285–1296.

41 Carrozza JP, Mumma M, Breall JA, *et al.* Randomized evaluation of the TriActiv balloon-protection flush and extraction system for the treatment of saphenous vein graft disease. *J Am Coll Cardiol.* 2005;**46**:1677–1683.

42 Stone GW, Rogers C, Hermiller J, *et al.* Randomized comparison of distal protection with a filter-based catheter and a balloon occlusion and aspiration system during percutaneous intervention of diseased saphenous vein aorto-coronary bypass grafts. *Circulation.* 2003;**108**:548–553.

43 Mak KH, Challapalli R, Eisenberg MJ, Anderson KM, Califf RM, Topol EJ. Effect of platelet glycoprotein IIb/IIIa receptor inhibition on distal embolization during percutaneous revascularization of aortocoronary saphenous vein grafts. *Am J Cardiol.* 1997;**80**:985–988.

44 Lincoff AM, Califf RM, Moliterno DJ, *et al.* Complementary clinical benefits of coronary-artery stenting and blockade of platelet glycoprotein IIb/IIIa receptors. *N Engl J Med.* 1999;**341**(5): 319–327.

45 Ramee SR, Schatz RA, Carrozza JP, *et al.* Results of the VeGAS I Pilot Study of the Possis coronary AngioJet, thrombectomy catheter. *Circulation.* 1996;**94**:I-619 [abstract].

46 Nakagawa Y, Matsuo S, Kimura T, *et al.* Thrombectomy with angiojet catheter in native coronary arteries for patients with acute or recent myocardial infarction. *Am J Cardiol.* 1999;**83**:994–999.

47 Limbruno U, Micheli A, De Carlo M, *et al.* Mechanical prevention of distal embolization during primary angioplasty: safety, feasibility, and impact on myocardial reperfusion. *Circulation.* 2003;**108**:171–176.

48 Yip HK, WU CJ, Chang HW, *et al.* Effect of the PercuuSurge GuardWire device on the integrity of microvasculature and clinical outcomes during transradial coronary intervention in acute myocardial infarction. *Am J Cardiol.* 2003;**92**:1331–1335.

49 Gick M, Jander N, Destechorn HP, *et al.* Randomized evaluation of the efforts of filter-based distal protection on myocardial perfusion and infarct size after primary percutaneous catheter intervention in myocardial infarction with and without ST-segment elevation. *Circulation.* 2005;**112**:1462–1469.

50 Brahmbhatt T, Marks DS, Cinquegrani M, Eastwood D. Improved angiographic and electrocardiographic, but not clinical outcomes, following coronary thrombectomy in patients with ST elevation

myocardial infarction: a meta-analysis. *Am J Cardiol.* TCT Supplement 98, October 2006; Suppl 61M:132.

51 Grube E, Schofer JJ, Webb J, *et al.* Evaluation of a balloon occlusion and aspiration system for protection from distal embolization during stenting in saphenous vein grafts. *J Invasive Cardiol.* 2002;**89**:941–945.

52 Napodano M, Pasquetto G, Sacca S, *et al.* Intracoronary thrombectomy improves myocardial reperfusion in patients undergoing direct angioplasty for acute myocardial infarction. *J Am Coll Cardiol.* 2003;**42**:1395–1402.

CHAPTER 29

Arrhythmia management in the cardiac catheterization laboratory

David S. Kwon¹ & Adam Strickberger²
¹Washington Hospital Center, Washington, DC, USA
²Georgetown University School of Medicine, Washington, DC, USA

Introduction

Patients present to the cardiac catheterization laboratory for emergent or elective evaluation with possible percutaneous intervention. In either scenario, a variety of cardiac arrhythmias may occur. Arrhythmias associated with hemodynamic instability are generally treated acutely and quickly according to the ACLS protocol (1,2), while arrhythmias associated without hemodynamic instability can be treated in many ways. In both situations, definitive therapy should be addressed after the procedure in the catheterization laboratory is completed.

General approach to arrhythmia management

Broadly, arrhythmias present as tachyarrhythmias or bradyarrhythmias. Either may cause hemodynamic instability, and the immediate concern for the interventional cardiologist is to protect cerebral and coronary perfusion. When needed, defibrillation, temporary pacing, or intravenous medications may be required to restore hemodynamic stability. An understanding of the arrhythmias and their associated hemodynamic effects that require immediate treatment, as opposed to treatment after the catheterization is completed, is necessary.

Pharmacology in the Catheterization Laboratory. Edited by Ron Waksman and Andrew E Ajani. © 2010 Blackwell Publishing, ISBN: 978-1-4051-5704-9.

Tachyarrhythmias

A tachyarrhythmia may or may not result in hemodynamic instability. Whether the rhythm responsible for hemodynamic collapse or instability is ventricular fibrillation, ventricular tachycardia, or supraventricular tachycardia is irrelevant to the emergency treatment, or the treatment required in the catheterization laboratory. When hemodynamic instability occurs, the next step is to stabilize the patient's hemodynamic status prior to continuing the procedure. According to the ACLS protocol, the first step is an external shock, perhaps followed by intravenous administration of amiodarone (3). Of course, catheter-induced ventricular tachycardia or ventricular fibrillation can occur. In this setting, removing the catheter(s) from the left and or right ventricle may be all that is required. If hemodynamic stability persists despite the tachycardia, then a variety of medical options are available including the intravenous administration of adenosine, beta blockers, amiodarone, or perhaps calcium channel blockers.

Bradyarrhythmias

Although asystole is a potential arrhythmia encountered in the cardiac catheterization laboratory, various degrees of atrioventricular (AV) block are more common in the catheterization laboratory. Some degree of AV block may be present at baseline, and higher degrees of AV block may arise as a consequence of coronary occlusion and acute myocardial infarction, such as with proximal RCA occlusions. In such cases, a ventricular escape rhythm may emerge. However, the acuity of the situation depends on whether the bradyarrhythmia, whether sinus, junctional, or ventricular in origin, is able to sustain an adequate blood pressure for cerebral and cardiac perfusion. Temporary transvenous pacing may be required.

At times, patients may present to the catheterization laboratory with evidence of a new left bundle branch block. Or the patient may have a history of cardiac valve repair or replacement. In these scenarios, the cardiologist should be particularly aware of the potential need for temporary pacing in order to avoid complications during or following the procedure. In addition, with the advent of alcohol septal ablation procedures for obstructive hypertrophic cardiomyopathy, temporary transvenous pacemakers are generally inserted prior to discharge from the catheterization laboratory as a routine precaution.

The basic medical approach to bradyarrhythmias depends on whether the patient has an adequate blood pressure. Atropine may be used and is beneficial in situations of excess vagal stimulation or to counteract medication effects, such as anesthesia used for intubation procedures. AV nodal blocking agents are generally avoided acutely until competent electrical conduction is verified.

Conclusions

While in the cardiac catheterization laboratory, patients may experience a variety of arrhythmias. While some are inherent to the underlying cardiac disorder, others may develop secondary to the acute clinical event or iatrogenically. Correct and rapid identification will provide patients with optimal care. If a patient requires emergent resuscitation, the interventional cardiologist should not hesitate to shock the patient or initiate intravenous medical therapy, as appropriate. The general approach is dictated by the ACLS protocol.

References

1 Cummins RO. *ACLS: Principles and Practice.* p. 1. Dallas: American Heart Association; 2003. ISBN 0-87493-341-2.

2 American Heart Association. 2005 American Heart Association Guidelines for cardiopulmonary resuscitation and emergency cardiovascular care. *Circulation.* 2005;**112**(24 Suppl):1703–1729.

3 Dager WE, Sanoski CA, Wiggins BS, Tisdale JE. Pharmacotherapy considerations in advanced cardiac life support. *Pharmacotherapy.* December 2006;**26**(12): 1703–1729.

CHAPTER 30

Tachyarrhythmias management

Dorinna D. Mendoza & Zayd A. Eldadah
Washington Hospital Center, Washington, DC, USA

Dysrhythmias are common in the setting of the cardiac catheterization laboratory. Those associated with acute myocardial infarction (AMI) can range in seriousness from benign premature beats to potentially lethal ventricular fibrillation. Cardiac catheterization itself, either right- or left-sided, can be complicated by arrhythmia. Serious arrhythmias occur in approximately 1% of all catheterizations. Prompt arrhythmia recognition and treatment is critical for successful management.

Tachyarrhythmias during AMI may be caused by reentry, enhanced automaticity, and triggered activity. Ischemia, heart failure, metabolic derangements, and fluctuations in autonomic tone can each be arrhythmogenic in the setting of AMI. In addition to these pathophysiologic causes, arrhythmias may be iatrogenic during procedures in the catheterization laboratory. Intracardiac catheter manipulation and contrast-induced myocardial ischemia are leading causes of iatrogenic arrhythmias.

Tachycardia accompanied by hypotension, heart failure, shortness of breath, shock, altered mental status, angina, or AMI should be treated with immediate cardioversion. In the absence of these signs and symptoms, a methodical approach to tachyarrhythmia diagnosis and management is the standard of care. It is necessary to determine the

type of arrhythmia and to ascertain the patient's left ventricular function, generally represented by the left ventricular ejection fraction (LVEF). Patients with LVEF <40% or signs of heart failure are at greatest risk for sudden cardiac death due to ventricular tachycardia or ventricular fibrillation.

Figure 30.1 presents a simple algorithm for tachycardia management and divides these rhythms into three categories (1):
• Atrial fibrillation and atrial flutter
• Narrow complex tachycardias
• Wide complex tachycardias

Atrial fibrillation and atrial flutter

When the electrocardiogram (ECG) demonstrates atrial fibrillation or atrial flutter, the initial evaluation should focus on the patient's clinical stability, left ventricular function, the presence of Wolff-Parkinson-White (WPW) syndrome, and the duration of the arrhythmia. First-line therapy in hemodynamically unstable patients is, of course, immediate cardioversion. When hemodynamics are tolerable, general management of atrial fibrillation is necessary. Three objectives must be satisfied for all patients: control of the ventricular response, minimization of thromboembolic risk, and restoration and maintenance of sinus rhythm in patients needing rhythm control.

Patients who are hemodynamically stable should be treated with drugs that slow the ventricular rate by impeding conduction through the

Pharmacology in the Catheterization Laboratory. Edited by Ron Waksman and Andrew E Ajani. © 2010 Blackwell Publishing, ISBN: 978-1-4051-5704-9.

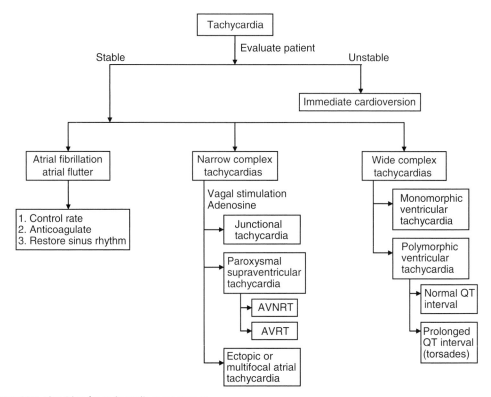

Figure 30.1 Algorithm for tachycardia management.

atrioventricular node. When left ventricular function is normal, the ventricular rate can be slowed with either a beta-blocker or a calcium channel blocker (class I recommendation) (2,3). Digoxin is a less desirable rate control agent. It acts by enhancing vagal tone but has a slow onset of action and is largely ineffective with increasing intrinsic heart rates. Intravenous amiodarone (class IIa) may be used when these therapies are ineffective, not tolerated, or contraindicated.

In the setting of AMI and atrial fibrillation, direct-current cardioversion is recommended for patients with severe hemodynamic compromise or intractable ischemia, or when adequate rate control cannot be achieved with pharmacological agents (class I). Intravenous administration of amiodarone is recommended to slow atrial fibrillation with rapid ventricular response and to improve left ventricular function in patients with AMI (class I). In patients with acute MI without clinical evidence of LV dysfunction, bronchospasm, or AV block,

intravenous beta blockers and nondihydropyridine calcium channel blockers are recommended to slow a rapid ventricular response to atrial fibrillation (class I). Additionally, in the absence of contraindications, anticoagulation is recommended for patients with atrial fibrillation and AMI (class I) (4).

In the presence of ventricular dysfunction with LVEF <40% or signs of heart failure, digoxin is the recommended drug for rate control (class IIb). Beta blockers, calcium channel blockers, or amiodarone may be employed as alternative or adjunctive therapies but should be used with caution in patients with clinical evidence of heart failure (class IIb).

In patients whose atrial fibrillation is asymptomatic, there is substantial debate over the benefit of restoring sinus rhythm versus simply controlling the ventricular response and minimizing the thromboembolic risk. The AFFIRM and RACE trials demonstrated noninferiority of a rate control strategy compared to a rhythm control strategy in predominantly elderly patients who were anticoagulated (5,6). However, multivariate analysis of patients in AFFIRM showed that the presence of sinus rhythm was associated with reduced mortality.

The approach to conversion of atrial fibrillation or atrial flutter is dependent upon the duration of the arrhythmia. Electric cardioversion is the preferred treatment for the restoration of sinus rhythm. Patients are at low risk for embolism if they do not have valvular heart disease, an enlarged left ventricle or heart failure, or a prior history of an embolic event (7). As such, cardioversion does not need to be delayed for chronic anticoagulation for those patients with normal left ventricular function and a duration of atrial fibrillation or atrial flutter <48 h. If electrical cardioversion is not feasible, not desirable, or is unsuccessful in restoring sinus rhythm, then pharmacologic conversion in patients with normal LV function may be achieved with amiodarone, ibutilide, flecainide, propafenone, or procainamide (class IIa). Alternative agents are sotalol and disopyramide (class IIb) (8–13). For those patients with impaired LV function and atrial fibrillation duration <48 h, electrical cardioversion is the preferred treatment, otherwise, intravenous amiodarone is the recommended pharmacologic therapy. Alternative agents are ibutilide or dofetilide.

When the duration of atrial fibrillation is >48 h or unknown, there is an increased risk of embolism from an atrial thrombus. Therefore, pharmacologic or electrical cardioversion should be delayed until at least 3 weeks of adequate anticoagulation with an INR of 2–3. After cardioversion, anticoagulation should be continued for at least 4 weeks because of atrial stunning and the potential risk for embolism despite electrical sinus rhythm. However, in patients who may benefit from immediate cardioversion, the presence of an intracardiac (most commonly left atrial appendage) thrombus may be excluded by transesophageal echocardiography followed by electrical cardioversion. Again, 4 weeks of warfarin should follow.

Patients with atrial fibrillation or atrial flutter associated with WPW generally have normal left ventricular function. Again, cardioversion is the preferred therapy for extremely rapid (e.g., >200 beats/min) or hemodynamically unstable rhythms. Antiarrhythmic drugs that directly affect accessory pathway conduction can be used in nonlife-threatening situations. Recommended agents include amiodarone, flecainide, propafenone, procainamide, or sotalol (14–17). Intravenous procainamide is the drug of choice for immediate effect. Drugs such as adenosine, beta blockers, calcium channel blockers, and digoxin slow conduction through the atrioventricular node and facilitate conduction through the accessory pathway, making them potentially harmful and thus contraindicated. Rapid, preexcited atrial fibrillation can degenerate to ventricular fibrillation with significant AV nodal blockade. Definitive therapy for atrial flutter and WPW, of course, is catheter ablation, which is curative.

Narrow complex tachycardias

Nonatrial fibrillation/flutter narrow complex tachycardias include atrioventricular nodal reentrant tachycardia (AVNRT), atrioventricular reciprocating tachycardia (AVRT), atrial tachycardia, and junctional tachycardia. Careful ECG analysis can indicate a specific diagnosis, which can guide therapy. If a diagnosis cannot be achieved readily, the use of adenosine or the application of vagal maneuvers to slow the heart rate can help elucidate the underlying arrhythmia. Adenosine should be avoided in patients with severe bronchial asthma. An ECG should be recorded during vagal maneuvers or drug administration because the response may aid in the diagnosis even if the arrhythmia does not terminate.

AVNRT and AVRT are the most common supraventricular tachycardias in adults. AVNRT results from a reentrant circuit in the territory of the AV node while AVRT involves reentry via an accessory pathway, which can traverse the tricuspid or mitral annulus and even occur near the AV node. These tachycardias typically manifest in a paroxysmal manner and can be highly symptomatic, although rarely life-threatening. In the setting of preserved LV function, AVNRT and AVRT can be treated with a nondihydropyridine calcium channel blocker, beta blocker, or digoxin. It is important to use extreme care with concomitant use of intravenous calcium channel blocker and beta blockers because of possible potentiation of hypotensive and/or bradycardic effects. If the arrhythmia persists, electric cardioversion should be performed. Should these therapies fail, amiodarone, sotalol, flecainide, propafenone, or disopyramide are recommended antiarrhythmic agents (class IIa) (18,19). In the setting of poor left ventricular function, digoxin, amiodarone, and diltiazem are recommended (class IIb). Electrical cardioversion should be avoided (20). Curative therapy of AVNRT and AVRT can be achieved by catheter ablation, which is the standard of care for these conditions.

Atrial tachycardia accounts for about 10% of all supraventricular tachycardias and is usually the result of a single ectopic atrial focus with enhanced automaticity. Because atrial tachycardias can result from other conditions or the use of catecholamines or theophylline, supportive measures and treatment of the underlying source are often effective. As cardioversion is ineffective in terminating arrhythmias due to enhanced automaticity, it should not be used in this situation. Recommended acute therapy for atrial tachycardia is intravenous administration of beta blockers or calcium channel blockers for either termination or to achieve rate control (21). Direct suppression of the tachycardia focus may be achieved with sotalol or amiodarone. Amiodarone, diltiazem, and digoxin are preferred for those with poor ventricular function (22). Again, definitive therapy of atrial tachycardia can also be achieved by catheter ablation.

Multifocal atrial tachycardia (MAT) must be distinguished from atrial fibrillation since both can present with an irregularly irregular rhythm. This arrhythmia is most commonly associated with underlying pulmonary disease but may result from metabolic or electrolyte derangements. Standard antiarrhythmic drugs are typically ineffective in MAT, so therapy should be directed at the underlying condition. Some success has been reported using calcium channel blockers, but beta blockers are usually contraindicated because of the presence of underlying pulmonary disease (23).

Junctional tachycardia is very rare in adults and usually due to enhanced automaticity from an ectopic focus in the atrioventricular junction. This can occur in the setting of digitalis toxicity or excess exogenous catecholamines or theophylline.

Withholding digitalis when junctional tachycardia is the only clinical manifestation of toxicity is usually adequate. If ventricular arrhythmias or high-grade heart block are observed, then treatment with digitalis-binding agents may be indicated (24). When the etiology of the junctional tachycardia is uncertain or if the arrhythmia persists after withdrawal of the causative agent, therapy with amiodarone, beta blockers, or calcium channel blockers is recommended with normal left ventricular function, while amiodarone is recommended in the setting of LVEF <40% (class IIa) (25,26). Catheter ablation can be curative.

Wide complex tachycardia

The differential diagnosis for wide complex tachycardia includes ventricular tachycardia, supraventricular tachycardia with aberrant conduction, or an antidromic AVRT (where the reentrant circuit travels from atrium to ventricle via the accessory pathway then returns to the atrium retrograde via the AV node).

Any wide complex tachycardia causing hemodynamic compromise must be treated immediately with electrical cardioversion. In the conscious patient, a brief trial of medications may be attempted in addition to a sedative or analgesic agent prior to cardioversion. Malignant ventricular arrhythmias remain the cause of most prehospital sudden deaths as a result of AMI.

In stable monomorphic ventricular tachycardia with normal left ventricular function, recommended pharmacologic therapy includes procainamide, sotalol, or amiodarone (class IIa). Intravenous amiodarone is not ideal for early conversion of stable monomorphic ventricular tachycardia, but may be reasonable for those patients who are hemodynamically unstable, refractory to conversion with countershock, or recurrent despite procainamide or other agents (27). Intravenous procainamide is more appropriate when early slowing of the ventricular tachycardia rate and termination of the monomorphic ventricular tachycardia are desired (28). Additionally, lidocaine might be reasonable for initial treatment of patients with stable sustained monomorphic ventricular tachycardia specifically associated with AMI (class IIb) (29). Recommended therapy in the patient with poor LVEF <40% is amiodarone or lidocaine (class IIb).

While polymorphic ventricular tachycardia is usually life-threatening and causes hemodynamic instability, it may be associated with a near normal blood pressure. Recommended pharmacologic therapy in this context is determined by the QT interval on the baseline ECG. With a prolonged QT interval, polymorphic ventricular tachycardia is termed torsades de pointes. This may be due to a congenital prolonged QT syndrome, or acquired from hypomagnesemia, hypokalemia, or drug therapy. The acute treatment of torsades de pointes includes withdrawal of any offending drugs and correction of electrolyte abnormalities (class I). Recommended therapies include magnesium, overdrive pacing, and isoproterenol as a temporizing measures prior to pacing, phenytoin, and lidocaine (30,31).

Polymorphic ventricular tachycardia with a normal QT interval is usually due to ischemia. Aggressive treatment of ischemia and correction of any electrolyte abnormalities is recommended. In the setting of recurrent polymorphic ventricular tachycardia with AMI, intravenous beta blockers are useful and improve mortality (32). Other recommended agents include lidocaine, amiodarone, procainamide, or sotalol (33,34).

Tachyarrhythmia is a common occurrence during cardiac catheterization. In patients with hemodynamic instability, immediate cardioversion is the treatment of choice. Most tachyarrhythmias, however, can be approached with drug therapy while in the laboratory. Rapid and effective therapy demands an understanding of the multiple possible etiologies and a familiarity with the pharmacologic armamentarium available. Catheter ablation is now the standard of care for long-term definitive management of most arrhythmias.

References

1 Guidelines 2000 for Cardiopulmonary Resuscitation and Emergency Cardiovascular Care. Part 6: advanced cardiovascular life support: 7D: the tachycardia algorithms. The American Heart Association in collaboration with the International Liaison Committee on Resuscitation. *Circulation.* 2000;**102**:I158.

2 Platia EV, Michelson EL, Porterfield JK, Das G. Esmolol versus verapamil in the acute treatment of atrial fibrillation or atrial flutter. *Am J Cardiol.* 1989; **63**:925.

3 Ellenbogen KA, Dias VC, Cardello FP, *et al.* Safety and efficacy of intravenous diltiazem in atrial fibrillation or atrial flutter. *Am J Cardiol.* 1995;**75**:45.

4 Fuster V, Ryden LE, Cannom DS, *et al.* ACC/AHA/ESC 2006 guidelines for management of patients with atrial fibrillation. *J Am Coll Cardiol.* 2006;**48**:854.

5 Wyse DG, Waldo AL, DiMarco JP, *et al.* A comparison of rate control and rhythm control in patients with atrial fibrillation. The atrial fibrillation follow-up investigation of rhythm management (AFFIRM) investigators. *N Engl J Med.* 2002;**347**:1825.

6 Van Gelder IC, Hagens VE, Bosker HA, *et al.* A comparison of rate control and rhythm control in patients with recurrent persistent atrial fibrillation. *N Engl J Med.* 2002;**347**:1834.

7 Weigner MJ, Caulfield TA, Danias PG, *et al.* Risk for clinical thromboembolism associated with conversion to sinus rhythm in patients with atrial fibrillation lasting less than 48 hours. *Ann Intern Med.* 1997;**126**:615.

8 Galve E, Rius T, Ballester R, *et al.* Intravenous amiodarone in treatment of recent-onset atrial fibrillation: results of a randomized, controlled study. *J Am Coll Cardiol.* 1996;**27**:1079.

9 Kafkas NV, Patsilinakos SP, Mertzanos GA, *et al.* Conversion efficacy of intravenous ibutilide compared with intravenous amiodarone in patients with recent-onset atrial fibrillation and atrial flutter. *Int J Cardiol.* 2007;**118**(3):321–325.

10 Reisinger J, Gatterer E, Lang W, *et al.* Flecainide versus ibutilide for immediate cardioversion of atrial fibrillation of recent onset. *Eur Heart J.* 2004;**25**:1318.

11 Kochiadakis GE, Igoumenidis NE, Simantirakis EN, *et al.* Intravenous propafenone versus intravenous amiodarone in the management of atrial fibrillation of recent onset: a placebo-controlled study. *Pacing Clin Electrophysiol.* 1998;**21**:2475.

12 Kochiadakis GE, Igoumenidis NE, Solomous MC, *et al.* Conversion of atrial fibrillation to sinus rhythm using acute intravenous procainamide infusion. *Cardiovasc Drugs Ther.* 1998;**12**:75.

13 Sung RJ, Tan HL, Karagounis L, *et al.* Intravenous sotalol for the termination of supraventricular tachycardia and atrial fibrillation and flutter: a multicenter, randomized, double-blind, placebo-controlled study. Sotalol Multicenter Study Group. *Am Heart J.* 1995;**129**:739.

14 Kuga K, Yamaguchi I, Sugishita Y. Effect of intravenous amiodarone on electrophysiologic variables and on the modes of termination of atrioventricular reciprocating tachycardia in Wolff-Parkinson-White syndrome. *Jpn Circ J.* 1999;**63**:189.

15 O'Nunain S, Garratt CJ, Linker NJ, *et al.* A comparison of intravenous propafenone and flecainide in the treatment of tachycardias associated with the Wolff-Parkinson-White syndrome. *Pacing Clin Electrophysiol.* 1991;**14**:2028.

16 Boahene KA, Klein GJ, Yee R, *et al.* Termination of acute atrial fibrillation in the Wolff-Parkinson-White syndrome by procainamide and propafenone: importance of atrial fibrillatory cycle length. *J Am Coll Cardiol.* 1990;**16**:1408.

17 Touboul P, Atallah G, Kirkorian G, *et al.* Effects of intravenous sotalol in patients with atrioventricular accessory pathways. *Am Heart J.* 1987;**114**:545.

18 Jordaens L, Gorgels A, Stroobandt R, *et al.* Efficacy and safety of intravenous sotalol for termination of paroxysmal supraventricular tachycardia. The Sotalol Versus Placebo Multicenter Study Group. *Am J Cardiol.* 1991;**68**:35.

19 Hellestrand KJ. Intravenous flecainide acetate for supraventricular tachycardias. *Am J Cardiol.* 1988;**62**:16D.

20 Blomström-Lundqvist C, Scheinman MM, Aliot EM, *et al.* ACC/AHA/ESC Guidelines for the Management of Patients with Supraventricular Arrhythmias. *J Am Coll Cardiol.* 2003;**42**:1493.

21 Steinbeck G, Hoffmann E. "True" atrial tachycardia. *Eur Heart J.* 1998;**19**(Suppl E):E10.

22 Wren C. Incessant tachycardias. *Eur Heart J.* 1998; **19**(Supple E):E32.

23 Schwartz M, Rodman D, Lowenstein SR. Recognition and treatment of multifocal atrial tachycardia: a critical review. *J Emerg Med.* 1994;**12**:353.

24 Storstein O, Hansteen V, Hatle L, *et al.* Studies on digitalis: XIII: a prospective study of 649 patients on maintenance treatment with digitoxin. *Am Heart J.* 1977;**93**:434.

25 Breslow MJ, Evers AS, Lebowitz P. Successful treatment of accelerated junctional rhythm with propranolol: possible role of sympathetic stimulation in the genesis of this rhythm disturbance. *Anesthesiology.* 1985;**62**:180.

26 Lee KL, Chun HM, Liem LB, *et al.* Effect of adenosine and verapamil in catecholamine-induced accelerated atrioventricular junctional rhythm: insights into the underlying mechanism. *Pacing Clin Electrophysiol.* 1999;**22**:866.

27 Zipes DP, Camm AJ, Borggrefe M, *et al.* ACC/AHA/ESC 2006 guidelines for management of patients with ventricular arrhythmias and the prevention of sudden cardiac death. *J Am Coll Cardiol.* 2006;**48**:1064.

28 Gorgels AP, van den Dool A, Hofs A, *et al.* Comparison of procainamide and lidocaine in terminating sustained monomorphic ventricular tachycardia. *Am J Cardiol.* 1996;**78**:43.

29 Nasir N, Taylor A, Doyle TK, *et al.* Evaluation of intravenous lidocaine for the termination of sustained monomorphic ventricular tachycardia in patients with coronary artery disease with or without healed myocardial infarction. *Am J Cardiol.* 1994;**74**:1183.

30 Tzivoni D, Banai S, Schuger C. Treatment of torsades de pointes with magnesium sulfate. *Circulation.* 1988; **77**:392.

31 Assimes TL, Malcolm I. Torsade de pointes with sotalol overdose treated successfully with lidocaine. *Can J Cardiol.* 1998;**14**:753.

32 Nademanee K, Taylor R, Bailey WE, *et al.* Treating electrical storm: sympathetic blockade versus advanced cardiac life support-guided therapy. *Circulation.* 2000;**102**:742.

33 2005 American Heart Association guidelines for cardiopulmonary resuscitation and emergency cardiovascular care. *Circulation.* 2005;**112**:IV1.

34 Kowley PR, Marinchak RA, Rials SJ, *et al.* Intravenous antiarrhythmic therapy in the acute control of in-hospital destabilizing ventricular tachycardia and fibrillation. *Am J Cardiol.* 1999;**84**:46R.

CHAPTER 31

Bradyarrhythmias management (intervention atropine, adrenaline, indications for temporary pacing wire)

Khan Pohlel¹ & Ziyad Ghazzal²
¹Athens Cardiology Group, Athens, Georgia, USA
²American University of Beirut, Beirut, Lebanon

Introduction

Arrhythmias can occur in the cardiac catheterization laboratory especially during percutaneous interventions. Bradyarrhythmias may present as an asymptomatic finding or may be potentially life-threatening. Different rhythms can present with bradycardia. These rhythms can range from sinus bradycardia to complete heart block, and may manifest with a narrow QRS complex (<0.12 ms) or with a wide QRS complex (>0.12 ms) especially in the presence of an escape beat.

Etiology

Bradycardia can result from decreased sympathetic tone or from an increase in vagal tone. Both the sinoatrial (SA) node and the atrioventricular (AV) node are richly innervated by the autonomic nervous system. The balance between the sympathetic and parasympathetic nervous systems determine the autonomic tone. Influences on the autonomic system can vary from intrinsic conduction disease or external factors affecting the conduction system. Increased vagal tone, ischemia, medications,

and electrolyte imbalances are common causes and should be identified and corrected.

Abnormal vagal tone requiring medical therapy occurs in approximately 3% of patients in the catheterization laboratory (1). Vasovagal reactions in the catheterization laboratory occur more commonly during the procedure, and occasionally following the procedure with removal of vascular sheaths. These events are usually ameliorated with normal saline infusion or intravenous atropine. Infrequently, vasopressors are required transiently for blood pressure support. One series showed by univariate analysis that vasovagal reactions in the catheterization laboratory were more common in men, with prolonged procedures, and those with multiple vascular access (1). Vasovagal reactions occur by two major mechanisms either centrally or reflex-mediated. The centrally mediated mechanism acts through pain or anxiety activation, and the reflex-mediated mechanism occurs through the Bezold-Jarisch reflex via vagal afferents (2).

Acute ischemia resulting in bradyarrhythmias occur via two predominant mechanisms. The Bezold-Jarisch reflex can arise from stimulation of receptors with nonmyelinated vagal afferent pathways on the inferoposterior left ventricle producing increased vagal tone (2). This reflex can also occur with reperfusion especially in the right coronary artery (3). Another manifestation of this reflex can

Pharmacology in the Catheterization Laboratory. Edited by Ron Waksman and Andrew E Ajani. © 2010 Blackwell Publishing, ISBN: 978-1-4051-5704-9.

be activated by vigorous left ventricular contraction in the setting of volume depletion. Occlusion of the blood supply to the SA or AV node from the right coronary artery during an inferior myocardial infarction often results in sinus bradycardia or sinus arrest, and varying degrees of AV block. Heart block can occur frequently in the setting of an inferior myocardial infarction. During the thrombolytic era it portended worst survival (4). Additionally, sinus bradycardia has been reported as a reperfusion arrhythmia during thrombolytics and percutaneous transluminal angioplasty in approximately 18% of the infarct patients with predominance in inferior infarcts (5). The importance has not been established since bradycardic reperfusion arrhythmias are relatively uncommon.

Atrioventricular block is usually transient and asymptomatic, but may require temporary pacing until the ischemia resolves. In the setting of an inferior myocardial infarct, AV block is frequently associated with an early critical clinical setting including symptomatic hypotension and more inhospital deaths. With anterior myocardial infarctions, the AV block can result from occlusion of the left anterior descending artery. The AV block is usually infranodal, and more malignant resulting in Mobitz Type II or third degree AV block. These forms of AV block are symptomatic and usually require permanent pacemaker therapy (6).

Angioplasty complications leading to acute vessel closures can result in bradyarrhythmias. Such complications as no-reflow, embolization, and dissection with threatened acute vessel closure may induce a spectrum of ischemic manifestations resulting in severe microvascular dysfunction. These may result in conduction disturbances, hypotension with or without cardiogenic shock, infarction, and death. No-reflow is more common after revascularization of thrombus-laden lesions, degenerate saphenous vein grafts and after Rotablator atherectomy. Episodes of no-reflow may respond to intracoronary verapamil, diltiazem, adenosine, or nitroprusside (Figure 31.1). Angioplasty induced spasm may infrequently respond to atropine in the setting of hypotension and bradycardia. The mechanism is thought to result from a paradoxical vasoconstriction of denuded arteries exposed to acetylcholine.

Standard ionic contrast agents are known to cause transient hypotension and bradycardia (7,8). These mechanisms are felt to be partly mediated by the direct dye effect and reflex effects on the pacemaker tissue. The origin of the vessel supplying these pacemaker tissues contribute to this effect (7). However, with the introduction of lower osmolality, nonionic contrast media, systemic hypotension, bradycardia, ST segment changes, QT prolongation, and T wave abnormalities are less frequently seen (8–10).

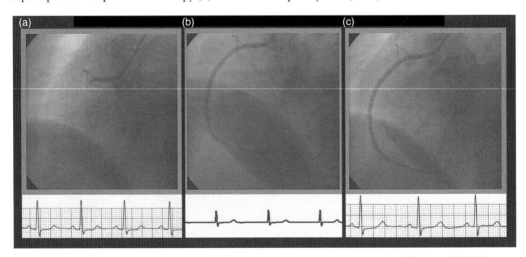

Figure 31.1 (a) Total occlusion of the proximal RCA with sinus rhythm. (b) After stenting, the proximal and mid-RCA segments, the distal RCA showed "slow-flow" on angiogram and a junctional bradycardic rhythm in the low 40's with hypotension. (c) Atropine was administered for the bradycardia and phenylephrine and fluids for the hypotension. Once the bradycardia and hypotension improved, intracoronary adenosine and later nitroglycerin were administered, resulting in TIMI 3 flow. The rhythm improved to normal sinus.

Common medications that can cause brady-cardia include beta-blockers, nondihydropyridine calcium-channel blockers, digoxin, class IA, IC, and III antiarrhythmics, and clonidine. Other reversible etiologies include hyperkalemia, increased vagal tone, and less commonly hypo-thermia, hypothyroidism, and sepsis. Coronary artery disease, postoperative cardiac surgery, and ischemia during acute myocardial infarction can intrinsically affect the conduction system and result in bradyarrhythmias. End-stage cardiomy-opathies, infiltrative cardiomyopathies such as amyloidosis, and sarcoidosis, collagen vascular disease, and myocarditis can also affect the con-duction system. These comorbidities should be considered for refractory bradyarrhythmias in the catheterization laboratory.

Treatment

Medical therapies for symptomatic bradyarrhyth-mias are limited to a few drugs. Atropine was first isolated in 1809 by Vaquelin, but its antivagal properties were later noted by Bezold and Bloebaum in 1867 (11). At usual therapeutic doses (0.5–1 mg IV bolus, maximum of 3 mg total), atropine prevents the effect of acetylcholine on the muscarinic receptors of the postganglionic para-sympathetic nerve endings thereby blocking vagal stimulation on the heart (11). These effects occur rapidly and peak after several minutes. Common adverse effects include nausea, constipation, urinary retention, mydriasis, and delirium. Severe bradycardia may paradoxically occur with doses less than 0.5 mg IV. The mechanism is unclear but postulated to be from either peripheral inhibi-tion of cholinesterase or vagal stimulation of the central nervous system, or the combination of the two (12). Given its rapid onset and availabil-ity in most catheterization laboratories, atropine is commonly the first line agent for symptomatic bradycardia.

Epinephrine is also effective in the treatment of symptomatic bradycardia. This catecholamine has potent effects on both alpha and beta-adrenergic agonist receptors. Once the beta-adrenergic recep-tors are stimulated, this results in an increased heart rate (chronotropy) and myocardial contrac-tility (inotropy), both important in the presence

of significant bradycardia (13). The usual recom-mended doses during these resuscitative efforts are 0.5–1 mg intravenous bolus and can be used alternatively with atropine. Prior to hemodynamic collapse, an infusion at 2–10 mcg/min intrave-nous may be helpful but is not recommended as the first line therapy. Common adverse reac-tions include tachycardia, palpitations, tremor, diaphoresis, hypertension, angina, and arrhyth-mias. Norepinephrine is another catecholamine that has similar physiologic effects as epinephrine, but has a more potent alpha-adrenergic effect relative to its beta-adrenergic effect. Its use for bradyarrhythmias is limited.

Isoproterenol is a synthetic catecholamine with pure beta-adrenergic receptor effects. It also has chronotropic and inotropic effects, resulting in an increased heart rate and myocardial contraction. Isoproterenol can be employed if a bradyarrhyth-mia is resistant to atropine such as in infranodal AV block especially if it is causing hemodynamic compromise. The usual dose is a 2–10 mcg/min infusion or in emergent situations a bolus of 0.02–0.06 mg IV can be given. Isoproterenol has a similar adverse effect profile as other catecho-lamines. Caution should be used in patients with myocardial ischemia due to intense myocardial stimulation, and in individuals with hypertrophic cardiomyopathy (14).

Dopamine is another catecholamine with alpha and beta-adrenergic receptor effects in addition to its dopaminergic effects. This is a naturally occurring compound that is the precursor to norepinephrine, hence the similar hemodynamic profile (15–17). It was first utilized as an agent for circulatory shock. Dopamine acts on the beta-adrenergic receptors, causing increased heart rates, and can be used as a second line agent for persistent bradycardia with the infusion at 2–10 mcg/kg/min intravenously. It is readily available in most cath-eterization laboratories.

Once pharmacologic therapy has been exhausted in the catheterization laboratory, a tem-porary transvenous pacemaker can be placed for refractory bradyarrhythmias. Symptomatic brady-cardia resulting in cerebral hypoperfusion with confusion, presycnope, or syncope, or resulting in hemodynamic instability is a primary indica-tion for pacemaker implantation. The transvenous pacemaker can be placed after vascular access is gained through the femoral, internal jugular, or subclavian vein. Prior reports have indicated the use of standard ionic contrast may decrease the ventricular fibrillation threshold and may cause more arrhythmias with right ventricular pacing (18). In this situation, placement of a right atrial pacing lead may alleviate these arrhythmias. Temporary pacing during percutaneous coronary interventions has been reported using a guide wire placed into the coronary artery with the external generator connected directly to the guide wire (19). This may be considered when vascular access has not been established, and pacing is needed immediately. Temporary pacing is preferred when the bradyarrhythmia is anticipated to be transient such as with inferior infarcts. Anterior myocardial infarcts commonly require permanent pacing after stabilization with a temporary pacemaker (6).

Special considerations

The AngioJet thrombectomy system (Possis Medical, Minneapolis, MN) has several applications in thrombus removal. Its use has been demonstrated for thrombus removal in acute coronary syndrome and has been relatively safe (20). However, a potential adverse effect from the device is the occurrence of bradyarrhythmias especially when used in the right coronary artery. These bradyarrhythmias are most often transient and cease with discontinuation of use. However, there are incidences of persistent significant heart block associated with its use even in the periphery (21), often requiring temporary pacing. The incidence of bradyarrhythmias ranging from sinus pause, asystole, to severe heart block is reportedly 20–26% with the AngioJet use (22). The mechanism of bradyarrhythmias is thought to occur during hemolysis of red blood cells releasing intracellular adenosine. However, pretreatment with intravenous aminophylline, a competitive inhibitor of adenosine receptor, was not as effective in preventing bradyarrhythmias as intracoronary aminophylline administration (22,23). Prophylactic placement of a temporary pacemaker should be considered prior to activating the AngioJet thrombectomy device.

Carotid angioplasty and stenting has also been associated with bradyarrhythmias. The procedure involves direct dilation at the carotid bulb invoking the parasympathetic reflexes that produces a slower pulse rate (24,25). The overall incidence of bradyarrhythmias with carotid angioplasty is variable but common (26,27). If significant, atropine is usually effective for the treatment of these bradyarrhythmias, but temporary pacemakers may be needed for persistent bradycardia.

References

1 Landau C, Lange RA, Glamann DB, Willard JE, Hillis LD. Vasovagal reactions in the cardiac catheterization laboratory. *Am J Cardiol*. 1994;**73**(1):95–97.

2 Mark AL. The Bezold-Jarisch reflex revisited: clinical implications of inhibitory reflexes originating in the heart. *J Am Coll Cardiol*. 1983;**1**(1):90–102.

3 Esente P, Giambartolomei A, Gensini GG, Dator C. Coronary reperfusion and Bezold-Jarisch reflex (bradycardia and hypotension). *Am J Cardiol*. 1983;**52**(3):221–224.

4 Berger PB, Ruocco NA Jr, Ryan TJ, Frederick MM, Jacobs AK, Faxon DP. Incidence and prognostic implications of heart block complicating inferior myocardial infarction treated with thrombolytic therapy: results from TIMI II. *J Am Coll Cardiol*. 1992; **20**(3):533–540.

5 Wehrens XH, Doevendans PA, Ophuis TJ, Wellens HJ. A comparison of electrocardiographic changes during reperfusion of acute myocardial infarction by thrombolysis or percutaneous transluminal coronary angioplasty. *Am Heart J*. 2000;**139**(3):430–436.

6 Gregoratos G, Abrams J, Epstein AE, *et al*. ACC/AHA/ NASPE 2002 Guideline Update for Implantation of Cardiac Pacemakers and Antiarrhythmia Devices— summary article: a report of the American College of Cardiology/American Heart Association Task Force on Practice Guidelines (ACC/AHA/NASPE Committee to Update the 1998 Pacemaker Guidelines). *J Am Coll Cardiol*. 2002;**40**(9):1703–1719.

7 Frink RJ, Merrick B, Lowe HM. Mechanism of the bradycardia during coronary angiography. *Am J Cardiol*. 1975;**35**(1):17–22.

8 Mancini GB, Bloomquist JN, Bhargava V, *et al*. Hemodynamic and electrocardiographic effects in man of a new nonionic contrast agent (iohexol): advantages over standard ionic agents. *Am J Cardiol*. 1983; **51**(7):1218–1222.

9 Piao ZE, Murdock DK, Hwang MH, Raymond RM, Scanlon PJ. Hemodynamic effects of contrast media during coronary angiography: a comparison of three nonionic agents to Hypaque-76. *Cathet Cardiovasc Diagn*. 1988;**14**(1):53–58.

10 Cooper MW, Reed PJ. Comparison of ionic and non-ionic contrast agents in cardiac catheterization: the effects of ventriculography and coronary arteriography on hemodynamics, electrocardiography, and serum creatinine. *Cathet Cardiovasc Diagn.* 1991;**22**(4):267–277.

11 Das G, Talmers FN, Weissler AM. New observations on the effects of atropine on the sinoatrial and atrioventricular nodes in man. *Am J Cardiol.* 1975;**36**(3):281–285.

12 Das G. Therapeutic review. Cardiac effects of atropine in man: an update. *Int J Clin Pharmacol Ther Toxicol.* 1989;**27**(10):473–477.

13 Otto CW, Yakaitis RW. The role of epinephrine in CPR: a reappraisal. *Ann Emerg Med.* 1984;**13**(9 Pt 2):840–843.

14 Ahlquist RP. Isoproterenol in cardiology. *Am Heart J.* 1973;**86**(2):149–151.

15 Loeb HS, Winslow EB, Rahimtoola SH, Rosen KM, Gunnar RM. Acute hemodynamic effects of dopamine in patients with shock. *Circulation.* 1971;**44**(2):163–173.

16 Talley RC, Goldberg LI, Johnson CE, McNay JL. A hemodynamic comparison of dopamine and isoproterenol in patients in shock. *Circulation.* 1969;**39**(3):361–378.

17 Schwarz R, Aviado DM. Drug action, reaction, and interaction. III. Dopamine for endotoxic shock. *J Clin Pharmacol.* 1976;**16**(2–3):88–98.

18 Gilchrist IC, Cameron A. Temporary pacemaker use during coronary arteriography. *Am J Cardiol.* 1987;**60**(13):1051–1054.

19 Mixon TA, Cross DS, Lawrence ME, Gantt DS, Dehmer GJ. Temporary coronary guidewire pacing during percutaneous coronary intervention. *Catheter Cardiovasc Interv.* 2004;**61**(4):494–500; discussion 502–503.

20 Nakagawa Y, Matsuo S, Kimura T, *et al.* Thrombectomy with AngioJet catheter in native coronary arteries for patients with acute or recent myocardial infarction. *Am J Cardiol.* 1999;**83**(7):994–999.

21 Fontaine AB, Borsa JJ, Hoffer EK, Bloch RD, So CR, Newton M. Type III heart block with peripheral use of the Angiojet thrombectomy system. *J Vasc Interv Radiol.* 2001;**12**(10):1223–1225.

22 Lee MS, Makkar R, Singh V, *et al.* Pre-procedural administration of aminophylline does not prevent AngioJet rheolytic thrombectomy-induced bradyarrhythmias. *J Invasive Cardiol.* 2005;**17**(1):19–22.

23 Murad B. Intracoronary aminophylline for heart block with AngioJet thrombectomy. *J Invasive Cardiol.* 2005;**17**(5):A4.

24 Harrop JS, Sharan AD, Benitez RP, Armonda R, Thomas J, Rosenwasser RH. Prevention of carotid angioplasty-induced bradycardia and hypotension with temporary venous pacemakers. *Neurosurgery.* 2001;**49**(4):814–820; discussion 820–822.

25 Mendelsohn FO, Weissman NJ, Lederman RJ, *et al.* Acute hemodynamic changes during carotid artery stenting. *Am J Cardiol.* 1998;**82**(9):1077–1081.

26 Nano G, Dalainas I, Bianchi P, *et al.* Ballooning-induced bradycardia during carotid stenting in primary stenosis and restenosis. *Neuroradiology.* 2006;**48**(8):533–536.

27 Mlekusch W, Schillinger M, Sabeti S, *et al.* Hypotension and bradycardia after elective carotid stenting: frequency and risk factors. *J Endovasc Ther.* 2003;**10**(5):851–859; discussion 860–861.

PART VII

Postprocedural pharmacotherapy

CHAPTER 32

Management of patients on long-term anticoagulation

Bryan P. Yan[1,2] & Andrew E. Ajani[3]
[1]Chinese University of Hong Kong, Hong Kong, China
[2]Prince of Wales Hospital, Hong Kong, China
[3]The Royal Melbourne Hospital, Melbourne, Australia

Background

Oral anticoagulants (OAC), such as warfarin, are commonly prescribed for patients at risk for arterial and venous thromboembolism. Perioperative management of patients receiving long-term OAC poses a clinical challenge. The risk of bleeding while maintaining anticoagulation needs to be balanced against the risk of thromboembolism with interruption of anticoagulation. Currently, there is little consensus on optimal management of patients on long-term OAC therapy undergoing surgery or invasive procedures such as percutaneous coronary interventions (PCI).

Several expert opinions and consensus groups recommend withholding OAC and institute bridging therapy with short-acting anticoagulants for most patients (1–6). The main patient groups that may require periprocedural alternatives to OAC include patients with prosthetic heart valves, atrial fibrillation, hypercoagulable states, and chronic venous thrombosis. The rationale for bridging therapy is to minimize the duration of subtherapeutic anticoagulation when OAC is discontinued before and after the procedure. The decision to bridge and how to bridge is based on an assessment

Pharmacology in the Catheterization Laboratory. Edited by Ron Waksman and Andrew E Ajani. © 2010 Blackwell Publishing, ISBN: 978-1-4051-5704-9.

of the perceived risk for bleeding and thrombosis, clinical consequences of a thrombotic or bleeding event, and the efficacy and safety of anticoagulants used for bridging. Alternatives to a bridging strategy include the use the radial approach or vascular closure devices for the femoral assess site in fully anticoagulated patients. This chapter aims to provide a clinical approach to risk stratification and recommendations for periprocedural strategies for patients on chronic anticoagulation undergoing PCI.

Risk of thromboembolism associated with interruption of anticoagulation

The risk of thrombosis with interruption of anticoagulation therapy is dependent on the indication for anticoagulation and patient risk factors (Table 32.1).

Mechanical heart valves

For patients with mechanical heart valves, the average rate of major thromboembolism in the absence of anticoagulation is estimated to be 8% per year. Anticoagulation reduces this risk by 80% (7). Thrombotic complications of mechanical heart valves are associated with significant mortality and morbidity (8). The risk of thromboembolism relates to the type of prosthetic heart valve, the valve site and associated risk factors (i.e., atrial fibrillation, prior embolic event or severe

Table 32.1 Thromboembolism risk characteristics.

Low risk	• Atrial fibrillation without a history of stroke or other risk factors • Bioprosthetic heart valves • Venous thrombosis >3 months
Intermediate / high risk	• Atrial fibrillation with history of stroke or risk factors (e.g., age >75 years, diabetes mellitus, congestive heart failure, hypertension, mitral stenosis) • Newer generation bileaflet heart valves in the aortic position • Venous thrombosis <3 months or >3 months with high-risk features (e.g., active malignancy, multiple venous thrombosis, hypercoagulable state)
Very high risk	• Older generation caged-ball or tilting-disk heart valves • Multiple mechanical heart valves • Mechanical heart valves in the mitral position with risk factors (e.g., atrial fibrillation, prior thrombotic events or severe left ventricular dysfunction) • Venous thrombosis <1 month with multiple risk factors

left ventricular dysfunction). Older generation mechanical heart valves in the mitral valve position carry the highest risk of thrombosis. The incidence of thromboembolism is two times higher with mitral than aortic valves (incidence rate per 100 patient-years (1.1 vs 2.7, $p < 0.05$) (7). Caged-ball type valves (e.g., Starr-Edwards) are associated with 1.5 times and twice the risk of thromboembolism compared to single tilting disk valves (e.g., Bjork Shiley, Medtronic Hall, Omnicarbon) and bileaflet valves (e.g., St Jude, Duromedics), respectively (7).

Atrial fibrillation

Patients with atrial fibrillation are generally considered to be at a relatively low risk of thromboembolism. Patients with nonvalvular atrial fibrillation who do not receive antithrombotic therapy have an average risk of systemic embolism of 4.5% per year (9). Embolic risk can be as high as 20% in patients with a history of stroke or in association with multiple risk factors for stroke, including congestive heart failure, hypertension, age >75 years, diabetes mellitus, and recent arterial embolism within 1 month (9,10).

Venous thromboembolism

The risk of recurrent thromboembolism following deep vein thrombosis or pulmonary embolism is highest within the first month of the initial event and the risk declines over the next 3 months (9). Anticoagulation therapy reduces the risk or recurrent thrombotic events by 80% (9). Independent risk factors for recurrent venous thromboembolism include increasing age and body mass index, active malignancy, and prolonged surgery (8).

Hypercoagulable state

Patients with inherited or acquired hypercoagulopathies who have had a recent thrombotic event are at high risk of perioperative complication when anticoagulation is interrupted (8,11). These disorders include prothrombin gene mutation, factor V Leiden mutation, antiphospholipid antibody syndrome, protein C deficiency, protein S deficiency, antithrombin III deficiency, and lupus anticoagulant antibodies.

Risk of bleeding associated with continuing anticoagulation

Nonsurgical invasive procedures such as PCI are associated with a low risk of major bleeding complications (4,12). Clinically significant access site complications occur in about 1–2% of anticoagulated patients undergoing PCI (13,14). The risk of bleeding is increased in female and elderly patients and in those with increased weight, prior history of bleeding and acquired coagulopathies (15). Procedural-related bleeding complications are higher with an activated clotting time >350 s during PCI (16). Increasing unfractionated heparin weight-indexed dose was independently associated with higher bleeding rates (odds ratio (OR) 1.04, 95% CI 1.02–1.07 for each 10 U/kg; $p = 0.001$) (16).

Bleeding complications may be as high as 15% with the use of adjuvant GP IIb/IIIa inhibitors (17). Vascular complications were not related to the size of the arterial sheath (15).

Recommendation for perioperative management of oral anticoagulation

The decision for perioperative thromboprophylaxis should be based on the perceived risks of bleeding and thromboembolism outlined above. In general, patients at intermediate to high risk of thromboembolism should receive perioperative bridging anticoagulation, whereas patients at low risk (<5% embolic risk per year) could be considered for conservative management without perioperative anticoagulation (1–6) (Table 32.2).

Bridging anticoagulation therapy

It takes approximately 4 days to reduce the international normalized ratio (INR) from a steady value of 2.0–3.0 to 1.5 after cessation of

warfarin OAC therapy. Patients are expected to have subtherapeutic INR for approximately 2 days before and 2 days after the procedure. Short-acting anticoagulants such as unfractionated heparin (UFH) or low-molecular-weight heparin (LMWH) are instituted during this time of subtherapeutic INR to maintain anticoagulation and to prevent thromboembolism.

Current guidelines from the American College of Chest Physicians and American Heart Association recommend that in patients at high-risk of thromboembolism, OAC should be withheld approximately 4 days prior to surgery or invasive procedure to allow the INR to normalize. Anticoagulation reversal with vitamin K should be avoided. Full-dose intravenous UFH or subcutaneous LMWH is given when INR falls below 2, approximately 2 days prior to procedure (5,6) (Table 32.3).

UFH can be continued up to or stopped 3–4 h before PCI. If LMWH was used for bridging, the last dose should be given at least 12 h before the procedure (unless LMWH is used for procedural anticoagulation, see Chapter 2). An activated clotting time (ACT) is measured at the beginning of

Table 32.2 Recommendation for perioperative management of anticoagulation therapy in relation to the risks of thromboembolism and bleeding in patients receiving long-term oral anticoagulation therapy.

	Low bleeding risk	High bleeding risk
Low thromboembolic risk	Continue OAC	Discontinue OAC No bridging therapy
Intermediate/high thromboembolic risk	Discontinue OAC Bridging therapy	Discontinue OAC ± bridging therapy

Abbreviation: OAC, oral anticoagulant.

Table 32.3 Protocol for perioperative management of patients on long-term anticoagulation at different levels of thromboembolic risk.

Day	INR	Oral anticoagulation	Low risk	High risk
			No bridging	Bridging anticoagulation
–4 to –5	>2	Discontinue		
–2 to –3	<2			Initiate UFH/LMWH
PCI	<1.5			Discontinue LMWH 12–24 or UFH 3–4 h pre-op
Post-PCI	<1.5	Resume day of PCI		Restart LMWH/UFH
2–4	>2			Stop bridging

Abbreviations: INR, international normalized ratio; LMWH, low-molecular weight heparin; PCI, percutaneous coronary intervention; UFH, unfractionated heparin.

the procedure and additional heparin bolus given as required to achieve target ACT (see Chapter 1).

Following PCI, OAC should be reinstated at the previous maintenance dose on the same day. Therapeutic doses of UFH or LMWH can be administered once hemostasis is achieved as early as 2 h after sheath removal (18,19). The use of bridging anticoagulation should be maintained until the INR is >2 (approximately 3 days after procedure). Intravenous heparin is restarted without a bolus.

There are a number of potential issues regarding the bridging strategy. Although widely practiced, periprocedural bridging therapy is only considered a grade 2C recommendation (i.e., risk/benefit unclear—observational studies—very weak recommendations) (5). This is due to the lack of randomized evidence comparing the relative benefits and risks after withdrawal of OAC therapy with and without periprocedural bridging therapy. Secondly, despite a low incidence of major bleeding with bridging therapy before and after invasive procedure, postoperative bleeding due to aggressive bridging anticoagulation may lead to temporary discontinuation of OAC therapy and a period of increased thromboembolic risk. Therefore, some clinicians opt for simply withholding OAC or continue OAC at a lower INR without bridging therapy. A strategy of continuing dose-reduced warfarin (targeting INR 1.5–2.0) for invasive procedures in patients with high thromboembolic risk is feasible but has not been validated in the PCI setting (20).

Unfractionated heparin vs low-molecular-weight heparin

Intravenous UFH has been the traditional perioperative anticoagulant. However, the use of UFH has a number of disadvantages including complexity of dosing, the need for monitoring of the activated partial thromboplastin time (aPTT) and the cost associated with hospitalization. Subcutaneous LMWH therapy offers advantages over UFH in terms of superior bioavailability, enhanced anti-Xa effects, and lower rates of heparin-induced thrombocytopenia (HITTS) than UFH (21). The predictable dose–response of LMWH obviates laboratory monitoring and facilitates outpatient administration. This strategy has the potential to substantially reduce health care costs.

Studies have shown that the two therapies are comparable in efficacy and safety as perioperative bridging anticoagulation (12,22,23). There were no significant differences in the incidence of thromboembolic events and bleeding complications between the two therapies. Patients receiving LMWH were hospitalized for a significantly shorter period (mean 4.3 vs 10.4 days, $p < 0.001$) (22). In a study comparing the time course in achieving effective anticoagulation after mechanical heart valve replacement, 87% of patients treated with LMWH had an anti-Xa activity within the range of efficacy (0.5–1 IU/mL) on the second day of treatment, whereas only 9% of UFH-treated patients had an aPTT value within the therapeutic range (1.5–2.5 times control, $p < 0.0001$ between the two groups) (24).

LMWH should be use cautiously in patients with severe renal impairment (creatinine clearance <30 mL/min) because of potential for drug accumulation and increase risk of bleeding. The safety of reduced dose LMWH in patients with severe renal impairment for periprocedural bridging is unproven. UFH may be a safer option in these patients.

Alternatives to bridging therapy

Alternatives to bridging therapy may be required in certain situations. For patients at the highest risk of thromboembolism, the risk of thrombotic complications if anticoagulation is interrupted may outweigh the concern of bleeding if anticoagulation is continued. Timely withdrawal of OAC and institution of bridging therapy may not be feasible in patients presenting with high-risk acute coronary syndromes or ST-elevation myocardial infarction and requiring urgent catheterization.

The femoral approach for PCI is generally contraindicated in fully anticoagulated patients with INR greater than 1.8 (25). Hemostasis by manual compression of the femoral artery, which lies deep in the pelvic fossa, may be ineffective. Alternatives to the femoral approach PCI in anticoagulated patients include the use of vascular closure devices for the femoral access site or the radial approach. The brachial approach should be avoided in anticoagulated patients because of the increased risk of median nerve compression by hematoma formation (26,27).

Radial artery approach

The use of radial approach is well established in PCI (see Chapter 21). The radial artery lies superficially in the fascia of the wrist and is therefore readily compressible and is anatomically separate from major nerves. A recent meta-analysis of 12 randomized trials involving 3,224 patients (1,155 patients for PCI) showed that vascular complications at the radial access site were significantly lower compared to the femoral approach (OR 0.20, 95% CI 0.09–0.42; $p < 0.0001$) (28).

A study by Hidick-Smith *et al.* showed that coronary angiography via the radial approach is safe and effective in 66 fully anticoagulated patients with INR> 2 but <4.5 (29). Using predominantly 6F sheaths (74%), success rate was 97%, with no failure of access and only one minor postprocedural hemorrhage. Immediate sheath removal postprocedure was safe despite therapeutic anticoagulation. Other studies have also shown minimal radial access site complications in patients at high risk of bleeding who underwent transradial access for primary and rescue PCI after failed thrombolysis for acute ST-elevation myocardial infarction (30,31).

Vascular closure devices

Vascular closure devices have emerged as alternatives to manual compression after PCI. A variety of suture- and collagen-based devices are currently available. These devices reduce time to hemostasis and allow for immediate sheath removal after PCI compared to manual compression (32–34). Complete hemostasis can be achieved after PCI in >90% of patients (34). However, the incidence of access site complications was similar between vascular closure device and manual compression.

A meta-analysis of 30 trials involving >37,000 patients demonstrated no difference in rates of access site complication between three vascular closure devices (Angio-Seal [Angio-Seal Daig, Minnetonka, MN], VasoSeal [VasoSeal Datascope Inc., Montvale, NJ], and Perclose [ProStar Plus or TecStar; Perclose, Redwood City, CA]) and manual compression in patients undergoing PCI (OR 1.11, 95% CI 0.94–1.333; $p = 0.22$) (33). In this study, the use of GP IIb/IIIa inhibitors was not associated with increased risk of bleeding with vascular closure devices. The risk of complications was similar regardless of sheath size (6–8 French) (33).

Although there is no evidence to support systematic use of vascular closure devices after PCI, the use of these devices in fully anticoagulated patients (INR > 1.8) undergoing PCI is an effective strategy to achieve access site hemostasis.

Key points

1 Optimal perioperative management of oral anticoagulation therapy needs to be based on assessment of the risk of thromboembolism and bleeding in an individual patient.

2 Patients at high or intermediate risk of thromboembolism should withhold oral anticoagulation therapy 4 days prior to procedure and use either intravenous unfractionated heparin or subcutaneous low-molecular-weight heparin as bridging anticoagulation during period of subtherapeutic INR (<2) before and after procedure.

3 Alternatively, percutaneous coronary intervention can be performed via the radial artery approach or with the use of vascular closure device for the femoral access site in fully anticoagulated patients.

4 Patients at low risk of thromboembolism can withhold warfarin 4 days prior to procedure without bridging therapy.

References

1 Spandorfer J. The management of anticoagulation before and after procedures. *Med Clin North Am.* 2001;**85**(5):1109–1116.

2 Douketis JD. Perioperative anticoagulation management in patients who are receiving oral anticoagulant therapy: a practical guide for clinicians. *Thromb Res.* 2002;**108**(1):3–13.

3 Jafri SM, Metha TP. Periprocedural management of anticoagulation in patients on extended warfarin therapy. *Semin Thromb Hemost.* 2004;**30**(6):657–664.

4 Dunn AS, Turpie AG. Perioperative management of patients receiving oral anticoagulants: a systematic review. *Arch Intern Med.* 2003;**163**(8):901–908.

5 Ansell J, Hirsh J, Poller L, Bussey H, Jacobson A, Hylek E. The pharmacology and management of the

vitamin K antagonists: the Seventh ACCP Conference on Antithrombotic and Thrombolytic Therapy. *Chest.* 2004;**126**(3 Suppl):204S–233S.

6 Hirsh J, Fuster V, Ansell J, Halperin JL, American Heart Association/American College of Cardiology Foundation guide to warfarin therapy. *Circulation.* 2003;**107**(12):1692–1711.

7 Cannegieter SC, Rosendaal FR, Briet E. Thromboembolic and bleeding complications in patients with mechanical heart valve prostheses. *Circulation.* 1994;**89**(2):635–641.

8 Heit JA. Perioperative management of the chronically anticoagulated patient. *J Thromb Thrombolysis.* 2001;**12**(1):81–87.

9 Kearon C, Hirsh J. Perioperative management of patients receiving oral anticoagulants. *Arch Intern Med.* 2003;**163**(20):2532–2533.

10 Fuster V, Ryden LE, Asinger RW, *et al.* ACC/AHA/ESC guidelines for the management of patients with atrial fibrillation: executive summary. A Report of the American College of Cardiology/American Heart Association Task Force on Practice Guidelines and the European Society of Cardiology Committee for Practice Guidelines and Policy Conferences (Committee to Develop Guidelines for the Management of Patients with Atrial Fibrillation): developed in Collaboration With the North American Society of Pacing and Electrophysiology. *J Am Coll Cardiol.* 2001;**38**(4):1231–1266.

11 Erkan D, Leibowitz E, Berman J, Lockshin MD. Perioperative medical management of antiphospholipid syndrome: hospital for special surgery experience, review of literature, and recommendations. *J Rheumatol.* 2002;**29**(4):843–849.

12 Douketis JD, Johnson JA, Turpie AG. Low-molecular-weight heparin as bridging anticoagulation during interruption of warfarin: assessment of a standardized periprocedural anticoagulation regimen. *Arch Intern Med.* 2004;**164**(12):1319–1326.

13 Bertrand ME, Legrand V, Boland J, *et al.* Randomized multicenter comparison of conventional anticoagulation versus antiplatelet therapy in unplanned and elective coronary stenting. The full anticoagulation versus aspirin and ticlopidine (fantastic) study. *Circulation.* 1998;**98**(16):1597–1603.

14 Leon MB, Baim DS, Popma JJ, *et al.* A clinical trial comparing three antithrombotic-drug regimens after coronary-artery stenting. Stent Anticoagulation Restenosis Study Investigators. *N Engl J Med.* 1998; **339**(23):1665–1671.

15 Waksman R, King SB, 3rd, Douglas JS, *et al.* Predictors of groin complications after balloon and new-device coronary intervention. *Am J Cardiol.* 1995;**75**(14):886–889.

16 Brener SJ, Moliterno DJ, Lincoff AM, Steinhubl SR, Wolski KE, Topol EJ. Relationship between activated clotting time and ischemic or hemorrhagic complications: analysis of 4 recent randomized clinical trials of percutaneous coronary intervention. *Circulation.* 2004; **110**(8):994–998.

17 Cote AV, Berger PB, Holmes DR, Jr, Scott CG, Bell MR. Hemorrhagic and vascular complications after percutaneous coronary intervention with adjunctive abciximab. *Mayo Clin Proc.* 2001;**76**(9):890–896.

18 Batchelor WB, Mahaffey KW, Berger PB, *et al.* A randomized, placebo-controlled trial of enoxaparin after high-risk coronary stenting: the ATLAST trial. *J Am Coll Cardiol.* 2001;**38**(6):1608–1613.

19 Zidar JP. Low-molecular-weight heparins in coronary stenting (the ENTICES trial). ENoxaparin and TIClopidine after Elective Stenting. *Am J Cardiol.* 1998;**82**(5B):29L–32L.

20 Larson BJ, Zumberg MS, Kitchens CS. A feasibility study of continuing dose-reduced warfarin for invasive procedures in patients with high thromboembolic risk. *Chest.* 2005;**127**(3):922–927.

21 Hirsh J, Warkentin TE, Shaughnessy SG, *et al.* Heparin and low-molecular-weight heparin: mechanisms of action, pharmacokinetics, dosing, monitoring, efficacy, and safety. *Chest.* 2001;**119**(1 Suppl):64S–94S.

22 Spyropoulos AC, Turpie AG, Dunn AS, *et al.* Clinical outcomes with unfractionated heparin or low-molecular-weight heparin as bridging therapy in patients on long-term oral anticoagulants: the REGIMEN registry. *J Thromb Haemost.* 2006;**4**(6):1246–1252.

23 Jaffer AK, Ahmed M, Brotman DJ, *et al.* Low-molecular-weight-heparins as periprocedural anticoagulation for patients on long-term warfarin therapy: a standardized bridging therapy protocol. *J Thromb Thrombolysis.* 2005;**20**(1):11–16.

24 Montalescot G, Polle V, Collet JP, *et al.* Low molecular weight heparin after mechanical heart valve replacement. *Circulation.* 2000;**101**(10):1083–1086.

25 Gohlke-Barwolf C, Acar J, Oakley C, *et al.* Guidelines for prevention of thromboembolic events in valvular heart disease. Study Group of the Working Group on Valvular Heart Disease of the European Society of Cardiology. *Eur Heart J.* 1995;**16**(10):1320–1330.

26 Kennedy AM, Grocott M, Schwartz MS, Modarres H, Scott M, Schon F. Median nerve injury: an underrecognised complication of brachial artery cardiac catheterisation? *J Neurol Neurosurg Psychiatry.* 1997;**63**(4):542–546.

27 Kiemeneij F, Laarman GJ, Odekerken D, Slagboom T, van der Wieken R. A randomized comparison of percutaneous transluminal coronary angioplasty by the radial, brachial and femoral approaches: the access study. *J Am Coll Cardiol.* 1997;**29**(6):1269–1275.

28 Agostoni P, Biondi-Zoccai GG, de Benedictis ML, *et al.* Radial versus femoral approach for percutaneous

coronary diagnostic and interventional procedures; systematic overview and meta-analysis of randomized trials. *J Am Coll Cardiol.* 2004;**44**(2):349–356.

29 Hildick-Smith DJ, Walsh JT, Lowe MD, Petch MC. Coronary angiography in the fully anticoagulated patient: the transradial route is successful and safe. *Catheter Cardiovasc Interv.* 2003;**58**(1):8–10.

30 Kassam S, Cantor WJ, Patel D, *et al.* Radial versus femoral access for rescue percutaneous coronary intervention with adjuvant glycoprotein IIb/IIIa inhibitor use. *Can J Cardiol.* 2004;**20**(14):1439–1442.

31 Cantor WJ, Puley G, Natarajan MK, *et al.* Radial versus femoral access for emergent percutaneous coronary intervention with adjunct glycoprotein IIb/IIIa inhibition in acute myocardial infarction–the RADIAL-AMI pilot randomized trial. *Am Heart J.* 2005;**150**(3):543–549.

32 Koreny M, Riedmuller E, Nikfardjam M, Siostrzonek P, Mullner M. Arterial puncture closing devices compared with standard manual compression after cardiac catheterization: systematic review and meta-analysis. *JAMA.* 2004;**291**(3):350–357.

33 Nikolsky E, Mehran R, Halkin A, *et al.* Vascular complications associated with arteriotomy closure devices in patients undergoing percutaneous coronary procedures: a meta-analysis. *J Am Coll Cardiol.* 2004;**44**(6):1200–1209.

34 Eggebrecht H, Haude M, Woertgen U, *et al.* Systematic use of a collagen-based vascular closure device immediately after cardiac catheterization procedures in 1,317 consecutive patients. *Catheter Cardiovasc Interv.* 2002;**57**(4):486–495.

CHAPTER 33

Indication for anticoagulation post-percutaneous coronary intervention

Roswitha Wolfram
Vienna General Hospital, Vienna, Austria

Introduction

Since its inception in the late 1970s, percutaneous coronary intervention (PCI) has evolved into an effective revascularization strategy for coronary artery disease with over a million procedures performed every year (1) in the United States alone. There is a huge body of evidence regarding anticoagulation and antithrombotic strategies before and during PCI, which is based on the experience of many randomized trials and summarized in international guidelines (2). In this chapter, we want to focus on the indications for anticoagulation post-PCI.

Glycoprotein (GP) IIb/IIIa inhibitors

In patients undergoing PCI, adjunct administration of GP IIb/IIIa inhibitors is known to consistently reduce thrombotic complications (EPIC, CAPTURE, EPILOG, EPISTENT, RESTORE, IMPACT-II, ESPRIT) (3). In most of these trials, utilization of GP IIb/IIIa inhibitors resulted in a significant reduction of the Combined endpoint of death, myocardial infarction (MI), and target vessel reintervention (TVR).

In a meta-analysis of all trials with abciximab, it was furthermore possible to show that abciximab given during and after PCI resulted in a reduction of subsequent mortality. The TARGET study compared two GP IIb/IIIa inhibitors, abciximab and tirofiban, at the time of PCI in patients with acute coronary syndromes (ACS) (4). Although abciximab appeared superior to tirofiban at 30 days (death and MI: 6.3% vs 9.3%, $P = 0.04$) and at 6 months (7.1% vs 9.6%, $P = 0.01$), outcomes were comparable at 1 year follow-up.

In PRISM-PLUS, the enrolled patients were high-risk patients, with unstable angina and "ischemic" ECG changes in the 12 h prior to enrolment (5). PRISM-PLUS compared three treatment arms. The regimen of tirofiban (same dose as in PRISM) without unfractionated heparin was discontinued because of an increased mortality rate in the first 345 patients (5).

PURSUIT was the largest GP IIb/IIIa inhibitor trial, including 10,948 patients with ACS and symptoms within 24 h prior to enrolment. The patients were randomized to an eptifibatide bolus followed by an infusion up to 72 h, or to placebo (6).

An analysis of the patients in CAPTURE (all patients underwent PCI) (7), and the subgroup of patients undergoing PCI in PURSUIT (6) and PRISM-PLUS (5), revealed a significant reduction of procedure-related events ($P = 0.001$). There was no additional treatment effect apparent at 30 days follow-up.

Furthermore data from CAPTURE and PARAGON-B (7,8) revealed that treatment with a GP IIb/IIIa inhibitors was particularly beneficial among patients admitted with elevated levels of cardiac troponin T or cardiac troponin I.

Pharmacology in the Catheterization Laboratory. Edited by Ron Waksman and Andrew E Ajani. © 2010 Blackwell Publishing, ISBN: 978-1-4051-5704-9.

Patients with elevated cardiac troponin levels seem to have active ongoing intracoronary thrombosis, which can be effectively reduced by powerful antiplatelet therapy.

Among 1,279 diabetic patients undergoing PCI during index hospitalization, the use of GP IIb/IIIa inhibitors was associated with a mortality reduction at 30 days, from 4.0% to 1.2% (95% confidence interval (CI): 0.14–0.69; $P = 0.002$) (9). This meta-analysis showed that the 30-day mortality benefit in patients with diabetes in the setting of UA/NSTEMI was greater in patients undergoing PCI (9). Thus, GP IIb/IIIa blockers are recommended, in particular in patients with diabetes and ACS.

The seventh ACCP Conference on Antithrombotic and Thrombolytic Therapy (10) recommends the following guidelines for the utilization of GP IIb/IIIa inhibitors in patients undergoing PCI.

1 For all patients undergoing PCI, particularly those undergoing primary PCI, or those with refractory UA or other high-risk features, use of a GP IIb/IIIa antagonist (abciximab or eptifibatide) is recommended (Grade 1A).

2 In patients undergoing PCI for STEMI, abciximab is recommended over eptifibatide (Grade 1B).

3 Administration of abciximab as a 0.25 mg/kg bolus followed by a 12-h infusion at a rate of 10 μg/min (Grade 1A) and eptifibatide as a double bolus (each of 180 μg/kg administered 10 min apart), followed by an 18-h infusion of 2.0 μg/kg/min is recommended (Grade 1A).

4 In patients undergoing PCI, we recommend against the use of tirofiban as an alternative to abciximab (Grade 1A).

5 For patients with NSTEMI/UA who are designated as moderate-to-high risk based on TIMI score, it is recommended that upstream use of a GP IIb/IIIa antagonist (either eptifibatide or tirofiban) is started as soon as possible prior to PCI (Grade 1A).

6 With planned PCI in NSTEMI/UA patients with an elevated troponin level, it is recommended that abciximab be started within 24 h prior to the intervention (Grade 1A).

Warfarin

Initially, antithrombotic regimens after PCI and stent implantation included aspirin, dipyridamole, dextran, IV heparin, and warfarin for 30 days in order to prevent subacute stent thrombosis (11,12). A number of randomized trials have later on shown that warfarin provided only little additional benefit over aspirin alone on early outcomes in patients treated with PCI and stent implantation. In the Stent Anti-thrombotic Regimen Study (13), patients were assigned to receive aspirin alone, aspirin plus warfarin, or dual antiplatelet therapy with aspirin plus ticlopidine. The primary end point of the study was a composite of death, target lesion revascularization, in-stent thrombosis, and MI at 30 days. The end point was met in 3.6% of patients in the aspirin alone group, 2.7% of patients in the aspirin plus warfarin group, and in 0.5% assigned to receive aspirin plus ticlopidine ($P = 0.001$ for the comparison of all three groups). A smaller trial including 164 patients compared the incidence of subacute thrombosis after provisional coronary stenting in patients receiving aspirin (100 mg/day) or aspirin plus warfarin. There was a trend toward better outcome in patients in the aspirin plus warfarin arm ($P = 0.09$) (14).

Five randomized trials have evaluated the potential long-term effectiveness of warfarin on the prevention of restenosis after PCI (15–19). The first trial included 110 patients, treated with angioplasty, who were randomized to receive either warfarin or placebo (16). Outcomes between the two groups regarding the occurrence of angiographic restenosis were comparable (16). Similar results were obtained from a study including 248 patients treated with aspirin (325 mg/d) or warfarin, which showed no benefit of warfarin over aspirin for the prevention of restenosis (15). In another trial (17), 191 patients undergoing uncomplicated PCI, with additional stent implantation in approximately 30%, were randomized to aspirin (100 mg/d) or to aspirin plus warfarin for 6 months. Again, restenosis rate at 6 months was comparable between the two groups (30% vs 33%) (17). The Balloon Angioplasty and Anticoagulation Study (18) evaluated 531 patients who were randomized to aspirin alone or to aspirin plus a coumarin derivative started 1 week prior to procedure, for 6 months angiographic outcomes. Like in the trials mentioned before, there was no difference between the two treatment arms (18). Recent studies such as the Intracoronary Stenting and Antithrombotic Regimen (ISAR) trial have shown that oral anticoagulation with warfarin, even in combination with aspirin, is inferior to dual antiplatelet therapy in the prevention of acute stent thrombosis (13,20–23).

Although warfarin apparently does not have an incremental benefit on clinical outcome after PCI, it is mandatory for patients with mechanical heart valves. Furthermore full anticoagulation with warfarin is recommended for 1–3 months post-STEMI in patients at high risk for emboli which include: left ventricular thrombus, left ventricular aneurysm, and a left ventricular ejection fraction (LVEF) <30% in the absence of thrombus (24).

For patients with atrial fibrillation (AF) or other indications for warfarin, the optimal approach post-PCI should be individualized depending on the calculated risk of thromboembolic vs bleeding complications while on full dual antiplatelet plus warfarin therapy. A recent study has suggested evidence based approaches to various clinical scenarios (25).

Recommendations for warfarin (10)

In patients who undergo PCI with no other indication for systemic anticoagulation therapy, the current guidelines recommend against routine use of warfarin (or other vitamin K antagonists) after PCI (Grade 1A) (26).

Unfractionated heparin (UFH)

Several randomized studies (27,28) have shown that prolonged heparin infusions after PCI do not reduce ischemic complications, and are associated with a higher rate of bleeding at the puncture site. Therefore routine use of IV heparin after PCI has been abandoned. Similar to the results from trials utilizing other antithrombotic agents, heparin failed to reduce the risk of restenosis after balloon angioplasty. In a randomized clinical trial (RCT) comparing heparin with dextrose, the intravenous application of heparin for 24 h after successful PCI showed no benefit regarding the reduction of angiographic restenosis (27) Another study enrolled 339 patients who were randomized to twice-daily subcutaneous (SC) heparin (12,500 IU) for 4 months after successful PCI or no heparin at all (29). Again outcomes were comparable between the two groups.

Based on the data obtained over the last years, routine use of UFH after uncomplicated PCI is

therefore no longer recommended (Grade 1A) (27,28,30–32) and may be associated with more frequent bleeding events (27), particularly when in combination with platelet GP IIb/IIIa inhibitors (27,28).

Low-molecular-weight heparin (LMWH)

A series of RCTs have recently shown that short-term administration of low-molecular-weight heparin (LMWH) after PCI does not significantly reduce the occurrence of early ischemic events. In the Antiplatelet Therapy alone vs Lovenox plus Antiplatelet therapy in patients at increased risk of Stent Thrombosis trial (33), 1,102 patients at increased risk of stent thrombosis (STEMI within 48 h, diffuse distal disease, large thrombus volume, acute closure, or residual dissection) were randomly assigned to receive either enoxaparin (40 or 60 mg, according to patients weight, SC q12h for 14 days) or placebo. All study patients received additional aspirin (325 mg/d) and ticlopidine (250 mg bid) for 14 days. The primary end point of the study was a 30-day composite of death, nonfatal MI, and urgent revascularization, which was met in 1.8% of patients receiving enoxaparin and in 2.7% of those receiving placebo ($P = $ NS). Table 33.1 summarizes RCTs investigating LMWH after PCI.

Direct thrombin inhibitors

The Hirudin in a European Trial vs Heparin in the Prevention of Restenosis After PTCA Study (42) enrolled 1,141 patients with UA undergoing PCI. All patients were treated with aspirin and were randomly assigned to receive a heparin bolus of 10,000 IU plus infusion of 15 IU/kg/h for 24 h; a hirudin bolus of 40 mg plus IV infusion of 0.2 mg/kg/h for 24 h; or a hirudin bolus of 40 mg followed by an IV infusion of 0.2 mg/kg/h for 24 h, followed by SC hirudin injections of 40 mg bid for another 3 days. The primary endpoint restenosis at 7 months was comparable between groups although hirudin was associated with a reduction in early (96-h) ischemic events.

The Bivalirudin Angioplasty Trial (43) compared bivalirudin with UFH in 4,098 patients with postinfarction angina or UA undergoing PCI. Patients were randomized to either receive high-dose heparin bolus (175 IU/kg bolus followed by a 15 IU/kg/h infusion for 18–24 h) or bivalirudin (1.0 mg/kg bolus followed by an infusion of

Table 33.1 Anticoagulation and restenosis after PCI[a]

Source	Year	Study design	Total No. of patients	Angiographic follow-up (No. of patients)	Stent use	Treatment	Pretreatment duration	Duration therapy	Restenosis rates, %
Warfarin									
Urban et al. (16)	1988	RCT	110	85	No	Warfarin (PT > 2.5 × normal)	None	5 months	29
						Placebo			37
Kastrati et al. (19)	1997	RCT	496	432	Yes	Warfarin (INR 3.5–4.5)	None	4 weeks	28.9
						Ticlopidine, 250 mg bid			26.8
Garachemani et al. (17)	2002	RCT	191	176	36	Warfarin (INR 2.5–4.0)	None	6 months	33
						Aspirin plus warfarin			30
Thornton et al. (15)	1984	RCT	248	178	No	Aspirin, 325 mg qd	24 h	6 months	27[b]
						Warfarin (to PT 2.5 × normal)			36
ten Berg et al. (18)	2003	RCT	531	480	34	Coumarin (INR 2.1–4.8)	7 days	6 months	38.9[c]
						Placebo			39.1
UFH									
Ellis et al. (27)	1989	RCT	416	255	No	UFH, 800–1,200 U/h	None	18–24 h	41
						Placebo			37
Brack et al. (29)	1995	RCT	339	299	No	UFH, 12,500 U bid	None	4 months	41[b]
						Placebo			51
LMWH									
Faxon et al. (34)	1994	RCT	458	357	No	Enoxaparin, 40 mg SQ qd	None	1 months	43
						Placebo			45
Cairns et al. (35)	1996	RCT	653	625	No	Enoxaparin, 30 mg bid	None	6 weeks	38
						Placebo			40.4

(Continued)

Table 33.1 Continued.

Source	Year	Study design	Total No. of patients	Angiographic follow-up (No. of patients)	Stent use	Treatment	Pretreatment duration	Duration therapy	Restenosis rates, %
Karsch et al. (36)	1996	RCT	625	514	No	Reviparin, 3,500 U bid	None	28 days	0.25[c]
						Placebo			0.29
Schmid et al. (37)	1993	RCT	41	37	No	Reviparin, 2,500 U bolus plus 5,000 U SC qd	None	21 days	18
						Reviparin, 5,000 U bolus plus 5,000 U SC qd	None	21 days	20
						Reviparin, 10,000 U bolus plus 10,000 U SC qd	None	21 days	9
						UFH, 10,000 U bolus plus 2,500 U SC qd	None	21 days	25
Lablanche et al. (38)	1997	RCT	354	269	No	Nadroparin, 6,150 U SQ qd	72 h	3 months	51.9
						Placebo			48.8
Amann et al. (39)	1993	Registry	20	20	No	Fraxiparin, 0.6 mL SQ qd	24 h	4 weeks	30
Grassman et al. (40)	2001	RCT	118	102	No	Certoparin, 80 mg SQ bid	NR	3 months	31
						Placebo	NR	3 months	49
Direct thrombin inhibitors									
Burchenal et al. (41)	1998	RCT	87	87	No	Bivalirudin bolus and infusion	None	36 h	62.2
						Heparin, 175 U/kg bolus			58
Serruys et al. (42)	1995	RCT	1,141	986	No	Hirudin, 40 mg bolus plus IV	None	24 h	0.32[c]
						Hirudin, 40 mg bolus plus IV plus SQ	None	72 h	0.26
						Heparin, 10,000 U bolus and infusion	None	24 h	0.26

[a]INR, international normalized ratio; PT, prothrombin time. Restenosis defined as >50% follow-up diameter stenosis unless indicated otherwise.

[b]Restenosis defined a loss of 50% of initial gain.

[c]Mean percentage stenosis at follow-up.

2.5 mg/kg/h infusion for 4 h, which was subsequently reduced to 0.2 mg/kg/h for another 14–20 h). There was no significant difference in restenosis between treatment groups at follow-up (Table 33.1).

Currently, there are no recommendations for the use of direct thrombin inhibitors after PCI available.

References

1 AHA. *Heart Disease and Stroke Statistics—2005 Update.* Dallas, Texas: AHA; 2004.

2 Smith SC, Jr, Jerilyn Allen RN, Blair SN, *et al.* AHA/ACC guidelines for secondary prevention for patients with coronary and other atherosclerotic vascular disease: 2006 update. Endorsed by the National Heart, Lung, and Blood Institute. *J Am Coll Cardiol.* 2006;**47**(10):2130–2139.

3 The EPIC Investigation. Use of a monoclonal antibody directed against the platelet glycoprotein IIb/IIIa receptor in high-risk coronary angioplasty. The EPIC Investigation. *N Engl J Med.* 1994;**330**(14):956–961.

4 Topol EJ, Moliterno DJ, Herrmann HC, *et al.* Comparison of two platelet glycoprotein IIb/IIIa inhibitors, tirofiban and abciximab, for the prevention of ischemic events with percutaneous coronary revascularization. *N Engl J Med.* 2001;**344**(25):1888–1894.

5 PRISM-PLUS Study Investigators. Inhibition of the platelet glycoprotein IIb/IIIa receptor with tirofiban in unstable angina and non-Q-wave myocardial infarction. Platelet Receptor Inhibition in Ischemic Syndrome Management in Patients Limited by Unstable Signs and Symptoms (PRISM-PLUS) study investigators. *N Engl J Med.* 1998;**338**(21):1488–1497.

6 PURSUIT Trial Investigators. Inhibition of platelet glycoprotein IIb/IIIa with eptifibatide in patients with acute coronary syndromes. The PURSUIT Trial Investigators. Platelet glycoprotein IIb/IIIa in unstable angina: receptor suppression using integrilin therapy. *N Engl J Med.* 1998;**339**(7):436–443.

7 Randomised placebo-controlled trial of abciximab before and during coronary intervention in refractory unstable angina: the CAPTURE Study. *Lancet.* 1997;**349**(9063):1429–1435.

8 Global Organization Network (PARAGON)-B Investigators. Randomized, placebo-controlled trial of titrated intravenous lamifiban for acute coronary syndromes. *Circulation.* 2002;**105**(3):316–321.

9 Roffi M, Chew DP, Mukherjee D, *et al.* Platelet glycoprotein IIb/IIIa inhibitors reduce mortality in diabetic patients with non-ST-segment-elevation acute coronary syndromes. *Circulation.* 2001;**104**(23):2767–2771.

10 Bhatt DL, Hirsch AT, Ringleb PA, Hacke W, Topol EJ. Reduction in the need for hospitalization for recurrent ischemic events and bleeding with clopidogrel instead of aspirin. CAPRIE investigators. *Am Heart J.* 2000;**140**(1):67–73.

11 Fischman DL, Leon MB, Baim DS, *et al.* A randomized comparison of coronary-stent placement and balloon angioplasty in the treatment of coronary artery disease. Stent Restenosis Study Investigators. *N Engl J Med.* 1994;**331**(8):496–501.

12 Serruys PW, de Jaegere P, Kiemeneij F, *et al.* A comparison of balloon-expandable-stent implantation with balloon angioplasty in patients with coronary artery disease. Benestent Study Group. *N Engl J Med.* 1994;**331**(8):489–495.

13 Leon MB, Baim DS, Popma JJ, *et al.* A clinical trial comparing three antithrombotic-drug regimens after coronary-artery stenting. Stent Anticoagulation Restenosis Study Investigators. *N Engl J Med.* 1998;**339**(23):1665–1671.

14 Machraoui A, Germing A, von Dryander S, *et al.* Comparison of the efficacy and safety of aspirin alone with coumadin plus aspirin after provisional coronary stenting: final and follow-up results of a randomized study. *Am Heart J.* 1999;**138**(4 Pt 1):663–669.

15 Thornton MA, Gruentzig AR, Hollman A, King 3rd, SB, Douglas JS. Coumadin and aspirin in prevention of recurrence after transluminal coronary angioplasty: a randomized study. *Circulation.* 1984;**69**(4):721–727.

16 Urban P, Buller N, Fox K, Shapiro L, Bayliss J, Rickards A. Lack of effect of warfarin on the restenosis rate or on clinical outcome after balloon coronary angioplasty. *Br Heart J.* 1988;**60**(6):485–488.

17 Garachemani AR, Fleisch M, Windecker S, Pfiffner D, Meier B. Heparin and coumadin versus acetylsalicylic acid for prevention of restenosis after coronary angioplasty. *Catheter Cardiovasc Interv.* 2002;**55**(3):315–320.

18 ten Berg JM, Kelder JC, Suttorp MJ, Verheugt FWA, Plokker HWT. A randomized trial assessing the effect of coumarins started before coronary angioplasty on restenosis: results of the 6-month angiographic substudy of the Balloon Angioplasty and Anticoagulation Study (BAAS). *Am Heart J.* 2003;**145**(1):58–65.

19 Kastrati A, Schühlen H, Hausleiter J, *et al.* Restenosis after coronary stent placement and randomization to a 4-week combined antiplatelet or anticoagulant therapy: six-month angiographic follow-up of the Intracoronary Stenting and Antithrombotic Regimen (ISAR) Trial. *Circulation.* 1997;**96**(2):462–467.

20 Popma JJ, Ohman EM, Weitz J, Lincoff AM, Harrington RJ, Berger P. Antithrombotic therapy in patients undergoing percutaneous coronary intervention. *Chest.* 2001;**119**(1 Suppl):321S–336S.

21 Urban P, Macaya C, Rupprecht HJ, *et al.* Randomized evaluation of anticoagulation versus antiplatelet therapy after coronary stent implantation in high-risk patients: the

multicenter aspirin and ticlopidine trial after intra-coronary stenting (MATTIS). *Circulation.* 1998;**98**(20): 2126–2132.

22 Schömig A, Neumann FJ, Kastrati A, *et al.* A randomized comparison of antiplatelet and anticoagulant therapy after the placement of coronary-artery stents. *N Engl J Med.* 1996;**334**(17):1084–1089.

23 CAPRIE Steering Committee. A randomised, blinded, trial of clopidogrel versus aspirin in patients at risk of ischaemic events (CAPRIE). CAPRIE Steering Committee. *Lancet.* 1996;**348**(9038):1329–1339.

24 Katz R, Purcell H. *Acute Coronary Syndrome.* In *Clinical Practice Series.* Livingstone: Elsevier Churchill; 2006.

25 Singer DE, Albers GW, Dalen JE, Go AS, Halperin JL, Manning WJ. Antithrombotic therapy in atrial fibrilla-tion: the Seventh ACCP Conference on Antithrombotic and Thrombolytic Therapy. *Chest.* 2004;**126**(3 Suppl):429S–456S.

26 Popma JJ, Berger P, Ohman EM, Harrington RA, Grines C, Weitz JI. Antithrombotic therapy during percutaneous coronary intervention: the Seventh ACCP Conference on Antithrombotic and Thrombolytic Therapy. *Chest.* 2004;**126**(3 Suppl):576S–599S.

27 Ellis SG, Roubin GS, Wilentz J, Douglas JS Jr, King SB 3rd. Effect of 18- to 24-hour heparin administration for prevention of restenosis after uncomplicated coronary angioplasty. *Am Heart J.* 1989;**117**(4):777–782.

28 Friedman HZ, Cragg DR, Glazier SM, *et al.* Randomized prospective evaluation of prolonged versus abbreviated intravenous heparin therapy after coronary angioplasty. *J Am Coll Cardiol.* 1994;**24**(5):1214–1219.

29 Brack MJ, Ray S, Chauhan A, *et al.* The Subcutaneous Heparin and Angioplasty Restenosis Prevention (SHARP) trial. Results of a multicenter randomized trial investigat-ing the effects of high dose unfractionated heparin on angiographic restenosis and clinical outcome. *J Am Coll Cardiol.* 1995;**26**(4):947–954.

30 Fail PS, Maniet AR, Banka VS. Subcutaneous heparin in postangioplasty management: compara-tive trial with intravenous heparin. *Am Heart J.* 1993; **126**(5):1059–1067.

31 Kong DF, Califf RM. Post-procedure heparin: boon or burden? *Am Heart J.* 1998;**136**(2):183–185.

32 Garachemani AR, Kaufmann U, Fleisch M, Meier B. Prolonged heparin after uncomplicated coronary inter-ventions: a prospective, randomized trial. *Am Heart J.* 1998;**136**(2):352–356.

33 Berger PB, Mahaffey KW, Meier SJ, *et al.* Safety and effi-cacy of only 2 weeks of ticlopidine therapy in patients at increased risk of coronary stent thrombosis: results from the Antiplatelet Therapy alone versus Lovenox plus Antiplatelet therapy in patients at increased risk

of Stent Thrombosis (ATLAST) trial. *Am Heart J.* 2002;**143**(5):841–846.

34 Faxon DP, Spiro TE, Minor S, *et al.* Low molecular weight heparin in prevention of restenosis after angi-oplasty. Results of Enoxaparin Restenosis (ERA) Trial. *Circulation.* 1994;**90**(2):908–914.

35 Cairns JA, Gill J, Morton B, *et al.* Fish oils and low-molecular-weight heparin for the reduction of restenosis after percutaneous transluminal coronary angioplasty. The EMPAR Study. *Circulation.* 1996;**94**(7):1553–1560.

36 Karsch KR, Preisack MB, Baildon R, *et al.* Low molecular weight heparin (reviparin) in percutaneous transluminal coronary angioplasty. Results of a ran-domized, double-blind, unfractionated heparin and placebo-controlled, multicenter trial (REDUCE trial). Reduction of Restenosis After PTCA, Early Administration of Reviparin in a Double-Blind Unfractionated Heparin and Placebo-Controlled Evaluation. *J Am Coll Cardiol.* 1996;**28**(6):1437–1443.

37 Schmid KM, Preisack M, Voelker W, Sujatta M, Karsch KR. First clinical experience with low molecular weight heparin LU 47311 (reviparin) for prevention of restenosis after percutaneous transluminal coronary angioplasty. *Semin Thromb Hemost.* 1993;**19**(Suppl 1): 155–159.

38 Lablanche JM, McFadden EP, Meneveau N, *et al.* Effect of nadroparin, a low-molecular-weight heparin, on clinical and angiographic restenosis after coronary balloon angioplasty: the FACT study. Fraxiparine Angioplastie Coronaire Transluminale. *Circulation.* 1997; **96**(10):3396–3402.

39 Amann FW, Neuenschwander C, Meyer BJ. Fraxiparin for prevention of restenosis after percutaneous trans-luminal coronary angioplasty. *Semin Thromb Hemost.* 1993;**19**(Suppl 1):160–163.

40 Grassman ED, Leya F, Fareed J, *et al.* A randomized trial of the low-molecular-weight heparin certoparin to pre-vent restenosis following coronary angioplasty. *J Invasive Cardiol.* 2001;**13**(11):723–728.

41 Burchenal JE, Marks DS, Tift Mann J, *et al.* Effect of direct thrombin inhibition with Bivalirudin (Hirulog) on restenosis after coronary angioplasty. *Am J Cardiol.* 1998;**82**(4):511–515.

42 Serruys PW, Herrman JP, Simon R, *et al.* A comparison of hirudin with heparin in the prevention of restenosis after coronary angioplasty. Helvetica Investigators. *N Engl J Med.* 1995;**333**(12):757–763.

43 Bittl JA, Strony J, Brinker JA, *et al.* Treatment with bivalirudin (Hirulog) as compared with heparin dur-ing coronary angioplasty for unstable or postinfarction angina. Hirulog Angioplasty Study Investigators. *N Engl J Med.* 1995;**333**(12):764–769.

CHAPTER 34

Clopidogrel use in patients requiring coronary artery bypass grafting

Nilesh U. Patel & Mark W. Connolly
St. Michael's Medical Center, Newark, NJ, USA

Introduction

Coronary artery bypass grafting (CABG) is one of the most common and extensively studied operations in the history of medicine with significant proven benefits in the treatment of ischemic heart disease. Clopidogrel and aspirin are given to patients before diagnostic angiography whenever a possibility of coronary stent implantation exists, and frequently patients are diagnosed with surgical disease. Additionally, many PCI patients on clopidogrel maintenance develop progressive coronary disease requiring CABG. Delaying surgery on patients with clopidogrel platelet inhibition to minimize bleeding has led to increased preoperative length of stay and hospital costs, and inconvenience to patients and families, creating a clinical quagmire.

Anti-platelet Therapy for Reduction Myocardial Damage during Angioplasty (ARMYDA-Reload) trial indicated individual variability to clopidogrel in as many as 30% of the patients on long-term clopidogrel maintenance therapy (1). Elevated plasma fibrinogen (≥ 375 mg/dL), diabetes mellitus, and obesity (BMI ≥ 25 kg/m²) are also associated with diminished platelet inhibition even on long-term clopidogrel therapy, resulting in

Pharmacology in the Catheterization Laboratory. Edited by Ron Waksman and Andrew E Ajani. © 2010 Blackwell Publishing, ISBN: 978-1-4051-5704-9.

increased adverse event rates after PCI (2,3). Super reloading up to 900 mg of clopidogrel on top of the 75 mg/day PCI maintenance (1) to achieve adequate platelet inhibition to cover such nonresponders poses significant potential surgical bleeding problems in patients referred for CABG. In patients with acute coronary syndromes, clopidogrel has been shown to be significantly beneficial in preventing major cardiac events (4). In the large multicenter Grace registry trial, 7.2% of patients needed surgical revascularization in the non-ST elevation myocardial infarction group, and the majority of them required surgery within 5 days (5). Most patients referred for CABG today have been recently loaded with high dose clopidogrel, or are on maintenance clopidogrel therapy post-PCI and reloaded, creating significant platelet inhibition.

CABG clopidogrel-related bleeding

Clopidogrel administration preoperatively with the potential of increased surgical bleeding and the potential increased risk of pre-CABG ischemic events in drug-eluting stent patients from withholding platelet inhibition therapy can be a clinical balancing act. A meta-analysis of 11 cohort studies (6,7) and other reports (8,9) have clearly shown recent clopidogrel administration within 5–7 days of surgery is associated with an increased chest drainage of 30–100%, increased in blood product usage, and a 2–5 times increase in the need for reexploration. Intraoperative transfusions contribute to the increased systemic inflammatory response after cardiac surgery, leading to significantly worse postoperative outcomes (10). Blood product transfusion in CABG patients is an independent risk factor for prolonged ICU and hospital length of stay (11), increased postoperative pneumonia (12), sternal wound infection (13), sepsis (14), and renal dysfunction (15). The National Heart, Lung, and Blood Institute defines transfusion-related acute lung injury (TRALI) as new acute lung injury occurring during or within 6 h after a blood transfusion (16). Transfusion-related acute lung injury (TRALI) has emerged as the leading cause of mortality in surgical patients. Perioperative CABG blood transfusion not only has short-term deleterious effects, but is also an independent risk factor for decreased 5-year survival (17).

The benefits of clopidogrel loading pre-PCI appear to outweigh the surgical bleeding risks (18), particularly, when considering the almost fourfold increased number of PCI compared to CABG procedures in the United States. Balancing the delaying of surgery to decrease surgical bleeding without adding further ischemic risk before surgery is a daily clinical dilemma. Since many patients undergo surgery with clopidogrel platelet inhibition, off-pump surgical techniques, cell-saver autotransfusion, and patient-specific strategies are used to optimize clinical results.

Clopidogrel-CABG strategy

The clopidogrel-CABG strategy developed between surgeons and cardiologists at our institution to minimize postoperative bleeding and pre-CABG ischemic events is as follows.

Stable patients

Stable patients on long-term clopidogrel therapy, or who received clopidogrel loading before angiography and require elective surgery, clinical symptoms and the severity of the coronary disease are evaluated. If a clopidogrel-loaded patient has minimal symptoms controlled with medical therapy, the coronary anatomy is noncritical and the risk of drug-eluting stent thrombosis is small (stent placed ≥12 months), we follow the Society of Thoracic Surgery Guidelines (19) of withholding clopidogrel for 5–7 days. Patients are sent home with specific instructions regarding new symptoms, and return in a week for elective surgery.

Semiurgent stable patients

In clinically stable patients requiring more urgent surgery due to severe critical coronary anatomy and/or recent drug-eluting stent (≤12 months) implantation, the optimum timing of surgery should be decided based on platelet studies such as the platelet $P2Y_{12}$ assay using aggregometry (veryfynow™, ACCUMETRICS, San Diego, CA) or platelet assay thromboelastogram (MARTAB, Mahwah, NJ). Due to large variability of platelet inhibition, knowing the individual platelet count and the percentage of platelets inhibited is critical for deciding surgical timing. If a patient's uninhibited platelet count is more than 100,000, surgery may be undertaken without significant increased bleeding. If total platelet count is low and/or high percentage of platelets are inhibited, clopidogrel is stopped, the patient is hospitalized for close observation and placed on heparin therapy until platelet inhibition decreases. The timing of the surgery is based upon serial follow-up platelet study results.

Unstable patients

Unstable patients requiring emergency surgery, intraoperative thromboelastogram or aggregometry with total platelet count serves as a guideline to counter excessive bleeding with targeted transfusion of platelet PRBC, FFP, or cryoprecipitate. Off-pump CABG has clearly proven beneficial with approximately 50% less postoperative bleeding and transfusion requirements compared to on-pump CABG by avoiding fibrinolysis, platelet dysfunction, thrombocytopenia, and the inflammatory response (20,21). Off-pump CABG is preferred in patients requiring CABG with significant clopidogrel-platelet inhibition. Use of aprotinin in patients who received clopidogrel <5 days and with normal renal function was shown to decrease postoperative bleeding and the number of transfusions in patients undergoing coronary artery bypass graft surgery (22), but this drug has been discontinued due to increased death and renal failure complications (23).

At our institution, a 25% decrease in blood products usage was achieved using the above strategies.

Graft occlusion

Despite the recent trend of total arterial revascularization, the saphenous vein remains the most common conduit of choice for most surgeons consisting of up to 70% of the total grafts (24). The biggest shortcoming of vein graft is early occlusion and sclerosis. Up to 15% of vein grafts occlude in the first year after bypass surgery and by 10 years, only 60% of grafts are patent (25). Late graft failures are due to progressive thickening of the media and intimal hyperplasia of which platelets play a major role (26). Clopidogrel, not only inhibits platelet activation and aggregation, but also has shown in animal modes to inhibit platelet-mediated intimal proliferation and medial hyperplasia (27). Many surgeons today prefer to have their patients on clopidogrel for 3–6 months postoperatively for potential graft patency benefits, particularly, with extensive coronary disease such as seen in diabetic mellitus patients. Clinical data does not exist at this time to support this strategy. CABG patients with severe, diffuse disease may benefit from lifelong clopidogrel therapy.

Newer drugs

Clopidogrel produces long-acting platelet inhibition and no short-acting platelet inhibitors are currently approved for maintenance of platelet inhibition before surgery. Newer platelet inhibitors such as Cangrelor, a potent, reversible and specific $P2Y_{12}$ purinorecepter antagonist, has shown rapid onset with short-acting effort in animal models, but needs clinical review to prove its safety and efficacy. The BRIDGE trial (Maintenance of platelet inhiBition with cangreloR after dIscontinuation of thienopyriDines in patients undergoing surGEry) will hopefully validate cangrelor use in CABG patients to minimize transfusion and hospital cost preoperatively.

Conclusion

Preoperative clopidogrel load in the drug-eluting stent era occurs in the majority of patients referred for CABG today with a substantial increased risk of perioperative bleeding and transfusion. Blood transfusions independently increase CABG mortality and morbidity. Institution-specific strategies, involving surgeons and cardiologists working together, with platelet inhibition analysis can improve patient results. Hopefully, the newer ultrashort-acting platelet inhibitors will further improve CABG outcomes in patients requiring platelet inhibition preoperatively.

References

1 Collet JP, Silvain J, Landivier A, et al. Dose effect of clopidogrel reloading in patients already on 75-mg maintenance dose: the Reload with Clopidogrel Before Coronary Angioplasty in Subjects Treated Long Term with Dual Antiplatelet Therapy (RELOAD) study. *Circulation.* 2008;**118**:1225–1233.

2 Lawrence A, Vachaspati P, Ahner K, et al. Elevated plasma fibrinogen and diabetes mellitus are associated with lowe inhibition of platelet reactivity with clopidogrel. *JACC.* 2008;**52**:1052–1059.

3 Bhatt Deepak. What makes platelets angry. Editorial comment. *JACC.* 2008;**52**:1060–1061.

4 The Clopidogrel in Unstable angina to prevent Recurrent Events (CURE) Trial Investigators. Effects of clopidogrel in addition to aspirin in patients with acute coronary syndromes without ST-segment elevation. *N Engl J Med.* 2001;**345**:494–502.

5 Fox KA, Anderson F, Jr, Dabbous O, et al. Intervention in acute coronary syndromes: do patients undergo intervention on the basis of their risk characteristics? The Global Registry of Acute Coronary Events (GRACE). *Heart.* 2007;**93**:177–182.

6 Bavry A, Lincoff A. Is clopidogrel cardiovascular medicine's double-edged sword? *Circulation.* 2006;**113**:1638–1640.

7 Purkayastha S, Athanasiou T, Malinovski V, et al. Does clopidogrel affect outcome after coronary artery bypass grafting? A meta-analysis. *Heart.* 2006;**92**:531–532.

8 Nurozler F, Kutlu T, Küçük F, et al. Impact of clopidogrel on postoperative blood loss after non-elective coronary bypass surgery. *Interact CardioVasc Thorac Surg.* 2005;**4**:546–549.

9 Shim J, Choi Y, Young J, et al. Effects of preoperative aspirin and clopidogrel therapy on perioperative blood loss and blood transfusion requirements in patients undergoing off-pump coronary artery bypass graft surgery. *J Thorac Cardiovasc Surg.* 2007;**134**:59–64.

10 Erik Fransen, Jos Maessen, Mieke Dentener, Nicole Senden, Wim Buurman. Impact of blood transfusions on inflammatory mediator release in patients undergoing cardiac surgery. *Chest.* 1999;**116**:1233–1239.

11 Michael W, Chu S, Richard W, et al. Does clopidogrel increase blood loss following coronary artery bypass surgery? *Ann Thorac Surg.* 2004;**78**:1536–1541.

12 Leal-Noval SR, Marquez-Vácaro JA, Garcia-Curiel A, et al. Nosocomial pneumonia in patients undergoing heart surgery. *Crit Care Med.* 2000;**28**:935–940.

13 Zacharias A, Habib RH. Factors predisposing to median sternotomy complications. Deep vs superficial infection. *Chest.* 1996;**110**:1173–1178.

14 Michalopoulos A, Stavridis G, Geroulanos S. Severe sepsis in cardiac surgical patients. *Eur J Surg.* 1998;**164**:217–222.

15 Ranucci, Pavesi, Mazza E, *et al.* Risk factors for renal dysfunction after coronary surgery: the role of cardiopulmonary bypass technique. *Perfusion.* 1994;**9**:319–326.

16 Toy P, Popovski M, Abraham E, et al. Transfusion-related acute lung injury: definition and review. *Crit Care Med.* April 2005;**33**(4):721–726.

17 Engoren M, Habib R, Zacharias A, *et al.* Effect of blood transfusion on long-term survival after cardiac operation. *Ann Thorac Surg.* 2002;**74**:1180–1186.

18 Yusuf S, Zhao F, Mehta S, *et al.* The CURE Trial Investigators. Effects of clopidogrel in addition to aspirin in patients with acute coronary syndromes without ST-segment elevation. *N Engl J Med.* 2001;**345**:494–502.

19 Ferraris VA, Ferraris SP, Saha SP, *et al.* Perioperative blood transfusion and blood conservation in cardiac surgery: the Society of Thoracic Surgeons and The Society of Cardiovascular Anesthesiologists clinical practice guideline. *Ann Thorac Surg.* 2007;**83**:S27–S86.

20 Levy J, Tanaka K. Inflammatory response to cardiopulmonary bypass. *Ann Thorac Surg.* 2003;**75**:S715–S720.

21 Valter C, Chiara G, Annalisa F, *et al.* Activation of coagulation and fibrinolysis during coronary surgery: on-pump versus off-pump techniques. *Anesthesiolgy.* November 2001;**95**:5.

22 Linden J, Lindvall G, Sartipy U. Aprotinin decreases postoperative bleeding and number of transfusions in patients on clopidogrel undergoing coronary artery bypass graft surgery. *Circulation.* August 30, 2005;**112**(9 Suppl):I276–I280.

23 Mangano D, Tudor I, Dietzel C. The risk associated with aprotinin in cardiac surgery. *N Eng J Med.* 2006;**354**:353–365.

24 Weintraub W, Jones E, Craver J, *et al.* Frequency of repeat coronary bypass or coronary angioplasty after coronary artery bypass surgery using saphenous venous grafts. *Am J Cardiol.* 1994;**73**:103–112.

25 Shah P, Gordon, Fuller J, *et al.* Factors affecting saphenous vein graft patency: clinical and angiographic study in 1042 symptomatic patients operated on between 1977 and 1999. *J Thorac Cardiovasc Surg.* 2003;**126**:1972–1977.

26 Jawien A, Bowen-Pope D, Lindner V, Schwrtz, *et al.* Platelet-derived growth factor promotes smooth muscle migration and intimal thickening in a rat model of balloon angioplasty. *J Clin Invest.* 1992;**89**:507–511.

27 Hollopeter G, Jantzen H, Vincent D, *et al.* Identification of the platelet ADP receptor targeted by antithrombotic drugs. *Nature.* 2001;**409**:202–207.

PART VIII

Anticoagulation anomalies

CHAPTER 35

Heparin-induced thrombocytopenia

Ignacio Cruz-Gonzalez, Maria Sanchez-Ledesma, &
Ik-Kyung Jang
Harvard Medical School, Boston, MA, USA

Introduction

Heparin is the most commonly used anticoagulant, with more than 1 trillion units used and 12 million patients treated annually (1,2). In cardiac catheterization, heparin is routinely used to prevent thromboembolic complications related to intraarterial catheter use.

The most common, well-recognized complication of heparin is hemorrhage, but a second and potentially more catastrophic complication is the development of heparin-induced thrombocytopenia. Heparin-induced thrombocytopenia (HIT; sometimes known as HIT type II) is a serious, immune-mediated complication of heparin therapy, often resulting in devastating thromboembolic outcomes.

Pathogenesis

HIT is caused by the antibodies, most frequently IgG, binding to the heparin–platelet factor 4 (PF4) complex. Heparin–PF4 antibodies activate platelets, causing the release of prothrombotic microparticles, platelet consumption, and thrombocytopenia (3,4). The microparticles in turn promote excessive thrombin generation, frequently resulting in

Pharmacology in the Catheterization Laboratory. Edited by Ron Waksman and Andrew E Ajani. © 2010 Blackwell Publishing, ISBN: 978-1-4051-5704-9.

thrombosis. The antibody–antigen complexes also interact with monocytes, leading to tissue factor production (5), and antibody-mediated endothelial injury may occur (6). Both of these latter processes may contribute further to thrombosis.

No distinguishing clinical or laboratory feature has yet been identified to predict which individual with heparin–PF4 antibodies will progress to HIT (7). But heparin–PF4 antibodies that fail to induce HIT appear to remain clinically significant in some patients. In some studies, the presence of heparin–PF4 antibodies in patients with acute coronary syndromes and normal platelet counts is associated with significantly higher rates of myocardial infarction at 30 days and with thrombotic outcomes at 1 year (8).

Incidence

The reported estimates of the frequency of HIT vary widely. As many as 10–20% of patients receiving unfractionated heparin will experience a fall in platelet count to less than the normal range or a 50% fall from the baseline. Most of these cases represent nonimmune type I disease. True immune-mediated HIT occurs in 0.5–5% of patients treated with heparin, depending on various factors, including the patient population and heparin type used (7,9–12). Despite variability in the frequency of HIT, patients of any age receiving any type of heparin at any dose by any route of administration can develop HIT (13,14).

Clinical manifestations

HIT typically occurs 5–14 days after the initiation of heparin therapy (15). But rapid-onset HIT and delayed-onset HIT are alternative presentations that are increasingly being recognized. Early onset of HIT (median time 10.5 h after the start of heparin administration) may be seen in about 30% of patients with persistent antibodies due to heparin therapy within the previous 3 months (16). In delayed-onset HIT, the thrombocytopenia occurs several days, possibly up to 3 weeks, after heparin has been stopped, often after hospital discharge (17).

The *thrombocytopenia* of HIT is typically moderate in severity, with median platelet counts of $50–80 \times 10^9$/L. This is in contrast to other immune-mediated thrombocytopenias such as idiopathic thrombocytopenic purpura and posttransfusion purpura where patients often present with platelet counts below 10,000/μL and clinical bleeding (18). Despite thrombocytopenia, bleeding is rare. Rather, HIT is strongly associated with thrombosis (16). Indeed, *thrombosis* often leads to the initial recognition of HIT. This risk persists well after platelet counts return to normal, which typically occurs within a week of stopping heparin (19–21).

Other complications of HIT include skin lesions and acute systemic reactions. Erythematous or necrotizing skin lesions occur at the heparin injection site in 10–20% of patients who develop heparin–PF4 antibodies during subcutaneous heparin therapy (22).

Diagnosis

The diagnosis of HIT is based on its typical clinical picture, that is, isolated thrombocytopenia in a patient treated for at least 5 days with a heparin product, or acute thrombosis associated with thrombocytopenia, and after other causes of thrombocytopenia have been excluded.

The "4 Ts" of HIT may be useful for assessing patients with suspected HIT and provide a catchy memory device for the salient clinical features of HIT (Table 35.1) (23).

Since the drop on platelet count is almost always present in HIT patients, routine monitoring of the platelet count is recommended for all patients receiving heparin therapy (15,24). A baseline platelet count before initiating heparin treatment is important to allow estimation of relative changes. In higher risk patients, the platelet count should be checked at least every day until day 14 of therapy (or until heparin is stopped). In lower-risk patients, monitoring should be at least every 2 or 3 days between days 4 and 14 while on heparin therapy (15).

Laboratory testing

The College of American Pathologists recommends heparin–PF4 antibody testing for patients in whom there is suspicion of HIT based on the temporal features of the thrombocytopenia or on the occurrence of new thrombosis during or soon after heparin treatment (25). Results from laboratory

Table 35.1 The "4 T's" assessment point system for patients with suspected HIT.

Category	2 Points	1 Point	0 Points
Thrombocytopenia	>50% fall, or nadir of $20–100 \times 10^9$/L	30–50% fall, or nadir of $10–19 \times 10^9$/L	<30% fall or nadir <10×10^9/L
Timing of platelet count fall	Days 5–10, or ≤1 day if heparin exposure within past 30 days	>Day 10 or unclear (but fits with HIT), or ≤1 day if heparin exposure within past 30–100 days	≤1 day (no recent heparin)
Thrombosis or other sequelae	Proven thrombosis, skin necrosis, or, after heparin bolus, acute systemic reaction	Progressive, recurrent, or silent thrombosis; erythematous skin lesions	None
Other cause for thrombocytopenia	None evident	Possible	Definite

Source: Adapted from Jang et al. (24).

tests for HIT antibodies may not be obtained for hours to days after being ordered. Because of the increased thrombotic risk early in the progression of HIT (26,27), appropriate therapy in a patient with suspected HIT must not be delayed pending laboratory results.

Antigenic and functional tests for heparin–PF4 antibodies are available yet often are labor intensive and time-consuming (25). The ELISA, an antigenic assay, has a sensitivity of 90%; however, it also detects antibodies that do not elicit HIT (false-positives) and has decreased specificity in certain populations such as cardiac surgery patients. Functional tests, including platelet aggregometry and the [14C] serotonin release assay, measure platelet activity in the presence of patient sera and heparin. Platelet aggregometry has a sensitivity of 35–85%, and acute-phase reactants can cause false-positives; its sensitivity and specificity can be improved by using washed platelets from normal donors (28). The serotonin-release assay is sensitive and specific (95%) yet is technically demanding, involves radioisotope, and is generally used as a confirmation test only.

Flow cytometric assays, including methods to detect platelet microparticle release and annexin V binding (29), are described that are strongly correlated with the serotonin release assay yet do not use radioisotope.

No single assay, however, has 100% sensitivity and specificity. Although testing becomes most effective when functional and antigen tests are done in combination and multiple samples are taken (30). This approach is often impractical and results are unlikely to be available in a timely manner.

Treatment

When HIT is suspected, all heparins must be avoided, including low-molecular-weight heparins, heparin flushes, heparin-coated catheters, and any other sources, and alternative anticoagulation must be initiated immediately. This treatment recommendation applies to HIT patients diagnosed with thrombocytopenia alone or with thromboembolism (15). In the absence of alternative anticoagulation, the risk of thrombosis is 5–10% per day in the first few days after stopping heparin, increasing to a total risk of 38–76% within a month (20). Appropriate treatment therefore requires immediately removing the trigger (stop heparin) as well as controlling the thrombin storm of HIT with appropriate alternative anticoagulation (Table 35.2).

In the specific setting of percutaneous coronary intervention (PCI), some considerations should be made.

Argatroban is an alternative anticoagulant approved for use in patients with or at risk for HIT who undergo PCI. The safety and efficacy of argatroban in this setting were evaluated in three similarly designed, multicenter, prospective

Table 35.2 Comparison of alternative anticoagulants.

Feature	Argratroban	Lepirudin
Mode of action	Direct thrombin inhibitor	Direct thrombin inhibitor
Molecular weight (Da)	526	6979
Cross-reactivity with HIT sera	No	No
Recommended dose	2 µg/kg per minute, adjusted to achieve aPTTs 1.5–3 times the baseline value (reduced dose if hepatic impairment) PCI[a]: 350 µg/kg initial bolus followed by 25 µg/kg per minute, adjusted to achieve ACTs of 300–450 s	0.4-mg/kg initial bolus followed by a 0.15-mg/kg per hour infusion, adjusted to achieve aPTT ratios of 1.5–2.5 (reduced dose if renal impairment)
Primary route of elimination	Hepatic	Renal
Elimination half-life	39–51 min	1.7 h
Monitoring	aPTT or ACT	aPTT or ECT
Antidote	None	None

[a]Reduced doses may be appropriate if used in combination with GP IIb/IIIa (32).

studies, and the combined-study data are reported (31).

Patients with clinically significant hepatic dysfunction were excluded. Overall, 91 patients with HIT or a history of HIT underwent 112 PCIs while receiving intravenous argatroban 25 µg/kg per minute following 350 µg/kg initial bolus, adjusted to achieve ACTs of 300–450 s. Among the 91 patients undergoing their first PCI on argatroban, subjective assessments of the satisfactory outcome of the procedure and adequate anticoagulation during PCI were achieved in 94.5% and 97.8%, respectively; 7.7% patients experienced the composite of death (no patient), myocardial infarction (four patients), or revascularization (four patients) within 24 h of PCI, and one (1.1%) patient had periprocedural major bleeding.

No unsatisfactory outcomes occurred in 21 patients who underwent repeated PCI on argatroban at a mean of 150 days later. Findings from a multicenter, prospective study evaluating argatroban and GP IIb/IIIa inhibition therapy in patients undergoing PCI, while not conducted specifically in HIT patients, suggest that a reduced dose of argatroban (perhaps a 300 µg/kg bolus, followed by a 15 µg/kg per minute infusion) provides adequate anticoagulation in combination with GP IIb/IIIa inhibition during PCI (32).

Bivalirudin has been evaluated in a prospective, open-label study of 52 patients with HIT undergoing PCI (2,33). Patients with severe renal impairment were excluded. Bivalirudin was administered as a 0.75 or 1.0 mg/kg bolus followed by a 1.75 or 2.5 mg/kg/h infusion for 4 h. The primary end point, major bleeding 48 h after discontinuation or until discharge, occurred in one (1.9%) patient. Procedural success (TIMI grade 3 flow and <50% stenosis) and clinical success (absence of death, emergency bypass surgery, or Q-wave infarction) occurred in 98% and 96% of patients, respectively. Furthermore, bivalirudin is indicated in the United States as an anticoagulant in patients with unstable angina undergoing percutaneous transluminal coronary angioplasty (34). And it is used in patients undergoing PCI with (or at risk of) heparin-induced.

Experience with lepirudin in patients with HIT undergoing PCI is limited to case reports and small, retrospective case series (35,36).

In the largest retrospective series (35), nine patients with a history of HIT or current HIT underwent ten interventional procedures with lepirudin anticoagulation and GP IIb/IIIa blockade. Procedural success (30% residual stenosis with TIMI 3 flow without death, myocardial infarction, or emergent revascularization within 30 days) was achieved in seven procedures, and one patient required transfusion.

Additional treatment considerations

Platelet transfusions should not be used for prophylaxis in HIT because they may exacerbate the hypercoagulable state, leading to additional thrombosis (15).

Thromboembolectomy or systemic or local thrombolysis, as adjunctive therapy to alternative parenteral anticoagulation, may be appropriate for selected patients with large-vessel arterial thromboembolism or severe pulmonary embolism, respectively (37).

GP IIb/IIIa inhibitors have been used successfully with alternative anticoagulants during PCI (37). However, these agents lack direct anticoagulant effects and do not inhibit Fc receptor–mediated activation of platelets by HIT antibody (37). Hence, GP IIb/IIIa inhibitors should not be used as a sole therapy for treating HIT.

Chronic anticoagulation

In patients with HIT initiation of warfarin must be delayed until adequate alternative parenteral anticoagulation has been provided and platelet counts have recovered substantially (to at least 100,000–109,000/mL or preferably 150,000–109,000/mL) (15). Warfarin should be started at the expected maintenance dose and not at a loading dose. Parenteral anticoagulation should be overlapped with warfarin for minimum of 5 days. When transitioning from a direct thrombin inhibitor, careful monitoring may be needed. Direct thrombin inhibitors prolong the INR (38), the extent of which depends on the drug and its concentration, the residual vitamin K-dependent protein activity, and the assay reagent (39).

Previously established relations with regard to bleeding risk and INRs during warfarin therapy are not fully applicable during direct thrombin inhibition. INRs >5 commonly occur during argatroban therapy and argatroban–warfarin cotherapy in HIT, without bleeding complications (38).

Guidelines for monitoring the transition from lepirudin (26) or argatroban (40) to oral anticoagulation have been published. Warfarin therapy is maintained for a minimum of 3–6 months (37).

Bleeding is a safety concern with any anticoagulant therapy. Direct thrombin inhibitors lack a specific antidote. In case of excessive levels of anticoagulation, with or without bleeding, the anticoagulant should be stopped or its dose decreased. With the direct thrombin inhibitors, anticoagulant effects decrease to baseline, typically within hours, in accordance with the drug's elimination half-life and the patient's organ function. Specifically, the half-life of argatroban (39–51 min) is increased with hepatic impairment (41) and the half-lives of lepirudin (1.7 h) and bivalirudin (36 min) are increased with renal impairment (42,43).

Hemodialysis or hemofiltration can sometimes reduce levels of lepirudin or bivalirudin; however, drug filtration characteristics vary considerably by filter type (44). Dialytic clearance of argatroban by high-flux membranes is clinically insignificant (45). Limited data exist on the use of recombinant factor VIIa as a nonspecific antidote for treating severe bleeding in patients with HIT (46).

Patients with a history of HIT

Patients with a history of HIT may not invariably have recurrent HIT on heparin reexposure (37). In addition, heparin has been tolerated for a brief period, such as during cardiac surgery, in patients in whom heparin–PF4 antibodies have fully waned (5). It is probably safe to rechallenge heparin after 3 months. However, until the risk of recurrent HIT in patients with a history of HIT is better defined, and because the consequences of recurrent HIT may be devastating, it is generally considered prudent to use an alternative anticoagulant to avoid reexposing these "at-risk" patients to heparin when possible (15,47).

Conclusions

In patients who had received heparin and developed a new thrombocytopenia and/or had a thromboembolic event is highly suspicious of HIT. But other causes of thrombocytopenia should always be ruled out. Measurement of PF4 heparin antibodies is warranted, although appropriate therapy in a patient with suspected HIT must not be delayed pending laboratory results. These patients should be treated with a direct thrombin inhibitor until their platelet counts recovered, and parenteral anticoagulation should be overlapped with warfarin for minimum of 5 days. It is recommended to maintain oral anticoagulation for 3–6 months. Patients with a history of HIT may not invariably have recurrent HIT on heparin reexposure, but because the consequences of recurrent HIT may be devastating, it is generally considered prudent to use an alternative anticoagulant to avoid reexposure.

References

1 Fahey VA. Heparin-induced thrombocytopenia. *J Vasc Nurs*. 1995;**467**(13):112–116.

2 Campbell KR, Mahaffey KW, Lewis BF, *et al*. Bivalirudin in patients with heparin-induced thrombocytopenia undergoing percutaneous coronary intervention. *J Invasc Cardiol*. 2000;**12**:14–19.

3 Chong BH, Fawaz I, Chesterman CN, Berndt MC. Heparin-induced thrombocytopenia: mechanism of interaction of the heparin-dependent antibody with platelets. *Br J Haematol*. 1989;**73**:235–240.

4 Warkentin TE, Hayward CPM, Boshkov LK, *et al*. Sera from patients with heparin-induced thrombocytopenia generate platelet-derived microparticles with procoagulant activity: an explanation for the thrombotic complications of heparin induced. *Blood*. 1994;**84**:3691–3699.

5 Arepally GM, Mayer IM. Antibodies from patients with heparin-induced thrombocytopenia stimulate monocytic cells to express tissue factor and secrete interleukin 8. *Blood*. 2001;**98**:1252–1254.

6 Cines DB, Tomaski A, Tannenbaum S. Immune endothelial-cell injury in heparin-associated thrombocytopenia. *N Engl J Med*. 1987;**316**:581–589.

7 Warkentin TE, Sheppard JI, Horsewood P, Simpson PJ, Moore JC, Kelton JG. Impact of the patient population on the risk for heparin induced thrombocytopenia. *Blood*. 2000;**96**:1703–1708.

8 Mattioli AV, Bonetti L, Sternieri S, Mattioli G. Heparin-induced thrombocytopenia in patients treated with unfractionated heparin: prevalence of thrombosis in a 1 year follow-up. *Ital Heart J*. 2000;**1**:39–42.

9 Verma AK, Levine M, Shalansky SJ, Carter CJ, Kelton JG. Frequency of heparin-induced thrombocytopenia in critical care patients. *Pharmacotherapy*. 2003;**23**:745–753.

10 Girolami B, Prandoni P, Stefani PM, *et al.* The incidence of heparininduced thrombocytopenia in hospitalized medical patients treated with subcutaneous unfractionated heparin: a prospective cohort study. *Blood*. 2003;**101**:2955–2959.

11 Yamamoto S, Koide M, Matsuo M, *et al.* Heparin-induced thrombocytopenia in hemodialysis patients. *Am J Kidney Dis*. 1996;**28**:82–85.

12 Martel N, Lee J, Wells PS. Risk for heparin-induced thrombocytopenia with unfractionated and low-molecular-weight heparin thromboprophylaxis: a meta-analysis. *Blood*. 2005;**106**:2710–2715.

13 Shuster TA, Silliman WR, Coats RD, Mureebe L, Silver D. Heparin induced thrombocytopenia: twenty-nine years later. *J Vasc Surg*. 2003;**38**:1316–1322.

14 Matsuo T, Tomaru T, Kario K, Hirokawa T, HIT Research Group of Japan. Incidence of heparin–PF4 complex antibody formation and heparin-induced thrombocytopenia in acute coronary syndrome. *Thromb Res*. 2005;**115**:475–481.

15 Warkentin TE, Greinacher A. Heparin-induced thrombocytopenia: recognition, treatment, and prevention: the Seventh ACCP Conference on Antithrombotic and Thrombolytic Therapy. *Chest*. 2004;**126**:311–337.

16 Warkentin TE, Levine MN, Hirsh J, *et al.* Heparin-induced thrombocytopenia in patients treated with low-molecular-weight heparin or unfractionated heparin. *N Engl J Med*. 1995;**332**:13301335.

17 Warkentin TE, Kelton JG. Delayed-onset heparin-induced thrombocytopenia and thrombosis. *Ann Intern Med*. 2001;**135**:502–506.

18 Lacey JV, Penner JA. Management of idiopathic thrombocytopenic purpura in the adult. *Semin Thromb Hemost*. 1977;**3**:160–174.

19 Lewis BE, Wallis DE, Leya F, Hursting MJ, Kelton JG. Argatroban anticoagulation in patients with heparin-induced thrombocytopenia. *Arch Intern Med*. 2003;**163**:1849–1856.

20 Hirsh J, Heddle N, Kelton JG. Treatment of heparin-induced thrombocytopenia: a critical review. *Arch Intern Med*. 2004;**164**:361–369.

21 Chong BH, Gallus AS, Cade JF, *et al.* Prospective randomized open-label comparison of danaparoid with dextran 70 in the treatment of heparin-induced thrombocytopenia with thrombosis. *Thromb Haemost*. 2001;**86**:1170–1175.

22 Warkentin TE. Heparin-induced skin lesions. *Br J Haematol*. 1996;**92**:494–497.

23 Warkentin TE, Aird WC, Rand JH. Platelet-endothelial interactions: sepsis, HIT, and antiphospholipid syndrome. *Hematology (Am Soc Hematol Educ Prog)*. 2003;**1**:497–519.

24 Jang IK, Hursting MJ. When heparins promote thrombosis: review of heparin-induced thrombocytopenia. *Circulation*. 2005;**111**:2671–2683.

25 Warkentin TE. Platelet count monitoring and laboratory testing for heparin-induced thrombocytopenia: recommendations of the College of American Pathologists. *Arch Pathol Lab Med*. 2002;**126**:1415–1423.

26 Greinacher A, Volpel H, Janssens U, *et al.* Recombinant hirudin (lepirudin) provides safe and effective anticoagulation in patients with heparin-induced thrombocytopenia: a prospective study. *Circulation*. 1999;**99**:73–80.

27 Greinacher A, Janssens U, Berg G, *et al.* Lepirudin (recombinant hirudin) for parenteral anticoagulation in patients with heparin-induced thrombocytopenia. *Circulation*. 1999;**100**:587–593.

28 Warkentin TE, Heddle NM. Laboratory diagnosis of immune heparininduced thrombocytopenia. *Curr Hematol Rep*. 2003;**2**:148–157.

29 Tomer A. A sensitive and specific functional flow cytometric assay for the diagnosis of heparin-induced thrombocytopenia. *Br J Haematol*. 1997;**98**:648–656.

30 Pouplard C, Amiral J, Borg J-Y, Laporte-Simitsidis S, Delahousse B, Gruel Y. Decision analysis for use of platelet aggregation test, carbon 14-serotonin release assay, and heparin–platelet factor 4 enzyme-linked immunosorbent assay for diagnosis of heparin-induced thrombocytopenia. *Am J Clin Pathol*. 1999;**111**:700–706.

31 Lewis BE, Matthai WH, Cohen M, Moses JW, Hursting MJ, Leya F. Argatroban anticoagulation during percutaneous coronary intervention in patients with heparin-induced thrombocytopenia. *Cathet Cardiovasc Interv*. 2002;**57**:177–184.

32 Jang IK, Lewis BE, Matthai WH, Kleiman NS. Argatroban anticoagulation in conjunction with glycoprotein IIb/IIIa inhibition in patients undergoing percutaneous coronary intervention: an open-label, nonran-domized pilot study. *J Thromb Thrombolysis*. 2004;**18**:31–37.

33 Mahaffey KW, Lewis BE, Wildermann NM, *et al.* The anticoagulant therapy with bivalirudin to assist in the performance of percutaneous coronary intervention in patients with heparin-induced thrombocytopenia (ATBAT) study: main results. *J Invasive Cardiol*. 2003; **15**:611–616.

34 Bittl JA, Chaitman BR, Feit F, Kimball W, Topol EJ. Bivalirudin versus heparin during coronary angioplasty for unstable or postinfarction angina: final report reanalysis of the Bivalirudin Angioplasty Study. *Am Heart J*. 2001;**142**:952–959.

35 Pinto DS, Sperling RT, Tu RM, Cohen DJ, Carrozza JP. Combination platelet glycoprotein IIb/IIIa receptor and lepirudin administration during percutaneous coronary

intervention in patients with heparin-induced thrombocytopenia. *Cathet Cardiovasc Interv.* 2003;**58**:65–68.

36 Manfredi JA, Wall RP, Sane DC, Braden GA. Lepirudin as a safe alternative for effective anticoagulation in patients with known heparin-induced thrombocytopenia undergoing percutaneous coronary intervention: case reports. *Cathet Cardiovasc Interv.* 2001;**52**:468–472.

37 Greinacher A, Warkentin TE. Treatment of heparin-induced thrombo-cytopenia: an overview. In: Warketin TE, Greinacher A, eds. *Heparin-Induced Thrombocytopenia*, 3rd ed. New York, NY: Marcel Dekker; 2004:335–370.

38 Hursting MJ, Lewis BE, Macfarlane DE. Transitioning from argatroban to warfarin therapy in patients with heparin-induced thrombocytopenia. *Clin Appl Thromb Hemost.* 2005;**11**:279–287.

39 Gosselin RC, Dager WE, King JH, *et al.* Effect of direct thrombin inhibitors, bivalirudin, lepirudin, and argatroban, on prothrombin time and INR values. *Am J Clin Pathol.* 2004;**121**:593–599.

40 Harder S, Graff J, Klinkhardt U, *et al.* Transition from argatroban to oral anticoagulation with phenprocoumon or acenocoumarol: effects on pro-thrombin time, activated partial thromboplastin time, and ecarin clotting time. *Thromb Haemost.* 2004;**91**:1137–1145.

41 Swan SK, Hursting MJ. The pharmacokinetics and pharmacodynamics of argatroban: effects of age, gender, and hepatic or renal dysfunction. *Pharmacotherapy.* 2000;**20**:318–329.

42 Vanholder R, Camez A, Veys N, Van Loo A, Dhondt AM, Rignoir S. Pharmacokinetics of recombinant hirudin in hemodialyzed end-stage renal failure patients. *Thromb Haemost.* 1997;**77**:650–655.

43 Fox I, Dawson A, Loynds P, *et al.* Anticoagulant activity of hirulog, a direct thrombin inhibitor, in humans. *Thromb Haemost.* 1993;**69**:157–163.

44 Fischer KG. Hirudin in renal insufficiency. *Semin Thromb Hemost.* 2002;**28**:467–482.

45 Murray PM, Reddy BV, Grossman EJ, *et al.* A prospective comparison of three argatroban treatment regimens during in end-stage renal disease. *Kidney Int.* 2004;**66**:2446–2453.

46 Stratmann G, diSilva AM, Tseng EE, *et al.* Reversal of direct thrombin inhibition after cardiopulmonary bypass in a patient with heparin-induced thrombocytopenia. *Anesth Analg.* 2004;**98**:1635–1639.

47 Warkentin TE, Kelton JG. Temporal aspects of heparin-induced thrombocytopenia. *N Engl J Med.* 2001;**344**:1286–1292.

CHAPTER 36

Thrombocytopenia, anemia, and transfusion of blood products in patients undergoing percutaneous coronary interventions

Eugenia Nikolsky[1] & Pravin Kahale[2]
[1]Cardiovascular Research Foundation, New York, NY, USA
[2]Adventist Wockhardt Hospital, Surat, India

The critical role of platelets in the pathogenesis of coronary artery disease (CAD) and response of platelets to balloon-mediated vascular injury after angioplasty or stent implantation have been well documented (1–3). Atherosclerotic plaque rupture and superimposed thrombus, resulting in limitation or interruption of coronary blood flow, represent the most common underlying cause of acute cardiac events (4,5). Platelets and thrombin play a fundamental role in thrombus formation, leading to acute coronary syndromes (1–5). Thrombin converts fibrinogen to fibrin, activate platelets, and mobilizes additional platelets into the platelet-rich thrombus.

Complex antiplatelet and antithrombotic regimens have significantly reduced incidence of ischemic complications related to percutaneous coronary intervention (PCI), but may result in serious side effects that need timely recognition and management. This chapter will review several complications related to periprocedural anticoagulation therapy.

Pharmacology in the Catheterization Laboratory. Edited by Ron Waksman and Andrew E Ajani. © 2010 Blackwell Publishing, ISBN: 978-1-4051-5704-9.

Heparin-induced thrombocytopenia

Unfractionated heparin (UFH) for many years was the only intraprocedural antithrombin agent. UFH inhibits factor IIa (thrombin) indirectly, via accelerating the action of antithrombin III, an enzyme that inactivates thrombin, factor IXa, and factor Xa. One of the important limitations of UFH is its formation of multimolecular complexes with a platelet surface glycoprotein (GP) known as platelet factor 4 (PF4). These complexes may initiate production of antibodies (mostly of IgG class) directed against PF4 and be a cause of immune-mediated heparin-induced thrombocytopenia (HIT).

On the basis of several principal differences, HIT has been divided into two types. HIT Type I is typically a benign condition, and as a rule, is limited to a mild drop in platelet count (to a nadir of $100 \times 10^9/L$ to $150 \times 10^9/L$) (6). It develops as a result of direct interaction between UFH and circulating platelets and typically does not increase propensity to bleeding. On the contrary, HIT type II is a potentially life-threatening condition that can result in a hypercoagulable state. It is an immune-mediated disorder that may present as an isolated heparin-induced thrombocytopenia (HIT) or as thrombocytopenia with thrombosis syndrome (HITTS), and is associated with significant mortality and morbidity. HIT type II is diagnosed based on clinical and immunologic criteria including a decrease in the platelet count to $<150 \times 10^9$/L or >50% below baseline values at least 5 days after the beginning of UFH therapy, resolution of thrombocytopenia after the cessation of UFH administration, exclusion of other possible reasons for thrombocytopenia, and the detection of heparin-dependent antiplatelet antibodies (6). Several assays for detecting HIT-induced antibodies have been proposed. However, no assay has provided 100% sensitivity and specificity, and, therefore, the confirmation of diagnosis requires using of at least two different methods. A negative testing for HIT antibodies using two sensitive assays usually rules out HIT, even if the clinical picture is suggestive of HIT (7). Given the reported time course of HIT, early recognition of HIT necessitates close monitoring of platelet counts starting on day 4 after initiation of UFH administration.

Development of immune-mediated HIT type II is associated with high risk of thromboembolic complications. Specifically, the overall risk of HIT-related thrombosis and mortality is approximately 75% and 30%, respectively (8,9).

Treatment of HIT

Type I HIT usually does not require special treatment, and platelet counts usually return to normal even if UFH is continued. The initial step in the treatment of immune-mediated HIT is discontinuation of UFH and avoidance of other potential sources of UFH (e.g., flush solutions and heparin-coated catheters and stents). High incidence of thrombotic events in patients with immune-mediated HIT necessitates anticoagulation with alternative agents.

Direct thrombin inhibitors (recombinant hirudin [lepirudin] and argatroban) are the treatment of choice in management of HIT and HITTS (Table 36.1). These agents are able to inactivate clot-bound as well as free thrombin, rapidly achieve a steady state and do not cross-react with HIT antibodies. Two prospective, multicenter trials, undertaken in Europe, HAT-1 (10) and HAT-2 (11), compared the efficacy of lepirudin vs historical controls in patients with confirmed HIT. In both studies, lepirudin provided rapid normalization of low platelet count or maintained normal platelet count in 88.7% (HAT-1) and 92.6% (HAT-2) of the patients. The incidence of the primary combined end point (new thromboembolic

Table 36.1 Approved direct thrombin inhibitors.

	Lepirudin (r-hirudin, Refludan®)	Argatroban	Bivalirudin (hirulog, angiomax)
Molecular weight	6979.5 Da	508.7 Da	2,180 Da
Elimination half-life, min	60–80 min	39–51 min	60 min
Clearance	Renal	Biliary secretion	Renal and proteolytic cleavage
Regimen of administration	Bolus 0.3–0.5 mg/kg IV, followed by IV infusion 0.12 mg/kg/h for 24 h or 0.24 mg/kg/h for 24 h followed by 0.04 mg/kg/h for 24 h	Start with continuous infusion at 2 µg/kg/min, titrate until steady-state aPTT is ×1.5–3.0 baseline value	Bolus 0.75 mg/kg IV, followed by IV infusion 1.75 mg/kg/h up to 4 h
Dosage adjustment	Infusion rate in patients with *renal impairment*: 0.075 mg/kg/h in patients with CrCl ≥45–60 mL/min and serum Cr 1.6–2.0 mg/dL; 0.045 mg/kg/h in patients with CrCl ≥30–44 mL/min, and serum Cr 2.1–3.0 mg/dL; and 0.0225 mg/kg/h in patients with CrCl ≥15–29 mL/min and serum Cr 3.1–6.0mg/dL	In patients with *hepatic impairment*: start with infusion at 0.5 µg/kg/min, titrate until steady-state aPTT is ×1.5–3.0 baseline value, but not to exceed 10 µg/kg/min or an aPTT >100s	In patients with *renal impairment*: infusion rate is reduced to 20% in patients with GFR 30–59 mL/min and CrCl 2.7 mL/min/kg, to 60% in patients with GFR 10–29 mL/min and CrCl 2.8 mL/min/kg, and to 90% in patients on dialysis and CrCl 1 mL/min/kg

complications, limb amputation, or death) at day 35 was 52.1% in the historical control group compared with 25.4% in HAT-1 and 31.9% in HAT-2 (10,11).

Argatroban treatment of patients with HIT has also been shown to improve clinical outcomes and slow disease progression compared with historical controls. The composite rates of death, amputation, or new thrombosis were significantly lower in argatroban-treated patients than in control group (25.6% vs 38.8% respectively, $p = 0.01$) (12). Mortality caused by thrombosis was also reduced significantly in both patients with HIT (0% vs 4.8%; $p = 0.005$) and patients with HITTS (0.7% vs 15.2%; $p < 0.001$) (12).

Direct thrombin inhibitors are also the anticoagulation regimen of choice in patients undergoing PCI who have previously been diagnosed with HIT or HITTS. Several trials and observational studies have demonstrated the feasibility and the efficacy of direct thrombin inhibitors in the PCI setting (12–16). In the pooled patent-based analysis from three prospective multicenter trials (ARD-216, ARG-310, and ARG-311) assessing the use of argatroban in 91 patients with HIT undergoing elective, urgent or emergent PCI, satisfactory outcome was obtained in 94.5% of the group treated with argatroban for the first time and 100% of the group treated with argatroban repeatedly (17). The majority of patients in each group were free from death, myocardial infarction, and emergent coronary bypass surgery (97.8% and 100%, respectively). Adequate anticoagulation was achieved in 97.8% and 100% of the patients, respectively. Major bleeding was uncommon in both groups (1.1% and 0%, respectively).

Prospective, multicenter, open-label ATBAT registry evaluated safety and efficacy of bivalirudin, a semisynthetic derivate of native hirudin (Table 36.1) in 52 patients with newly diagnosed HIT (37%), history of HIT (43%) or HITTS (21%) undergoing PCI (18). In this registry, two patients had platelet drop of 40–50%, but absolute platelet count did not decrease to lower than 75×10^9/L. No patients developed thrombocytopenia less than 50×10^9/L, and no patients had bleeding or thrombotic complications (18).

Thrombocytopenia related to platelet glycoprotein IIb/IIIa receptor blockade

Adjunctive therapy with platelet GP IIb/IIIa inhibitors is an established therapeutic modality for the prevention of early ischemic complications and urgent target vessel revascularization in high-risk patients undergoing PCI. However, these drugs can also cause thrombocytopenia (19). The large-scale clinical trials assessing safety and efficacy of GP IIb/IIIa inhibitors have defined thrombocytopenia as mild, severe, or profound when nadir platelet counts decreased to less than 100×10^9/L, 50×10^9/L, and 20×10^9/L, respectively (20–22). In a pooled analysis from several trials assessing GP IIb/IIIa inhibitors, the rates of both mild and severe thrombocytopenia were higher in patients given abciximab (4.2% and 1%, respectively) than the small-molecule IIb/IIIa inhibitors (2.3% and 0.3%, respectively) (23). Moreover, when compared with placebo, only abciximab was associated with an excess of mild and severe thrombocytopenia; rates of thrombocytopenia in patients treated with small-molecule inhibitors were close to those of the placebo group (23,24). In the double-blind, randomized, multicenter Do Tirofiban and Reopro Give Similar Efficacy Outcomes (TARGET) trial, in which tirofiban and abciximab were compared in 4,089 patients with stable or acute coronary syndromes undergoing PCI, thrombocytopenia developed in 2.4% of patients treated with abciximab and 0.5% of patients treated with tirofiban (25). Profound thrombocytopenia in this study developed only in patients treated with abciximab (0.9%).

Abciximab-induced thrombocytopenia is of immune origin. Abciximab induces the formation of human antichimeric antibodies (HACA). This immune response is believed to increase platelet consumption and leads to the greater incidence of thrombocytopenia seen with abciximab than other GP IIb/IIIa inhibitors. In the Evaluation of 7E3 for the Prevention of Ischemic Complications (EPIC) trial, HACA developed within the first 12 weeks of exposure to abciximab in 5.8% of the patients, and slightly higher in the bolus-plus infusion group than in the bolus-only arm (6.5% and 5.2%, respectively) (19,26). In contrast to the abciximab group, none of the patients in the placebo group developed HACA (19).

In the EPIC trial, older age, lower weight, and lower baseline platelet count independently predicted thrombocytopenia in patients treated with abciximab (19). In the same trial, the highest rates of thrombocytopenia have been observed also in patients treated concomitantly with abciximab and full-dose heparin.

Readministration of abciximab does not increase overall rate of thrombocytopenia (5.0%), however, profound thrombocytopenia ($<20 \times 10^9$/L) is observed with an increased rate (2.0%) (26). There is no evidence of the greater incidence of thrombocytopenia after administration of abciximab among patients who formerly were exposed to tirofiban or eptifibatide (27).

Time course of IIb/IIIa inhibitor-induced thrombocytopenia

In the EPIC trial, among patients treated with abciximab, the mean time to the development of thrombocytopenia was 12 h (one-third of the patients developed thrombocytopenia 2 h after an abciximab bolus and one-half of the patients developed thrombocytopenia 12 h after the bolus), and the mean duration of thrombocytopenia was 2.2 days (19). In the TARGET trial, the mean time to onset of thrombocytopenia was 24 h, with no cases occurring later than 48 h after PCI in patients treated with either abciximab or tirofiban (25). However, in some cases, thrombocytopenia may occur either very early (90 min after the exposure to abciximab) (28) or very late (5–7 days) after abciximab or tirofiban (29,30). Patients with readministration of abciximab have an increased incidence of delayed (beyond 48 h) thrombocytopenia with a nadir platelet count between 5 and 7 days and a prolonged restoration of >7 days (26).

Clinical implications of GP IIb/IIIa inhibitor-induced thrombocytopenia

In the pooled analysis from three randomized trials (EPIC, EPILOG, and EPISTENT), thrombocytopenia was associated with an increased incidence of death (Figure 36.1) and bleeding events (31). Namely, in the abciximab group, patients that developed thrombocytopenia compared to patients without thrombocytopenia had sixfold higher

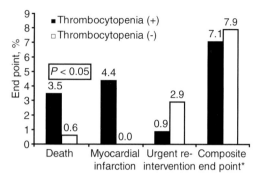

Figure 36.1 Ischemic end point events in patients with and without thrombocytopenia from a pooled analysis from the EPIC, EPILOG, and EPISTENT trials (31). Patients undergoing coronary artery bypass surgery are not included. *Composite end point includes death, myocardial infarction, and urgent reintervention.

rates of 30-day death (3.5% vs 0.6%, respectively, $P < 0.05$) and major bleeding (15.9% vs 2.7%, respectively) (31) and as a result, a significantly higher requirement for blood product transfusions (32.7% vs 4.7%). Still, compared to patients with thrombocytopenia in the placebo arm, abciximab-treated patients with thrombocytopenia had lower rates of major bleeding (15.9% and 46.2%, respectively) and any transfusion (32.7% and 61.5%, respectively). Similarly, in the TARGET trial, patients with vs without thrombocytopenia had higher rates of severe bleeding (5.1% vs 0.7%, $P = 0.001$), blood product transfusions (6.1% vs 1.4%, $P = 0.001$), 30-day death (2.0% vs 0.4%; $P=0.02$), and target vessel revascularization (12.2% vs 6.6%; $P = 0.04$) (25).

Though there are no strict recommendations for the management of thrombocytopenia related to administration of GP IIb/IIIa inhibitors, discontinuation of the drug has been recommended if the platelet count decreases to $<60 \times 10^9$/L, and platelet transfusion is advocated when the platelet count falls to $<20 \times 10^9$/L.

True thrombocytopenia in patients treated with abciximab must be distinguished from a benign laboratory condition termed pseudothrombocytopenia that is a consequence of the agglutinating effect of the ethylenediaminetetraacetate (EDTA) used as an anticoagulant in many blood collecting test tubes The incidence of pseudothrombocytopenia is approximately 2% among abciximab-treated patients, and in contrast to true thrombocytopenia, prognosis of patients with pseudothrombocytopenia do not differ from patients with normal platelet counts (32). To differentiate pseudothrombocytopenia from true thrombocytopenia, either a peripheral blood smear should be examined or the blood drawn for platelet counts should be collected in a heparin-coated tube.

Impact of preexisting anemia on outcomes of patients treated with PCI

Anemia is a frequent comorbid condition in patients with coronary artery disease (CAD). The prevalence of anemia defined by WHO (hemoglobin value <13 g/dL for men and <12 g/dL for women, or hematocrit <39% for men and <36% for women) in contemporary PCI series is as great as approximately 20% in men and 30% in women (33–35). The mechanisms underlying the detrimental influence of anemia on outcomes of patients with CAD are probably multifactorial. Populations with anemia are typically older, more frequently women and more frequently have serious comorbid conditions including diabetes, chronic renal insufficiency, chronic inflammatory diseases, and neoplasms all of which have a negative impact on prognosis (34,35). Anemia may increase myocardial oxygen demand through a secondary increase in cardiac output, dilatation and hypertrophy of cardiac chambers, and increase in plasma catecholamine levels (36–39). Anemia of chronic disease may be a marker of more advanced atherosclerosis and is known to be mediated by inflammatory cytokines (40). Depletion of nitric oxide, an endothelium-derived relaxing factor, which is essential for oxygen exchange in patients with low hemoglobin, has been hypothesized as a cause of myocardial ischemia (41). Differences in pharmacological treatments may also be a factor worsening prognosis in patients with anemia. Specifically, anemic patients are less likely to be treated with aspirin, β-blockers, and statins, all of which are have positive impact on survival (35).

In the retrospective cohort analysis of inhospital and long-term mortality in 689 males undergoing elective PCI within a 2-year period, the lowest quintile of hemoglobin was independently associated

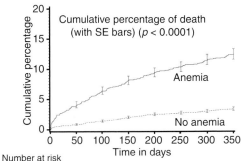

Figure 36.2 One-year survival after percutaneous coronary intervention in patients with and without anemia in patients treated with percutaneous coronary interventions. Reprodued from Nikolsky *et al.* (34).

with significantly higher all-cause and cardiac death (42). In another series of 6,929 consecutive patients treated with PCI in a large tertiary center during a 5-year period, patients with vs without anemia had significantly higher rates of inhospital death (1.9% vs 0.4%) including cardiac death (1.2% vs 0.3%), and lower 1-year survival (88.2% vs 96.5%) (Figure 36.2) (34). After adjustment for potential confounders, lower baseline hematocrit was identified as an independent predictor of 1-year mortality (odds ratio = 0.94 per 1% increase in hematocrit, 95% CI 0.91–0.97) (34). In a multicenter retrospective study of 48,851 patients with non-ST elevation myocardial infarction treated with PCI, baseline anemia was associated with significantly increased inhospital mortality in both men (3.0% vs 0.8%) and women (2.4% vs 1.5%) (43). In a study examining the outcomes of 78,974 Medicare beneficiaries ≥65 years old hospitalized for acute myocardial infarction, anemia was an independent correlate of 30-day mortality (44). In the analysis from the Myocardial Infarction Data Acquisition System, 1-year mortality was higher in patients after acute myocardial infarction with concomitant anemia compared to those without; however, the difference in mortality became insignificant after controlling for co-morbid conditions (45). Finally, in the multicenter, randomized the Controlled Abciximab and Device Investigation to Lower Late Angioplasty Complications (CADILLAC) trial of contemporary mechanical reperfusion strategies in acute myocardial infarction, patients with vs without

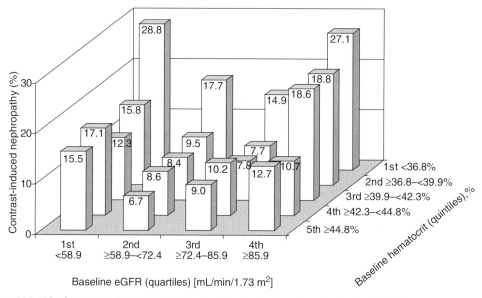

Figure 36.3 Risk of contrast-induced nephropathy in relation to baseline hematocrit and eGFR (47).

baseline anemia had strikingly higher mortality during index hospitalization (4.6% vs 1.1%), at 30 days (5.8% vs 1.5%), and at 1 year (9.4% vs 3.5%) (all $P < 0.001$) (35). Rates of disabling stroke were also higher in patients with baseline anemia both at 30 days (0.8% vs 0.1%, $P = 0.005$) and at 1-year (2.1% vs 0.4%, $P = 0.0007$) (35). In several trials, anemia was an independent predictor of inhospital and 1-year mortality (34,35,46). In the pooled analysis from 16 Thrombolysis in Myocardial Infarction (TIMI) clinical trials, in the subset of patients with ST-elevation myocardial infarction, cardiovascular mortality increased in patients with hemoglobin levels <14 g/dL, with an adjusted OR of 1.21 (95% CI 1.12–1.30, $P < 0.001$) for each 1-g/dL decrement in hemoglobin compared with control (patients with hemoglobin values of 14–15 g/dL) (46).

One study highlighted the negative impact of baseline anemia and of procedure-related blood loss in the development of CIN in patients undergoing PCI (47). A significant and independent relationship has been described between lower hematocrit and increased risk of contrast induced nephropathy (CIN): rates of CIN steadily increased as baseline hematocrit quintile decreased (from 10.3% in the highest quintile to 10.6%, 11.8%, 13.3%, and 23.3% in the lower quintiles, respectively; χ^2 for trend $P < 0.0001$). Despite significant interaction between

the baseline hematocrit and eGFR, the effect of lower eGFR was modified by higher hematocrit (Figure 36.3). By multivariable analysis, lower baseline hematocrit was identified as an independent predictor of CIN; each 3% decrease in baseline hematocrit resulted in a significant increase in the odds of CIN. A procedure-related drop in hematocrit also independently predicted CIN irrespective of baseline hematocrit, though being especially detrimental in patients with a lower hematocrit level (Figure 36.4) (47).

Impact of blood transfusion on outcomes of patients treated with PCI

Despite the widespread use of red blood cell (RBC) transfusion, there is very limited evidence to guide transfusion decisions in patients with CAD. Improved survival in patients with CAD after RBC transfusions has not been prospectively demonstrated, and the majority of data currently available examining outcomes after RBC transfusions are from retrospective series with conflicting results. In a series on patients with acute myocardial infarction, the impact of RBC transfusion appeared to be different in patients with lower vs higher hematocrit or hemoglobin values that preceded

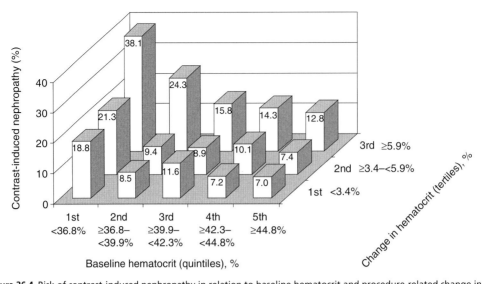

Figure 36.4 Risk of contrast-induced nephropathy in relation to baseline hematocrit and procedure-related change in hematocrit (47).

transfusion (44,46). In retrospective analysis on 78,974 Medicare beneficiaries ≥65 years old with acute myocardial infarction, RBC transfusion was associated with lower 30-day mortality among patients whose hematocrit values on admission were ≤30.0% but with increased 30-day mortality for patients whose hematocrit values were ≥36.1% (44). In a patient-level pooled analysis on 41,637 patients with acute coronary syndromes from 16 Thrombolysis In Myocardial Infarction (TIMI) trials, among 25,419 patients with ST elevation myocardial infarction, transfusion was associated with a decreased risk of cardiovascular death when the baseline hemoglobin was <12 g/dL (adjusted OR 0.42, 95% CI 0.20–0.89) but not when hemoglobin was ≥12 g/dL (adjusted OR 1.42, 95% CI 0.94–2.17) (46). However, in the same study, among 14,503 patients with non ST elevation myocardial infarction, RBC transfusion appeared to be associated with an increased risk of the composite end point of death, MI, and recurrent ischemia (adjusted OR 1.54), regardless of the baseline hemoglobin (46). Furthermore, in a study on 4,470 critically ill patients, an increase in hemoglobin in a subgroup of anemic patients with cardiac disease was associated with improved survival (48), while in the multicenter randomized Transfusion Requirement in Critical Care (TRICC) trial, 30-day mortality did not differ significantly in subgroup

of critically ill normovolemic patients with known cardiovascular disease assigned to restrictive transfusion strategy (transfused when hemoglobin was <7 g/dL, with hemoglobin was maintained between 7 and 9 g/dL) or liberal transfusion strategy (transfused when hemoglobin was <10 g/dL, with hemoglobin was maintained between 10 and 12 g/dL) (20.5% and 22.9%, respectively) (49). Two other retrospective studies also failed to show any survival benefit in patients with known CAD treated with RBC transfusion (50,51). On the contrary, in the pooled analysis from three large international trials of patients with acute coronary syndromes (the GUSTO IIb, PURSUIT, and PARAGON B trials) including 24,112 patients, those who received RBC transfusions compared to patients who did not had significantly higher rates of 30-day death (8.0% vs 3.1%, P < 0.001) and MI (25.2% vs 8.2%, P < 0.001) (50). In this analysis, after adjustment for baseline characteristics, bleeding and transfusion propensity, and nadir hematocrit, RBC transfusion was strongly associated with a hazard ratio for death of 3.9 (50). Similarly, in the Can Rapid risk stratification of Unstable Angina Patients Suppress Adverse Outcomes with Early Implementation of the American College of Cardiology/American Heart Association Guidelines (CRUSADE) National Quality Improvement Initiative that included a broad sampling of U.S. practices, after adjustment for potential confounders patients receiving RBC transfusions were 67% more likely to die and 44% more likely to experience either death or myocardial infarction during index hospitalization compared to those not transfused (51). Finally, in CADILLAC trial, short- and long-term outcome of patients undergoing contemporary mechanical reperfusion strategies for acute myocardial infarction and treated with blood transfusion (3.9% of the study population) was significantly worse compared to the patients who did not receive blood transfusion (52). Specifically, patients treated with RBC transfusion due to preceding moderate or severe bleeding event (group 1) or in the absence of bleeding (group 2) had strikingly higher rates of inhospital, 30-day, and 1-year mortality, disabling stroke, reinfarction, and composite of major adverse cardiac events regardless of preceding bleeding event. After adjustment for potential confounders including blood transfusion propensity score, RBC transfusion was identified as independent predictor of mortality at 30 days (hazard ratio 4.71 [1.97, 11.26], $p = 0.0005$), and at 1 year (hazard ratio 3.16 [1.66, 6.03], $p = 0.0005$) (52).

It is an important question whether RBC transfusion is a surrogate marker of increased comorbidities as well as complicated and less successful PCI or RBC transfusion itself may worsen prognosis of patients undergoing PCI. There are several possible ways in which RBC transfusion can produce adverse outcomes. Transfusion of RBC presents a large inflammatory stimulus and may contribute to the inflammatory state (53–56). Cytokine levels have been shown a 15-fold increase with a single RBC transfusion after coronary artery bypass grafting (54). Additional studies are required to explore the mechanism, and determine the optimal threshold for RBC transfusion in patients with undergoing PCI for stable and acute coronary syndromes. Randomized studies are needed to establish the optimal threshold for RBC transfusion and to evaluate safety of RBC transfusion compared to other alternative treatments.

References

1 Steele PM, Chesebro JH, Stanson AW, *et al*. Balloon angioplasty. Natural history of the pathophysiological response to injury in a pig model. *Circ Res*. 1985;**57**:105–112.

2 Merhi Y, Guidoin R, Provost P, Leung TK, Lam JY. Increase of neutrophil adhesion and vasoconstriction with platelet deposition after deep arterial injury by angioplasty. *Am Heart J*. 1995;**129**:445–451.

3 Fuster V, Badimon L, Badimon JJ, Chesebro JH. The pathogenesis of coronary artery disease and the acute coronary syndromes. *N Engl J Med*. 1992;**326**:242–250.

4 Burke AP, Farb A, Malcom GT, Liang YH, Smialek J, Virmani R. Coronary risk factors and plaque morphology in men with coronary disease who died suddenly. *N Engl J Med*. 1997;**336**:1276–1282.

5 Yamagishi M, Terashima M, Awano K, *et al*. Morphology of vulnerable plaque: insights from follow-up of patients examined by intravscular ultrasound before an acute coronary syndrome. *J Am Coll Cardiol*. 2000;**35**:106–111.

6 Warkentin TE, Kelton JG. Temporal aspects of heparin-induced thrombocytopenia. *N Engl J Med*. 2001;**344**:1286–1292.

7 Brieger DB, Mak KH, Kottke-Marchant K, Topol EJ. Heparin-induced thrombocytopenia. *J Am Coll Cardiol*. 1998;**31**:1449–1159.

8 Warkentin TE, Hayward CP, Boshkov LK, *et al*. Sera from patients with heparin-induced thrombocytopenia generate platelet-derived microparticles with procoagulant activity: an explanation for the thrombotic complications of heparin-induced thrombocytopenia. *Blood*. 1994;**84**:3691–3699.

9 Warkentin TE. Heparin-induced thrombocytopenia: IgG-mediated platelet activation, platelet microparticle generation, and altered procoagulant/anticoagulant balance in the pathogenesis of thrombosis and venous limb gangrene complicating heparin-induced thrombocytopenia. *Transfus Med Rev*. 1996;**10**:249–258.

10 Greinacher A, Volpel H, Janssens U, *et al*. Recombinant hirudin (lepirudin) provides safe and effective anticoagulation in patients with heparin-induced thrombocytopenia: a prospective study. *Circulation*. 1999;**99**:73–80.

11 Greinacher A, Janssens U, Berg G, *et al*. Lepirudin (recombinant hirudin) for parenteral anticoagulation in patients with heparin-induced thrombocytopenia. Heparin-Associated Thrombocytopenia Study (HAT) investigators. *Circulation*. 1999;**100**:587–593.

12 Lewis BE, Wallis DE, Leya F, Hursting MJ, Kelton JG; Argatroban-915 Investigators. Argatroban anticoagulation in patients with heparin-induced thrombocytopenia. *Arch Intern Med*. 2003;**163**:1849–1856.

13 Matsuo T, Koide M, Kario K. Development of argatroban, a direct thrombin inhibitor, and its clinical application. *Semin Thromb Hemost*. 1997;**23**:517–522.

14 Bittl JA, Chaitman BR, Feit F, Kimball W, Topol EJ. Bivalirudin versus heparin during coronary angioplasty for unstable or postinfarction angina: final report reanalysis of the Bivalirudin Angioplasty Study. *Am Heart J.* 2001;**142**:952–959.

15 Lincoff AM, Kleiman NS, Kottke-Marchant K, *et al.* Bivalirudin with planned or provisional abciximab versus low-dose heparin and abciximab during percutaneous coronary revascularization: results of the Comparison of Abciximab Complications with Hirulog for Ischemic Events Trial (CACHET). *Am Heart J.* 2002;**143**:847–853.

16 Lincoff AM, Bittl JA, Harrington RA, *et al.* Bivalirudin and provisional glycoprotein IIb/IIIa blockade compared with heparin and planned glycoprotein IIb/IIIa blockade during percutaneous coronary intervention: REPLACE-2 randomized trial. *JAMA.* 2003;**289**:853–863.

17 Lewis BE, Matthai WH, Jr, Cohen M, *et al.* Argatroban anticoagulation during percutaneous coronary intervention in patients with heparin-induced thrombocytopenia. *Catheter Cardiovasc Interv.* 2002;**57**:177–184.

18 Mahaffey KW, Lewis BE, Wildermann NM *et al.* The anticoagulant therapy with bivalirudin to assist in the performance of percutaneous coronary intervention in patients with heparin-induced thrombocytopenia (ATBAT) Study: main results. *J Invasive Cardiol.* 2003;**15**:611–616.

19 Berkowitz SD, Sane DC, Sigmon KN, *et al.* Occurrence and clinical significance of thrombocytopenia in a population undergoing high-risk percutaneous coronary revascularization. Evaluation of c7E3 for the Prevention of Ischemic Complications (EPIC) Study Group. *J Am Coll Cardiol.* 1998;**32**:311–319.

20 Topol EJ, Califf RM, Weisman HF, *et al.* Randomised trial of coronary intervention with antibody against platelet IIb/IIIa integrin for reduction of clinical restenosis: results at six months. The EPIC Investigators. *Lancet.* 1994;**343**(8902):881–886.

21 Platelet glycoprotein IIb/IIIa receptor blockade and low-dose heparin during percutaneous coronary revascularization. The EPILOG Investigators. *N Engl J Med.* 1998;**339**:1861–1863.

22 Randomised placebo-controlled and balloon-angioplasty-controlled trial to assess safety of coronary stenting with use of platelet glycoprotein-IIb/IIIa blockade. The EPISTENT Investigators. Evaluation of Platelet IIb/IIIa Inhibitor for Stenting. *Lancet.* 1998;**352**(9122):87–92.

23 Dasgupta H, Blankenship JC, Wood GC, Frey CM, Demko SL, Menapace FJ. Thrombocytopenia complicating treatment with intravenous glycoprotein IIb/IIIa receptor inhibitors: a pooled analysis. *Am Heart J.* 2000;**140**:206–211.

24 The ESPRIT Investigators. Enhanced Suppression of the Platelet IIb/IIIa Receptor with Integrilin Therapy. Novel dosing regimen of eptifibatide in planned coronary stent implantation (ESPRIT): a randomised, placebo-controlled trial. *Lancet.* 2000;**356**(9247):2037–2044.

25 Merlini PA, Rossi M, Menozzi A, *et al.* Thrombocytopenia caused by abciximab or tirofiban and its association with clinical outcome in patients undergoing coronary stenting. *Circulation.* 2004;**109**:2203–2206.

26 Tcheng JE, Kereiakes DJ, Lincoff AM, *et al.* Abciximab re-administration: results of the ReoPro Re-administration Registry. *Circulation.* 2001;**104**:870–875.

27 Lev EI, Osende JI, Richard MF, *et al.* Administration of abciximab to patients receiving tirofiban or eptifibatide: effect on platelet function. *J Am Coll Cardiol.* 2001;**37**:847–855.

28 Vahdat B, Canavy I, Fourcade L, *et al.* Fatal cerebral hemorrhage and severe thrombocytopenia during abciximab treatment. *Cathet Cardiovasc Interv.* 2000;**49**:177–180.

29 Kaluski E, Leitman M, Khiger I, Cotter G. Delayed thrombocytopenia following abciximab therapy. *Int J Cardiovasc Interv.* 2001;**4**:151–155.

30 Sharma S, Bhambi B, Nyitray W, *et al.* Delayed profound thrombocytopenia presenting 7 days after use of abciximab (ReoPro). *J Cardiovasc Pharmacol Ther.* 2002;**7**:21–24.

31 Kereiakes DJ, Berkowitz SD, Lincoff AM, *et al.* Clinical correlates and course of thrombocytopenia during percutaneous coronary intervention in the era of abciximab platelet glycoprotein IIb/IIIa blockade. *Am Heart J.* 2000;**140**:74–80.

32 Sane DC, Damaraju LV, Topol EJ, *et al.* Occurrence and clinical significance of pseudothrombocytopenia during abciximab therapy. *J Am Coll Cardiol.* 2000;**36**:75–83.

33 McKechnie RS, Smith D, Montoye C, *et al.* Prognostic implication of anemia on in-hospital outcomes after percutaneous coronary intervention. *Circulation.* 2004;**110**:271–277.

34 Nikolsky E, Mehran R, Aymong ED, *et al.* Impact of anemia on outcomes of patients undergoing percutaneous coronary interventions. *Am J Cardiol.* 2004;**94**:1023–1027.

35 Nikolsky E, Aymong ED, Halkin A, *et al.* Impact of anemia in patients with acute myocardial infarction undergoing primary percutaneous coronary intervention: analysis from the Controlled Abciximab and Device Investigation to Lower Late Angioplasty Complications (CADILLAC) trial. *J Am Coll Cardiol.* 2004;**44**:547–553.

36 Takahashi M, Kurokawa S, Tsuyusaki T, Kikawada R. Studies of hyperkinetic circulatory state in chronic anemia (Article in Japanese). *J Cardiol.* 1990;**20**:331–339.

37 Cannella G, La Canna G, Sandrini M, *et al.* Renormalization of high cardiac output and of left ventricular size following long-term recombinant human erythropoietin treatment of anemic dialyzed uremic patients. *Clin Nephrol.* 1990;**34**:272–278.

38 Amin MG, Tighiouart H, Weiner DE, *et al.* Hematocrit and left ventricular mass: the Framingham Heart study. *J Am Coll Cardiol.* 2004;**43**:1276–1282.

39 Dillmann E, Johnson DG, Martin J, Mackler B, Finch C. Catecholamine elevation in iron deficiency. *Am J Physiol.* 1979;**237**:R297–R300.

40 Means RT. Pathogenesis of the anemia of chronic disease: a cytokine-mediated anemia. *Stem Cells.* 1995;**13**:32–37.

41 McMahon TJ, Moon RE, Luschinger BP, *et al.* Nitric oxide in the human respiratory cycle. *Nat Med.* 2002; **8**:711–717.

42 Reinecke H, Trey T, Wellmann J, *et al.* Haemoglobin-related mortality in patients undergoing percutaneous coronary interventions. *Eur Heart J.* 2003;**24**:2142–2150.

43 McKechnie RS, Smith D, Montoye C, *et al.* Prognostic implication of anemia on in-hospital outcomes after percutaneous coronary intervention. *Circulation.* 2004; **110**:271–277.

44 Wu WC, Rathore SS, Wang Y, Radford MJ, Krumholz HM. Blood transfusion in elderly patients with acute myocardial infarction. *N Engl J Med.* 2001; **345**:1230–1236.

45 Al Falluji N, Lawrence-Nelson J, Kostis JB, *et al.* Effect of anemia on 1-year mortality in patients with acute myocardial infarction. *Am Heart J.* 2002;**144**:636–641.

46 Sabatine MS, Morrow DA, Giugliano RP, *et al.* Association of hemoglobin levels with clinical outcomes in acute coronary syndromes. *Circulation.* 2005;**111**:2042–2049.

47 Nikolsky E, Mehran R, Lasic Z, *et al.* Low hematocrit predicts contrast-induced nephropathy after percutaneous coronary interventions. *Kidney Int.* 2005;**67**:706–713.

48 Hebert PC, Wells G, Tweeddale M, *et al.* Does transfusion practice affect mortality in critically ill patients? Transfusion Requirements in Critical Care (TRICC) Investigators and the Canadian Critical Care Trials Group. *Am J Respir Crit Care Med.* 1997;**155**:1618–1623.

49 Hebert PC, Wells G, Blajchman MA, *et al.* A multicenter, randomized, controlled clinical trial of transfusion requirements in critical care. Transfusion Requirements in Critical Care Investigators, Canadian Critical Care Trials Group. *N Engl J Med.* 1999;**340**:409–417.

50 Rao SV, Jollis JG, Harrington RA, *et al.* Relationship of blood transfusion and clinical outcomes in patients with acute coronary syndromes. *JAMA.* 2004;**292**:1555–1562.

51 Yang X, Alexander KP, Chen AY, *et al.* The implications of blood transfusions for patients with non-ST-segment elevation acute coronary syndromes: results from the CRUSADE National Quality Improvement Initiative. *J Am Coll Cardiol.* 2005;**46**:1490–1495.

52 Nikolsky E, Mehran R, Sadeghi M, *et al.* Prognostic Impact of Blood Transfusion after Primary Angioplasty for Acute Myocardial Infarction: Analysis from the CADILLAC trial. *JACC Cardiovasc Interv.* 2009;**2**:624–632.

53 Zallen G, Moore EE, Ciesla DJ, Brown M, Biffl WL, Silliman CC. Stored red blood cells selectively activate human neutrophils to release IL-8 and secretory PLA2. *Shock.* 2000;**13**:29–33.

54 Fransen E, Maessen J, Dentener M, Senden N, Buurman W. Impact of blood transfusions on inflammatory mediator release in patients undergoing cardiac surgery. *Chest.* 1999;**116**:1233–1239.

55 Biedler AE, Schneider SO, Seyfert U, *et al.* Impact of alloantigens and storage-associated factors on stimulated cytokine response in an in vitro model of blood transfusion. *Anesthesiology.* 2002;**97**:1102–1109.

56 Twomley KM, Rao SV, Becker RC. Proinflammatory, immunomodulating, and prothrombotic properties of anemia and red blood cell transfusions. *J Thromb Thrombolysis.* 2006;**21**:167–174.

CHAPTER 37

Antiplatelet therapy resistance: Definition, diagnosis, and clinical implications

Saurabh Gupta[1] & Peter J. Casterella[2]
[1]Oregon Health & Science University, Portland, OR, USA
[2]Seattle Cardiology, Seattle, WA, USA

Introduction

Antiplatelet therapy with aspirin 75–325 mg/day, in the absence of contraindications, offers protection against myocardial infarction, stroke, and death. Significant benefit is evident among patients with acute coronary syndromes, such as unstable angina or acute myocardial infarction (AMI), patients undergoing coronary and peripheral percutaneous intervention, and those with chronic ischemic vascular disease, or cerebrovascular disease. With regards to safety, efficacy and cost effectiveness, aspirin has demonstrated the best risk–benefit ratio of any available therapy for AMI. In the Second International Study of Infarct Survival (ISIS-2) involving more than 17,000 patients presenting within 24 h of onset of AMI, aspirin compared to placebo was associated with a 23% reduction in vascular mortality, 49% reduction in reinfarction, and 46% reduction in nonfatal stroke at 5-week follow-up. There was no increase in hemorrhagic stroke or gastrointestinal bleeding in the aspirin-treated group, and only a small increase in minor bleeding (1). The early survival advantages conferred by fibrinolytic therapy and aspirin are maintained for at least 10 years (2).

Pharmacology in the Catheterization Laboratory. Edited by Ron Waksman and Andrew E Ajani. © 2010 Blackwell Publishing, ISBN: 978-1-4051-5704-9.

The benefit of aspirin after percutaneous coronary intervention (PCI) is quite well established. Early studies in the setting of balloon angioplasty showed significant reductions in adverse clinical outcomes with aspirin compared to placebo (3,4). More recently, in the setting of coronary stenting, dual antiplatelet therapy with aspirin and the thienopyridine ticlopidine was demonstrated to be superior to aspirin alone, or aspirin and warfarin in reducing the incidence of cardiac events, and hemorrhagic and vascular complications (5).

Ticlopidine, while efficacious as an antiplatelet therapy, is associated with frequent side effects including rash and gastrointestinal upset and also the rare but potentially life-threatening occurrence of neutropenia. Clopidogrel is an alternative thienopyridine agent with similar therapeutic effects compared to ticlopidine, but a better safety and side effect profile. Clopidogrel is a prodrug, which undergoes activation by the cytochrome P450 3A4 system becoming an irreversible inhibitor of the platelet $P2Y_{12}$ receptor. Clopidogrel has demonstrated significant benefits across a wide spectrum of coronary artery disease clinical scenarios. In the CURE trial of patients with non-ST-elevation acute coronary syndrome, clopidogrel plus aspirin therapy compared to aspirin alone was associated with a 20% reduction in the combined clinical end point of death, MI, or stroke (6). The PCI-CURE substudy of patients within the CURE trial, undergoing PCI, demonstrated the long-term benefits of upstream clopidogrel therapy in patients who ultimately underwent PCI. Patients receiving clopidogrel pretreatment prior to PCI experienced a 31% reduction in cardiovascular death or myocardial infarction during 1-year follow-up (7). Similarly, in patients presenting with ST-elevation myocardial infarction (STEMI), the addition of clopidogrel to aspirin and fibrinolytic therapy improves infarct-related artery patency and reduces ischemic complications (8).

The benefits of an early loading dose of clopidogrel prior to PCI have been demonstrated in several clinical trials. The TARGET trial compared abciximab and tirofiban in the setting of PCI with coronary stenting. In TARGET, clopidogrel pretreatment prior to PCI was associated with a significant reduction of death and MI regardless of the type of GP IIb/IIIa inhibitor used (9). In the CREDO trial, a 300 mg loading dose of clopidogrel, given at least 6 h prior to PCI, resulted in 3% absolute reduction, and 39% relative reduction in the incidence of the composite end point of 1-month death, myocardial infarction, and urgent target vessel revascularization (10).

Glycoprotein (GP) IIb-IIIa inhibitors attach to the platelet IIb-IIIa receptor, competing with fibrinogen, and provide near-complete inhibition of platelet aggregation. GP IIb-IIIa inhibitors are parenteral agents given as an intravenous bolus followed by a continuous infusion. Several studies have demonstrated significant benefits of GP IIb-IIIa inhibitor therapy in the setting of acute coronary syndromes and PCI (11). Early trials with oral GP IIb-IIIa inhibitors failed to demonstrate a significant clinical benefit. As such, the use of these agents is currently limited to parenteral administration during inhospital management of acute coronary syndromes and patients undergoing PCI.

Platelet resistance: Definitions, incidence, prevalence, and clinical significance

Definition of platelet resistance

Platelet resistance is best defined as the lack of the desired pharmacologic effect of an antiplatelet medication. However, the definition is complicated by the absence of standardized methods of platelet function assessment and the use of multiple assays

and agonists. The occurrence of an ischemic clinical event while on antiplatelet therapy, although reflective of treatment failure, does not necessarily indicate that resistance is present. In order to understand the concept of platelet resistance, one must first understand the nomenclature associated with platelet aggregation testing. Light transmission aggregometry and point-of-care platelet function assays typically express results as percent aggregation. The assessment of platelet function *after* administration of platelet inhibitors may be expressed as residual platelet aggregation, or as level of platelet inhibition, which is the inverse of residual aggregation. The most widely accepted definition of ASA resistance is ≥70% residual platelet aggregation with 10 μM ADP stimulation, or ≥20% residual platelet aggregation with 0.5 mg/mL arachadonic acid stimulation (12). With clopidogrel, a less than 10% change in 5 μM ADP-mediated platelet aggregation compared to baseline defines the presence of clopidogrel resistance (13).

Platelet resistance does not appear to be an "all or none" phenomenon. Some patients appear to be nearly completely resistant to aspirin, clopidogrel, or both agents, while others have a partial but incomplete response of their platelets to these agents. While clopidogrel dosing is consistent, the optimal dose of aspirin has not been established. Additionally, it is unclear whether "one-size-fits-all" dosing of clopidogrel is appropriate, and it has been postulated that some individuals may require a higher maintenance dose of clopidogrel to achieve the desired platelet inhibitory effect.

Aspirin resistance: Incidence and clinical implications

The incidence of aspirin resistance varies from 15% to 60% of patients with vascular disease depending upon the definition and assay used (12). The etiology of aspirin resistance is poorly understood and likely involves clinical, cellular, and genetic factors (Figure 37.1) (14). Patients with aspirin resistance or partial responders have an increased risk of ischemic events (15). Gum and colleagues assessed 326 patients with clinically stable coronary artery disease (CAD). The incidence of aspirin resistance was 5.2%, and was associated with a significantly increased risk of myocardial infarction or stroke (24% with aspirin resistance vs 10% without

Clinical factors

- Non-absorption
- Interaction with NSAIDs
- Acute coronary syndrome
- Congestive heart failure
- Hyperglycemia
- Catecholamine surge

Cellular factors

- Insufficient suppression of COX-1
- Over-expression of COX-2 mRNA
- Erythrocyte induced platelet activation
- Increased norepinephrine
- Generation of 8-iso-PGF 2α
- Resolvins

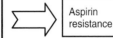

Aspirin resistance

Genetic polymorphisms

- COX-1
- GP IIIa receptor
- Collagen receptor
- vWF receptor
- P2Y$_1$ single nucleotide

Figure 37.1 Factors contributing to aspirin resistance. Reproduced from Bhatt (14) with permission from The American College of Cardiology Foundation.

aspirin resistance, hazard ratio 3.12, $p = 0.03$) (16). Despite pretreatment with clopidogrel, patients with aspirin resistance have an increased risk of myonecrosis following nonurgent PCI (17).

Clopidogrel resistance: Incidence and clinical implications

The prevalence of clopidogrel resistance varies from 15% to 30% of patients with CAD depending upon clinical scenario, test assay, and clopidogrel dose (13,18,19). A number of extrinsic and intrinsic factors have been hypothesized as operative in the etiology of clopidogrel resistance (Table 37.1) (19). Serebruany and colleagues evaluated 544 individuals receiving clopidogrel and observed wide variability in platelet aggregation response to 5 μmol/L of adenosine diphosphate following a normal distribution curve (Figure 37.2) (20). Clopidogrel resistance has been associated with adverse clinical outcomes in a variety of clinical scenarios. Up to 25% of STEMI patients undergoing primary PCI with stenting are resistant to

Table 37.1 Potential mechanisms of clopidogrel resistance (19).

Extrinsic factors
- Dose: Does the optimal dose vary amongst individual patients and in different clinical scenarios (i.e., ACS vs stable CAD)?
- Drug–drug interactions (i.e., lipitor)
- CYP3A4 activity
- Variable pro-drug absorption
- Variable active metabolite clearance

Intrinsic factors
- P2Y$_{12}$ receptor variability in numbers or affinity for drug
- Increased intrinsic ADP levels
- Up-regulation of other platelet activation pathways

clopidogrel and have an increased risk of adverse cardiovascular events including stent thrombosis (21). Patients with unstable angina undergoing PCI have a lower inhibition of platelet aggregation

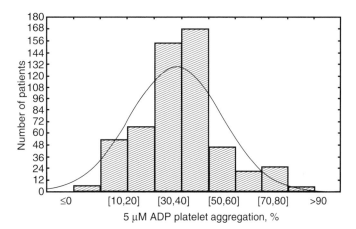

Figure 37.2 Distribution of 5 μmol of adenosine diphosphate (ADP)-induced residual platelet aggregation in 544 patients after receiving clopidogrel therapy (20).

following clopidogrel loading (22). These findings suggest that patients presenting with acute coronary syndromes (STEMI, non-ST-Elevation MI, and unstable angina) are a subgroup of patients with an increased likelihood of clopidogrel resistance.

Among patients undergoing percutaneous coronary interventions, those with high pretreatment platelet reactivity are most likely to demonstrate resistance to clopidogrel (13). Baseline platelet aggregation measured before elective coronary stenting in patients receiving a 600 mg loading dose of clopidogrel correlates with periprocedural outcomes (23). A review of published analyses shows that approximately 50% of patients are resistant to either ASA, clopidogrel, or both agents.

Treatment modifications in patients with platelet resistance

The optimal treatment of ASA resistance remains unclear. It has been theorized that an increased aspirin dose may overcome resistance in some patients, especially those who are partial responders. However, while some small *in vitro* studies showed that increasing the dose of aspirin may overcome biological resistance, several large trials have demonstrated no significant difference in clinical outcomes with varying doses of ASA (24). Therefore it seems unlikely that increasing the dose of aspirin will be an effective approach to the aspirin-resistant individual. There is *in vitro* evidence suggesting that aspirin-resistant patients may benefit from clopidogrel due to their increased platelet sensitivity to adenosine diphosphate (ADP) (19,25). It has also been proposed that

the use of a loading dose of clopidogrel may prevent adverse events in aspirin-resistant patients undergoing PCI. However, Chen *et al.* demonstrated that aspirin-resistant patients pretreated with 300 mg of clopidogrel prior to PCI still had a greater than two-fold increase in the incidence of CK-MB elevation following PCI (17). Additionally, Lev and colleagues reported that 47% of aspirin-resistant individual demonstrated concurrent clopidogrel resistance as well (26). Thus, it seems unlikely that the use of clopidogrel in aspirin-resistant patients will be a suitable therapeutic option.

Similar to the scenario with aspirin resistance, the optimal therapeutic adjustment in the setting of clopidogrel resistance has yet to be determined. Gurbel and colleagues demonstrated that following PCI, a 300-mg loading dose of clopidogrel, followed by 75-mg daily maintenance dose is associated with an incidence of resistance of 63% at 2 h, 31% at 2 and 5 days, and 15% at 30 days. The declining incidence of resistance over time suggests that a higher loading and/or maintenance dose might overcome resistance in some individuals (13). In a subsequent study, Gurbel *et al.* demonstrated superior levels of platelet inhibition in the first 24 h after PCI with a 600 mg vs 300 mg loading dose of clopidogrel (27). It would be naïve however to conclude that simply raising the dose progressively will overcome all clopidogrel resistance. Price and colleagues reported that a 900-mg dose of clopidogrel provides no benefit in terms of magnitude or time to maximal platelet inhibition compared with a 600-mg dose, but both are superior to a 300-mg dose (28).

In the setting of PCI, a potential way to combat both aspirin and clopidogrel resistance is the use of a parenteral glycoprotein (GP) IIb-IIIa antagonist. These agents block the platelet GP IIb-IIIa receptor, resulting in near-complete inhibition of platelet aggregation. Prior clinical studies of the GP IIb-IIIa inhibitor class showed significant reductions in major adverse cardiac events, leading to the widespread use of these agents in the late 1990s and early 2000 era of PCI. However, recent studies such as the REPLACE 2 (29) and ISAR REACT (30) trials suggest that not all PCI patients require aggressive antiplatelet therapy. Subsequently, utilization of GP IIb-IIIa inhibitors during PCI has declined in recent years. However, the recently completed ISAR REACT 2 trial showed that ACS patients undergoing PCI benefit from the addition of a GP IIb-IIIa antagonist to baseline therapy with aspirin, clopidogrel 600 mg loading dose, and intravenous heparin during PCI (31). It has also been demonstrated that ACS patients are more likely to manifest platelet resistance. Thus it seems plausible that a bona fide indication for the use of GP IIb-IIIa inhibitors may be the presence of platelet resistance. This premise is currently under investigation in the RESISTOR (Research Evaluation to Study Individuals who Show Thromboxane or P2Y$_{12}$ Receptor Resistance) trial. In this study, elective PCI patients undergo preprocedure platelet function testing with the Accumetrics Verify Now™ point-of-care assay. Those patients demonstrating platelet resistance are then randomized to GP IIb-IIIa inhibitor therapy with eptifibatide vs placebo with a primary end point analysis of myonecrosis as assessed by cardiac biomarker elevations.

Future directions in the management of platelet resistance

Effectively dealing with and resolving the clinical challenges posed by platelet resistance hinges upon several critical issues including:

1 The need for standardized, convenient and easily interpretable point-of-care platelet function assays;

2 Development of standardized terminology and nomenclature to define platelet resistance and to characterize platelet function response to inhibitory therapies; and

3 Development of new pharmacologic therapeutic agents to address the shortcomings of aspirin and clopidogrel.

Light transmission platelet aggregometry (LTA) has been the gold standard of platelet function analysis for decades. However, this technology is tedious, time-consuming, and not available in all hospital institutions. Furthermore, results of LTA are not immediately available, and thus cannot be used to guide acute therapies in the catheterization laboratory setting. Recently, point-of-care platelet function tests have become available and are analogous to an activated clotting time (ACT) in that results are immediately available to guide therapy. To integrate the results of such assays into patient management, it will be necessary to standardize features such as agonist type and strength used to test specific antiplatelet agents, and nomenclature of reporting test results. The ideal platelet function test will use whole blood (no requirement for specimen preparation), will accurately assess platelet responsiveness even in the setting of baseline therapy with antiplatelet medications, and will provide results in 10 min or less.

Measurements of individual responsiveness to antiplatelet therapy provide the potential for individualized therapy. The results of the EXCELSIOR study represent an important contribution to our understanding of the impact of platelet reactivity on clinical outcomes in patients undergoing routine PCI and underscore the fact that uniform dosing of antiplatelet therapies may not achieve optimal platelet inhibition. In this study, despite pretreatment with a 600-mg clopidogrel loading dose, ~40% of patients demonstrated suboptimal platelet inhibition, and an increased risk of adverse outcomes. Eventually, prospective, randomized clinical trials will determine if monitoring of platelet function response to therapy and subsequent adjustment of antiplatelet therapy translates into improved clinical outcomes (32).

Newer pharmacologic agents may demonstrate better efficacy and a lower incidence of resistance compared to the current standard of care of aspirin and clopidogrel. Prasugrel is a third generation thienopyridine that has demonstrated greater potency, more rapid onset, more consistent platelet inhibition, and a lower incidence of resistance compared to clopidogrel (33). Prasugrel has been evaluated vs clopidogrel in the setting of PCI in the TRITON TIMI 38 study and in other trials and has recently been approved by the FDA. Other novel agents such as cangrelor and AZD6140 are rapid, reversible $P2Y_{12}$ inhibitors that are direct inhibitors as opposed to prodrugs.

Conclusions

- Antiplatelet therapy resistance is common and conveys an increased risk of adverse outcomes with ACS and PCI.
- Resistant patients may require more potent antiplatelet therapies (i.e., GP IIb-IIIa antagonists) or higher doses of oral antiplatelet therapies to optimize outcomes.
- Standardized methods of platelet function testing and interpretation, along with integration of point-of-service testing may assist in individualizing antiplatelet therapy to improve outcomes in patients with platelet resistance.
- Dose adjustments of existing regimens based upon the platelet function response to therapy, and the advancement of new agents with a more reliable pharmacologic effect, and reduced incidence of resistance may assist in combating the deleterious effects of antiplatelet therapy resistance.

References

1 Randomised trial of intravenous streptokinase, oral aspirin, both, or neither among 17,187 cases of suspected acute myocardial infarction: Isis-2. Isis-2 (second international study of infarct survival) collaborative group. *Lancet.* 1988;**2**:349–360.

2 Baigent C, Collins R, Appleby P, Parish S, Sleight P, Peto R. Isis-2: 10 year survival among patients with suspected acute myocardial infarction in randomised comparison of intravenous streptokinase, oral aspirin, both, or neither. *BMJ.* 1998;**316**:1337–1343.

3 Schwartz L, Bourassa MG, Lesperance J, *et al.* Aspirin and dipyridamole in the prevention of restenosis after percutaneous transluminal coronary angioplasty. *N Engl J Med.* 1988;**318**:1714–1719.

4 Barnathan ES, Schwartz JS, Taylor L, *et al.* Aspirin and dipyridamole in the prevention of acute coronary thrombosis complicating coronary angioplasty. *Circulation.* 1987;**76**:125–134.

5 Schomig A, Neumann F-J, Kastrati A, *et al.* A randomized comparison of antiplatelet and anticoagulant therapy

6 Yusuf S, Zhao F, Mehta SR, *et al.* The clopidogrel in unstable angina to prevent recurrent events trial I. Effects of clopidogrel in addition to aspirin in patients with acute coronary syndromes without ST-segment elevation. *N Engl J Med.* 2001;**345**:494–502.

7 Mehta SR, Yusuf S, Peters RJG, *et al.* Effects of pretreatment with clopidogrel and aspirin followed by long-term therapy in patients undergoing percutaneous coronary intervention: the pci-cure study. *Lancet.* 2001;**358**:527–533.

8 Sabatine MS, Cannon CP, Gibson CM, *et al.* Addition of clopidogrel to aspirin and fibrinolytic therapy for myocardial infarction with ST-segment elevation. *N Engl J Med.* 2005;**352**:1179–1189.

9 Chan AW, Moliterno DJ, Berger PB, *et al.* Triple antiplatelet therapy during percutaneous coronary intervention is associated withimproved outcomes including one-year survival: results from the do tirofiban and reoprogive similar efficacy outcome trial (target). *J Am Coll Cardiol.* 2003;**42**:1188–1195.

10 Steinhubl SR, Berger PB, Mann Iii JT, *et al.* Early and sustained dual oral antiplatelet therapy following percutaneous coronary intervention: a randomized controlled trial. *JAMA.* 2002;**288**:2411–2420.

11 Nguyen CM, Harrington RA. Glycoprotein iib/iiia receptor antagonists: a comparative review of their use in percutaneous coronary intervention. *Am J Cardiovasc Drugs.* 2003;**3**:423–436.

12 Gum PA, Kottke-Marchant K, Poggio ED, *et al.* Profile and prevalence of aspirin resistance in patients with cardiovascular disease. *Am J Cardiol.* 2001;**88**:230–235.

13 Gurbel PA, Bliden KP, Hiatt BL, O'Connor CM. Clopidogrel for coronary stenting: response variability, drug resistance, and the effect of pretreatment platelet reactivity. *Circulation.* 2003;**107**:2908–2913.

14 Bhatt DL. Aspirin resistance: More than just a laboratory curiosity. *J Am Coll Cardiol.* 2004;**43**:1127–1129.

15 Grotemeyer KH, Scharafinski HW, Husstedt IW. Two-year follow-up of aspirin responder and aspirin non responder. A pilot-study including 180 post-stroke patients. *Thromb Res.* 1993;**71**:397–403.

16 Gum PA, Kottke-Marchant K, Welsh PA, White J, Topol EJ. A prospective, blinded determination of the natural history of aspirin resistance among stable patients with cardiovascular disease. *J Am Coll Cardiol.* 2003;**41**:961–965.

17 Chen W-H, Lee P-Y, Ng W, Tse H-F, Lau C-P. Aspirin resistance is associated with a high incidence of myonecrosis after non-urgent percutaneous coronary intervention despite clopidogrel pretreatment. *J Am Coll Cardiol.* 2004;**43**:1122–1126.

18 Muller I, Besta F, Schulz C, Massberg S, Schonig A, Gawaz M. Prevalence of clopidogrel non-responders among patients with stable angina pectoris scheduled for elective coronary stent placement. *Thromb Haemost.* 2003;**89**:783–787.

19 Nguyen TA, Diodati JG, Pharand C. Resistance to clopidogrel: a review of the evidence. *J Am Coll Cardiol.* 2005;**45**:1157–1164.

20 Serebruany VL, Steinhubl SR, Berger PB, Malinin AI, Bhatt DL, Topol EJ. Variability in platelet responsiveness to clopidogrel among 544 individuals. *J Am Coll Cardiol.* 2005;**45**:246–251.

21 Matetzky S, Shenkman B, Guetta V, *et al.* Clopidogrel resistance is associated with increased risk of recurrent atherothrombotic events in patients with acute myocardial infarction. *Circulation.* 2004;**109**:3171–3175.

22 Soffer D, Moussa I, Harjaim KJ, *et al.* Impact of angina class on inhibition of platelet aggregation following clopidogrel loading in patients undergoing coronary intervention: do we need more aggressive dosing regimens in unstable angina? *Catheter Cardiovasc Interv.* 2003;**59**:21–25.

23 Hochholzer W, Trenk D, Bestehorn H-P, *et al.* Impact of the degree of peri-interventional platelet inhibition after loading with clopidogrel on early clinical outcome of elective coronary stent placement. *J Am Coll Cardiol.* 2006;**48**:1742–1750.

24 Collaborative meta-analysis of randomised trials of antiplatelet therapy for prevention of death, myocardial infarction, and stroke in high risk patients. *BMJ.* 2002;**324**:71–86.

25 Macchi L, Christiaens L, Brabant S, *et al.* Resistance to aspirin in vitro is associated with increased platelet sensitivity to adenosine diphosphate. *Thromb Res.* 2002;**107**:45–49.

26 Lev EI, Patel RT, Maresh KJ, *et al.* Aspirin and clopidogrel drug response in patients undergoing percutaneous coronary intervention: the role of dual drug resistance. *J Am Coll Cardiol.* 2006;**47**:27–33.

27 Gurbel PA, Bliden KP, Zaman KA, Yoho JA, Hayes KM, Tantry US. Clopidogrel loading with eptifibatide to arrest the reactivity of platelets: results of the clopidogrel loading with eptifibatide to arrest the reactivity of platelets (CLEAR PLATELETS) study. *Circulation.* 2005;**111**:1153–1159.

28 Price MJ, Coleman JL, Steinhubl SR, Wong GB, Cannon CP, Teirstein PS. Onset and offset of platelet inhibition after high-dose clopidogrel loading and standard daily therapy measured by a point-of-care assay in healthy volunteers. *Am J Cardiol.* 2006;**98**:681–684.

29 Lincoff AM, Bittl JA, Harrington RA, *et al.* Bivalirudin and provisional glycoprotein IIb/IIIa blockade compared with heparin and planned glycoprotein iib/iiia blockade during percutaneous coronary intervention: replace-2 randomized trial. *JAMA.* 2003;**289**:853–863.

30 Kastrati A, Mehilli J, Schuhlen H, *et al.* A clinical trial of abciximab in elective percutaneous coronary intervention after pretreatment with clopidogrel. *N Engl J Med.* 2004;**350**:232–238.

31 Kastrati A, Mehilli J, Neumann FJ, *et al.* Abciximab in patients with acute coronary syndromes undergoing percutaneous coronary intervention after clopidogrel pretreatment: the ISAR_REACT 2 randomized trial. *JAMA.* 2006;**295**:1531–1538.

32 Alfonso F, Angiolillo DJ. Platelet function assessment to predict outcomes after coronary interventions: hype or hope? *J Am Coll Cardiol.* 2006;**48**:1751–1754.

33 Jernberg T, Payne CD, Winters KJ, *et al.* Prasugrel achieves greater inhibition of platelet aggregation and a lower rate of non-responders compared with clopidogrel in aspirin-treated patients with stable coronary artery disease. *Eur Heart J.* 2006;**27**:1166–1173.

CHAPTER 38

Reversal of anticoagulation: Protamine

Bengt Lindblad & Jan Holst
University Hospital MAS, Malmö, Sweden

Introduction

Adequate anticoagulation is a cornerstone in vascular procedures. For a long time, unfractionated heparin (UH) has been the substance of choice to minimize the risk of thrombotic complications. Both anticoagulation and the possibility to reverse it has been a prerequisite for treatment of deep vein thrombosis, development of cardiovascular surgery, hemodialysis, and endovascular interventions. Reversal is normally achieved with intravenous administration of protamine, a strongly basic heterogeneous protein (average molecular weight 4.5 kDa). Physiologically protamine is bound to sperm nucleic acids, where it plays an integral role during spermatogenesis through chromatin compaction. Recent research has focused on many facets of protamine biology, among others involvement of protamine in male fertility (1).

Miescher characterized in 1868 a strongly basic compound—protamine—from the sperm of salmon. Later two-thirds of the protein molecule was found to consist of arginine. This and other substances (heparin, hexadimethrine) were during the 1930s tested as anticoagulants. Heparin was the most effective anticoagulant and found to be neutralized by both protamine and hexadimethrine (2).

Pharmacology in the Catheterization Laboratory. Edited by Ron Waksman and Andrew E Ajani. © 2010 Blackwell Publishing, ISBN: 978-1-4051-5704-9.

Occasionally when using protamine (one case in a thousand), a severe and even fatal hemodynamic catastrophic reaction can be seen, including varying degree of systemic hypotension, bradycardia, and bronchoconstriction. Reactions that are more moderate are more frequent. The frequency of these reactions from different materials in given in Table 38.1 (3–8). The frequencies of adverse reactions to protamine reported are varying—from 0% up to 92% of cases. A difference is seen depending of type of procedure; after endovascular procedures, it is probably infrequent, though well-made studies are few.

The intention of this review is to summarize present knowledge, alternatives for anticoagulation reversal, and give some practical advice on how to avoid or reduce these reactions.

Mechanism of action—reversal of heparinization

Heparin induces anticoagulation in at least two principally different ways; firstly, and most importantly, through antithrombin (AT) and secondly by the release of endothelial-bound tissue factor pathway inhibitor (TFPI) (9). Heparin and AT forms a complex, which inhibits the catalytic activity of thrombin (FIIa) and FXa and other proteins in the coagulation cascade. The activity of AT is augmented 1000-fold when complexed to heparin. TFPI in the presence of FXa inhibits the FVIIa-Tissue Factor complex. This complex is

Table 38.1 Haemodynamic adverse response to protamine reversal of anticoagulation.

Authors	Type of procedure	No of patients	Frequency of adverse hemodynamic response (percent)
Welsby et al. 2005	CABG	6,771	52% (Systemic BP decrease of 20%)
Welsby et al. 2005	CABG	5,649	92% (PAP increase of 20%)
Welsby et al. 2005	CABG	6,846	One fatal response
Stewart et al. 1984	PCI	651	1.1% (one fatal)
Stewart et al. 1984	PCI + DM (NPH-insulin treated)	15	27%
Ducas et al. 2002	PCI	429	0%
Vincent et al. 1991	PCI	3,341	0.1%
Wakefield et al. 1994	Peripheral arterial surgery	38,121	4.9%
Dorman et al. 1995	Peripheral arterial surgery	120	0%

the principal initiator of the coagulation cascade *in vivo*.

Protamine has stronger affinity to heparin than AT has. Thus protamine causes dissociation of the heparin–AT complex and heparin consequently binds to protamine. The newly formed protamine–heparin complexes, which are devoid of anticoagulant properties, is subsequently deposited in the kidney and broken down by the reticuloendothelial system (10).

Protamine is effective (completely and permanently) in reversing unfractionated heparin's (UH) anti-FIIa and anti-FXa activity (Table 38.2) (11). Standard unfractionated heparin is exceedingly being replaced by low-molecular-weight heparins (LMWH) as anticoagulant agents, mainly because of better pharmacodynamic properties, especially when given subcutaneously, improved safety and a lesser need for monitoring. Since it is often used in cardiac patients, the knowledge that protamine can be used for reversal in these patients is important. The different LMWHs are not identical. One should look upon this group of substances as brothers/cousins and not twins.

Three principally different aspects regarding reversal of LMWH should be considered:

1 They all have different ratios of shorter vs longer chains. Previously this difference was considered to be the most important reason for the well documented incomplete ability for protamine to neutralize the different LMWHs. Newer data indicate that it is the degree of sulfatation that is the discriminating factor. Reduced sulfate charge, not molecular mass, is the principal reason that

Table 38.2 The capability of protamine to reverse UH and different LMHWs measured as the anti-FIIa and anti-FXa activity.

Type of heparin	Anti-FIIa activity (%)	Anti-FXa activity (%)
UH	100	100
Reviparin	>84	37
Enoxaparin	>87	46
Nadroparin	>89	51
Dalteparin	>93	59
Tinzaparin	>96	81

Source: Adapted from *in vivo* data from Holst *et al.* (11) and from *in vitro* data by Crowther (12).

protamine is unable to fully reverse LMWH induced anticoagulation (Table 38.2) (12).

2 For pharmacokinetic reasons, LMWH is usually given as a subcutaneous injection. The purpose of such administration is to give a graded release of the substance during a long period of time. This is reflected by also after protamine reversal a return of the anticoagulant activity of subcutaneously administered LMHW. Repeated doses of protamine may be required since the half-life of protamine is short (5 min to 2 h).

3 Finally, protamine can by itself be anticoagulative (see below), this applies that "overdose of protamine" should be avoided also for the neutralization of UH.

Protamine reversal of heparinization also gives a dramatic reduction in plasma TFPI levels. TFPI released by heparins both UH and LMWH (tinzaparin) remains in the circulation only as long as heparin is present and shows essentially the same pharmacokinetic pattern as unfractionated heparin (11).

Protamine dose

Firstly, it must at all times be calculated individually. Depending on the different commercially available preparations of protamine sulfate, the neutralizing capacity toward UH may differ. But generally 1 mg protamine sulfate neutralizes between 100 and 140 IU UH, measured as anti-FIIa activity. The biological half-life of UH is about 90 min and is dependent of liver and kidney functions. It is therefore important to know which anticoagulant was given, when and how the anticoagulant was administrated and patient comorbidities. Especially since the potentially difficult side effects are related to the protamine dose, never larger doses than required should be given. Maybe it should be preferentially administered in a peripheral vein instead of having a high concentration in the pulmonary circulation?

Should the neutralizing effect of protamine be monitored?

This naturally depends on if heparinization is monitored and the reason for reversal and type of heparin used. From our experience, in the angiosuite, we have found it satisfactory to use a simple bedside monitoring device (Activated Clotting Time, ACT, Hemocrone Jr, Int Technodyne Corp) for monitoring the level of UH induced anticoagulation. In normal procedures, we avoid the use of protamine, but if required we are using low calculated protamine dose with ACT-monitoring. If LMWH is needed to be reversed ACT or aPTT (which primarily reflects the anti-FIIa activity) is clearly of lesser use. In those cases, anti-FXa activity needs to be monitored but in an emergency situation normally not possible to analyze promptly.

Direct effect on hemostasis of protamine

Protamine itself can have anticoagulant effects because of tissue factor inhibition and more importantly due to effect on platelets. Twenty percent of patients treated with protamine develop relative thrombocytopenia (2). Late bleeding after initially adequate reversal can occur, especially after the use of heart–lung machine but whether this is due to a "heparin rebound" effect or to protamine anticoagulant effect is not clear. In peripheral vascular surgery patients, protamine reversal of heparinization did even increase the amount of bleeding (9).

Immunological reactions

Type I and III immunological reactions according to Coombs and Gell's classification could cause the anaphylactoid reactions seen from protamine (13). Type I reactions refers to a sudden, potentially life-threatening, systemic condition mediated by highly reactive molecules released from mast cells and basophils. Mediators include histamine, platelet-activating factor, and products of arachidonic acid metabolism. Release of mediators depends typically upon the interaction of antigen with specific antibodies of the IgE class (reagines) that are bound to the mast cells and basophils. Such a reaction can induce urticaria, skin rash and generalized priritus, but also hemodynamic collapse (2,10,13).

Antibodies of other immunoglobulin classes (IgG, IgM) are also thought to mediate anaphylaxis on occasion. By definition, IgG and IgM antibodies are formed due to prior exposure to the same or a closely related antigen. Anaphylaxis results from widespread release of vasoactive mediators that will enter the circulation. Thus, anaphylaxis mediated by IgG and IgM antibodies is an expression of allergy that is systemic. At a cellular level, the reaction begins within seconds of exposure to the inciting antigen. However, depending upon the degree of sensitization (IgE, IgG and IgM protamine-antibody formation are seen), and presumably upon the rate with which the antigen (protamine infusion) enters the circulation, symptoms may not be expressed for minutes or even a few hours. Classic symptoms include pallor and then diffuse erythema, urticaria and itching, subcutaneous edema, edema and spasm of the larynx, bronchoconstriction, tachycardia, hypotension, and hypovolemic shock.

The clinical presentation of anaphylaxis can also be produced by intravascular antigen–antibody reactions that activate the complement system and other cascade systems. In this case, the antibodies may be of the IgG or IgM class. Peptides that are split from activated complement components act on mast cells and basophils to induce the release of the same vasoactive mediators (10). This reaction is recognized most clearly after intravenous administration of antigen; it has been hypothesized to occur rarely after intramuscular or subcutaneous injection but more commonly after rapid infusion (within 1–5 min) of large amounts of the antigen into the venous circulation, especially the pulmonary circulation.

The immune response to protamine is IgE-, IgG-, and IgM-mediated and is achieved since protamine used for heparin reversal is a nonhuman protein. Patients at increased risk for immunologic response (Table 38.3) are diabetic patients treated with protamine-containing insulin where protamine was added to insulin preparations (in neutral protamine Hagedorn [NPH] and protamine–zinc insulins) to delay insulin absorption and thereby prolong their pharmacologic effect. Protamine–insulin diabetic patients have developed antibodies to IgE in over 50% and IgG in over 90% (13). Also having an increased risk are those earlier treated with intravenous protamine at cardiovascular procedures. Intracutaneous allergy tests with protamine may be helpful in identifying a possible IgE- and IgG-mediated response in selected cases, however, these tests must be interpreted with caution because they do not necessarily predict an immunological reaction and do not identify all patients at risk. Many patients without detected antibodies still have adverse acute protamine reactions (2,10).

Fish allergy has been speculated to be a possible risk factor in some case reports of acute protamine sensitivity, but data is not convincing, and there is

Table 38.3 Increased risk for development of adverse reaction to protamine.

1. Earlier adverse reaction to protamine administration
2. Diabetic patient treated with protamine-insulin(?)
3. Positive immunologic testing for protamine(?)
4. Earlier cardiovascular procedure and protamine administration??
5. Vasectomy patients???

in vitro evidence for lack of immunologic cross-reactivity between commercially available salmon extracts (derived predominantly from salmon muscle tissue) and protamine (13).

After vasectomies, men have been shown to develop IgE and other antibodies to protamine and similar human proteins, presumably because of immunologic responses to systemic absorption of sperm that can be seen after vasectomy. Such men are probably at increased risk for adverse protamine reactions (10). Because anaphylaxis to intravenous protamine apparently may occur also by a variety of nonantibody-mediated mechanisms, immunologic testing to detect elevated levels of IgE or IgG antibodies to protamine (available from several immunologic reference laboratories) does not identify all patients at risk for having anaphylaxis induced by protamine.

Nonimmunological reactions

Nonimmunological reactions may include cell–membrane interactions and interactions with the cascade systems, especially the complement system (2,10). Protamine infusion does reduce thrombin uptake on endothelial surfaces, and thrombin-induced platelet aggregation is reduced and red cells are lyzed. Additionally, membrane transport of calcium is reduced and all these cell membrane interactions lead to release of vasoactive enzymes, especially from neutrophils and basophils. Increased release of, for example, bradykinin, endothelin-1, thromboxane A2, histamine release from basophils, toll-like receptor stimulation (TLR 7 and 8 were protamine with an affinity for nucleoid material bound to e.g., m-RNA, which binds to TLR and initiates an anaphylactoid reaction (14)), follistatin release from endothelial cells are some reported cell-membrane-induced effects. These cell membrane interactions and release of vasoactive substances can induce even the severe fatal adverse reactions to protamine that thus can be seen without immunologic changes or complement activation. It has been shown that nitric oxide levels are increased in the pulmonary circulation after protamine administration. Endothelial cell ATP-production is reduced and this effect is potentiated by heparin administration before protamine is given.

It has been suggested that complement activation via the classic pathway and C3 and C5 activation should be one major cause for the adverse nonimmunologic reactions. Most of these studies regarding complement activation are, however, made on patients undergoing cardiopulmonary bypass, where the procedure in itself gives complement activation. Neither experimentally in complement depleted dogs nor in humans undergoing peripheral vascular surgery have we been able to document complement consumption (10).

How to minimize the risk for adverse reactions—clinical recommendations for endovascular procedures

Be aware of the risk of adverse reactions to protamine. Do not use it routinely—use it selectively. Heparin administration has a short half-life of around 70–90 min. This implies that the dose given for reversal of heparinization should be calculated and the short half-life of intravenous administered heparin taken into account.

Another problem is that in some centres after endovascular procedure, one maintains the introducer for a while and this sheath is often removed by others than those performing the procedure. Even if these personnel have been trained to remove the sheet and apply pressure at the puncture site, this is even better achieved by the interventionist who made the puncture. The compression can be more precise and adjusted to catheter size, other pharmacological treatment given and so on. We often, after the initial manual compression, add a fem-stop equipment using which a applied "balloon-like" compression is applied on the puncture site with a "girdle-like frame" around the pelvis-hip region. This should also by placed by the responsible interventionist and a pressure initially chosen individually and reduced after an individual time scheme.

Additionally, few coronary interventions are performed with initial micropuncture of the femoral artery to obtain the best possible puncture site in the common femoral artery, if used, that will allow optimal compression. Since many of endovascular-treated patients have several hemostatic-interfering drugs, it seems also rational to use some type of

closure device of the puncture site depending on introducer size and the quality of the femoral artery at the puncture site. Use of closure device shall not replace manual compression nor can protamine reversal of anticoagulation replace good manual compression.

Be even more restrictive to use protamine if the patient has earlier been exposed to protamine by either protamine-containing insulin or cardiac or vascular procedures were protamine was used. In patients with previous exposure to protamine, the determination of antibodies to protamine will delineate a risk group for adverse reaction. However, many of those having IgE or IgG antibodies against protamine still may show no adverse reaction to protamine. Thus reliable identification of those who will suffer from an anyphylactic/anyphylactoid reaction is not possible. In cardiac surgery and sometimes in vascular surgery, reversal of anticoagulation is required. In endovascular patients, a very restrictive use of protamine reversal is recommended.

In the selected group of patients where protamine administration is needed, a slow intravenous infusion is recommended. Hypovolemia is normally not a problem in endovascular patients but should be minimized prior to protamine is given. If adverse response to protamine is achieved, volume substitution and alpha-stimulating catecholamines may be necessary.

Alternatives to protamine

Alternative use other than protamine for heparin reversal should be considered in patients that earlier have had adverse reactions to protamine administration (Table 38.3). It could also be considered when heparinization reversal is required in diabetic patients with a history of protamine-containing insulin use, as well as in other patients at increased risk for reactions from protamine. One alternative that should be considered is autoreversal of lower dose heparinization. Other alternatives are the use of heparin-bound catheters, heart bypass pump circuits (to avoid need for protamine reversal), but for endovascular procedures only limited material is available with heparin coating. Pharmacologically reversal of heparinization is also possible with hexadimethrine (polybrene), heparinase, or platelet factor 4 (15). Platelet factor 4 and heparinase currently are investigational agents and are difficult to obtain. Hexadimethrine (polybrene) is a quarternary ammonium polycationic salt that has been used for reversal of heparinization for example during cardiac surgery (2,10). However, hexadimethrine has since many years been replaced by protamine, mainly because of hexadimethrines potential nephrotoxicity.

A novel low-molecular-weight protamine has experimentally been shown to be less toxic than standard protamine. In humans, this LMW-protamine was as effective as regular protamine to reverse heparinization and decreased the count of platelets less than standard protamine. Nevertheless, both regular and LMW-protamine decreased platelet aggregation to the same extent (16).

In the event that it is not possible to use one or more of the above alternatives, consideration might be given to prophylaxis with antihistamines and corticosteroids before protamine administration, as is used to prevent anaphylactoid reactions to radiographic contrast agents. However, there are no controlled, prospective studies that demonstrate that this approach is reliable; experimentally it is of no value.

New anticoagulants and its reversal

New pharmacological agents that are more specific anticoagulants than unfractionated heparin or low-molecular-weight heparin has become available. This is covered elsewhere and will only briefly be discussed since most do not have agents that will reverse their effect. These new anticoagulants are developed with the target of affecting one single coagulation factor and have predictable dose–response relationships. These include direct thrombin inhibitors and factor Xa inhibitors (17). Three parenteral direct thrombin inhibitors, argatroban, bivalirudin, and lepirudin, have FDA approval for the management of heparin-induced thrombocytopenia (HIT)-patients undergoing percutaneous coronary interventions. Ximelagatran, an oral prodrug of the direct thrombin inhibitor melagatran, showed efficacy in the prevention and treatment of venous thromboembolism as well as stroke prevention in patients with atrial fibrillation.

However, due to liver toxicity, it did not receive FDA approval and has been taken off market. A number of oral direct factor Xa inhibitors as well as other oral direct thrombin inhibitors are in clinical development for the prevention and treatment of thrombosis. Fondaparinux is a synthetic pentasaccharide, which binds to antithrombin, but still selectively inhibiting factor Xa. It has shown efficiency in treatment of deep venous thrombosis and especially to prevent postoperative thrombosis in hip surgery patients. Recently, a large study including over 20,000 patients compared fondaparinux (prophylactic dose 2.5 mg) with enoxaparin (full dose 1 mg/kg) in patients with unstable angina (18). It was found that death at 30 days were lower (295 vs 352 deaths, $p < 0.02$) in the fondaparinux group in which also major bleeding at 9 days were reduced (217 vs 412 bleeding events, $p < 0.001$). If emergent surgery or PCI is required, no agent for reversal of this specific anticoagulation is known.

Of the other specific substances for inhibition of Factor IIa and Xa that are under evaluation, importantly none of them have an agent reversing the effect acquired on anticoagulation.

RNA oligonucleotide aptamers have been produced with specific effects on Factor IIa, IXa, and Xa and importantly has a specific antidote (nucleic acid sequence binding selectively to the aptamer) that quickly halt the anticoagulant effect. In humans, the anticoagulative effect as well as a complete reversal by the antidote has been reported (19). Aptamers and its antidote seems to have a potential that other new anticoagulants do not have.

References

1 Oliva R. Protamines and male infertility. *Hum Reprod Update.* 2006;**12**:417–435.

2 Lindblad B. Protamine sulphate: a review of its effects, hypersensitivity and toxicity. *Eur J Vasc Surg.* 1989;**3**:195–201.

3 Welsby IJ, Newman MF, Philips-Bute B, Messier RH, Kakkis ED, Stafford-Smith M. Hemodynamic changes after protamine administration: association with mortality after coronary artery bypass surgery. *Anesthesiology.* 2005;**102**:308–314.

4 Stewart WJ, McSweeney SM, Kellett MA, Faxon DP, Ryan TJ. Increased risk of severe protamine reactions in

NPH insulin-dependent diabetics undergoing cardiac catheterization. *Circulation.* 1984;**70**:788–792.

5 Ducas J, Chan MC, Miller A, Kashour T. Immediate protamine administration and sheath removal following percutaneous coronary intervention: a prospective study of 429 patients. *Catheter Cardiovasc Interv.* 2002; **56**:196–199.

6 Vincent GM, Janowski M, Menlove R. Protamine allergy reactions during cardiac catheterization and cardiac surgery: risk in patients taking protamine-insulin preparations. *Cathet Cardiovasc Diagn.* 1991;**23**:164–168.

7 Wakefield TW, Lindblad B, Stanley JC, *et al.* Heparin and protamine use in peripheral vascular surgery: a comparison between surgeons of the Society for Vascular Surgery and the European Society for Vascular Surgery. *Eur J Vasc Surg.* 1994;**8**:193–198.

8 Dorman BH, Elliott BM, Spinale FG, *et al.* Protamine use during peripheral vascular surgery: a prospective randomized trial. *J Vasc Surg.* 1995;**22**:248–255.

9 Holst J, Lindblad B, Bergqvist D, Hedner U, Nordfang O, Ostergaard P. The effect of protamine sulphate on plasma tissue factor pathway inhibitor released by intravenous and subcutaneous unfractionated and low molecular weight heparin in man. *Thromb Res.* 1997;**86**:343–348.

10 Wakefield TW, Stanley JC. Intraoperative heparin anticoagulation and its reversal. *Semin Vasc Surg.* 1996;**9**: 296–302.

11 Holst J, Lindblad B, Bergqvist D, *et al.* Protamine neutralization of intravenous and subcutaneous low-molecular-weight heparin (tinzaparin, Logiparin). An experimental investigation in healthy volunteers. *Blood Coagul Fibrinolysis.* 1994;**5**:795–803.

12 Crowther MA, Berry LR, Monagle PT, *et al.* Mechanisms for the failure of protamine to inactivate low-molecular-weight-heparin. *Br J Haemost.* 2002;**116**:178–186.

13 Weiss ME, Nyhan D, Peng ZK, *et al.* Association of protamine IgE and IgG antibodies with life-threatening reactions to intravenous protamine. *N Engl J Med.* 1989; **320**:886–892.

14 Scheel B, Teufel R, Probst J, *et al.* Toll-like receptor-dependent activation of several human blood cell types by protamine-condensed mRNA. *Eur J Immunol.* 2005;**35**:1557–1566.

15 Dehmer GJ, Fisher M, Tate DA, Teo S, Bonnem EM. Reversal of heparin anticoagulation by recombinant platelet factor 4 in humans. *Circulation.* 1995;**91**:2188–2194.

16 Hulin MS, Wakefield TW, Andrews PC, *et al.* A novel protamine variant of heparin anticoagulation in human blood *in vitro. J Vasc Surg.* 1997;**26**:1043–1048.

17 Schulman S, Bijsterveld NR. Anticoagulants and their reversal. *Transfus Med Rev.* 2007;**21**:37–48.

18 Yusuf S, Mehta SR, Chrolavicius S, *et al.* Effects of fondaparinux on mortality and reinfarction in patients with acute ST-segment elevation myocardial infarction: the OASIS-6 randomized trial. *JAMA.* 2006;**295**: 1519–1530.

19 Dyke CK, Steinhubl SR, Kleiman NS, *et al.* First-in-human experience of an antidote-contorlled anticoagulant using RNA aptamer technology. A phase 1a pharmacodynamic evaluation of a drug-antidote pair for controlled regulation of factor IXa activity. *Circulation.* 2006;**114**:2490–2497.

CHAPTER 39

Thrombocytopenia post-percutaneous coronary intervention: Glycoprotein IIb/IIIa-induced

Ronen Gurvitch & Jeffrey Lefkovits
The Royal Melbourne Hospital, Melbourne, Victoria, Australia

Introduction

Atherosclerotic plaque rupture is the cornerstone of acute coronary syndromes, culminating in thrombus formation and adverse clinical events (1,2). Platelets play a central role in this process via aggregation and contribution to clot formation. During percutaneous coronary intervention (PCI), mechanical plaque disruption occurs and this too can result in predominantly platelet-rich thrombus formation, periprocedural cardiac enzyme elevation, and adverse clinical sequelae. The platelet glycoprotein (GP) IIb/IIIa receptor is the final common pathway, leading to platelet aggregation (3). Accordingly, much focus has been directed toward agents that inhibit this receptor. Clinical trials have shown significant benefits with these agents, with reductions in periprocedural myocardial infarction and late clinical adverse outcomes (4–6).

Three GP IIb/IIIa receptor inhibitors are currently approved for clinical use—abciximab (ReoPro®—Eli Lilly, Johnson & Johnson), eptifibatide (Integrilin®—Schering Corporation, Kenilworth, NJ) and tirofiban (Aggrastat®—Merck Sharp & Dohme, NJ, Whitehouse Station). Abciximab is a chimeric monoclonal antibody directed against the GP IIb/IIIa receptor, whereas tirofiban and eptifibatide are high-affinity nonantibody receptor inhibitors. In the setting of PCI, abciximab and eptifibatide usage is highly effective and is associated with significantly improved clinical outcomes. However, there is also a small but significant risk of adverse events that include bleeding, thrombocytopenia, pulmonary haemorrhage, and anaphylactic reactions.

Results of large randomized trials show that all three available GP IIb/IIIa receptor inhibitors cause thrombocytopenia in 0.5–6% of patients, leading to significant hemorrhagic complications and potential reductions in their overall net clinical benefit (4,5,7–10). However, accurate assessment of the increased risk of thrombocytopenia with these drugs is clouded by the frequent coadministration of other antithrombotic agents such as heparin and clopidogrel, and other concomitant procedures such as intra-aortic balloon counter pulsation or coronary graft surgery. The interrelationship of platelet GP IIb/IIIa receptor blockade and thrombocytopenia has important clinical implications, and this chapter will focus on this specific problem, its pathogenesis and diagnosis, differential diagnosis, monitoring, and approach to treatment.

Pathogenesis and incidence of thrombocytopenia

Abciximab

Abciximab is derived from the Fab fragment of the chimeric human murine monoclonal antibody c7E3.

Pharmacology in the Catheterization Laboratory. Edited by Ron Waksman and Andrew E Ajani. © 2010 Blackwell Publishing, ISBN: 978-1-4051-5704-9.

It binds primarily to the platelet GP IIb/IIIa receptor, but can also bind to Mac-1 and vitronectin receptors. Results of clinical trials have indicated that abciximab use is associated with rates of thrombocytopenia (platelets $<100 \times 10^9/L$) between 2.5% and 6%, and severe thrombocytopenia (platelets $<50 \times 10^9/L$) in 0.4–1.6% of patients (5,11–13).

Abciximab-induced thrombocytopenia typically occurs within 24 h of administration and occasionally within 30 min, suggesting an immune process (8,9). One possibility for such rapid occurrence of thrombocytopenia is the presence of naturally occurring antibodies against neoepitopes that may be exposed during normal platelet function (14–16). Human antichimeric antibodies (HACA) were noted in up to 19% of patients after the repeated administration of abciximab (17,18), supporting an immune-mediated mechanism for abciximab-related thrombocytopenia. Significantly higher concentrations of IgG and/or IgM were seen in patients with severe thrombocytopenia during repeated exposure to the drug. These HACA antibodies may also react with abciximab-inhibited platelets and lead to increased platelet consumption (17). In a pooled analysis by Dasgupta *et al.*, abciximab was associated with increased rates of both mild thrombocytopenia (4.2% vs 2.0%; $p < 0.01$) and severe thrombocytopenia (1.0% vs 0.4%; $p = 0.01$) compared with placebo. In contrast, the same analysis demonstrated that the small-molecule GP IIb/IIIa inhibitors tirofiban and eptifibatide were not associated with a statistically significant increase in thrombocytopenia (7).

Eptifibatide

Eptifibatide is a synthetic cyclic heptapeptide that binds to the GP IIb/IIIa receptor and reversibly inhibits platelet aggregation. The reported incidence of profound thrombocytopenia ($<20 \times 10^9/L$) appears less than for abciximab. In the ESPRIT trial, only 0.2% developed this complication (0% placebo) (19), while the PURSUIT trial reported a rate of any thrombocytopenia ($<100 \times 10^9/L$) of 6.8%, which was similar to the placebo rate of 6.7% (20).

Although the drug is not derived from an antibody source, Bougie *et al.* described a number of cases of severe thrombocytopenia with eptifibatide

use where an immune-mediated process was implicated (14). The study showed that thrombocytopenia was associated with antibodies specific for ligand-occupied receptors (drug-dependent) and that these IgG antibodies can occur naturally in a small proportion of healthy people. As such, patients may develop thrombocytopenia even on first exposure to the drug.

Tirofiban

This nonpeptide molecule mimics the geometric and stereotactic characteristics of the GP IIb/IIIa receptor binding site and reversibly inhibits platelet aggregation. Its role in PCI is less well-established. However, in the RESTORE trial of 2,139 patients undergoing PCI who were randomized to receive either tirofiban or placebo, there were no differences in rates of thrombocytopenia between the two groups (1.5% vs 1.2% respectively, $p = 0.7$) (21). In the PRISM—PLUS trial, there was a trend toward more thrombocytopenia ($<90 \times 10^9/L$) with tirofiban compared with placebo (1.8% vs 1.2%, $p = 0.06$), in high-risk patients with acute coronary syndromes. However, there was no difference in the rates of severe thrombocytopenia ($<50 \times 10^9/L$) (0.5% vs 0.3%, $p = 0.39$) (22).

Timing of thrombocytopenia

Glycoprotein IIb/IIIa inhibitor-induced thrombocytopenia usually develops in the first few hours of treatment. Abciximab therapy in particular, has also been associated with very rapid reactions within 30 min but this is extremely rare (8,23). Delayed thrombocytopenia after 5 or 7 days has also been seen with abciximab therapy (24,25). This may be a result of the long receptor half-life, which may stimulate weaker preformed antibodies at higher titers (26).

Clinical sequelae

In most cases, thrombocytopenia does not result in significant adverse events and responds to platelet transfusion. In a pooled analysis by Dasgupta *et al.*, 42 patients with thrombocytopenia were analyzed—23 with severe and 19 with profound thrombocytopenia. Although some had counts less than $10 \times 10^9/L$, no major bleeding complications were reported (7). However, other trials have found that clinically significant bleeding can occur in patients who develop thrombocytopenia, resulting in adverse clinical outcomes (9,10,27). In the TARGET trial, thrombocytopenia developed more frequently with abciximab than with tirofiban (2.4% vs 0.5%) (10), and patients with thrombocytopenia had more frequent severe bleeding (5.1 vs 0.7%, $p < 0.001$), received more blood transfusions (6.1% vs 1.4%, $p < 0.001$) and had higher incidence of death, myocardial infarction, and target vessel revascularization at 30 days (12.2% vs 6.6%, $p < 0.04$). The development of thrombocytopenia may also lengthen hospital stay (28), and is associated with worse long-term outcomes (29). An increase in ischemic adverse events has been found at follow-up, yet the mechanism for this remains unclear.

The main independent risk factors for development of thrombocytopenia are age >65 years, low initial platelet count ($<180 \times 10^9$/L), and low body mass index (9,10).

Diagnosis

Timing of platelet counts

It is imperative that the diagnosis of thrombocytopenia is made as soon as possible given the possible adverse clinical sequelae. As thrombocytopenia can occur within the first few hours of administration, platelet counts should be assessed prior to treatment and within 1–4 h of treatment commencement. Counts should be repeated after 12 h and then twice daily if prolonged treatment is administered. In the case of abciximab, delayed thrombocytopenia is also possible and it is therefore recommended that a platelet count be checked again a few days after administration.

Criteria for diagnosis of thrombocytopenia

The principles of the diagnosis of GP IIb/IIIa receptor inhibitor-induced thrombocytopenia are the following:
- Laboratory confirmation of the platelet count
- Exclude pseudothrombocytopenia
- Exclude other causes such as heparin-induced thrombocytopenia (HIT), thrombotic thrombocytopenic purpura (TTP), and other drug causes of thrombocytopenia

Laboratory confirmation

If a platelet count $<100 \times 10^9$/L is noted or there is a fall in counts to <50% of baseline, the test should be repeated urgently to confirm the result. The platelet count should be repeated in a tube with a different anticoagulant such as sodium citrate.

Pseudothrombocytopenia

Pseudothrombocytopenia results from an *in vitro* phenomenon of platelet clumping, leading to a falsely low platelet count. It is critical to exclude the presence of clumping when low platelet counts are found, as it may otherwise result in the inappropriate cessation of therapy. In a review of four large abciximab trials, the incidence of pseudothrombocytopenia was 2.1%, and it accounted for 36% of cases of low platelet counts during abciximab therapy (30). The main offending collecting tube anticoagulant was ethylenediaminetetraacetic acid (EDTA), while a small number of cases also occurred in the presence of sodium citrate. Apart from presence of certain anticoagulants such as EDTA, factors that enhance the occurrence of pseudothrombocytopenia include a prolonged time interval between blood drawn and laboratory assessment and low temperatures (31,32). Unlike true thrombocytopenia, pseudothrombocytopenia is not associated with any adverse outcomes (30). Although pseudothrombocytopenia has been reported in patients receiving placebo therapy in abciximab trials, there are no reports of this condition in association with eptifibatide or tirofiban therapy to date.

Differential diagnosis

Apart from pseudothrombocytopenia, the main differential diagnoses to consider when a low platelet count is encountered include the following.

Heparin-induced thrombocytopenia syndrome (HIT)—type I and type II

Type I HIT occurs in about 25% of patients within the first 2 days of commencing heparin treatment and results from a proaggregatory action of heparin on platelets (33,34). There is usually only a small fall in platelet counts (usually to $100–150 \times 10^9$/L) not necessitating cessation of heparin. Type II HIT is an immune-mediated event occurring within 4–14 days of commencing heparin therapy or within a few hours of reexposure. The fall in platelet count can be profound ($<20 \times 10^9$/L) and the condition is associated with thrombotic events in both arteries and veins. It is diagnosed with positive HIPA and antiplatelet factor 4 assays (35–37).

The distinction between GP IIb/IIIa inhibitor-induced thrombocytopenia and type II HIT is particularly important. While the former is associated with bleeding and may require platelet transfusion, the latter causes thrombosis that may be exacerbated by replacement therapy. If thrombocytopenia occurs early (<24 h) in a patient with no prior heparin exposure in the last few months and both antiplatelet factor 4 antibody and HIPA assays are negative, then type II HIT is unlikely.

Clopidogrel-induced thrombotic thrombocytopenic purpura (TTP)/hemolytic uremic syndrome (HUS)

Although the pivotal trials of clopidogrel in cardiovascular disease did not record any cases of TTP-HUS, the subsequent widespread use of the drug has been associated with a number of cases cited in postmarketing reports (38–41).

The syndrome is characterized by fluctuating neurological abnormalities, fever, and renal insufficiency. Microangiopathic hemolytic anemia is the hallmark of the disorder and is defined as nonimmune hemolysis with prominent red cell fragmentation or schistocytes that can be observed on a peripheral blood film. These features help distinguish it from GP IIb/IIIa inhibitor-induced thrombocytopenia.

Other medications

Several drugs have been implicated in causing thrombocytopenia, with some of the more common ones being ezetimibe, quinine, frusemide, and a number of antibiotics.

Treatment

The treatment of GP IIb/IIIa inhibitor-induced thrombocytopenia is controversial and can depend on the severity of thrombocytopenia and presence or absence of bleeding. The cornerstones of therapy are discontinuation of the offending agent and platelet transfusion (Table 39.1).

Table 39.1 Recommended approach to management according to platelet counts.

Platelet count ($\times 10^9$/L)	Recommended approach to management
100–150	• Monitor count every 2 h
50–100	• Repeat count from a tube with a different anticoagulant, e.g., citrate, and perform blood film
	• Monitor count every 2 h
	• HIT antibodies
20–50	• Repeat count from a tube with a different anticoagulant, e.g., citrate, and perform blood film
	• HIT antibodies
	• Monitor count every 2 h
	• Stop GP IIb/IIIa inhibitor + heparin
	• Continue aspirin and clopidogrel
	• If bleeding (unlikely):
	○ reverse heparin with protamine
	○ stop aspirin and clopidogrel
	○ transfuse platelets
<20	• Repeat count from a tube with a different anticoagulant, e.g., citrate, and perform blood film
	• HIT antibodies
	• Stop GP IIb/IIIa inhibitor + heparin
	• Stop aspirin and clopidogrel
	• Reverse heparin with protamine
	• If bleeding—transfuse platelets
	• If $<10 \times 10^6$—transfuse platelets

For confirmed platelet counts between 50 and $100 \times 10^9/L$, consideration should be given to stopping the GP IIb/IIIa inhibitor. The platelet count should be repeated in 2 h and if it continues to drop or if any bleeding occurs, GP IIb/IIIa blockade should be stopped (42). Cessation of the drug infusion is usually enough to allow the platelet count to recover. For counts $<50 \times 10^9/L$, it is recommended that both the GP IIb/IIIa inhibitor and heparin should be stopped. If bleeding occurs, heparin can be reversed with protamine and a platelet transfusion should be administered.

For counts $<10–20 \times 10^9/L$, antiplatelet agents such as aspirin and clopidogrel should all be withheld, together with the cessation of the GP IIb/IIIa inhibitor and reversal of heparin. Designating a specific platelet count level at which to administer prophylactic platelet transfusion (without bleeding) is controversial. While no randomized data are available in this population, in patients with leukaemia, limiting prophylactic platelet transfusions to patients with platelet counts of $<10 \times 10^9/L$ has been shown to be as safe and more cost-effective compared with the traditional approach of using a cutoff value of $<20 \times 10^9/L$ (43–45). However, once bleeding occurs, platelet transfusion should be considered with any level of significant thrombocytopenia.

Steroids and intravenous gamma globulin

Although corticosteroids and intravenous immunoglobulin (IVIG) have been considered standard therapy in immune thrombocytopenia, evidence for their use in the setting of GP IIb/IIIa blockade is limited (46–50). Kereiakes *et al.* reported on four cases of abciximab-induced thrombocytopenia with bleeding complications—two treated with platelet transfusions only, one with transfusion and IVIG, and one with IVIG without concomitant platelet transfusion. They noted that whereas platelet transfusion resulted in rapid and sustained increments in platelet counts, recovery of platelet count was not improved by IVIG therapy. In the patient with IVIG treatment only, very slow platelet count recovery took place (>48 h) (50). Other investigators have also reported on the use of IVIG, but did not provide information regarding dose or response to therapy (14). There are no reports on the efficacy of steroids in this setting and further data are needed to determine the utility of these therapies in the setting of GP IIb/IIIa inhibitor-induced thrombocytopenia.

Readministration of drug

The ReoPro Re-Administration Registry (R^3) was the largest of a number of trials assessing the efficacy and safety of abciximab readministration (18,51). A total of 1,343 patients undergoing PCI and receiving abciximab for at least a second time were studied. Patients with thrombocytopenia following initial administration were excluded.

The overall rate of thrombocytopenia after abciximab readministration was similar to rates of thrombocytopenia in randomized trials of first-time abciximab treatment. However, those patients who developed thrombocytopenia with drug readministration were more likely to develop profound falls in platelet counts ($<20 \times 10^9/L$) (18). Furthermore, those who received abciximab within 1 month of a previous treatment had a higher risk of developing thrombocytopenia (16.5%) and profound thrombocytopenia (12.2%). In another report evaluating readministration, the incidence of profound thrombocytopenia was 4% in those reexposed to abciximab, but was 12% if reexposed within 2 weeks (52).

The R^3 also measured HACA titers before and after readministration. A positive HACA before readministration (5.6% of study participants) was associated with higher risk of thrombocytopenia (14.1% vs 4.4%, $p = 0.002$) and profound thrombocytopenia (5.6% vs 1.6%, $p = 0.036$). Whether HACA titres prereadministration may assist in risk stratification regarding future thrombocytopenia requires further evaluation.

There are no published data available to date on the risks of readministration of tirofiban or eptifibatide, and only scant information regarding potential cross-reactions among different GP IIb/IIIa inhibitors. While there have been reports of abciximab-associated thrombocytopenia after tirofiban-related thrombocytopenia, others have suggested that the administration of a different GP IIb/IIIa inhibitor appears safe (23,53).

Summary

Despite significant clinical benefits of GP IIb/IIIa receptor blockade during PCI, GP IIb/IIIa inhibitor-induced thrombocytopenia is a well-recognized phenomenon with potentially serious adverse clinical outcomes. Patients receiving this form of antiplatelet therapy must be closely monitored for the development of this complication. Early detection and immediate cessation of the GP IIb/IIIa inhibitor is usually all that is required for treatment, with spontaneous recovery of the platelet count ensuing in the majority of cases. Other antiplatelet agents such as aspirin and clopidogrel may also need to be withheld temporarily until platelet counts recover. In a small minority of cases with severe falls in platelet count or active bleeding, platelet transfusion may be necessary. However, currently there are no convincing data to support the use of other therapies such as steroids or intravenous immunoglobulin.

References

1 Kristensen SD, Ravn HB, Falk E. Insights into the pathophysiology of unstable coronary artery disease. *Am J Cardiol.* 1997;**80**(5A):5E–9E.

2 Falk E, Shah PK, Fuster V. Coronary plaque disruption. *Circulation.* 1995;**92**(3):657–671.

3 Plow EF, Ginsberg MH. Cellular adhesion: GPIIb-IIIa as a prototypic adhesion receptor. *Prog Hemost Thromb.* 1989;**9**:117–156.

4 Use of a monoclonal antibody directed against the platelet glycoprotein IIb/IIIa receptor in high-risk coronary angioplasty. The EPIC Investigation. *N Engl J Med.* 1994;**330**(14):956–961.

5 Platelet glycoprotein IIb/IIIa receptor blockade and low-dose heparin during percutaneous coronary revascularization. The EPILOG Investigators. *N Engl J Med.* 1997;**336**(24):1689–1696.

6 Blankenship JC, Tasissa G, O'Shea JC, *et al.* Effect of glycoprotein IIb/IIIa receptor inhibition on angiographic complications during percutaneous coronary intervention in the ESPRIT trial. *J Am Coll Cardiol.* 2001;**38**(3):653–658.

7 Dasgupta H, Blankenship JC, Wood GC, Frey CM, Demko SL, Menapace FJ. Thrombocytopenia complicating treatment with intravenous glycoprotein IIb/IIIa receptor inhibitors: a pooled analysis. *Am Heart J.* 2000;**140**(2):206–211.

8 Berkowitz SD, Harrington RA, Rund MM, Tcheng JE. Acute profound thrombocytopenia after C7E3 Fab (abciximab) therapy. *Circulation.* 1997;**95**(4):809–813.

9 Berkowitz SD, Sane DC, Sigmon KN, *et al.* Occurrence and clinical significance of thrombocytopenia in a population undergoing high-risk percutaneous coronary revascularization. Evaluation of c7E3 for the Prevention of Ischemic Complications (EPIC) Study Group. *J Am Coll Cardiol.* 1998;**32**(2):311–319.

10 Merlini PA, Rossi M, Menozzi A, *et al.* Thrombocytopenia caused by abciximab or tirofiban and its association with clinical outcome in patients undergoing coronary stenting. *Circulation.* 2004;**109**(18):2203–2206.

11 Randomised placebo-controlled trial of abciximab before and during coronary intervention in refractory unstable angina: the CAPTURE Study. *Lancet.* 1997;**349**(9063):1429–1435.

12 Montalescot G, Barragan P, Wittenberg O, *et al.* Platelet glycoprotein IIb/IIIa inhibition with coronary stenting for acute myocardial infarction. *N Engl J Med.* 2001;**344**(25):1895–1903.

13 Stone GW, Grines CL, Cox DA, *et al.* Comparison of angioplasty with stenting, with or without abciximab, in acute myocardial infarction. *N Engl J Med.* 2002;**346**(13):957–966.

14 Bougie DW, Wilker PR, Wuitschick ED, *et al.* Acute thrombocytopenia after treatment with tirofiban or eptifibatide is associated with antibodies specific for ligand-occupied GPIIb/IIIa. *Blood.* 2002;**100**(6):2071–2076.

15 Billheimer JT, Dicker IB, Wynn R, *et al.* Evidence that thrombocytopenia observed in humans treated with orally bioavailable glycoprotein IIb/IIIa antagonists is immune mediated. *Blood.* 2002;**99**(10):3540–3546.

16 Aster RH, Curtis BR, Bougie DW. Thrombocytopenia resulting from sensitivity to GPIIb-IIIa inhibitors. *Semin Thromb Hemost.* 2004;**30**(5):569–577.

17 Aster RH. Immune thrombocytopenia caused by glycoprotein IIb/IIIa inhibitors. *Chest.* 2005;**127**(2 Suppl): 53S–59S.

18 Tcheng JE, Kereiakes DJ, Lincoff AM, *et al.* Abciximab readministration: results of the ReoPro Readministration Registry. *Circulation.* 2001;**104**(8):870–875.

19 Novel dosing regimen of eptifibatide in planned coronary stent implantation (ESPRIT): a randomised, placebo-controlled trial. *Lancet.* 2000;**356**(9247):2037–2044.

20 Inhibition of platelet glycoprotein IIb/IIIa with eptifibatide in patients with acute coronary syndromes. The PURSUIT Trial Investigators. Platelet glycoprotein IIb/IIIa in unstable angina: receptor suppression using integrilin therapy. *N Engl J Med.* 1998;**339**(7):436–443.

21 Effects of platelet glycoprotein IIb/IIIa blockade with tirofiban on adverse cardiac events in patients with unstable angina or acute myocardial infarction undergoing

coronary angioplasty. The RESTORE Investigators. Randomized Efficacy Study of Tirofiban for Outcomes and REstenosis. *Circulation.* 1997;**96**(5):1445–1453.

22 Inhibition of the platelet glycoprotein IIb/IIIa receptor with tirofiban in unstable angina and non-Q-wave myocardial infarction. Platelet Receptor Inhibition in Ischemic Syndrome Management in Patients Limited by Unstable Signs and Symptoms (PRISM-PLUS) study investigators. *N Engl J Med.* 1998;**338**(21):1488–1497.

23 Simon BC, Herzum M, Klisch A, *et al.* Acute severe thrombocytopenia after c7E3 Fab (abciximab) therapy in a patient with unstable angina and stenting of the right coronary artery. Occurrence of subacute stent thrombosis and safe readministration of the GPIIb/IIIa inhibitor tirofiban. *Int J Cardiovasc Interv.* 2000;**3**(3):185–188.

24 Jenkins LA, Lau S, Crawford M, Keung YK. Delayed profound thrombocytopenia after c7E3 Fab (abciximab) therapy. *Circulation.* 1998;**97**(12):1214–1215.

25 Reddy MS, Carmody TJ, Kereiakes DJ. Severe delayed thrombocytopenia associated with abciximab (ReoPro) therapy. *Catheter Cardiovasc Interv.* 2001;**52**(4):486–488.

26 Curtis BR, Divgi A, Garritty M, Aster RH. Delayed thrombocytopenia after treatment with abciximab: a distinct clinical entity associated with the immune response to the drug. *J Thromb Haemost.* 2004;**2**(6):985–992.

27 Kereiakes DJ, Berkowitz SD, Lincoff AM, *et al.* Clinical correlates and course of thrombocytopenia during percutaneous coronary intervention in the era of abciximab platelet glycoprotein IIb/IIIa blockade. *Am Heart J.* 2000;**140**(1):74–80.

28 George BJ, Eckart RE, Shry EA, Simpson DE. Glycoprotein IIb/IIIa inhibitor-associated thrombocytopenia: clinical predictors and effect on outcome. *Cardiology.* 2004;**102**(4):184–187.

29 McClure MW, Berkowitz SD, Sparapani R, *et al.* Clinical significance of thrombocytopenia during a non-ST-elevation acute coronary syndrome. The platelet glycoprotein IIb/IIIa in unstable angina: receptor suppression using integrilin therapy (PURSUIT) trial experience. *Circulation.* 1999;**99**(22):2892–2900.

30 Sane DC, Damaraju LV, Topol EJ, *et al.* Occurrence and clinical significance of pseudothrombocytopenia during abciximab therapy. *J Am Coll Cardiol.* 2000;**36**(1):75–83.

31 Schrezenmeier H, Muller H, Gunsilius E, Heimpel H, Seifried E. Anticoagulant-induced pseudothrombocytopenia and pseudoleucocytosis. *Thromb Haemost.* 1995;**73**(3):506–513.

32 Bizzaro N. EDTA-dependent pseudothrombocytopenia: a clinical and epidemiological study of 112 cases, with 10-year follow-up. *Am J Hematol.* 1995;**50**(2):103–109.

33 Chong BH, Berndt MC. Heparin-induced thrombocytopenia. *Blut.* 1989;**58**(2):53–57.

34 Chong BH, Fawaz I, Chesterman CN, Berndt MC. Heparin-induced thrombocytopenia: mechanism of interaction of the heparin-dependent antibody with platelets. *Br J Haematol.* 1989;**73**(2):235–240.

35 Warkentin TE, Levine MN, Hirsh J, *et al.* Heparin-induced thrombocytopenia in patients treated with low-molecular-weight heparin or unfractionated heparin. *N Engl J Med.* 1995;**332**(20):1330–1335.

36 Warkentin TE. Heparin-induced thrombocytopenia. Pathogenesis, frequency, avoidance and management. *Drug Saf.* 1997;**17**(5):325–341.

37 Brieger DB, Mak KH, Kottke-Marchant K, Topol EJ. Heparin-induced thrombocytopenia. *J Am Coll Cardiol.* 1998;**31**(7):1449–1459.

38 Bennett CL, Connors JM, Carwile JM, *et al.* Thrombotic thrombocytopenic purpura associated with clopidogrel. *N Engl J Med.* 2000;**342**(24):1773–1777.

39 Zakarija A, Bandarenko N, Pandey DK, *et al.* Clopidogrel-associated TTP: an update of pharmacovigilance efforts conducted by independent researchers, pharmaceutical suppliers, and the Food and Drug Administration. *Stroke.* 2004;**35**(2):533–537.

40 Hankey GJ. Clopidogrel and thrombotic thrombocytopenic purpura. *Lancet.* 2000;**356**(9226):269–270.

41 Paradiso-Hardy FL, Papastergiou J, Lanctot KL, Cohen EA. Thrombotic thrombocytopenic purpura associated with clopidogrel: further evaluation. *Can J Cardiol.* 2002;**18**(7):771–773.

42 Patel S, Patel M, Din I, Reddy CV, Kassotis J. Profound thrombocytopenia associated with tirofiban: case report and review of literature. *Angiology.* 2005;**56**(3):351–355.

43 Wandt H, Frank M, Ehninger G, *et al.* Safety and cost effectiveness of a 10 × 10(9)/L trigger for prophylactic platelet transfusions compared with the traditional 20 × 10(9)/L trigger: a prospective comparative trial in 105 patients with acute myeloid leukemia. *Blood.* 1998;**91**(10):3601–3606.

44 Rebulla P, Finazzi G, Marangoni F, *et al.* The threshold for prophylactic platelet transfusions in adults with acute myeloid leukemia. Gruppo Italiano Malattie Ematologiche Maligne dell'Adulto. *N Engl J Med.* 1997;**337**(26):1870–1875.

45 Heckman KD, Weiner GJ, Davis CS, Strauss RG, Jones MP, Burns CP. Randomized study of prophylactic platelet transfusion threshold during induction therapy for adult acute leukemia: 10,000/microL versus 20,000/microL. *J Clin Oncol.* 1997;**15**(3):1143–1149.

46 McMillan R. Classical management of refractory adult immune (idiopathic) thrombocytopenic purpura. *Blood Rev.* 2002;**16**(1):51–55.

47 Andersen JC. Response of resistant idiopathic thrombocytopenic purpura to pulsed high-dose dexamethasone therapy. *N Engl J Med.* 1994;**330**(22):1560–1564.

48 George JN. Diagnosis, clinical course, and management of idiopathic thrombocytopenic purpura. *Curr Opin Hematol.* 1996;**3**(5):335–340.

49 George JN, Woolf SH, Raskob GE, *et al.* Idiopathic thrombocytopenic purpura: a practice guideline developed by explicit methods for the American Society of Hematology. *Blood.* 1996;**88**(1):3–40.

50 Kereiakes DJ, Essell JH, Abbottsmith CW, Broderick TM, Runyon JP. Abciximab-associated profound thrombocytopenia: therapy with immunoglobulin and platelet transfusion. *Am J Cardiol.* 1996;**78**(10):1161–1163.

51 Dery JP, Braden GA, Lincoff AM, *et al.* Final results of the ReoPro readministration registry. *Am J Cardiol.* 2004;**93**(8):979–984.

52 Madan M, Kereiakes DJ, Hermiller JB, *et al.* Efficacy of abciximab readministration in coronary intervention. *Am J Cardiol.* 2000;**85**(4):435–440.

53 Dorsch MP, Montague D, Rodgers JE, Patterson C. Abciximab-associated thrombocytopenia after previous tirofiban-related thrombocytopenia. *Pharmacotherapy.* 2006;**26**(3):423–427.

PART IX

Systemic pharmacotherapy for in-stent restenosis

CHAPTER 40

Is oral rapamycin plus bare metal stents a feasible alternative to drug-eluting stents? Lessons learned from Argentina observational and randomized studies (ORAR I, II, and III trials)

Alfredo E. Rodriguez

Buenos Aires School of Medicine, Buenos Aires, Argentina

Introduction

The "problem" of coronary restenosis

Since the introduction of coronary angioplasty, restenosis of the target lesion has been the main limitation of this procedure. Acute vessel recoil, chronic remodeling, and intimal hyperplasia were the mechanisms involved in this process (1–4). However, after the introduction of stents in the daily practice during interventional procedures, intimal hyperplasia become the only mechanism associated with the pathophysiology of in-stent restenosis (5–9). Therefore, its prevention should be related with therapies, which inhibit smooth muscle cell proliferation.

Since the introduction of drug-eluting stents (DES) for percutaneous coronary interventional procedures, angiographic and clinical parameters of coronary restenosis have strikingly decreased during the first years of follow-up. Several randomized studies comparing bare metal stents (BMS) vs

Pharmacology in the Catheterization Laboratory. Edited by Ron Waksman and Andrew E Ajani. © 2010 Blackwell Publishing, ISBN: 978-1-4051-5704-9.

FDA-approved DES designs, sirolimus-eluting stent (SES), and paclitaxel-eluting stent (PES) in patients with low-risk coronary lesions demonstrated a significant reduction in coronary restenosis, which translated into lower target vessel revascularization (TVR) and target lesion revascularization (TLR) rates (10–17). Following approval, we have witnessed a widespread use of DES technology to include higher-risk patients and complex lesions such as overlapping stents for long lesions, bifurcating lesions and left main stenosis including patients with nonsevere obstructive coronary disease (18–20).

However, after 4 years of carrying out an almost unselected, systematic use of these devices in the United States and in many countries all over the world, the angiographic and clinical improvement of the rate of restenosis has not been translated into a reduction of the two strongest and most powerful cardiac events, that is, myocardial infarction and death.

Moreover, recently worrisome data showed a significant increase of such hard events with the use of DES in determined clinical circumstances and/or lesion or procedural characteristics (18,19).

Additionally, through the years, we have also learned that angiographic coronary restenosis after percutaneous coronary interventions (PCI) is a prevalent but also a "soft" and clinically irrelevant event. This concept is supported by the results of several randomized studies comparing a variety of percutaneous approaches that have shown a significant reduction in angiographic and clinical parameters of restenosis after implantation. These studies consistently failed to show any reduction in cardiac mortality and/or myocardial infarction (21,22). In randomized studies comparing BMS vs plain optimal balloon angioplasty (POBA), provisional vs universal stenting (9,10,23–25), POBA vs coronary bypass surgery (CABG), BMS vs CABG or lately BMS vs DES (26–31), restenosis and TVR reduction are not associated with similar reductions of death and/or myocardial infarction. Even though from a patient's point of view, restenosis is not an irrelevant event, we also know since the beginning of PCI that coronary restenosis is a nonlife-threatening event; otherwise, it would have been impossible for percutaneous interventions to be a feasible alternative to CABG.

Moreover, excluding the diabetic population, all individual randomized studies have shown no significant differences at midterm follow-up in death and/or nonfatal myocardial infarction between CABG and POBA or BMS (25–27). In addition, the long-term follow-up of DES Pivotal trials (Taxus and SIRIUS) once again demonstrated that restenosis is a benign event. Pooled analysis from those randomized studies over 4 years reported an extremely lower restenosis rate with DES as compared to BMS. However, this lower restenosis rate failed to translate into any advantage in the incidence of death and/or nonfatal myocardial infarction (32,33).

If we take into account the aforementioned findings as we search for therapies with the potential to reduce restenosis, we cannot accept any increase (not even few) in "hard" cardiac events (death and myocardial infarction) as a price to pay to achieve such a target. The disturbing observation that stent thrombosis could appear late and very late, beyond 1, 2, or more years after stent deployment, means that dual antiplatelet therapy should be taken for 1 or more years or perhaps indefinitely. Recent data from the Basket Late Trial, Duke Registry, and ERACI III trials stressed the role of clopidogrel discontinuation after DES implantation. These studies showed significantly higher incidence of death and MI in patients where clopidogrel was discontinued (34,35).

Systemic immunosuppressive therapies in the treatment of restenosis

Sirolimus and sirolimus analogues in experimental and clinical data

Animal data suggest that the degree of neointimal proliferation formed after stent implantation is mediated by smooth muscle cell proliferation and occurs during the first 2 weeks after the initial vascular injury (36). The relative success of nonpolymeric-based drug delivery stents using short-time release of medications support the concept that sustained release of antiproliferative agents may not be necessary to maintain a biological effect (37). The inflammatory response after coronary artery stenting is deeply involved in the pathophysiology of in-stent restenosis (ISR), linking the vascular injury induced by coronary stenting with the intimal smooth muscle cell migration/proliferation that culminates in ISR (38). It is well known that PCI alters the systemic expression of inflammatory markers, especially when stents are implanted. In agreement with that, matrix metalloproteinase (MMP-9) plays important roles in every biological process where extracellular matrix turnover or repair is involved including restenosis. Thus MMP-9 was recognized as a factor present in patients with coronary restenosis after PCI and plays a key role in the process of coronary restenosis (39).

Sirolimus is an immunosuppressant agent with antiproliferative, antimigratory, and anti-inflammatory properties. Gallo was the first to report animal data showing a significant reduction of neointimal hyperplasia with the systemic infusion of rapamycin (40). After that, several preclinical studies have demonstrated the ability of systemically administered sirolimus or its analogues in reducing smooth muscle cell proliferation occurring after vascular injury (35,39–41). In agreement with this, a marked reduction of MMP-9 in patients after bare metal stent implantation was reported with oral sirolimus therapy (39).

More recently, other antiproliferative drugs such Everolimus or Paclitaxel, used systemically, have been shown a significant reduction of neointimal hyperplasia in animal data. Additionally, local delivery of paclitaxel nanoparticles was associated recently with a significant reduction of in-stent restenosis (42).

Rapamycin (Rapamune, Wyeth-Ayerst Laboratories) is a natural macrocyclic lactone with a potent immunosuppressive and antiproliferative effect that was approved by the FDA for the prophylaxis against renal transplant rejection.

The anti-inflammatory and antiproliferative effects of rapamycin was based on its ability to inhibit the TOR kinase (target of rapamycin), an essential component in the pathways of the cell cycle progression (36,40,41). Several nonrandomized pilot studies in *de novo* lesions have been reported in recent years with the systemic use of rapamycin.

The clinical and angiographic results of these studies are described in Table 40.1. As we can see in the table, even though some differences in study design are found, similar clinical and angiographic long-term outcome data was obtained. As we can see in Table 40.1, angiographic restenosis, from these pilot studies, was in the order of a single digit, with a late loss around of 0.6 mm. All these numbers compared to the average restenosis rate of control arm from more recent DES trials means a reduction of 81% of in-stent restenosis and a 42% reduction of late loss, also with a significant reduction of MACCE.

We obtained several results from these pilot trials (44–47). First, angiographic in-stent binary restenosis was approximately 10%. Second, a high maintenance dose did not improve angiographic follow-up results and in contrast was associated with higher side effects.

As ORBIT study shows, with 2 mg per day, ORBIT investigators (45) found 40% of minor and moderate side effects, compared with 66% when they used 5 mg per day during 30 days.

A small pilot trial from Brazil also confirmed these positive results, reporting 6.6% of in-stent restenosis with 0.61 mm of late loss and with no target lesion revascularization or any major events after 2 years of follow-up (48).

Furthermore, side effects were minor or moderate in almost all studies, and they are attributed to the maintenance doses used in these studies. At the present time, it is clear that it is not reasonable to give more than 3 mg per day as a maintenance dose and no longer than 14 days (45). With high maintenance doses, similar final angiographic results were obtained but with poor clinical tolerance as we mentioned above with the ORBIT trial.

Third, a key issue for this therapy is to give the immunosuppressive drug before the PCI procedure was performed. Coronary stent deployment should be performed under the effects of immunosuppressive therapy.

Lastly, in patients with in stent restenosis, even though the first pilot trial reported negative results in a small high-risk population with restenosis after brachyterapy failure (47,49), the only randomized

Table 40.1 Angiographic and clinical outcome at follow-up of oral rapamycin studies (Published until 2005).

	OSIRIS[a] (n = 99)	ORAR I[b] (n = 76)	ORBIT (2 mg)[b] (n = 30)	ORBIT (5 mg)[b] (n = 30)
Binary Restenosis (%)				
In-stent	—	6.2[c]	7.1	6.9
In-lesion	22.1	10.4[c]	4.8	6.9
Late Loss (mm)	0.49 + 0.54	0.63 + 0.22[c]	0.60 + 0.56	0.68 + 0.56
Stent Thrombosis (%)	0	0	0	0
TVR (%)	15.2	15	16.7	20.6
MACCE (%)	18.2	20	24	20

[a]In-stent restenosis (43).

[b]*De novo* lesions (44,45).

[c]All stents were deployed *successfully*.

data in this population was reported by the OSIRIS trial (50), and showed a significant reduction of clinical and angiographic parameters of restenosis ($p = 0.005$) using a loading dose of oral rapamycin of 12 mg started 48 h before the PCI procedure followed by 2 mg per day during 7 days after (50). Angiographic restenosis and need for target lesion revascularization were reduced by 50% and 40%, respectively, with the use of oral sirolimus therapy (Table 40.1).

Oral rapamycin in *de novo* lesions: lessons learned from Argentina ORAR studies

ORAR I pilot trial

From December 2001 though February 2003, 76 patients with a clinical indication for PCI in a novo coronary lesion were included in this protocol. The procedures were performed at the cardiac catheterization laboratories of the Cardiovascular Research Center in Buenos Aires, Argentina (44,46).

Among these 76 patients, 109 bare coronary stents were deployed in 103 *de novo* lesions in an equal number of major native epicardial vessels. Patients with in-stent restenosis, bifurcation lesions, vein graft lesions, lesion length 20 mm, acute myocardial infarction in the previous 72 h, poor left ventricular function (ejection fraction <35%), renal failure defined as creatinine concentration >2 mg, or under immunosuppressive treatment were excluded from the study.

This observational study was performed in two phases. In Phase I, rapamycin was given orally as a loading dose of 6 mg at the time of PCI followed by a daily dose of 2 mg/day for 28 days, starting immediately after successful stent deployment.

In Phase II, a daily dose of 180 mg of diltiazem was added; diltiazem associated with oral rapamycin in patients after renal transplant increased blood concentration of the drug with low side effects (51).

It has been shown that coadministration of a single dose of diltiazem with rapamycin leads to higher rapamycin exposure. The mean whole blood rapamycin area under the plasma concentration in time curve increased 60% and maximum concentration increased 43%. Coadministration also decreased the renal clearance of rapamycin,

presumably by inhibiting the first pass metabolism of rapamycin (51,52).

Rapamycin blood concentrations were measured in all patients in Phase I, after the third week of treatment. However, as the immunosuppressive effect of the drug has been shown to be optimal within 4 days after treatment, in Phase II, they were measured earlier, during the first week (41,53,54).

A lipid profile (cholesterol, high-density lipoprotein, low-density lipoprotein, and triglycerides) and complete blood count were determined before and after 4 weeks of treatment for all the patients.

Results

Baseline demographic, clinical, and angiographic characteristics of the patient population are described in Table 40.2. Mean age was 63 years. More than 60% of patients presented with unstable angina; 20% were diabetic, 23% had a previous AMI, and more than 80% had class B or C lesions according to the American College of Cardiology/ American Heart Association classification.

Hospital and 30-day results

All stents were deployed successfully. One patient, who developed subacute artery closure few hours after the procedure, presented the only adverse event during hospitalization. During the first month, 19 patients (25%) had minor side effects, six patients in Phase I (18%) and 13 in Phase II (31%) but only three discontinued the medication (3.9%), one in Phase I and two in Phase II. The most frequent side effects were diarrhea (7.8%) and skin rash (9.2%). There were no changes in white cell count or cholesterol concentration relative to baseline, whereas triglyceride concentrations tended to be higher than at baseline. Additionally, sirolimus blood concentration was significantly higher in Phase II than in Phase I (9.3 ng/mL vs 6.2 ng/mL, $p = 0.0002$).

Late clinical and angiographic follow-up

Clinical follow-up was obtained for all patients during 1 year after PCI. Angiographic follow-up 6.8 ± 1.1 months after the procedure was available for 82% of the arteries treated (85 of 103), 90% in Phase I (44 of 49) and 76% (41 of 54) in Phase II.

Table 40.2 Baseline, clinical and angiographic characteristics.

Characteristics	Overall (76 patients/ 103 arteries)	>8 ng/mL (44 patients/ 58 arteries)	<8 ng/mL (32 patients/ 45 arteries)	P
Female	6/76 (8%)	2/44 (4.5%)	4/32 (12.5%)	ns
Hypertension	47/76 (62%)	23//44 (52%)	24/32 (75%)	ns
High Cholesterol	47/76 (62%)	28/44 (64%)	19/32 (59%)	ns
Diabetes	15/76 (20%)	5/44 (11.3%)	10/32 (31%)	ns
Stroke	0	0	0	ns
Current Smoker	18/76 (24%)	12/44 (27%)	6/32 (19%)	ns
Previous AMI	17/76 (22.3%)	10/44 (23%)	7/32 (22%)	ns
Unstable Angina IIB- IIIB-C	52/76 (68.4%)	29/44 (66%)	24/32 (75%)	ns
ACC/AHA morphology				
Type A	16/103 (16%)	8/58 (14%)	8/45 (18%)	ns
Type B1	28/103 (27%)	15/58 (26%)	13/45 (29%)	ns
Type B2	29/103 (28%)	17/58 (29%)	12/45 (27%)	ns
Type C	30/103 (29%)	18/58 (31%)	12/45 (27%)	ns
Target artery (%)				
LMCA	6/103 (6%)	4/58 (7%)	2/45 (4.4%)	ns
LAD	57/103 (55%)	32/58 (55%)	25/45 (56%)	ns
LCX	23/103 (22%)	12/58 (21%)	12/45 (27%)	ns
RCA	17/103 (17%)	10/58 (17%)	6/45 (13%)	ns

Abbreviations: LMCA, left main coronary artery; LAD, left anterior descending; LCX, left circumflex; RCA, right coronary artery.

Source: Modified from Rodriguez A *et al.* (44).

Table 40.3 Baseline and follow up quantitative coronary angiography data.

	Rapamycin blood concentration		p value
	>8 ng/mL (n = 48)	<8 ng/mL (n = 37)	
Reference diameter (mm)	3.0 (0.49)	3.15 (0.48)	NS
MLD post (mm)	2.79 (0.48)	2.9 (0.50)	NS
MLD follow-up (mm)	2.16 (0.62)	1.71 (0.59)	0.05
Late loss (mm)	0.60 (0.56)	1.1 (0.61)	0.031
Net gain (mm)	1.4 (0.61)	1.0 (0.63)	0.021
In-stent restenosis	6.2%	22%	0.041
In-segment restenosis	10.4%	22%	NS

Data are mean (SD) or percentage.

Abbreviation: MLD, minimum luminal diameter.

Source: Modified from Rodriguez A *et al.* (44).

During the 1 year of follow-up, cumulative frequency of MACCE occurred in 15 of 76 of patients (20%): 13 target vessel revascularizations, one repeat PCI and stenting in a nontarget vessel, and one myocardial infarction (this patient also had an emergency PCI after the initial procedure).

In Table 40.3, quantitative coronary angiography data of the 85 lesions with follow-up angiography are presented. At follow-up, the MLD of lesions in patients with a high rapamycin blood concentration was significantly larger than in those with lower concentrations of the drug. The analysis of late loss and net gain with rapamycin concentrations also showed a significant difference in favor of patients with high rapamycin concentrations (Table 40.3). Angiographic binary in-stent restenosis was also significantly lower in the group with rapamycin high concentrations (6.2% vs 22%, $p = 0.041$). During the first week of treatment, Pearson test showed a linear correlation between late loss at follow-up and rapamycin blood concentration ($r = 20.826$, $p = 0.008$). Multivariate logistic regression analysis identified that reference vessel size (-2.206, $p = 0.008$) and rapamycin blood concentration (-0.243, $p < 0.036$) are the only independent predictors of angiographic restenosis at follow-up.

ORAR II randomized trial

Patient population and study design

After the end of the two observational studies, we organized the first randomized comparison study with oral sirolimus treatment in patients after bare metal stent implantation in de novo coronary lesions.

Thus, from September 2003 to September 2004, 100 patients with severe stenosis in de novo coronary artery were enrolled and included in the ORAR II randomized protocol (55).

Inclusion criteria was similar to our previous pilot study (44,46), patients with clinical indication of percutaneous coronary revascularization were randomized if they had a de novo severe stenosis in a native coronary artery, lesion suitable for stent, reference vessel size between 2.5 and 4.0 by visual estimation, and candidate for coronary bypass surgery.

Patients were excluded if they had acute myocardial infarction 48 h prior to randomization, rapamycin allergy, clopidogrel or aspirin intolerance, significant bleeding in the last 6 months, stroke or transient ischemic attack in the last 12 months, severe concomitant illness, recent major bleeding requiring transfusion, major blood dyscrasias, participation in another trial that do not allow a follow-up angiogram, patients with dyslipemia of difficult treatment, patients with thrombocytopenic disease, patients with chronic total occlusion or in stent restenosis lesions, and patients not amenable to sign the informed consent allowed

to a follow-up angiogram. In contrast with the previous ORAR pilot, now lesion length was not an exclusion criterion and multiple stents in the same vessel as well overlapping stent were allowed.

The protocol of this nonindustry sponsor study was approved by the Ethics Committee of the Argentine Society of Cardiac Angiography and Interventions and by the Argentina National Regulatory Agency for Drug, Food and Medical Technology. During the study, an Independent Safety Monitoring Committee adjudicated the clinical adverse events.

All eligible patients were randomized to control or oral rapamycin group. In the oral rapamycin arm, we modified the therapeutic scheme in relation to our previous pilot studies, patients in ORAR II, received a loading dose of 6 mg, at least 2 h before stent implantation, followed by 3 mg day for a total of 14 days. Diltiazem sustained release 180 mg a day and was added to sirolimus regimen in order to achieve a higher sirolimus blood concentrations (51). Blood samples were drawn to measure sirolimus blood levels and were taken at 7 days after the oral loading dose of sirolimus. In addition, serum creatine, cholesterol, triglycerides, red and white blood cell and platelet counts were measured before and at the end of sirolimus treatment. Coronary angiography was scheduled between 6 to 9 months after the initial PCI procedure.

PCI was performed using standard techniques (6,46). All 100 patients received one or more identical close cell stent design. Same stent design was used in order to avoid potential bias with stent selection in both groups. All patients received 325 mg/day of aspirin indefinitely and clopidogrel as a loading dose of 300 mg in the day of the procedure and 75 mg/day thereafter for 1 month. Statins were given to all patients indefinitely.

The primary end point of the study was to compare the angiographic binary restenosis rate and late loss determined by an independent core laboratory blinded to treatment allocation. Angiographic binary restenosis was defined as >50% residual stenosis in the target lesion in the follow-up angiography. In patient with multiple lesions, lesions were counted separately. Secondary end points were target lesion, target vessel revascularization, target vessel failure, and major adverse cardiovascular events. Target lesion and target vessel revascularization were performed in the presence of angiographic restenosis and symptoms and signs of myocardial ischemia. A major adverse cardiovascular event was defined as death, myocardial infarction, stroke, and target vessel revascularization at 1 year of follow-up. Target vessel failure was defined as death, nonfatal myocardial infarction, and target vessel revascularization during the entire follow-up period (55).

Results

Between September 2003 and September 4, 2004, 100 patients were randomized, 50 patients in control (55 arteries and 59 lesions) and 50 patients in oral sirolimus arm (60 arteries and 66 lesions). A total of 132 stents were deployed, 61 in control and 71 in oral sirolimus; small stent size (2.5 mm) was deployed in 44.7% of the lesions.

Baseline demographic, clinical, angiographic characteristics among both groups are described in Table 40.4. Treated diabetes was more frequent in oral sirolimus group $p = 0.056$. Hospital and 30-day outcome in both groups were similar. During the course of treatment with oral sirolimus, 26% of the patients had side effects; however, none of them were major. The most frequent side effect was mouth ulceration (16%). Only two patients (3.9%) discontinued the treatment, 3 and 8 days

Table 40.4 Baseline demographic, clinical and angiographic characteristics.

Characteristics	Oral sirolimus + BMS group (n = 50)	Control group (n = 50)	P value
Age (years)	64.6 ± 9.1	65.1 ± 8.3	Ns
Male sex (%)	88	94	Ns
Diabetes mellitus (%)	24	8	0.056
Hyperlipidemia (%)	92	92	Ns
Hypertension (%)	92	82	Ns
Stroke (%)	0	0	Ns
Renal failure	0	0	Ns
Current smoker (%)	24	18	Ns
Previous myocardial infarction (%)	22	38	Ns
Non Q type	0	0.5	Ns
Q type	22	36	Ns
Stable angina	0	2	Ns
Unstable angina	76	54	Ns
Target artery (%)			
RCA	20	27.2	Ns
LAD	53.3	40	Ns
LCX	25	32.7	Ns
LM	1.6	0	Ns
MVD	86	88	Ns
ACC-AHA class (%)[a]			
A	4.5	5	Ns
B1	25.7	35.5	Ns
B2	46.9	39	Ns
C	22.7	20.3	Ns

Abbreviations: RCA, Right coronary artery; LCX, Left Circumflex coronary artery, LAD, Left anterior descending artery; LM, Left Main; MVD, Multiple Vessel Disease; BMS, Standard Stent.

[a]ACC denotes American College of Cardiology and AHA American Heart Association.

Source: Modified from Rodriguez A, *et al*. (55).

Table 40.5 Side effects with oral sirolimus therapy.

Symptoms	ORAR I (n = 76)	ORAR II (n = 50)	OSIRIS[a] (n = 99)	ORBIT	
				(n = 30) (2 mg)	(n = 30) (5 mg)
Nausea and vomiting	1	0	0	2	1
Gum Sores	4	8	0	4	6
Diarrhoea	6	3	1	5	6
Pneumonia	0	0	0	0	0
Rash	7	1	0	2	10
Leucopenia	0	0	0	0	2
Hepatic dysfunction	0	0	0	0	1
Fatigue	0	0	0	0	1
Elevated triglycerides	0	0	0	0	1
Fever	2	0	0	0	0
Constipation	2	0	0	0	0
Gastritis	1	0	0	0	0
Insomnia	1	0	0	0	0
Headache	1	0	0	0	0
Otitis	0	0	1	0	0
Allergic reaction	1	0	2	0	0
Overall (%)	19 (25)	13 (26)	4(4)	13 (43)	20 (66)
Drug discontinuation (%)	3 (3.9)	2 (4)	4(4)	4 (13)	10 (33.3)

[a]Only severe side effects.

Source: From References 44,45,50,55.

after the first doses. Overall adverse side effects of ORAR I, II (44,55), ORBIT (45), and OSIRIS (50) are described in Table 40.5.

After rapamycin treatment, during the first 30 days, white blood counts showed a significant transient changes, however, severe leucopoenia was not seen in any case.

Hospital and follow-up results of ORAR II randomized are described in Table 40.6. One-year clinical follow-up was obtained in all patients in both groups. After hospital discharge during the follow-up, there were two deaths (4%) in control group (both cardiac), while two patients in oral sirolimus (4%) died during follow-up (one due to colon cancer and the other after an elective coronary bypass surgery). After hospital discharge, there was no documented nonfatal myocardial infarction or stroke in both groups. Angiographically proven or clinically suspected stent thrombosis was not seen in any patient treated with oral sirolimus therapy.

The rate of clinically driven target lesion or target vessel revascularization was significantly lower in oral sirolimus compared with control. Target vessel revascularization was 5/60 (8.3%) vs 21/55 (38%) [$p < 0.001$] and target lesion revascularization was 5/66 (7.6%) vs 22/59 (37.2%) [$p < 0.001$]. Target vessel failure and major adverse cardiovascular events were also improved with oral sirolimus therapy ($p = 0.01$ and $p = 0.031$; Table 40.6).

In Figure 40.1 are described survival curves of freedom from target vessel revascularization (3,A) and freedom from Major Adverse Cardiovascular Events (3,B) showing significantly better outcome in those patients treated with oral sirolimus. The numbers represent a 80% reduction of target vessel revascularization and 55% reduction of major adverse cardiovascular events compared to control.

Baseline and follow-up angiographic data are shown in Table 40.7. At 9 months, the binary in-stent restenosis rate was 12% for the rapamycin group and 34.6% for the control group ($p = 0.015$). The in-segment analysis showed a restenosis rate of 12% and 42.8% for the rapamycin and control group respectively ($p = 0.001$). As shown in Figure 40.2,

Table 40.6 Hospital and follow up results of ORAR II.

Variable	Oral sirolimus+ BMS group (n = 50)	BMS group (n = 50)	P value
In Hospital events (%)			
Death	0	0	Ns
Myocardial Infarction	4	2	Ns
Stroke	2	2	Ns
Target-lesion revascularization	0	0	ns
Target-vessel revascularization	0	0	ns
Target-vessel failure	4	2	ns
Any major adverse cardiac and cardiovascular event	6	2	ns
At follow up (%)			
Death	4	4	ns
Myocardial Infarction	4	2	ns
Stroke	2	2	ns
Target-lesion revascularization	7.6	37.2	<0.001
Target-vessel revascularization	8.3	38	<0.001
Target-vessel failure	18	44	0.009
Any major adverse cardiac and cardiovascular event	20	44	0.018

Source: Modified from Rodriguez *et al*. (55).

(a)

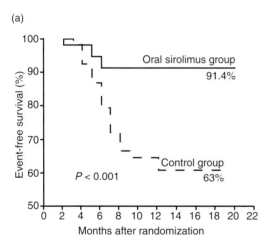

(b)

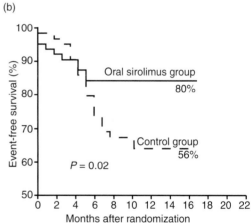

Figure 40.1 Kaplan–Meier curves showing event-free survival from target vessel revascularization (a), and major adverse cardiovascular events (b) for the global follow-up.

The p values were calculated using the log-rank test. (*Source*: Adapted from Reference (52).)

the use of oral rapamycin reduced the risk of binary restenosis by 65% within the stent and by 72% in the analysis segment.

With the oral therapy, in-stent late loss was reduced from 1.41 mm in control vs 0.73 mm in oral rapamycin group, and in segment from 1.13 mm in control vs 0.66 mm in oral rapamycin group, meaning a reduction of 48% and 43% in stent and in segment late loss, respectively.

Multivariate analysis (Table 40.8) showed that randomization to control group was the only independent predictor of restenosis (odds ratio OR 6.01; 95% CI: 2.19–16.46, $p < 0.0001$). The relative reduction in the risk of restenosis among patients who received oral rapamycin was independent of diabetes mellitus status, vessel location, and the length and diameter of the lesion or stent.

Table 40.7 Results of quantitative coronary angiography.

Variable	Oral sirolimus + BMS group (n = 50)	BMS group (n = 50)	P value
Diameter of reference vessel (mm)	2.8 ± 0.63	2.81 ± 0.45	1
Minimal luminal diameter (mm)			
Before procedure	1.03 ± 0.43	0.98 ± 0.48	0.571
After procedure	2.7 ± 0.37	2.62 ± 0.38	0.171
At 270 days	2.04 ± 0.70	1.47 ± 0.76	0.0002
Stenosis (% of luminal diameter)			
Before procedure	66.5 ± 12.2	65.68 ± 14.66	0.755
After procedure	11.7 ± 5.6	11.3 ± 7.27	0.726
At 270 days	32.7 ± 20.15	55.76 ± 25.01	0.001
Lesion length (mm)	13.35 ± 6.33	12.79 ± 4.28	0.144
Stent length (mm)	15.7 ± 2.62	16 ± 2.78	0.149
Net gain (mm)	0.97 ± 0.62	0.49 ± 0.88	0.007
Late luminal loss (mm)	0.66 ± 0.59	1.13 ± 0.72	0.0002
Restenosis (%)[a]			
In segment (n = 99)	12(6/50)	42.8(21/49)	0.001
In stent (n =99)	12(6/50)	34.6(17/49)	0.015

[a]Modified from Rodriguez A *et al.* (55).

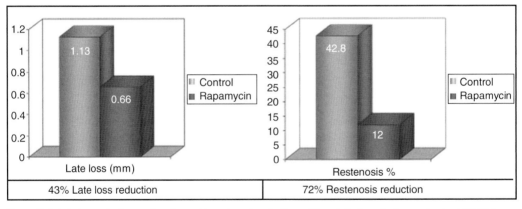

Figure 40.2 Late loss reduction and angiographic restenosis reduction with oral sirolimus in the randomized ORAR II study (52).

Clinical implications of the ORAR II randomized study

This prospective, randomized, and controlled trial in patients with *de novo* lesions demonstrated a significant reduction of angiographic binary restenosis and late loss when patients were allocated to oral sirolimus arm, and both end points were determined by blind operators. Clinical safety and efficacy parameters of restenosis such as target vessel, target lesion revascularization, and major

adverse cardiovascular events at follow-up were also significantly improved with oral sirolimus therapy. As we can see in Table 40.9, compared with control group, ORAR II active patients had similar degree of reduction of in stent restenosis, TLR, and MACCE than those obtained with DES in major recent randomized trials (43,56). Furthermore, the population sample analyzed in the present study represents a relatively high-risk population involving B2/C lesions (~70%), small vessels (44.7%), and lesions longer than 18 mm (53%).

Table 40.8 Multivariate logistic regression analysis: predictors of restenosis of ORAR II randomized.

Variable	Odds ratio	95% CI	P value
Rapamycin treatment	0.163	0.060–0.447	0.0002
Diabetes	0.401	0.084–1.915	0.252
Dislipemia	0.570	0.225–1.444	0.236
Previous AMI	1.367	0.515–3.627	0.530
Unstable angina	0.596	0.252–1.406	0.237
Lesion class ACC/AHA			
A	0.893	0.089–8.945	0.923
B1	0.636	0.241–1.682	0.362
B2	1.493	0.632–3.527	0.360
C	0.988	0.365–2.673	0.981
Reference diameter <2.9 mm	2.334	0.963–5.66	0.061
Lesion length >15 mm	1.26	0.4–4.0	0.68
Right coronary Artery	1.36	0.51–3.62	0.53
Left anterior descending coronary	0.42	0.16–1.06	0.06
Left circumflex coronary	1.75	0.69–4.44	0.23

ACC/AHA, American College of Cardiology, American Heart Association.

Source: From Rodriguez *et al.* (55) with permission from Elsevier.

Table 40.9 Reduction of binary restenosis, TLR and MACCE. Comparison between randomized DES trials and ORAR II study.

Variable	Restenosis (%)	Restenosis reduction (%)	TLR (%)	TLR reduction (%)	MACCE (%)	MACCE reduction (%)
SIRIUS	9	75	4	75	8	62
E-SIRIUS	5.9	86	4	81	8	64
TAXUS II	11	75	4.7	62	11	50
TAXUS IV	7.9	70	3	73.5	8.5	43
TAXUS V	19	45	8.6	45	15	29
ORAR II	12	72	8.3	75	20	50

Source: From References 12,14–16, 55, 57.

Also, overlapping (7%) and multiple stent implantations per treated vessel (17%) were also allowed in the study.

DES has been extensively studied in several randomized studies (10–17) and has been associated with a significant reduction of restenosis and late loss compared to bare stents. In fact, late loss during the first year of follow-up showed only minor increase of minimal luminal diameter with DES therapy, and these numbers (10–17) are lower than the one presented here, meaning that local therapy achieved high immunosuppressive effects. However, efficacy of reducing clinical and angiographic restenosis should be balanced with the higher risk of late stent thrombosis with DES, including higher incidence of death and myocardial infarction, which was recently reported in several studies. In these studies, the incidence of stent thrombosis with DES was higher than bare metal stents in determined subset of patients/lesions characteristics such as those with multiple vessel stenting, overlapping, bifurcations, diabetes, ST myocardial infarction etc. In contrast, as we will discuss later, no patient included in oral sirolimus therapy suffered confirmed or suspected stent thrombosis after hospital discharge.

Cost-effective comparison with drug eluting stents

The randomized controlled ORAR III study

Observational nonrandomized comparison among DES or bare metal stent plus oral sirolimus demonstrated 1-year similar safety/efficacy profile but with a significantly lower cost with the oral sirolimus therapy (58). Thus, after the completion of 1-year follow-up of our randomized ORAR II study, we moved to the third version of ORAR studies: the randomized cost-effective comparison with DES.

This last version, ORAR III, was a randomized, multicenter, and controlled comparison among patients with *de novo* coronary lesions treated with oral rapamycin plus bare metal stent implantation vs DES.

Previous randomized studies and registries with DES in a nonselect, real world population reported 1-year incidence of TVR and repeat revascularization procedures similar to that reported with oral sirolimus therapy. Furthermore, in our previous ORAR II, the incidence of TLR and TVR was completely equivalent to those presented by the ERACI III study with similar patient population, treated either with sirolimus or paclitaxel eluting stents. In the DES arm of ERACI III (31), TVR at 1 year was 8.8% quite comparable to 8.3% with the oral sirolimus arm of ORAR II (55).

The above numbers and similar safety and efficacy end points with both revascularization strategies formed the basis of the new randomized comparison using oral sirolimus therapy.

Patient selection and study design

From January 2006 to September 2007, in three hospitals of Buenos Aires, Argentina, 200 patients meeting clinical or angiographic inclusion criteria were randomized to BMS plus OR (100 patients) or DES (100 patients). Similar exclusion criteria used in our previous studies was also present in this protocol (Figure 40.3). In agreement with those protocols, patients with acute myocardial infarction in the last 24 h, in-stent restenosis, or previous PCI in the last 6 months were excluded.

The primary end point was to compare the overall costs between DES vs oral rapamycin (OR) plus bare metal stents (BMS) at 1, 2, 3, and 5 years of follow-up. The secondary end point was to assess the differences in incidence of safety parameters defined as major adverse cardiovascular events (MACCE) including death from any cause, acute myocardial infarction (AMI), and stroke. Efficacy parameter was analyzed as target vessel revascularization (TVR) and target lesion revascularization (TLR), both of which are specifically excluded from MACCE definition.

Death was defined as cardiac, noncardiac, and unexplained. OR was given as a bolus of 10 mg the day before PCI followed by daily doses of 3 mg plus diltiazem during 13 days after. In DES arm, stent designs were Taxus (Boston Scientific), Endeavor

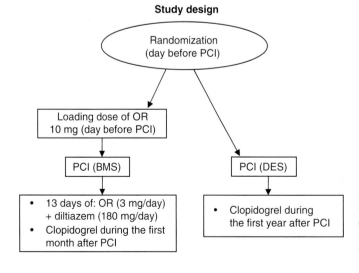

Study design

Figure 40.3 Flow chart of ORAR III trial (56). *Abbreviations*: PCI, percutaneous coronary intervention; OR, oral rapamycin; BMS, bare metal stent; DES, drug eluting stent.

(Medtronic), or Cypher (Jonhson & Jonhson). In BMS, any stent with thin struts was allowed. Cost analysis was conducted by the Economic Department of Argentina National Ministry of Health and included hospital cost, procedural, devices cost, honorarium, medications including oral sirolimus therapy and follow-up cost. Antiplatelet therapy was prescribed for 1 month in OR and for 1 year in DES group. All cost was estimated in U.S. dollars. An Independent Safety Committee adjudicated all clinical adverse events.

Baseline demographic, clinical, and angiographic characteristics of both groups showed no significant difference (diabetic 30%). High proportion of complex and multiple vessels lesions in both groups was seen. The number of stents deployed in OR group and DES are 171 and 176, respectively.

In hospital and 30-day outcome, there were no significant differences in the incidence of any specified safety and efficacy end points whereas the initial cost analysis showed significant differences among both revascularization strategies and in favor of oral sirolimus treatment.

Six months follow-up for the first 140 patients included in the study was recently reported (Table 40.10) and showed similar clinical outcome with both revascularization strategies with significant cost saving in oral rapamycin group ($5483 per patient with oral therapy vs $7615 per patient with DES; $p = 0.0001$).

All clinical and cost-saving end points of the study will be measured at 1, 2, 3, and 5 years of follow-up, and the first available report of the entire population at 1 year will be released in the first quartile of the year 2008.

Conclusions

Since the end of year 2001, we conducted four studies testing the systemic approach of restenosis prevention with oral sirolimus therapy. After more than 5 years, several take-home messages emerge from these experiences.

Firstly, in the two observational studies, we demonstrated that there was a linear correlation among follow-up late loss and sirolimus blood concentration measured during the first week of treatment, meaning that it was unnecessary to give the drug for more than 14 days after the procedure. In these two pilot experiences, high sirolimus blood concentration was associated with low restenosis and late loss.

Secondly, in the first randomized study, ORAR II, we modified the loading and daily dose of the drug. Sirolimus oral administration scheme was different than we previously reported (46): the bolus was given before intervention, the daily dose was 3 mg instead 2 mg, and only for 14 days. It is not clear what will be the ideal moment to begin the oral treatment. However, taking into account the concept that immunosuppressive effects of sirolimus achieved optimal levels after 4 days of treatment, a preintervention loading dose will obtain better results, especially in those patients at high risk of restenosis.

Table 40.10 Results from the first 140 patients.

	OR + BMS (n = 70 patients)	DES (n = 70 patients)	P value
Hospital results			
Death	0% (0/70)	0% (0/70)	ns
MI (Q & non Q)	4.3% (3/70)	1.4% (1/70)	ns (0.63)
TVR	0% (0/70)	0% (0/70)	ns
MACCE	4.3% (3/70)	1.4% (1/70)	ns (0.63)
Cumulative results at 6.4 months (±3.4) of follow up			
Death	0% (0/70)	4.3% (3/70)	ns (0.25)
MI (Q & non Q)	4.3% (3/70)	5.7% (4/70)	ns (0.98)
TVR	4.3% (3/70)	4.3% (3/70)	ns
MACCE	4.3% (3/70)	10% (7/70)	ns (0.37)

Abbreviations: MI, Acute Myocardial Infarction; MACCE, Major Adverse Cardiovascular Events; TVR, Target Vessel Revascularization.

Thirdly, in the last randomized experience, ORAR III (58), we would investigate if systemic prevention of restenosis in patients with *de novo* lesions will be a cost-effective strategy compared to DES treatment. In this last version of ORAR trial, in comparison to the previous one, we increase sirolimus loading dose and the treatment was initiated 1 day before PCI in all patients. If, the final and complete results of this trial would be positive for the systemic strategy compared to DES, which would mean that this less expensive therapy would be an alternative to DES in a wide spectrum of patients undergoing PCI with *de novo* coronary lesions.

Lastly, taking into account new independent data with DES reporting high incidence of stent thrombosis, which was associated with unpredicted late mortality and nonfatal myocardial infarction (32,33,59,60,61), we should recognize that only one patient from our total cohort of 226 patients treated with oral sirolimus and included either in the observational or randomized studies (ORAR, ORAR II, and ORAR III) (44,55,58) developed clinically possible suspected stent thrombosis (0.4%) after hospital discharge and with a clinical restenosis rate (TVR and TLR) of 7–10%. Therefore, all these findings suggested that this therapy would provide our patients with a safe and dependable PCI procedure, which was the major goal and dream of any percutaneous interventional technique (62).

References

1 Rodríguez A, Santaera O, Larribau M, Sosa MI, Palacios IF. Early decrease in minimal luminal diameter after successful percutaneous transluminal coronary angioplasty predicts late restenosis. *Am J Cardiol.* 1993;**71**:1391–1395.

2 Rensing BJ, Hermans WRM, Beatt KJ, *et al.* Quantitative angiographic assessment of elastic recoil after percutaneous transluminal coronary angioplasty. *Am J Cardiol.* 1990;**66**:1039–1044.

3 Rodríguez A, Palacios I, Fernández M, Larribau M, Giraudo M, Ambrose J. Time course and mechanism of early luminal diameter loss after percutaneous transluminal coronary angioplasty. *Am J Cardiol.* 1995;**76**:1131–1134.

4 Mintz G, Popma J, Pichard A, *et al.* Arterial remodeling after coronay angioplasty. A serial intravascular ultrasound study. *Circulation.* 1996;**94**:35–44.

5 Kimura T, Nosaka H, Yokol H, Iwabuchi M, Nobuyoshi M. Serial angiographic follow up after Palmaz-Schatz stent implantation comparison with conventional balloon angioplasty. *J Am Coll Cardiol.* 1993;**21**:1557–1563.

6 Rodríguez A, Santaera O, Larribau M, *et al.* Coronary stenting decreases restenosis in lesions with early loss in luminal diameter 24 hours after successful PTCA. *Circulation.* 1995;**91**:1397–1402.

7 Serruys PW, Jaegere P, Kiemeneij F, *et al.* A comparison of balloon expandable stent implantation with balloon angioplasty in patients with coronary artery disease. *N Engl J Med.* 1994;**331**:489–495.

8 Fischman D, Leon M, Baim D, *et al.* A randomized comparison of coronary stent and balloon angioplasty in the treatment of coronary artery disease. *N Engl J Med.* 1994;**331**:496–501.

9 Rodríguez A, Ayala F, Bernardi V, *et al.* Optimal Coronary Balloon Angioplasty with Provisional Stenting versus Primary Stent (OCBAS). Immediate and long-term follow up results. *J Am Coll Cardiol.* 1998;**32**:1351–1357.

10 Sousa JE, Costa MA, Abizaid AC, *et al.* Sustained suppression of neointimal proliferation by sirolimus-eluting stents one-year angiographic and intravascular ultrasound follow-up. *Circulation.* 2001;**104**:2007–2011.

11 Morice MC, Serruys PW, Sousa JE, *et al.* A randomized comparison of sirolimus-eluting stent with a standard stent for coronary revascularitation. *N Eng J Med.* 2002;**346**:1773–1780.

12 Moses JW, Leon MB, Popma JJ, *et al.* Sirolimus-eluting stents versus standard stents in patients with stenosis in a native coronary artery. *N Engl J Med.* 2003;**349**:1315–1323.

13 Grube E, Silber S, Hauptmann KE, *et al.* TAXUS I. Six- and twelve month results from a randomized, double-blind trial on a slow-release paclitaxel-eluting stent for *de novo* coronary lesions. *Circulation.* 2003;**107**:38–42.

14 Colombo A, Drzewiecki J, Banning A, *et al.* Randomized study to assess the effectiveness of slow- and moderate-release polymer based paclitaxel-eluting stents for coronary artery lesions. TAXUS II Study Group. *Circulation.* 2003;**108**:788–794.

15 Stone GW, Ellis SG, Cox DA, *et al.* A polymer-based, paclitaxel-eluting stent in patients with coronary artery disease. *N Engl J Med.* 2004;**350**:221–231.

16 Schofer J, Schluter M, Gershlick AH, *et al.* Sirolimus-eluting stents for treatment of patients with long atherosclerotic lesions in small coronary arteries. Double-blind, randomized controlled trial. (E-SIRIUS). *Lancet.* 2003;**362**:1093–1099.

17 Schampaert E, Cohen EA, Schluter M, *et al.* The Canadian study of the sirolimus-eluting stent in the treatment of patients with long *de novo* lesions in small

native coronary arteries (C-SIRIUS). *J Am Coll Cardiol.* 2004;**43**:1110–1115.

18 Spertus JA, Kettelksmp R, Vance C, *et al.* Prevalence, predictors, and outcomes of premature discontinuation of thienopyridine therapy after drug-eluting stent placement. Results from the PREMIER Registry. *Circulation.* 2006;**113**(25):2803–2809.

19 Iakovou I, Schmidt T, Bonizzoni E, *et al.* Incidence, predictors and outcome of thrombosis after successful implantation of drug-eluting stents. *JAMA.* 2005;**293**:2126–2130.

20 Rodríguez-Granillo G, Valgimigli M, Ong AT, *et al.* Paclitaxel eluting stents for treatment of angiographically non-signicant atheroscloríct lesions. *Int J Cardiovasc Intervent.* 2005;**7**(2):68–71.

21 Fischman DL, Leon MB, Baim DS, *et al.* The Stent Restenosis Study Investigators. A randomized comparison of coronary stent and balloon angioplasty in the treatment of coronary artery disease. *N Engl J Med.* 1994;**331**:496–501.

22 Al Suwaidi J, Holmes DR, Salam AM, *et al.* Impact of coronary artery stents on mortality and nonfatal myocardial infaction: meta-analysis of randomized trials comparing strategy of routine stenting with that of balloon angioplasty. *Am Heart J.* 2004;**147**:815–822.

23 Lagerqvist B, James SK, Stenestraud IJ, *et al.* Long-term outcomes with drug-eluting stents versus bare-metal stents in Sweden. SCAAR Study Group. *N Engl J Med.* 2007;**356**(10):1009–1019.

24 Di Mario C, Moses JW, Anderson TJ, *et al.* Randomized comparison elective stent implantatation and coronary balloon angioplasty guided by online quantitative angiography and intracoronary Doppler. DESTINI Study Group (Doppler Endpoint Stenting International Investigation). *Circulation.* 2000;**102**:2938–2944.

25 Dangas G, Ambrose JA, Rehmann D, *et al.* Balloon optimization versus stent study (BOSS): provisional stenting and early recoil after balloon angioplasty. *Am J Cardiol.* 2000;**85**:957–961.

26 Pocock SJ, Henderson RA, Rickards AF, *et al.* Meta-analysis of randomized trials comparing angioplasty with bypass surgery. *Lancet.* 1995;**346**:1184–1189.

27 Mercado N, Wijns W, Serruys PW, *et al.* One year outcome of coronary artery bypass graft surgery versus percutaneous coronary intervention with multiple stenting for multisystem disease: a metaanalysis of individual patient dta from randomized clinical trials. *J Throrac Cardiovasc Surg.* 2005;**130**:512–519.

28 Rodríguez AE, Baldi J, Fernández Pereira C, *et al.* ERACI II Investigators. Five years follow up of the Argentina Randomized trial of coronary angioplasty with stenting vs. coronary bypass surgery in patients with multiple vessel disease (ERACI II). *J Am Coll Cardiol.* 2005;**46**:582–588.

29 Serruys PW, Ong AT, Van Herwerden LA, *et al.* Five year outcome alter coronary stenting versus bypass surgery for the tratment of multivessel disease. The final analysis of the Arterial Revascularization Therapies Study (ARTS) randomized study. *J Am Coll Cardiol.* 2005;**46**:575–578.

30 Serruys PW, Ong AT, Morice MC, *et al.* On behalf of the ARTS II investigators. Arterial Revascularization Therapies Study (ARTSII): sirolimus eluting stents for treatment of patients with multiple vessel *de novo* coronary artery lesions. *Eurointervention.* 2005;**2**:147–156.

31 Rodríguez A, Maree AO, Grinfeld L, *et al.* Revascularization strategies of coronary multiple vessel disease in the drug-eluting stent era: one year follow-up results of the ERACI III trial. *Eurointervention.* 2006;**2**:53–60.

32 Spaulding C, Daemen J, Boersma E, *et al.* A pooled analysis of data comparing sirolimus-eluting stents with bare-metal stents. *N Engl J Med.* 2007;**356**:989–997.

33 Daemen J, Wenaweser P, Tsuchida K, *et al.* Early and late coronary stent thrombosis of sirolimus eluting and paclitaxel eluting stents in routine clinical practice: data from a large two institutional cohort study. *Lancet.* 2007;**369**:667–678.

34 Mc Fadden E, Stabile E, Regar E, *et al.* Late thrombosis in drug-eluting coronary stent after discontinuation of antiplatelet therapy. *Lancet.* 2004;**364**:1419–1421.

35 Pfisterer M, Brunner-La Rocca HP, Buser PT, *et al.* BASKET-LATE Investigators. Late clinical event after clopidogrel discontinuation my limit the benefit of drug-eluting stents: an observational study of drg-eluting versus bare-metal stents. *J Am Coll Cardiol.* 2006;**48**(12):2584–2591.

36 Poon M, Marx SO, Gallo R, *et al.* Rapamycin inhibits vascular smooth muscle cell migration. *J Clin Invest.* 1996;**82**:2277–2283.

37 Park SJ, Shim WH, Ho DS, *et al.* A paclitaxel eluting stent for the prevention of coronary restenosis. *N Engl J Med.* 2003;**348**:1537.

38 Kornowoski R, Hong MK, Tio FO, *et al.* In-stent restenosis: contributions of inflammatory responses and arterial injury to neointimal hyperplasia. *J Am Coll Cardiol.* 1998;**31**:224.

39 Ge J, Shen C, Liang C, *et al.* Elevated matrix metalloproteinase expression after stent implantatantion is associated with restenosis. *Int J Cardiol.* 2006;**112**(1):85–90.

40 Gallo R, Padurean A, Jayaraman T, *et al.* Inhibition of intimal thickening after balloon angioplasty in porcine coronary arteries by targeting regulators of the cell cycle. *Circulation.* 1999;**99**:2164–2470.

41 Burke SE, Lubbers NL, Chen YW, *et al.* Neointimal formation after balloon-induced vascular injury in Yucatan minipigs is reduced by oral rapamycin. *J Cardiovasc Pharmacol.* 1999;**33**:829–835.

42 Rodriguez AE, Fernandez-Pereira C. Systemic immunosuppressive therapy with oral sirolimus plus bare metal

srtent implantation: the missing alternative to prevent coronary restenosis after percutaneous coronary interventions. *Recent Patents Cardiovasc Drug Disc.* 2008;3:201–208.

43 Stone GW, Ellis SG, Cannon L, *et al.* Comparison of a polymer-based paclitaxel-eluting stent with a bare metal stent in patients with complex coronary artery disease: a randomized controlled trial. *JAMA.* 2005;**294**:1215–1223.

44 Rodríguez A, Rodríguez Alemparte M, Vigo C, *et al.* Role of oral rapamycin to prevent restenosis in patients with *de novo* lesions undergoing coronary stent therapy. Results of the Argentina single center study (ORAR Trial). *Heart.* 2005;**91**(11):1433–1437.

45 Waksman R, Ajani A, Pichard A, *et al.* Oral Rapamycin to inhibit restenosis after stenting of *de novo* coronary lesions. The oral rapamune to inhibit restenosis (ORBIT) study. *J Am Coll Cardiol.* 2004;**44**:1386–1392.

46 Rodríguez A, Rodríguez Alemparte M, Vigo C, *et al.* Pilot study of oral rapamycin to prevent restenosis in patients undergoing coronary stent therapy. Argentina single center study. *J Invasive Cardiol.* 2003;**15**:581–584.

47 Rodríguez A, Fernández Pereira C, Rodríguez Alemparte M. Oral rapamycin in the treatment of diffuse proliferative in-stent restenosis in a patient with small reference vessel. *J Invasive Cardiol.* 2003;**15**:515–518.

48 Chaves AJ, Sousa AG, Mattos L, *et al.* Pilot study with an intensified oral sirolimus regimen for the prevention of in-stent restenosis in *de novo* lesions. *Catheter Cardiovasc Interv.* 2005;**66**:535–540.

49 Brara P, Moussavian M, Grise M, *et al.* Pilot trial of oral rapamycin for recalcitrant restenosis. *Circulation.* 2003;**107**:1722–1724.

50 Hausleiter J, Kastrati A, Mehilli J, *et al.* Randomized, double blind, placebo controlled trial of oral sirolimus for restenosis prevention in patients with in stent restenosis. The oral sirolimus to inhibit recurrent in stent stenosis trial (OSIRIS). *Circulation.* 2004;**110**:790–795.

51 Bottiger Y, Sawe J, Brattstrom C, *et al.* Pharmacokinetic interaction between single oral dose of diltiazem and sirolimus in healthy volunteers. *Clin Pharmacol Ther.* 2001;**69**:32–40.

52 Jhonson RW, Kreis H, Oberbauer R, *et al.* Sirolimus allows early cyclosporine withdrawal in renal transplantation resulting in improved renal function and lower blood pressure. *Transplantation.* 2001;**72**:777–786.

53 Farb A, Jhon M, Acampado E, *et al.* Oral everolimus inhibits in-stent neointimal growth. *Circulation.* 2002; **106**:2379–2384.

54 Dong-Woon K, Jin-Sook K, Young-Gyu K, *et al.* Novel oral formulation of Paclitaxel inhibits neointimal hyperplasia in a rat carotid artery injury model. *Circulation.* 2004;**109**:1558–1563.

55 Rodriguez A, Granada J, Rodriguez-Alemparte M, *et al.* Oral rapamycin after coronary bare-metal stent implantation to prevent restenosis: the Prospective, Randomized Oral Rapamycin in Argentina (ORAR II). *J Am Coll Cardiol.* 2006;**47**(8):1522–1529.

56 Dawkins KD, Grube E, Guagliumi G, *et al.* Clinical efficacy of polymer-based paclitaxel-eluting stents in the treatment of complex, long coronary artery lesions from a multicenter, randomized trial: support for the use of drug-eluting stents in contemporary clinical practice. *Circulation.* 2005;**112**:3306–3313.

57 Stone GW, Ellis SG, Cannon L, *et al.* TAXUS V Investigators. Comparison of a polymer-based paclitaxel-eluting stent in patient with complex coronary artery disease: a randomized controlled trial. *JAMA.* 2005;**294**(10):1215–1223.

58 Rodriguez A, Mieres J, Rodriguez-Granillo AM, *et al.* Is oral rapamycin plus bare metal stents a feasible alternative to drug eluting stent to prevent restenosis? A cost effective follow up analysis from the randomized, controlled ORAR III study. European Society Congress, Vienna, Austria, 2007.

59 Rodriguez A, Mieres J, Fernandez-Pereira C, *et al.* Coronary stent thrombosis in current drug eluting stent era: insights from ERACI III trial. *J Am Coll Cardiol.* 2006;**47**:205–207.

60 Kaiser C, Brunner-La Rocca HP, Buser PT, *et al.* Incremental cost-effectiveness of drug-eluting stents compared with a third-generation bare-metal stent in real-world setting: randomized Basel Stent Kosten Effektivitas Trial (BASKET). *Lancet.* 2005;**366**(9489):921–929.

61 Fernandez-Pereira C, Mieres J, Vigo C, *et al.* Cost effectiveness in patients treated with drug eluting stents vs bare metal stents and oral rapamycin. *Am J Cardiol.* 2006;**96**(7 Suppl-331) (Abst):114.

62 Rodriguez A, Rodriguez-Granillo G, Palacios I. Late stent thrombosis: the Damocles sword of drug eluting stents? *Eurointervention.* 2007;**2**:512–517.

CHAPTER 41

Systemic paclitaxel for prevention of restenosis

Neil P. Desai
Abraxis BioScience, LLC, Los Angeles, CA, USA

Introduction

Paclitaxel, a potent antiproliferative and cytotoxic drug that was originally isolated from the bark of the Pacific yew (*Taxus brevifolia*), is widely used to treat breast, ovarian, and lung cancers. Paclitaxel causes G2/M cell-cycle arrest and inhibits cell migration by stabilizing microtubules and disrupting the normal microtubule reorganization process (1). The microtubule damage and mitotic arrest subsequently trigger apoptosis by promoting the phosphorylation and downregulation of antiapoptotic protein Bcl-2 (2,3). In addition to its application in antitumor chemotherapy, paclitaxel has been investigated for the prevention of restenosis following percutaneous transluminal coronary angiography or stenting. *In vitro*, paclitaxel inhibits vascular smooth muscle cell (VSMC) proliferation, migration, and extracellular matrix formation, thus blocking all the essential steps required for restenosis (4).

Paclitaxel as a systemic agent for cancer treatment was first approved for marketing in December 1992 (Taxol®, Bristol-Myers Squibb Co., Princeton, NJ). This version of paclitaxel contains the solvents Cremophor® EL (BASF Aktiengesellschaft, Ludwigshafen, Germany) and ethanol as diluents to increase drug solubility. Because these components

can cause severe hypersensitivity, including anaphylactic reactions (5,6), patients must be premedicated with steroids and antihistamines before intravenous administration of Taxol. A novel nanoparticle albumin-bound version of paclitaxel (*nab*-paclitaxel, ABI-007, Abraxane®; Abraxis BioScience, Inc., Los Angeles, CA) was approved for the treatment of metastatic breast cancer in January 2005 with significantly improved efficacy and a favorable safety profile (7,8). The Cremophor-based and albumin-based formulations are the only currently marketed versions of systemically administered paclitaxel.

The only other approved and marketed use of paclitaxel is on coronary stents (Taxus®, Boston Scientific Corp., Natick, MA, and CoStar®, Conor Medsystems, LLC, Menlo Park, CA) for local delivery to treated lesions. The paclitaxel–stent combination was first approved for marketing in March 2004. Although there has been much enthusiasm over the use of paclitaxel- and other drug-eluting stents (DES) in the clinic owing to large reductions in restenosis rates and in the need for repeat revascularization compared to bare-metal stents (9), recent concerns of late stent thrombosis (10–13) due to impaired healing of the neointima and reendothelialization (14,15) as well as a report of increased mortality (16) have caused a major shift in the use of DES worldwide. In a statement issued by FDA in January 2007, the Circulatory System Devices Panel of the Medical Devices Advisory Committee agreed that DES are associated

Pharmacology in the Catheterization Laboratory. Edited by Ron Waksman and Andrew E Ajani. © 2010 Blackwell Publishing, ISBN: 978-1-4051-5704-9.

with a small increase in stent thrombosis compared with bare-metal stents (17). The panel cautioned that there is an expected increased risk in adverse events, including stent thrombosis, death, or myocardial infarction (MI) in off-label use of DES in more complex patients, which could represent at least 60% of current DES use. The panel suggested longer duration of antiplatelet therapy and inclusion of the information in the DES labeling.

Preclinical and human autopsy data have clearly shown that DES significantly inhibit neointimal growth but can also cause delayed healing and endothelialization, leading to intimal fibrin deposits, intraintimal hemorrhage, localized aneurysms, sudden thrombotic occlusion, and increased inflammation at the stent site (18,19). This is believed to be due to the long-term presence of drug and polymer at the stent site (14,18,19). Systemic delivery of paclitaxel might resolve some of these issues by reducing exposure to the drug and polymer. In addition, systemic treatment in conjunction with the available bare-metal stent platforms could overcome the restricted choice of DES platforms, geographic miss, and cost of multiple DES, as well as prolonged antiplatelet therapy with drugs like clopidogrel, particularly for patients with multivessel disease.

Systemic paclitaxel therapies for prevention of restenosis

Preclinical studies

In one of the first studies to describe the systemic application of paclitaxel to prevent restenosis in an animal model, Sollott and coworkers (20) used intraperitoneal injection of paclitaxel dissolved in dimethylsulfoxide/Cremophor EL/ethanol. This study showed a 70% reduction in neointimal area in rat carotid arteries 11 days after balloon catheter denudation injury.

Studies with novel albumin-based nanoparticles of paclitaxel (*nab*-paclitaxel) showed that concentrations of paclitaxel as low as 0.01 μM significantly inhibited proliferation and migration of rabbit smooth muscle cells *in vitro* (21). In a rabbit bilateral iliac stenting model of restenosis, a single intra-arterial infusion of *nab*-paclitaxel at the time of stenting was well tolerated, and doses of 2.5–5.0 mg/kg produced a dose-dependent

reduction in neointimal proliferation at 4 weeks, with significantly lower intimal thickness of the treatment groups vs the controls (0.09 ± 0.01 mm vs 0.13 ± 0.01 mm, $P \leq 0.02$) (22). A repeat intravenous dose of *nab*-paclitaxel 3.5 mg/kg at 28 days after stenting resulted in sustained reduction of neointimal thickness at 90 days (0.09 ± 0.01 mm vs 0.18 ± 0.03 mm for negative control, $P \leq 0.009$) with nearly complete neointimal healing (22). These studies demonstrated the ability of a single systemic dose at time of stenting to produce an antirestenotic effect as well as the ability of repeat administration for sustained neointimal suppression. Mechanistic studies showed that the transcytosis of *nab*-paclitaxel across the endothelial cells is facilitated by the binding of albumin–paclitaxel complex to the endothelial gp60 receptor and caveolar transport (8). The accumulation of *nab*-paclitaxel in interstitial space is mediated by SPARC (secreted protein, acidic and rich in cysteine), an albumin-binding protein that is overexpressed in tumors and at sites of inflammation and injury (23). These studies may help in understanding why a single systemic dose of *nab*-paclitaxel may deliver sufficient paclitaxel to the vessel wall to suppress restenosis.

A series of animal studies by Scheller *et al.* demonstrated the feasibility of adding paclitaxel to contrast medium to prevent restenosis (24–27). In cell culture, a brief (3-min) exposure to 14.6 μM paclitaxel formulated in the contrast medium iopromide 370 (Ultravist®, Bayer Schering Pharma AG, Berlin, Germany) inhibited the proliferation of VSMC for more than 12 days. In a porcine coronary stent model, intracoronary delivery of paclitaxel–iopromide demonstrated superior efficacy over intravenous administration in preventing neointimal growth. At 28 days, intracoronary paclitaxel–iopromide at 13.6 mg showed a significant reduction in diameter stenosis (13 ± 12% vs 55 ± 13% for controls, $P < 0.001$), late lumen loss (0.82 ± 0.54 mm vs 1.94 ± 0.35 mm for controls, $P < 0.001$), neointimal area (by 56%), and neointimal thickness (by 62%), while allowing healing of the stented segment (25).

Several other preclinical studies were conducted to test the intracoronary delivery of paclitaxel with porous (28), microporous (29), and double-balloon (30) catheters in rabbit carotid arteries injured by electrical stimulation. In a study by Axel *et al.*, administration of Taxol through a microporous balloon catheter with 0.4- and 0.8-μm pore diameters significantly reduced neointimal thickness (0.11 ± 0.04 mm vs 0.14 ± 0.09 mm for controls, $P = 0.04$) and diameter stenosis (26 ± 8% vs 34 ± 20% for controls, $P = 0.01$) at 28 days (29). A study by Herdeg *et al.* showed that intracoronary delivery of paclitaxel dissolved in ethanol with a double-balloon catheter significantly reduced the diameter restenosis at 8 weeks (20.5 ± 5.3% vs 43.1 ± 17.3% of balloon-dilated animal controls, $P = 0.0012$) (30). A four-arm animal study by Herdeg *et al.* directly compared three-balloon catheter systems (porous, microporous, and double-balloon) in intracoronary paclitaxel treatment for restenosis. The results from this study favored the double-balloon approach (28).

Oral paclitaxel is also being studied as an alternative approach of systemic delivery. The oral bioavailability of paclitaxel is very low due to the efficient transport of the drug by the intestinal drug efflux pump *p*-glycoprotein (pgp). This pgp pump can be inhibited by cyclosporine and the calcium-channel blocker verapamil. An oral formulation of paclitaxel and verapamil analogue KR-30031 was shown to enhance the absorption of paclitaxel to achieve a plasma concentration high enough for restenosis therapy (31). In a rat carotid artery model with balloon injury, the oral paclitaxel treatment showed significantly increased angiographic minimum luminal diameter (MLD) and reduced neointimal formation compared with the control group at 11 days, indicating the potential benefit of oral paclitaxel in the prevention of in-stent restenosis (31).

Clinical studies
Albumin-based nanoparticle paclitaxel (*nab*-paclitaxel): The SNAPIST trials
The relatively low toxicity of Abraxane® in cancer treatment allowed for the exploration of *nab*-paclitaxel, under the name Coroxane™ (Abraxis BioScience, Inc., Los Angeles, CA), as a potential therapy for restenosis. In an initial clinical trial by Margolis *et al.* (32) for treatment of coronary restenosis (Systemic NAnoparticle Paclitaxel for In-STent Restenosis [SNAPIST-I]), 23 patients received *nab*-paclitaxel (Coroxane™)

intravenously at doses of 10, 30, 70, or 100 mg/m^2 within 30 min following deployment of a bare-metal stent in a *de novo* coronary artery lesion (n = 7, 5, 6, and 5, respectively). The results demonstrated that systemic *nab*-paclitaxel was well tolerated, with no significant adverse events at doses below 70 mg/m^2 in this patient population. Reversible, mild-to-moderate alopecia occurred in patients treated at the higher dose levels (70 and 100 mg/m^2). One patient at 100 mg/m^2 had neutropenia (grade 3) and neuropathy (grade 2), and one patient at 70 mg/m^2 had neutropenia (grade 2). At 6 months, the 10- and 100-mg/m^2 dose groups each had two target lesion revascularizations (TLR) and two binary restenoses. In contrast, the 30- and 70-mg/m^2 dose groups had no major adverse cardiac events (MACE) or binary restenoses, and the in-segment angiographic late lumen loss in these groups was encouraging (0.46 ± 0.16 mm and 0.30 ± 0.12 mm, respectively).

Based on the safety results from SNAPIST-I, the SNAPIST-II study by McDonald *et al.* (33) was initiated to compare the safety and efficacy of one vs two doses of *nab*-paclitaxel in patients with up to two stented lesions in coronary arteries. Seventy-six patients were randomly assigned to IV treatment with either one dose of *nab*-paclitaxel 35 mg/m^2 immediately after stenting or one dose at stenting plus a second dose 2 months later. Primary endpoints were safety and MACE (death, MI, coronary artery bypass grafting [CABG], TLR, and target vessel revascularization [TVR]) at 2 months. Secondary end points were MACE, quantitative coronary angiography (QCA), and intravascular ultrasound (IVUS) evaluation of restenosis at 6 months and MACE at 12 months. The patient population was fairly typical for patients with *de novo* lesions ≤25 mm. QCA at baseline showed reference vessel diameter 2.90 ± 0.54 mm, lesion length 10.16 ± 3.49 mm, MLD 1.08 ± 0.47 mm before stenting, and MLD 2.77 ± 0.44 mm after stenting. Adverse events in this study attributed to *nab*-paclitaxel were mostly mild, with reports of nausea (6.6%), fatigue (5.3%), lymphopenia (3.9%), and mild hair loss on the scalp or body (3.9%). Only one event (gastrointestinal bleeding) was considered a possibly drug-related serious toxicity. No cardiac deaths, MIs, or CABG procedures were reported during the 12-month follow-up period. No statistically significant differences in angiographic or ultrasound findings were observed at 6 months or in MACE, TLR, or TVR at 2, 6, or 12 months between the single- and double-dose groups. At 6 months for all patients, QCA in-segment analysis showed late loss of 0.52 ± 0.38 mm and a binary restenosis rate of 12.8%. IVUS analysis showed a percent volume obstruction of 22.8 ± 14.7%. For all 76 patients, no MACE was observed at 2 months; MACE at 6 months included 6.6% TLR (5/76) and 9.2% TVR (7/76), and MACE at 12 months included 7% TLR (5/71) and 9.8% TVR (7/71). No early or late stent thrombosis was reported in any of the SNAPIST studies.

Additional studies with *nab*-paclitaxel in the SNAPIST series are ongoing to explore the potential of systemic paclitaxel treatment in both *de novo* and in-stent restenosis coronary lesions. These studies will investigate different doses and schedules, as well as intracoronary and intravenous routes of administration. In addition, *nab*-paclitaxel is being explored for the treatment of lesions in the superficial femoral artery (SFA) in conjunction with balloon angioplasty in the PARS (Paclitaxel Assisted Revascularization of the SFA) trial.

Taxol intracoronary administration through a porous balloon: The TAXIC trial

In a recent study by Reifart *et al.* (TAXIC trial) (34), 77 patients with diffuse in-stent restenosis were treated with low intracoronary doses of Taxol delivered through a porous balloon catheter with 16–24 holes of approximately 100 μm in diameter. Taxol was delivered through the balloon at a total dose of about 0.9–1.2 mg given in 10 mL of a 1:1:1 mixture of saline:contrast media:patient's blood at a balloon inflation pressure of 3–4 bar for 60 s. Mean lesion length was 28.37 mm, percent diameter stenosis was 80.7% before the procedure, and MLD was 2.63 mm after the procedure. At 6-month follow-up, the percent diameter stenosis for these patients was 41.3%, the binary angiographic restenosis rate was 31%, and TVR was 22% (17/77). Angiographic restenosis rates in the TAXIC trial compared favorably with those seen in the randomized studies of brachytherapy such as the Long WRIST (38.3%) (35) and START (28.8%) (36) trials. When compared with DES studies for in-stent restenosis, the angiographic restenosis rates for the DES were lower than those seen in the TAXIC trial: 21.7% for Taxus and 14.3% for a sirolimus-eluting stent (Cypher®, Cordis Corp., Miami Lakes, FL) (37). No safety issues were noted with the administration of systemic paclitaxel in this study.

Intracoronary administration of paclitaxel dissolved in contrast media: The THUNDER trial

Tepe *et al.* (38) enrolled 154 patients into a three-arm randomized study (THUNDER) to investigate the use of paclitaxel in femoropopliteal lesions for the prevention of restenosis. The three study arms included control angioplasty alone with an uncoated balloon (*n* = 54), angioplasty followed by intra-arterial administration of approximately 17 mg paclitaxel in 100 mL contrast media (PCM; *n* = 52) and angioplasty with a paclitaxel-coated balloon (Paccocath, Bavaria Medizin Technologie GmbH, Germany; *n* = 48), with similar average preprocedure lesion lengths (7.3, 6.7, and 6.5 cm, respectively). Among other inclusion criteria, patients had an occlusion or stenosis of greater than 2 cm and a Rutherford score of 3–5. Study participants had an average of 1.7 lesions treated, and the mean degree of stenosis before the procedure ranged from 87.7% to 90.7% in the three arms. At 6-month follow-up, patients in the Paccocath arm had significantly reduced mean late lumen loss ($P < 0.01$) and a significantly better binary restenosis rate ($P < 0.01$) compared with controls with uncoated balloons, whereas the systemic PCM group showed no significant improvement. Patients in the control arm had mean Rutherford scores of 3.1 at baseline and 1.6 at 6-month follow-up, compared with 3.4 and 2.0 in the PCM arm and 3.4 and 1.2 in the Paccocath arm. The TLR rate (6.3%) in the Paccocath arm was also reduced compared with 29.6% in the control arm and 25% in the PCM arm.

In this study, paclitaxel dissolved in contrast media and administered systemically showed no advantage over the control angioplasty group. Studies using paclitaxel dissolved in contrast media in the porcine coronary model (24,25) did show significant improvement with intracoronary administration but not with intravenous administration. It is possible in this clinical study, due to the high velocity of blood flow through the femoral artery, there was insufficient contact time between paclitaxel in contrast media and the arterial wall to allow adequate drug penetration to treated lesions. As a result, the outcomes appear to be similar to those obtained with intravenous administration in the porcine study. Contrast media also may increase the solubility of paclitaxel sufficiently to prevent or reduce partitioning to the vessel wall.

Summary

Systemic delivery of paclitaxel has the potential to overcome some of the risks associated with prolonged local exposure to cytotoxic antiproliferative drugs released by DES. *In vitro* and *in vivo* studies have demonstrated that prolonged drug exposure is unnecessary, and restenosis can be inhibited by short exposure to systemic paclitaxel at a dose far lower than that used in cancer therapy, thus with less expected toxicity. The intravenous dose for *nab*-paclitaxel is 35 mg/m^2 in SNAPIST-II study compared to intravenous antitumor doses of 175 mg/m^2 for Taxol (39) and 260 mg/m^2 for *nab*-paclitaxel (7), and the intracoronary dose for restenosis therapy is even lower with 1.2 mg (~6 mg/m^2) of paclitaxel dose in TAXIC trial (34). Although paclitaxel dissolved in contrast media does not appear to show any benefit in the femoropopliteal artery, other preclinical and clinical studies have suggested the safety and efficacy of systemic paclitaxel delivery. *nab*-Paclitaxel, a novel paclitaxel already approved for metastatic breast cancer, has shown promise in restenosis therapy in animal studies and early clinical trials. The enhanced endothelial transcytosis of albumin-bound paclitaxel (8) may have some advantages relative to paclitaxel dissolved in contrast media alone or Cremophor-based paclitaxel.

If proved successful in larger clinical studies, systemic therapies with paclitaxel may be used with any of the currently available stents designed for different types of lesions. Systemic therapies also may be effective after angioplasty, regardless of whether a stent is used. The systemic availability of paclitaxel would make it suitable for stenting single or multiple lesions, short or long lesions, and lesions in bifurcations, thus reducing the high cost of DES, especially for patients with multivessel

disease. Systemic delivery also allows for treatment of the entire vessel, eliminating edge effects, and avoids issues related to the proper delivery of the drug often raised with possible underdeployed DES. It is postulated that stent struts free of the antiproliferative agents used in DES may undergo more rapid healing and reendothelialization, thus avoiding the current safety issues of DES related to late stent thrombosis. Furthermore, systemic delivery of paclitaxel has the advantage of possible repeat dosing, allowing indefinite treatment if required and management of restenosis in both peripheral and cardiac applications.

Acknowledgement

Dr. Shihe Hou's expert editorial and writing assistance of this manuscript is greatly appreciated.

References

1 Schiff PB, Horwitz SB. Taxol stabilizes microtubules in mouse fibroblast cells. *Proc Natl Acad Sci USA*. 1980;77(3):1561–1565.

2 Srivastava RK, Srivastava AR, Korsmeyer SJ, *et al*. Involvement of microtubules in the regulation of Bcl2 phosphorylation and apoptosis through cyclic AMP-dependent protein kinase. *Mol Cell Biol*. 1998;18(6):3509–3517.

3 Chadebech P, Brichese L, Baldin V, Vidal S, Valette A. Phosphorylation and proteasome-dependent degradation of Bcl-2 in mitotic-arrested cells after microtubule damage. *Biochem Biophys Res Commun*. 1999;262(3):823–827.

4 Wiskirchen J, Schober W, Schart N, *et al*. The effects of paclitaxel on the three phases of restenosis: smooth muscle cell proliferation, migration, and matrix formation: an in vitro study. *Invest Radiol*. 2004;39(9):565–571.

5 Gelderblom H, Verweij J, Nooter K, Sparreboom A. Cremophor EL: the drawbacks and advantages of vehicle selection for drug formulation. *Eur J Cancer*. 2001;37(13):1590–1598.

6 Weiss RB, Donehower RC, Wiernik PH, *et al*. Hypersensitivity reactions from taxol. *J Clin Oncol*. 1990; 8(7):1263–1268.

7 Gradishar WJ, Tjulandin S, Davidson N, *et al*. Phase III trial of nanoparticle albumin-bound paclitaxel compared with polyethylated castor oil-based paclitaxel in women with breast cancer. *J Clin Oncol*. 2005;23(31):7794–7803.

8 Desai N, Trieu V, Yao Z, *et al*. Increased antitumor activity, intratumor paclitaxel concentrations, and endothelial

cell transport of cremophor-free, albumin-bound paclitaxel, ABI-007, compared with cremophor-based paclitaxel. *Clin Cancer Res.* 2006;**12**(4):1317–1324.

9 Stone GW, Ellis SG, Cox DA, *et al*. A polymer-based, paclitaxel-eluting stent in patients with coronary artery disease. *N Engl J Med.* 2004;**350**(3):221–231.

10 Ellis SG, Colombo A, Grube E, *et al*. Incidence, timing, and correlates of stent thrombosis with the polymeric paclitaxel drug-eluting stent: a TAXUS II, IV, V, and VI meta-analysis of 3,445 patients followed for up to 3 years. *J Am Coll Cardiol.* 2007;**49**(10):1043–1051.

11 Kawaguchi R, Angiolillo DJ, Futamatsu H, *et al*. Stent thrombosis in the era of drug eluting stents. *Minerva Cardioangiol.* 2007;**55**(2):199–211.

12 Pfisterer M, Brunner-La Rocca HP, Buser PT, *et al*. Late clinical events after clopidogrel discontinuation may limit the benefit of drug-eluting stents: an observational study of drug-eluting versus bare-metal stents. *J Am Coll Cardiol.* 2006;**48**(12):2584–2591.

13 Ong AT, McFadden EP, Regar E, *et al*. Late angiographic stent thrombosis (LAST) events with drug-eluting stents. *J Am Coll Cardiol.* 2005;**45**(12):2088–2092.

14 Virmani R, Kolodgie FD, Farb A. Drug-eluting stents: are they really safe? *Am Heart Hosp J.* 2004;**2**(2):85–88.

15 Joner M, Finn AV, Farb A, *et al*. Pathology of drug-eluting stents in humans: delayed healing and late thrombotic risk. *J Am Coll Cardiol.* 2006;**48**(1):193–202.

16 Camenzind E, Steg P, Wijns W. Safety of Drug Eluting Stents: A meta-analysis of first generation drug eluting stent programs. In *European Society of Cardiology 2006 World Congress (WCC)*. Barcelona, Spain, September 2–6, 2006.

17 *Update to FDA Statement on Coronary Drug-Eluting Stents, January 4, 2007*. Available at http://www.fda.gov/cdrh/news/010407.html.

18 van der Giessen WJ, Lincoff AM, Schwartz RS, *et al*. Marked inflammatory sequelae to implantation of biodegradable and nonbiodegradable polymers in porcine coronary arteries. *Circulation.* 1996;**94**(7):1690–1697.

19 van der Hoeven BL, Pires NM, Warda HM, *et al*. Drug-eluting stents: results, promises and problems. *Int J Cardiol.* 2005;**99**(1):9–17.

20 Sollott SJ, Cheng L, Pauly RR, *et al*. Taxol inhibits neointimal smooth muscle cell accumulation after angioplasty in the rat. *J Clin Invest.* 1995;**95**(4):1869–1876.

21 John MC, Khurana C, Kolodgie FD, *et al*. A novel preparation of systemic paclitaxel reduces in-stent restenosis in the rabbit. *J Am Coll Cardiol.* 2002;**39**(Suppl 1):5–5(1).

22 Kolodgie FD, John M, Khurana C, *et al*. Sustained reduction of in-stent neointimal growth with the use of a novel systemic nanoparticle paclitaxel. *Circulation.* 2002;**106**(10):1195–1198.

23 Carver LA, Schnitzer JE. Caveolae: mining little caves for new cancer targets. *Nat Rev Cancer.* 2003;**3**(8):571–581.

24 Scheller B, Speck U, Romeike B, *et al*. Contrast media as carriers for local drug delivery. Successful inhibition of neointimal proliferation in the porcine coronary stent model. *Eur Heart J.* 2003;**24**(15):1462–1467.

25 Scheller B, Speck U, Schmitt A, Bohm M, Nickenig G. Addition of paclitaxel to contrast media prevents restenosis after coronary stent implantation. *J Am Coll Cardiol.* 2003;**42**(8):1415–1420.

26 Scheller B, Speck U, Schmitt A, *et al*. Acute cardiac tolerance of current contrast media and the new taxane protaxel using iopromide as carrier during porcine coronary angiography and stenting. *Invest Radiol.* 2002;**37**(1):29–34.

27 Speck U, Scheller B, Abramjuk C, *et al*. Inhibition of restenosis in stented porcine coronary arteries: uptake of Paclitaxel from angiographic contrast media. *Invest Radiol.* 2004;**39**(3):182–186.

28 Herdeg C, Oberhoff M, Siegel-Axel DI, *et al*. Paclitaxel: a chemotherapeutic agent for prevention of restenosis? Experimental studies in vitro and in vivo. *Z Kardiol.* 2000;**89**(5):390–397.

29 Axel DI, Kunert W, Goggelmann C, *et al*. Paclitaxel inhibits arterial smooth muscle cell proliferation and migration in vitro and in vivo using local drug delivery. *Circulation.* 1997;**96**(2):636–645.

30 Herdeg C, Oberhoff M, Baumbach A, *et al*. Local paclitaxel delivery for the prevention of restenosis: biological effects and efficacy in vivo. *J Am Coll Cardiol.* 2000;**35**(7):1969–1976.

31 Kim DW, Kwon JS, Kim YG, *et al*. Novel oral formulation of paclitaxel inhibits neointimal hyperplasia in a rat carotid artery injury model. *Circulation.* 2004;**109**(12):1558–1563.

32 Margolis J, McDonald J, Heuser R, *et al*. Systemic Nanoparticle Paclitaxel (nab-Paclitaxel) for In-stent Restenosis I (SNAPIST-I): a First-in-Human Safety and Dose-finding Study. *Clin Cardiol.* 2007;**30**:165–170.

33 McDonald JE, Klinke P, Fung A, *et al*. Systemic Nanoparticle Albumin-Bound Paclitaxel (nab-Paclitaxel) for the Prevention of In-Stent Restenosis (SNAPIST-II): a randomized comparison of single dose and single dose plus repeat dose at 2 months [abstract 574]. In *Transcatheter Cardiovascular Therapeutics (TCT) 2006*. October 22–27, 2006: Washington DC.

34 Reifart N, Paclitaxel locally for instent restenosis. In *Interventional Cardiology 2007, 22nd Annual International Symposium: Comprehensive Approach to the Percutaneous Management of Structural Heart Disease and Coronary and Peripheral Vascular Disease*. March 11–16, 2007: Snowmass Village, Colorado.

35 Waksman R, Cheneau E, Ajani AE, *et al.* Intracoronary radiation therapy improves the clinical and angiographic outcomes of diffuse in-stent restenotic lesions: results of the Washington Radiation for In-Stent Restenosis Trial for Long Lesions (Long WRIST) Studies. *Circulation.* 2003;**107**(13):1744–1749.

36 Popma JJ, Suntharalingam M, Lansky AJ, *et al.* Randomized trial of 90Sr/90Y beta-radiation versus placebo control for treatment of in-stent restenosis. *Circulation.* 2002;**106**(9):1090–1096.

37 Kastrati A, Mehilli J, von Beckerath N, *et al.* Sirolimus-eluting stent or paclitaxel-eluting stent vs balloon angioplasty for prevention of recurrences in patients with coronary in-stent restenosis: a randomized controlled trial. *JAMA.* 2005;**293**(2):165–171.

38 Tepe G. Local paclitaxel for prevention of restenosis in femoro-popliteal lesion: analysis of the 6-month data of paclitaxel coated balloons, paclitaxel in the contrast media and plain balloon angioplasty. In *Interventional Cardiology 2007, 22nd Annual International Symposium: Comprehensive Approach to the Percutaneous Management of Structural Heart Disease and Coronary and Peripheral Vascular Disease.* March 11–16, 2007: Snowmass Village, Colorado.

39 Nabholtz JM, Gelmon K, Bontenbal M, *et al.* Multicenter, randomized comparative study of two doses of paclitaxel in patients with metastatic breast cancer. *J Clin Oncol.* 1996;**14**(6):1858–1867.

CHAPTER 42

Systemic pharmacotherapy for in-stent restenosis: Steroids

Valeria Ferrero & Flavio Ribichini

Ospedale Civile Maggiore, Verona, Italy

Abstract

It is broadly accepted that the central mechanism at the basis of the whole pathophysiologic process of restenosis is inflammation, triggered by vascular injury and activated through autocrine or paracrine mediators. Steroids exert beneficial effects on platelet function, on smooth muscle cells (SMC) proliferation, and on collagen synthesis as well as inflammatory cells migration and activation, thus interfering with several steps of the cascade, leading to neointima formation and subsequent late lumen loss.

Initial experiences with systemic administration of glucocorticoids after percutaneous coronary interventions (PCI) failed to confirm the expected benefits of this treatment, likely due to inadequate dose and pharmacokinetic calculations. Conversely, a high-dose immunosuppressive treatment with oral prednisone demonstrated remarkable clinical and angiographic results when prednisone was given orally at a dose of 1 mg/kg for 10 days, 0.5 mg/kg for 20 days and 0.25 mg/kg for 15 days. This treatment reduced the incidence of clinical vascular events at 1 year compared to controls (relative risk 0.34, 95% CI: 0.12–0.96, $p = 0.006$) and the incidence of angiographic restenosis below 10% in different clinical and angiographic subsets. Secondary effects of a short steroid treatment are generally minor, predictable and reversible: gastric pain, water, and salt retention and worsened hypertension manifest in nearly 10% of patients. The addition of diuretics and antiacids before discharge, and the upgrading of the antihypertensive medication thereafter, if needed, are useful preventive measures to control these temporary disorders. Routine blood cell count 4 weeks after PCI is advised in patients assuming thienopyridines associated to prednisone to rule out infrequent hematological dyscracias.

Emerging evidence supports this strategy as a convenient and safe alternative to more expensive and complex revascularization procedures as drug-eluting stent (DES) implantation or cardiac surgery, provided that the treatment is reserved to selected candidates. The recent concerns referred to the long-term safety of first generation DES, and the yet undetermined duration of the dual antiplatelet treatment, further supports the need for a simple pharmacological treatment that can be applied, however, in a large percentage of patients currently treated with PCI. Multicenter randomized studies aimed at defining the efficacy and safety of the oral prednisone treatment compared to metallic stents and DES are needed to better establish efficacy and limits of this treatment.

Restenosis after angioplasty: Pathophysiology and treatment perspectives

With the exception of the oral administration of immunosuppressor rapamycin (1,2), practically

Pharmacology in the Catheterization Laboratory. Edited by Ron Waksman and Andrew E Ajani. © 2010 Blackwell Publishing, ISBN: 978-1-4051-5704-9.

all systemic drug approaches aimed at limiting the restenosis process failed to achieve this almost elusive goal, including several drugs bearing anti-inflammatory properties. This failure may reflect the limited effects of some compounds, inappropriate dosage, and pharmacokinetics, or just the different biological efficacy of drugs in the experimental setting in animals compared to the biology of the human disease.

It was not until the advent of the DES technology that a real breakthrough in the prevention of restenosis was achieved. However, despite the unarguable efficacy of first generation DES, reluctances related to the long-term efficacy and safety of these devices increase over time (3). Furthermore, a local form of therapy as DES is cannot address the ubiquitous nature of the atherosclerotic vascular disease. In fact, the major theoretical advantage of a systemic treatment is its potential for being effective independently of the technical limitations of catheter-based interventions and the locally delivered drug treatment.

It is broadly accepted that the central mechanism at the basis of the whole pathophysiologic process of restenosis is inflammation, triggered by vascular injury and activated through autocrine or paracrine mediators (4). Continued inflammation results in increased number of macrophages and lymphocytes, which both emigrate from the blood and multiply within the lesion. Activation of these cells leads to the release of hydrolytic enzymes, cytokines, chemokines, and growth factors, which can induce further damage and eventually cause restenosis after (PCI) (5).

Rationale of the use of glucocorticoids as antirestenotic agents

Inflammation is a key target for a nonspecific antirestenosis treatment, and glucocorticoids are the most effective and well known anti-inflammatory agents. In fact, steroids exert beneficial effects on platelet function, on SMC proliferation and on collagen synthesis as well as inflammatory cells migration and activation, thus interfering with several steps of the cascade, leading to neointima formation and subsequent late lumen loss (6,7).

Mechanisms of action

Glucocorticoids are potent immunosuppressive and anti-inflammatory agents. In particular, glucocorticoids affect the number, distribution, and function of all types of leukocytes (T and B lymphocytes, granulocytes, macrophages, and monocytes), causing lymphocytopenia (mainly T lymphocytes depletion) and inhibition of the accumulation of monocytes and macrophages, neutrophils, and eosinophils at the sites of inflammation (6). In nonlymphoid cells, steroids cause a decrease in the production of vasoactive and chemoattractant factors and lypolytic and proteolytic enzymes. This results in inhibition of neutrophil adhesion to endothelial cells, prevention of macrophage differentiation, and downregulation of endothelial function and inhibition of the production of leukotrienes and prostaglandins, modifying the capillary and membrane permeability (8).

Side effects

Side effects corticosteroids are grouped according to their relative potencies in Na^+ retention, effects on carbohydrate metabolism, and anti-inflammatory effect (Table 42.1). In general these same properties are able to develop undesirable effect after a sustained treatment. Steroids increase blood glucose levels and can worsen the metabolic control in diabetic patients by stimulating the liver to form glucose from amino acids and by stimulating the deposition of glucose as liver glycogen. In the periphery, steroids reduce glucose utilization, augment protein breakdown, and activate lipolysis providing amino acids for gluconeogenesis. In the kidney, corticosteroids enhance the reabsorption of Na^+ on distal and collecting tubes and increase the excretion of K^+ and H^+. Consequently, they induce volume expansion, increase of plasma Na^+ concentration, hypokalemia, and alkalosis, mechanisms that chronically may cause hypertension with consequences on the cardiovascular system. In the bone, glucocorticoids decrease density by multiple mechanisms, including diminished gastrointestinal absorption and increased excretion of Ca^+ in the kidney, and inhibiting bone formation by suppressive effects on osteoblasts (8). Their association with ulcers and gastric bleeding is debated. Due to the concomitant administration of aspirin and thyenopiridine after PCI, a short prophylactic

Table 42.1 Effects and relative potency of glucocorticoids.

Possible side-effects (8)	Relative anti-inflammatory potency	Relative Na$^+$ retention potency	Half-life	Dose equivalence to cortisol
Hyperglycemia: By stimulating the liver to form glucose from amino acids and by stimulating the deposition of glucose as liver glycogen. In the periphery, steroids reduce glucose utilization, augment protein breakdown, and activate lipolysis providing amino acids for gluconeogenesis.	Cortisol 1	1	8–12 h	20 mg
Hypertension: Enhanced reabsorption of Na$^+$ on distal and collecting renal tubes and increased excretion of K$^+$ and H$^+$. Volume expansion, increase of plasma Na$^+$ concentration, hypokalemia and alkalosis.	Prednisone PREDNISOLONE 4	0.8	12–36 h	5 mg
Delayed healing after necrosis: the inhibition of cell factors that generate the inflammatory response such as vasoactive and chemoattractive substances, and the secretion of lipolytic and proteolytic factors and extravasation of leukocytes to areas of necrosis cause decreased fibrosis and delayed tissue healing.	Triamcinolone 5	0	12–36 h	4
Osteoporosis: reduced gastrointestinal absorption and increased excretion of Ca$^+$ in the kidney, and inhibition of bone formation by suppressive effects on osteoblasts.	Dexamethasone Betameathasone 25	0	38–72 h	0.75 mg

regimen with histamine 2-receptor antagonists or proton pump inhibitors may be indicated.

Steroids after percutaneous myocardial revascularization: clinical results

Systemic treatment

Because of the importance of inflammation in the mechanisms of restenosis, anti-inflammatory therapy with steroids after PCI has been experimented previously (9–11). In particular, two randomized, placebo-controlled studies showed that a single i.v. infusion of 1.0 g of methylprednisolone given 2–24 h before PCI is not able to influence restenosis after PCI compared to placebo (9,10). Previously, a small randomized study has shown a nonsignificant reduction of the recurrence of angina at 1.2 years with steroids (24%) compared to placebo (39%) using a higher-dose treatment started with 125 mg of methylprednisolone i.m. the night before and morning of PCI, followed by 60 mg day of oral prednisone for 1 week (11). Such negative results discouraged cardiologist to pursue the antirestenosis steroid strategy. The low dosage and too short length of the steroid treatment used in these studies are likely the main reasons for their lack of efficacy.

The administration of a short cycle of high-dose prednisone treatment to prevent restenosis after PCI yielded remarkable clinical and angiographic results in the high-dose IMmunosuppressive therapy for the Prevention of REStenosis after coronary artery Stent implantation (IMPRESS) studies (12,13). The first IMPRESS study was a randomized single-blinded study performed in 86 patients undergoing single bare metal stent (BMS) implantation and starting the oral prednisone treatment after 72 h of PCI and evidence of elevation of the C-reactive protein (CRP) levels in plasma. Patients were then randomized to either placebo ($n = 43$) or oral prednisone ($n = 43$) according to the treatment scheme depicted in the Figure 42.1, briefly, prednisone was given orally at a dose of 1 mg/kg for

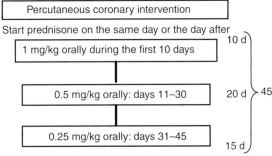

Oral prednisone treatment to prevent restenosis

Percutaneous coronary intervention

Start prednisone on the same day or the day after

1 mg/kg orally during the first 10 days — 10 d

0.5 mg/kg orally: days 11–30 — 20 d ⎫ 45

0.25 mg/kg orally: days 31–45 — 15 d ⎭

At hospital discharge associate:
Diuretics (25–50 mg of furosemide)
Anti-acids (20–40 mg of proton pump inhibitor)
At 4 weeks
Check blood cells count to rule out side effects of thienopyridines
Assess treatment compliance and side-effects
Up-grade anti-hypertensive treatment if needed
Eventually withdraw diuretics, anti-acids and thienopyridine if not
otherwise indicated

Figure 42.1 High-dose prednisone treatment scheme.

10 days, 0.5 mg/kg for 20 days and 0.25 mg/kg for 15 days. This dosage was chosen from the immunosuppressive protocol utilized for heart transplantation (7). Dual antiplatelet treatment was maintained for only 1 month. The angiographic results at 6 months and the clinical results at 1 year are shown in Table 42.2.

The IMPRESS 2/MVD study is a registry that included 86 consecutive patients with multivessel coronary artery disease (CAD) treated with multiple PCI. Patients with high CRP levels 48 h after PCI and no contraindications were prescribed high-dose oral prednisone at hospital discharge. No restriction instead was used for the clinical presentation of angina, the angiographic characteristics of the coronary lesions, and the PCI strategy, except the use of DES. The scheme of the steroid treatment was the same as that used in the IMPRESS randomized trial. The results of the study are shown in the Table 42.2. Of note, the clinical and angiographic efficacy of the prednisone treatment in this difficult population of patients with diffuse multivessel CAD was very similar to that observed in patients treated with single vessel intervention, resulting in a significant relative risk reduction of encountering vascular events at 1 year (death, infarction, or recurrence of angina) in prednisone-treated patients vs controls (0.34, 95% CI = 0.12–0.96, $p = 0.006$).

Recently, the effects of the same therapeutic scheme have been tested in the challenging setting of coronary bifurcation lesions (14). The IMPRESS-Y (bifurcation) study enrolled 25 patients treated on 58 lesions placed at sites of vessel bifurcation. Despite the known suboptimal outcome of PCI in this type of lesions using either conventional BMS or DES, the administration of high-dose oral prednisone after optimal lesion preparation and provisional stenting yielded encouraging clinical and angiographic results, as shown in Table 42.2.

The monitoring of outcome of patients enrolled in the IMPRESS studies at the long-term has confirmed the safety and efficacy of this treatment (15).

It must be acknowledged that in all the IMPRESS studies, the potential undesirable effects of high-dose steroids refrained the investigators from treating some specific subgroups of patients. In particular, patients with diabetes mellitus, infectious diseases, a recent transmural myocardial infarction (MI), or a relevant history of gastritis or peptic ulcer were excluded from the studies. Table 42.3 details the exclusion criteria applied in these studies.

Local stent elution of steroids
The administration of glucocorticoids locally, at the site of vascular injury with a DES technology has been tested using a commercially available

Table 42.2 Clinical and angiographic results of the IMPRESS studies.

Clinical endpoint at 12 months	Impress SVD (12)			IMPRESS 2 MVD (13)			IMPRESS Y (14)
	Prednisone	Control	p	Prednisone	Control	p	Prednisone
Death	—	—	1	—	2 (4.7%)	0.2	—
Myocardial infarction	—	1 (2%)	0.3	—	2 (4.7%)	0.2	—
TVR	3 (7%)	14 (35%)	0.001	3 (7%)	10 (23.3%)	0.03	2 (8%)
Combined end point	3 (7%)	16 (40%)	0.0004	3 (7%)	13 (30.2%)	0.006	2 (8%)
Angiographic endpoint at 6–8 months							
Restenosis rate (%)	3 (7%)	14 (36%)	0.0007	4/104 (3.8%)	NA	—	5/58 (8.6%)
Late luminal loss (mm)	0.39 ± 0.56	0.85 ± 0.64	0.001	0.61 ± 0.35	NA	—	0.36 ± 0.6 (MB) 0.47 ± 0.46 (SB)

Abbreviations: MB, main branch; NA, non analyzed; SB, side branch; TVR, target vessel revascularization.

Table 42.3 Contraindications to the use of high-dose prednisone after PCI.

1. Diabetes mellitus
2. Recent (<3 weeks) transmural (Q-wave) myocardial infarction
3. Peptic ulcer or history of gastric bleeding
4. Infectious diseases (consider also local processes like gingivitis, hepers, etc.)
5. Osteoporosis and bone demineralization (advanced age, generally >80)
6. Severe, uncontrolled hypertension

dexamethasone-eluting stent (Dexamet™, Abbott Vascular Devices, Galway, Ireland), a stainless steel stent, coated with phosphorylcholine and loaded with 0.5 μg of dexamethasone/mm^2 of stent surface. According to the manufacturer indications, 80% of the drug content is released from the polymer within 3–4 h of stent deployment and is completely delivered within 1 week. The local elution of a potent anti-inflammatory agent at the plaque level represents the theoretical background for the use of a dexamethasone-DES in patients with acute coronary syndromes (ACS) due to the predominant role that inflammation plays in the cellular mechanisms of unstable plaques (4).

The Dexamethasone Eluling Stent Italian REgistry (DESIRE) is a multicentre study performed with Dexamet™ (16). The study assessed the 6-month outcome of patients with non-ST elevation ACS treated according to an "early-invasive strategy" by means of PCI with implantation of Dexamet™ in a nation-wide, prospective, registry conducted on 334 patients. DESIRE yielded a low rate of subacute stent thrombosis at 30 days (0.6%), MI (2.1%) and ischemia-driven TVR (8.5%), with a global 11.5% incidence of the composite primary end point. As a DES study, the BMS-like angiographic findings reported in this study (33% restenosis rate, 0.95 ± 0.64 mm late loss) excluded a significant antiproliferative effect of this device, as previously suggested in smaller observations (17). This may indicate a suboptimal formulation of the drug concentration and release, with insufficient pharmacological effect in the arterial wall.

Differences of local vs systemic administration of glucocorticoids

Unlike other drug families, the systemic efficacy of steroids may be superior to the local delivery because of important systemic effects that can modulate the restenosis process. In fact, steroids act on the monocyte/macrophages cell lines inhibiting monocyte production and transformation into mature macrophages. This would cause a limited availability of monocytes able to enter the injured vessel wall to mediate the reparative processes that leads to neointimal growth. Furthermore, high doses of steroids are known to inhibit the monocyte-derived release of interleukins and other cytokines that act as potent mediators of inflammation (7). These agents recall inflammatory cells, activated platelets, and proliferative SMC, leading to restenosis. Steroids thus have the potential for blocking the restenosis process at a primitive stage compared to antiproliferative drugs, such as the cytostatic or cytotoxic drugs currently used in local treatments with DES technology (18). Moreover, unlike such drugs released form current DES, steroids do not prevent reendothelialization, thus allowing for a safe tissue covering of the metallic struts, as recently demonstrated in the experimental animal model (19). The beneficial effects of the systemic administration of the drug are therefore less likely to be achieved with local delivery of low doses of steroids at the artery wall site.

Side effects and clinical recommendations
Side effects of the short-term steroid treatment and possible long-term vascular effects

The secondary effects of the steroid treatment are generally minor, predictable, and reversible. The nature and the causes of these adverse effects are briefly summarized in Table 42.1. In the high-dose IMPRESS studies (12,13), gastric pain (4.7%), water, and salt retention with edema (1.2%), and worsened hypertension (4.7%) were observed in 11% of patients. The addition of diuretics and anti-acids before discharge and the upgrading of the antihypertensive medication thereafter, if needed, are useful preventive measures to control these temporary disorders (20). In the IMPRESS lowered-dose study the occurrence of such side effects of prednisone was not prevented despite a 50% reduction of the dose (21).

A brief comment is dedicated to the possible detrimental actions that a steroid treatment may cause in the cardiovascular system in the long term as a consequence of the effects on the glucose, water, and salt, and lipid metabolisms (8). Available analyses have been performed retrospectively in patients with important comorbidities being the indication to the steroid treatment, comorbidities that incorporate strong confounding variables for the assessment of the long-term clinical outcome (22). A short-term steroid exposure as that tested in the IMPRESS trials (45 days) is unlikely to develop permanent vascular damage through long-acting mechanisms as those involved in atherosclerosis progression (15).

Possible occurrence of neutropenia

"Unexpected" severe neutropenia or "agranulocytosis" (absolute neutrophil count $<0.5 \times 10^9$/L) was diagnosed at the time of routine blood cells counting, performed 28 days after PCI in three cases out of our whole experience of prednisone treatment. In all cases, treatment with prednisone (tapered at this time to 0.25 mg/kg/day) and thienopyridines was withdrawn and a progressive increment of the neutrophil counting was observed with return to basal levels within 10 days (23).

High doses of corticosteroids are used to treat aplastic anemia and drug-induced neutropenia (24) and prednisone is not a known cause of neutropenia. Neutropenia is instead, an uncommon but recognized undesirable effect of antiplatelet drugs (25). In particular, ticlopidine can induce blood dyscrasias in 0.8–2.3% of patients (mainly thrombocytopenia) through direct reversible myelosuppression (25). However, neutropenia is a very rare complication of thienopyridines, ranging between 0.1% and 0.2%, with agranulocytosis occurring in 0.05% of cases.

Thienopyridines are inactive *in vitro* and require hepatic biotransformation for pharmacological activity, which is mainly catalyzed by CYP3A4 (26). Glucocorticoids induce CYP2B, CYP2C, and CYP3A subfamilies *in vivo* and *in vitro*. In human hepatocyte cultures, prednisolone induces CYP3A4 through an enhanced expression of nuclear and

glucocorticoid receptors (27). Therefore, we hypothesize that prednisone, by increasing CYP3A4 activity, may enhance the formation of the active thienopyridine metabolite, possibly amplifying the risk of its side effects (23).

Recommendations

A word of caution is thus added to report a rare and unexpected side effect of thienopyridines when given in association with prednisone. Until the mechanisms leading to neutropenia in this setting are clarified, we would rather discourage the simultaneous use of DES and prednisone. Indeed, patients receiving DES need long-term double antiplatelet therapy with aspirin and thienopyridine, and premature discontinuation after PCI (e.g., due to neutropenia) increases dramatically the risk of DES thrombosis, a dreadful event that often is a cause of MI or death (28). Conversely, patients receiving BMS do not need prolonged dual antiplatelet treatment and can be safely treated with aspirin alone after 4 weeks of PCI. The exclusion of patients as detailed in Table 42.3 may avoid treatment-related complications and warrants the safety of this treatment. Furthermore, the therapeutic scheme reported in the high-dose IMPRESS studies should be considered as a bottomline, below which the treatment loses efficacy (21).

Conclusions

Modern pathophysiologic insides of the inflammation-related pathways of restenosis give renewed credit to glucocorticoids as antirestenotic agents. The administration of an immunosuppressive therapeutic scheme in selected patients has demonstrated promising perspectives of this systemic treatment to prevent restenosis, despite initial disappointing experiences likely due to inadequate dose and pharmacokinetic calculations.

Emerging evidence supports this strategy as a convenient and safe alternative to more expensive and complexes revascularization procedures as DES implantation or cardiac surgery, provided that the treatment is focused on selected candidates. The latest concerns referred to the long-term safety of first generation DES, and the yet undetermined duration of the dual antiplatelet treatment (3) further support the need for a simple pharmacological treatment that can be applied, however, in a large percentage of patients currently treated with PCI.

The advantages of a systemic treatment to prevent atherosclerosis progression after percutaneous vascular injury compared to a catheter-based, locally delivered treatment are evident, due to its simplicity and the potential for overcoming the technical limitations of stenting. However, appropriately sized randomized trials are needed to establish definitively the efficacy and the limitations of this treatment. Results of a large multicentre study of this kind are expected in the upcoming years (29).

Acknowledgment

The authors have no conflict of interest regarding the opinions expressed in this chapter and did not receive grants or financial support from the industry or form any other source. We thank Prof. Sandra Brunelleschi, from the Department of Medical Science, Laboratory of Experimental Pharmacology, of the Università del Piemonte Orientale, Novara, Italy, for her valuable assistance and continuous support.

References

1 Waksman R, Ajani AE, Pichard A, *et al.* Oral rapamycin to inhibit restenosis after stenting of de novo coronary lesions: the Oral Rapamune to Inhibit Restenosis (ORBIT) study. *J Am Coll Cardiol.* 2004; **44**:1386–1392.

2 Hausleiter J, Kastrati A, Mehilli J, *et al.* Randomized, double-blind, placebo-controlled trial of oral sirolimus for restenosis prevention in patients with in-stent restenosis. *Circulation.* 2004;**110**:790–795.

3 Nordmann AJ, Briel M, Bucher HC. Mortality in randomized controlled trials comparing drug-eluting stents vs. bare metal stents in coronary artery disease: a meta-analysis. *Eur Heart J.* 2006;**23**:2784–2814.

4 Welt FG, Rogers C. Inflammation and restenosis in the stent era. *Arterioscler Thromb Vasc Biol.* 2002;**22**: 1769–1776.

5 Ross R. Atherosclerosis. An inflammatory disease. *N Engl J Med.* 1999;**340**:115–126.

6 MacDonald RG, Panush RS, Pepine CJ. Rationale for use of glucocorticoids in modification of restenosis after percutaneous transluminal coronary angioplasty. *Am J Cardiol.* 1987;**60**:56B–60B.

7 Lindenfeld JA, Miller GG, Shakar SF, *et al.* Drug therapy in the heart transplant recipient. Part II: immunosuppressive drugs. *Circulation.* 2004;**110**:3858–3865.

8 Schimmer BP, Parker KL. Adrenocorticotropic hormone:adrenocortical steroids and their synthetic analogs; inhibitors of the synthesis and actions of adrenocortical hormones. In: Hardman JG, Limbird LE, eds. *Goodman & Gilman's The Pharmacological Basis of the Disease*, 10th Edition. New York: The McGraw-Hill Companies, Inc.

9 Pepine CJ, Hirshfeld JW, Macdonald RG, *et al.* A controlled trial of corticosteroids to prevent restenosis after coronary angioplasty. *Circulation.* 1990;**81**: 1753–1761.

10 Lee CW, Chae J, Lim H, *et al.* Prospective randomized trial of corticosteroids for the prevention of restenosis after intracoronary stent implantation. *Am Heart J.* 1999;**138**:60–63.

11 Stone GW, Rutherford BD, McConahay DR, *et al.* A randomized trial of corticosteroids for the prevention of restenosis in 102 patients undergoing repeat coronary angioplasty. *Catheter Cardiovasc Diagn.* 1989;**18**:227–231.

12 Versaci F, Gaspardone A, Tomai F, *et al.* Immunosuppressive therapy for the prevention of restenosis after coronary artery stent implantation (IMPRESS Study). *J Am Coll Cardiol.* 2002;**40**:1935–1942.

13 Ribichini F, Tomai F, Ferrero V, *et al.* Immunosuppressive oral prednisone after percutaneous interventions in patients with multi-vessel coronary artery disease. The IMPRESS-2/MVD Study. *Eurointervention.* 2005; **2**:173–180.

14 Ribichini F, Ferrero V, Rognoni A, *et al.* Percutaneous treatment of coronary bifurcations: lesion preparation before provisional bare metal stenting and subsequent immunosuppression with oral prednisone. The IMPRESS-Y Study. *J Interv Cardiol.* 2007;**20**:114–121.

15 Ferrero V, Tomai F, Versaci F, *et al.* Long-term results of immunosuppressive oral prednisone after coronary angioplasty in non-diabetic patients with elevated C-reactive protein levels. *EuroIntervention* 2009;**5**:250–254.

16 Ribichini F, Tomai F, Paloscia L, *et al.* Steroid-eluting stents in patients with acute coronary syndromes. The DESIRE: Dexamethasone Eluting Stent Italian REgistry. *Heart.* 2007;**93**:598–600.

17 Hoffmann R, Langenberg R, Radke P, *et al.* Evaluation of a high-dose dexamethasone-eluting stent. *Am J Cardiol.* 2004;**94**:193–195.

18 Costa MA, Simon DI. Molecular basis of restenosis and drug-eluting stents. *Circulation.* 2005;**111**:2257–2273.

19 Ribichini F, Joner M, Ferrero V, *et al.* Effects of oral prednisone after stenting in a rabbit model of established atherosclerosis. *J Am Coll Cardiol* 2007;**50**:176–85.

20 Ferrero V, Ribichini F, Pesarini G, *et al.* Therapeutic potential of glucocorticoids in the pre-vention of restenosis after coronary angioplasty. *Drugs* 2007;**67**:1243–55.

21 Ferrero V, Ribichini F, Rognoni A, *et al.* Comparison of efficacy and safety of lowered-dose to higher-dose oral prednisone after percutaneous coronary intervention. The IMPRESS-LD Study. *Am J Cardiol.* 2007;**99**:1082–1086.

22 Wei L, MacDonald TM, Walker BR. Taking glucocorticoids by prescription is associated with subsequent cardiovascular disease. *Ann Intern Med.* 2004;**141**:764–770.

23 Ribichini F, Ferrero V, Feola M, *et al.* Neutropenia in patients treated with thienopyridines and high-dose oral prednisone after percutaneous coronary interventions. *J Interven Cardiol* 2007;**20**:209–13.

24 Bhatt V, Saleem A. Review: drug-induced neutropenia. Pathophysiology, clinical features, and management. *Ann Clin Lab Sci.* 2004;**34**:131–137.

25 Quinn MJ, Fitzgerald DJ. Ticlopidine and clopidogrel. *Circulation.* 1999;**100**:1667–1672.

26 Pereillo JM, Maftouh M, Andrieu A, *et al.* Structure and stereochemistry of the active metabolite of clopidogrel. *Drug Metab Dispos.* 2002;**30**:1288–1295.

27 Pascussi JM, Gerbal-Chaloin S, Drocourt L, *et al.* The expression of CYP2B6, CYP2C9 and CYP3A4 genes: a tangle of networks of nuclear and steroid. *Biochim Biophys Acta.* 2003;**1619**:243–253.

28 Iakovou I, Schmidt T, Bonizzoni E, *et al.* Incidence, predictors, and outcome of thrombosis after successful implantation of drug-eluting stents. *JAMA.* 2005;**293**:2126–2130.

29 Ribichini F, Tomai F, De Luca G, *et al.* A multicenter, randomized study to test immunosuppressive therapy with oral prednisone for the prevention of restenosis after percutaneous coronary interventions: cortisone plus BMS or DES versus BMS alone to eliminate restenosis (CEREA-DES) – study design and rationale. *J Cardiovasc Med.* 2009;**10**:192–199.

CHAPTER 43

Oral agents to prevent in-stent restenosis (oral sirolimus and glitazones)

Pramod Kumar Kuchulakanti

Wockhardt Heart Center, Hyderabad, India

Introduction

Percutaneous coronary angioplasty and stenting are currently the standard treatment modality for atherosclerotic coronary artery disease. Improvements in stent design, lower strut thickness, optimization of stent apposition by high-pressure deployment, and reduction of stent thrombosis with oral antiplatelet agents etc., established this modality as safe and durable therapy to treat patients with coronary artery disease. However, in stent restenosis (ISR) that is, reoccurrence of luminal narrowing due to neointimal hyperplasia has emerged as a significant disadvantage of this technology affecting a quarter or more of stent-treated patients overall and up to one half of patients with long lesions or multiple stented sites (1). Several methods were attempted to prevent and treat ISR including administration of oral agents, intracoronary brachytherapy and currently local administration of drugs by way of drug-eluting stents. Majority of the studies to prevent ISR with oral agents are associated with negative or inconsistent results and only a few agents with positive results (Table 43.1).

The relevance of oral agents to prevent ISR

Each year, approximately more than 1 million patients are undergoing treatment with stents for coronary artery disease (2) and with ISR rates of 20–30% with bare metal stents (3,4), the population requiring repeat revascularization procedures is very high. The introduction of drug-eluting stents has decreased this incidence, but not eliminated the problem (5). Oral agents may be considered an attractive alternative strategy to prevent ISR for the following reasons:

1 They are simple to administer.

2 Local delivery of drugs in the form of drug-eluting stents is associated with neointimal catch up (6), late stent malapposition (7), and safety issues such as late stent thrombosis (8).

3 Possibility of targeting multiple causes that incite restenosis such as inflammation, smooth muscle cell proliferation, and reendothelialization.

4 Possibility of drug withdrawal or change over in case of adverse effects.

Pathology of ISR and targets for prevention

Inflammation plays a key role in coronary artery disease and other manifestations of atherosclerosis (9). Balloon angioplasty fractures the plaque and stents act as scaffolding and prevents elastic recoil and vascular remodeling (10). Although stents

Pharmacology in the Catheterization Laboratory. Edited by Ron Waksman and Andrew E Ajani. © 2010 Blackwell Publishing, ISBN: 978-1-4051-5704-9.

Table 43.1 Oral agents tested in clinical studies and the outcomes.

Oral agent	Not beneficial	Beneficial
Antiplatelet and antithrombotic drugs	Aspirin, dipyridamole, ticlopidine Warfarin, Vapiprost, Sulotroban	Cilastozole
Antianginal drugs	Calcium channel antagonists, Beta blockers	—
ACE inhibitors and angiotensin receptor blockers	Cilazapril, fosinopril, enalapril	Valsartan
Growth factor antagonist	Trapidil	—
Antiallergic drug	Tranilast	Tranilast
Antifibrotic drug	Colchicine	—
HMG-CoA reductase inhibitors	Lovastatin, fluvastatin, simvastatin	Probucol, Pravastatin
Vitamins and Nutritional supplements	α-Tocopherol, ω-3 Fatty Acids	Folic Acid
Nitric Oxide donor	Molsidomine	—
Serotonin receptor antagonist	Ketanserin	—
Anti proliferative agents	—	Sirolimus
Thiozolidendiones	—	Pioglitazone, Rosiglitazone, Troglitazone
Cortocosteroids	—	Prednisolone
Others	—	Pemirolast Sarproglate

are effective in reducing restenosis by these two mechanisms, they cause restenosis by additional mechanism—neointimal hyperplasia.

Recent research has demonstrated that inflammation plays an important role in the development of ISR (11). Within 10–15 min of stent implantation, leucocytes are recruited at the site of injury. Leukocyte invasion (mainly macrophages and T lymphocytes) is associated with massive deposition of activated platelets. Activated platelets express adhesion molecules such as P-selectin and glycoprotein Gp Ibα, which attach to circulating leucocytes via platelet receptors. Cytokines released from vascular smooth muscle cells and resident leucocytes induce migration of leucocytes across the platelet-fibrin layer and into the tissue. Growth factors are released from platelets, leucocytes, and vascular smooth muscle cells (VSMCs), and influence the proliferation and migration of VSMCs from the media into the denuded intimal area. These mitogenic stimuli act at cellular DNA level known as cell cycle (12). The cell cycle consists of four phases—resting phase, G_0, the dividing phase, or interphase, G_1, which leads to the phase of DNA synthesis, the S phase, and final M phase. Once stimulated, the cells undergo proliferation and in

less than 4 weeks, a new intima with minimal extra cellular matrix covers the stent struts.

Studies in the past investigated a variety of oral agents for their efficacy in decreasing restenosis, but only a few agents were reported to be beneficial (13). Brachytherapy guided the direction for prevention of restenosis by focusing on antiproliferative therapy by targeting the cell cycle. On the basis of current understanding of the mechanisms of ISR, the oral agents to prevent ISR are grouped into five classes, and some agents may have more than one mechanism of action (14):

1 Anti-inflammatory and immunomodulators
2 Antiproliferative agents
3 Inhibitors of VSMC migration
4 Agents promoting reendothelialization
5 Vitamins, antioxidants, and others

The present chapter focuses on oral sirolimus and glitazones in the prevention of ISR.

Oral sirolimus for prevention of ISR

Sirolimus—mechanism of action

Sirolimus, obtained from *Streptomyces hygroscopicus*, is a macrolide antibiotic with anti-inflammatory and immunosuppressive effects. It binds to the FK506 binding protein and this complex binds to mammalian Target of Rapamycin (mTOR) kinase, a cell cycle regulatory protein, thereby inhibiting mTOR action. The mTOR inhibition prevents cell cycle progression from late G1 phase to S phase (15). Systemic administration of rapamycin was shown to significantly reduce the arterial proliferative response after balloon angioplasty in animal models (16) and subsequently stent-based local delivery of rapamycin was developed, which met with significant success in terms of reduction of ISR and repeat revascularization in randomized clinical studies (17,18). Encouraged by these results and evidence of oral sirolimus slowing the progression of cardiac transplantation vasculopathy (19), clinical studies were undertaken to test if oral sirolimus is useful to prevent and treat ISR (Table 43.2).

Clinical studies

The clinical studies with oral sirolimus included de novo and ISR lesions. Among them, the most were open label (21–25,27) and only two were randomized (26,28). Studies by Waksman (22), Rodriguez (20,25–26), and Hausleiter (28) showed beneficial effect while other studies were negative. The inconsistency among the results of these studies could be due to variations in the loading dose, maintenance dose, duration of therapy, initiation of the loading dose before or after percutaneous coronary intervention, and side effects leading to withdrawal of drug. The loading dose varied between 4 and 24 mg and the daily maintenance dose between 2 and 5 mg The duration of therapy was between 1 and 4 weeks. Most investigators initiated the oral drugs immediately post-PCI or up to 12 h post-PCI. The incidence of side effects was 10–80% and discontinuation of drug due to side effects was 10–50% of the study patients. The late loss varied between 0.6 and 1.4 ± 1.1 mm for de novo lesions and 0.49 ± 0.54 mm for ISR lesions. The binary restenosis was 7.1–40% for de novo lesions and a very high 22.1–86.7% in ISR lesions. Rapamycin levels were not measured in all studies and some studies have shown correlation with lower late loss if the blood levels were >8 ng/mL.

Lessons from positive studies

What lessons can be learnt from the positive studies? First, the optimal rapamycin dose to prevent restenosis is not known. The dose used in pilot studies is based on the FDA-recommended dose for renal transplant patients. It may be important to have effective drug levels in the circulation at the time of PCI. Further, it is known that immunosuppressive effects of oral administration of rapamycin are optimal after 4 days of treatment. The positive results obtained by Hausleiter *et al.* could be attributable to administering high dose of rapamycin 2 days prior to PCI.

Second, effective drug levels should be achieved in the blood. It was shown by Hausleiter *et al.*, that rapamycin levels on the day of PCI correlate with late loss and Rodriguez *et al.* have shown blood rapamycin level of >8 ng/mL correlated with late loss at follow-up. Consistent with these early observations, in the subsequent study by Hausleiter *et al.*, rapamycin levels on the day of PCI were 10.0 ± 8.5 and 18.1 ± 5.2 ng/L in the groups loaded with 8 and 24 mg and significant reduction in late loss and ISR was demonstrated in the high-dose group with rapamycin blood levels 10.0 ± 5.0 ng/L on day 3 after PCI.

Third, duration of oral therapy should be sufficient to inhibit the inflammation and proliferative reactions, which occur in the initial 1–2 weeks. It is probable that a shorter duration of intense therapy may be more effective than a low dose administered over a longer period.

Fourth, compliance with the drug is important until at least first 1–2 weeks. The most important side effects that precluded continuation of the drug were oral ulcers, esophagitis, diarrhea, leucopenia, thrombocytopenia, hypertriglyceridemia. In the study by Brara *et al.*, with highest number of patients (50%) discontinued therapy, the duration before discontinuation of therapy was 14.5 ± 6.5 days showing 1–2 weeks of therapy is tolerable to almost all patients.

Summary—role of oral Sirolimus

In summary, oral sirolimus therapy appears to be beneficial in small randomized and open label studies. Further larger studies by modifying the protocols to high loading dose at least 2–4 days before PCI and continuing maintenance dose for

Table 43.2 Published studies conducted with oral sirolimus to prevent restenosis and the results.

| Author | Year | Study design | N | Dose | | Duration | Late loss (mm) | ISR | Conclusion |
				Loading	Maintenance				
De novo lesions									
Rodriguez et al. (20)	2003	Open label	34[a]	6 mg	2 mg/day	4 weeks	0.9	18.5%	Beneficial
Guardo et al. (21)	2004	Open label	15	5 mg	2 mg/day	4 weeks	1.4 ± 1.1	40%	Not beneficial
Waksman et al. (22)	2004	Open label	60	5 mg	2 or 5 mg/day	4 weeks	0.60 ± 0.54	7.1%	Beneficial
Brito et al. (23)	2005	Open label	12[b]	15 mg	5 mg/day	4 weeks	0.67 ± 0.45	11.1%	Not beneficial
Chaves et al. (24)	2005	Open label	15	15 mg	5 mg/day	4 weeks	0.61 ± 0.31	13%	Not beneficial
Rodriguez et al. (25)	2005	Open label	76	6 mg	2 mg/day	4 weeks	0.60	15%	Beneficial
Rodriguez et al. (26)	2006	Randomized	100	6 mg	3 mg/day	2 weeks	0.73 ± 0.40	11.6%	Beneficial
ISR lesions									
Brara et al. (27)	2003	Open label	22	6 mg	2 mg/day	4 weeks	N/A	86.7%	Not beneficial
Hausleiter et al. (28)	2004	Randomized	300	6 or 24 mg	2 mg/day	1 week	0.49 ± 0.54	22.1%	Beneficial

[a]Included 12 lesions with ISR.
[b]Included 8 lesions with ISR.

1–2 weeks achieving optimal rapamycin levels to >8 ng/mL may establish the role of oral sirolimus firmly.

Oral glitazones for prevention of ISR

Glitazones—mechanism of action

Glitazones, also known as thiozolidenidones (TZDs) are oral drugs used to treat patients with diabetes mellitus because of their ability to lower fasting and postprandial glucose concentrations as well as free fatty acid concentrations. Glitazones act as insulin sensitizers and have favorable effect on increasing high-density lipoproteins.

Recent evidence indicates important role for glitazones in atherosclerosis and restenosis. To understand this, we should know what peroxisome proliferator activator receptors (PPARs) are. PPARs are a subfamily of the 48-member nuclear-receptor superfamily and regulate gene expression in response to ligand binding. Three PPARs have been identified to date namely—α, δ (also known as β), and γ. After ligand binding, PPARs undergo conformational changes and regulate gene transcription by DNA-dependent transactivation and DNA-independent transrepression that may explain the anti-inflammatory actions of PPARs (29). Various fatty acids serve as endogenous ligands; certain drugs such as fibrates act as ligands for PPAR-α and glitazones are selective ligands of PPAR-γ. There are three glitazones—troglitazone, the first drug introduced and withdrawn due to hepatotoxicity, and two currently available drugs, namely, rosiglitazone and pioglitazone.

Clinical studies have demonstrated that beneficial effects of glitazones are not solely explained by their ability to control diabetes. There are several other mechanisms by which they may provide salutary effects in atherosclerosis and restenosis (30). These mechanisms are—inhibition of VSMC proliferation by blocking G1 to S transition in the cell cycle and inhibition of VSMC migration from the media to the intima (31). They also exhibit anti-inflammatory effects on the macrophages. Further they reduce the plasma and vascular tissue levels of plasmiogen activator inhibitor 1 (PAI-1), which is linked to accelerated atherosclerosis and restenosis after balloon-induced injury. Preclinical studies

with troglitazone (32) and pioglitazone (33) have demonstrated efficacy in reducing neointimal proliferation, thus leading to clinical studies.

Clinical studies

As with other oral agents to prevent restenosis, there are a limited number of studies with glitazones (Table 43.3). Most of the studies were positive (34–39) except the study by Osman using rosiglitazone (40), which did not show any benefit with glitazones in reducing restenosis. In the studies by Takagi et al. using troglitazone (34,35) and pioglitazone (36), the authors have demonstrated that in patients with impaired glucose tolerance (34) and type 2 diabetes mellitus (35,36). These agents significantly reduced intimal area and neointimal index by serial intravascular ultrasound measurement at 6 months follow-up. The glycemic control as measured by Hb A1 C and the fasting blood glucose levels were similar between control group and glitazone group at 6 months follow-up. Interestingly, there was no relation between neointimal index and glycemic control at follow-up, suggesting independent effect of glitazones on reduction of neointimal proliferation. Glitazone therapy was initiated 24–48 h before PCI studies with troglitazone and 8 ± 2 days in the study using pioglitazone.

In a study which included only 16 patients (rosiglitazone, $n = 8$; placebo, $n = 8$), Osman et al. have concluded that oral rosiglitazone was not beneficial in reducing ISR and was not associated with significant reduction of neo intimal volume by IVUS (37). In this study, rosiglitazone was administered within 6 h of PCI.

Choi et al. have studied effect of rosiglitazone 8 mg administered 1 day before PCI, followed by 4 mg daily for 6 months in 95 diabetic patients and found significant reduction in ISR (17.6% vs 38.2%, $p = 0.03$) compared to control group (38). In their study, there was significant reduction of hs-CRP in the rosiglitazone group compared to control group (from 2.92 ± 1.98 to 0.62 ± 0.44 mg/L, $P < 0.001$ vs from 2.01 ± 1.33 to 1.79 ± 1.22 mg/L, $P = NS$), suggesting a role for the anti-inflammatory effects of rosiglitazone.

The beneficial effects of glitazones were shown in nondiabetic patients in the study by Marx et al. (39). In this randomized, double-blind, placebo-controlled

Table 43.3 Published studies with oral Glitazones to prevent restenosis and the results.

Author	Drug	Year	Study design	N (study drug)	Diabetic status	Dose	Duration	ISR	Conclusion
Takagi (34)	Troglitazone	2000	Randomized	28	IGT	400 mg	6 months	—	Beneficial
Takagi (35)	Troglitazone	2002	Randomized	27	Type 2 DM	400 mg	6 months	23%	Beneficial
Takagi (36)	Pioglitazone	2003	Randomized	23	Type 2 DM	30 mg	6 months	19%	Beneficial
Osman (40)	Rosiglitazone	2004	Randomized	8	Type 2 DM	4 mg, 8 mg	6 months	25%	Not beneficial
Choi (37)	Rosiglitazone	2004	Randomized	47	Type 2 DM	8 mg, 4 mg	6 months	17.6%	Beneficial
Marx (38)	Pioglitazone	2005	Randomized	25	Non diabetic	30 mg	6 months	3.4%	Beneficial
Nishio (39)	Pioglitazone	2006	Randomized	26	Type 2 DM	30 mg	6 months	7.7%	Beneficial
Katayama (41)	Pioglitazone	2007	Randomized	14	Non diabetic	30 mg	6 months	0%	Beneficial

study, 50 patients (pioglitazone, $n = 25$; placebo, $n = 25$) were treated with 30 mg/day dose of pioglitazone or matching placebo, commenced before PCI and continued for 6 months. In this study population of nondiabetic patients, pioglitazone treatment did not significantly change fasting blood glucose, fasting insulin, or glycosylated hemoglobin levels, as well as lipid parameters. In contrast, pioglitazone treatment significantly reduced neointima volume within the stented segment, total plaque volume, and importantly the binary restenosis rate when compared to placebo (3.4% vs 32.3%, $P < 0.01$). This study underscores the direct influence of pioglitazone on the neointimal suppression independent of metabolic effects.

Nishio *et al.* have studied the effect of pioglitazone in 26 diabetic patients compared to 28 diabetic patients in control group and demonstrated that late luminal loss (0.30 ± 0.66 vs 1.43 ± 1.04, $p = 0.0008$) and in-stent restenosis (7.7% vs 57.1%, $p = 0.005$) were significantly less in the pioglitazone group than in the control group at 6 months follow-up (40). Insulin, homeostasis model assessment of insulin resistance, eNOS, and leptin at follow-up were significantly reduced in the pioglitazone group compared with the control group, suggesting that pioglitazone helps improving endothelial function and thereby reducing restenosis.

In the latest published study, Katayama *et al.* have studied 28 nondiabetic patients with metabolic syndrome (pioglitazone, $n = 14$; control, $n = 14$) who underwent coronary stenting and reported 0% restenosis in pioglitazone group compared to control group (41).

The authors concluded the beneficial effect of pioglitazone to improved insulin resistance and decreased visceral fat accumulation.

Lessons from positive studies

Lindsay *et al.* have shown that preprocedural hyperglycemia is shown to be associated with increased restenosis in diabetic patients (42). It is also known that optimal glycemic control determined by preprocedural HbA1c was associated with reduced rates of target vessel revascularization (43). Therefore, it is intuitive to know that glitazones will be beneficial in reducing ISR by way of optimizing glycemic control. However, there was no significant difference in either fasting glucose levels

or HbA1C at baseline and at 6-month follow-up in almost all the studies with oral glitazones compared to control group. Further, beneficial effect of glitazones was also shown in nondiabetic patients and in nondiabetic patients with metabolic syndrome. This clearly shows that glitazones are able to reduce ISR by mechanisms other than glycemic control alone. As discussed earlier, direct effect of glitazones on VSMCs might be a potential beneficial effect. Additional mechanisms explored in the above discussed studies are—reduced hs-CRP with rosiglitazone (38), reduced eNOS and leptin concentrations with pioglitazone (40), and decreased insulin resistance and visceral fat accumulation with pioglitazone (41).

The initiation of glitazone therapy varied among the studies from 2 days pre-PCI to 1 week post-PCI. Loading dose was not administered for the possible fear of hypoglycemia. All the studies used glitazones for 6 months following PCI. Tolerance to glitazones was excellent except very few patients withdrawn due to dizziness and skin rash.

Summary—role of oral glitazones

In summary, oral glitazone therapy appears to be beneficial in small randomized and open label studies. However, larger studies are needed to establish the role of glitazones in prevention of ISR.

Conclusions

In conclusion, oral sirolimus and oral glitazone therapy appears to be a promising option for the reduction of ISR. However, large-scale randomized, double-blind, placebo-controlled studies are needed to establish this modality of therapy for prevention of ISR.

References

1 Kastrati A, Schomig A, Elezi S, *et al.* Predictive factors of restenosis after coronary stent placement. *J Am Coll Cardiol.* 1997;**30**:1428–1436.

2 Heart disease and Stroke Statistics: 2007 Update, A Report from the AmericanHeart Association Statistics Committee and Stroke Statistics Subcommittee. Dallas, TX. Available at http//www.americanheart.org. Accessed on 5 April 2007.

3 Fischman DL, Leon MB, Baim DS, *et al.* A randomized comparison of coronary stent placement and balloon

angioplasty in the treatment of coronary artery disease. *N Engl J Med.* 1994;**331**:496–501.

4 Serruys PW, de Jaegere P, Kiemeneij F, *et al.* A comparison of balloon-expandable stent implantation with balloon angioplasty in patients with coronary artery disease. *N Engl J Med.* 1994;**331**:489–495.

5 Waksman R. Drug eluting stents: from bench to bed. *Cardiovasc Radiat Med.* 2002;**3**:226–241.

6 Farb A, Heller PF, Shroff S, *et al.* Pathological analysis of local delivery of Paclitaxel via a polymer-coated stent. *Circulation.* 2001;**104**:473–479.

7 Hong MK, Mintz GS, Lee CW, *et al.* Late stent malapposition after drug-eluting stent implantation: an intravascular ultrasound analysis with long-term follow-up. *Circulation.* 2006;**113**:414–419.

8 Bavry AA, Kumbhani DJ, Helton TJ, *et al.* Late stent thrombosis of Drug eluting stents- a Meta analysis of randomized clinical trials. *Am J Med.* 2007;**119**:1056–1061.

9 Hansson GK. Inflammation, atherosclerosis and coronary artery disease. *N Engl J Med.* 2005;**352**:1685–1695.

10 Hoffman R, Mintz GS, Dussaillant GR, *et al.* Patterns and mechanisms of in-stent restenosis: a serial intravascular ultrasound study. *Circulation.* 1996;**94**:1247–1254.

11 Gaspardone A, Versaci F. Coronary stenting and inflammation. *Am J Cardiol.* 2005;**96**(suppl):65L–70L.

12 Kutryk MJB, Serruys PW. Antirestenosis alternatives in the new millennium. In: Waksman R, ed. *Vascular Brachytherapy*, Third Edition. New York: Futura Publishing Co.; 2002:55–62, Chapter 6.

13 Faxon DP. Systemic drug therapy for restenosis: "*de javu all over again*". *Circulation.* 2002;**106**:2296–2298.

14 Kuchulakanti P, Waksman R. Therapeutic potential of oral anti proliferative agents in the prevention of coronary restenosis. *Drugs.* 2004;**64**:2379–2388.

15 Poon M, Badimon JJ, Fuster V. Overcoming restenosis with sirolimus: from alphabet soup to clinical reality. *Lancet.* 2002;**359**:619–622.

16 Gallo R, Padurean A, Jayaraman T, *et al.* Inhibition of intimal thickening after balloon angioplasty in porcine coronary arteries by targeting regulators of the cell cycle. *Circulation.* 1999;**99**:2164–2170.

17 Morris ML, Serruys PW, Sousa JE, *et al.* Randomized study with the sirolimus-coated Bx velocity balloon-expandable stent in the treatment of patients with de novo native coronary artery lesions. *N Engl J Med.* 2002;**346**:1773–1780.

18 Moses JW, Leon MB, Popma JJ, *et al.* Sirolimus-eluting stents versus standard stents in patients with stenosis in a native coronary artery. *N Engl J Med.* 2003;**349**:1315–1323.

19 Mancini D, Pinney S, Burkhoff D, *et al.* Use of rapamycin slows progression of cardiac transplantation vasculopathy. *Circulation.* 2003;**108**:48–53.

20 Rodríguez AE, Alemparte MR, Vigo CF, *et al.* Pilot study of oral rapamycin to prevent restenosis in patients undergoing coronary stent therapy: argentina single center study (ORAR Trial). *J Invasive Cardiol.* 2003;**15**:581–584.

21 Guarda E, Marchant E, Fajuri A, *et al.* Oral rapamycin to prevent human coronary stent restenosis: a pilot study. *Am Heart J.* 2004;**148**:e9.

22 Waksman R, Ajani AE, Pichard AD, *et al.* Oral Rapamycin to inhibit restenosis after stenting of de novo coronary lesions, the Oral Rapamune to inhibit restenosis (ORBIT) study. *J Am Coll Cardiol.* 2004;**44**:1386–1392.

23 Brito FS Jr, Rosa WCM, Arruda JA, *et al.* Efficacy and safety of oral sirolimus to inhibit in-stent intimal hyperplasia. *Catheter Cardiovasc Interv.* 2005;**64**:413–418.

24 Chaves AJ, Sousa AG, Mattos LA, *et al.* Pilot study with an intensified oral sirolimus regimen for the prevention of in-stent restenosis in de novo lesions: a serial intravascular ultrasound study. *Catheter Cardiovasc Interv.* 2005;**66**:535–540.

25 Rodríguez AE, Alemparte MR, Vigo CF, *et al.* Role of oral rapamycin to prevent restenosis in patients with de novo lesions undergoing coronary stenting: results of the Argentina single centre study (ORAR trial). *Heart.* 2005;**91**:1433–1437.

26 Rodríguez AE, Granada JF, Alemparte MR, *et al.* Oral rapamycin after coronary bare-metal stent implantation to prevent restenosis the prospective, randomized oral rapamycin in Argentina (ORAR II) study. *J Am Coll Cardiol.* 2006;**47**:1522–1529.

27 Brara PS, Moussavian M, Grise MA, *et al.* Pilot trial of oral rapamycin for recalcitrant restenosis. *Circulation.* 2003;**107**:1722–1724.

28 Hausleiter J, Kastrati A, Mehilli J, *et al.* Randomized, double-blind, placebo-controlled trial of oral sirolimus for restenosis prevention in patients with in-stent restenosis. The Oral Sirolimus to Inhibit Recurrent In-stent Stenosis (OSIRIS) trial. *Circulation.* 2004;**110**:790–795.

29 Yki-Järvinen H. Thiozolidinediones. *N Engl J Med.* 2004;**351**:1106–1118.

30 Pakala R, Rha SW, Kuchulakanti P, *et al.* Peroxisome proliferator-activated receptor-γ its role in atherosclerosis and restenosis. *Cardiovasc Radiat Med.* 2004;**5**:44–48.

31 Bruemmer D, Law RE. Thiozolidinedione regulation of smooth muscle cell proliferation. *Am J Med.* 2003;**115**:87S–92S.

32 Law RE, Meehan WP, Xi XP, *et al.* Troglitazone inhibits vascular smooth muscle cell growth and intimal hyperplasia. *J Clin Invest.* 1996;**98**:1897–1905.

33 Yoshimoto T, Naruse M, Shizume H. Vasculo-protective effects of insulin sensitizing agent pioglitazone in neointimal thickening and hypertensive vascular hypertrophy. *Atherosclerosis.* 1999;**145**:333–340.

34 Takagi T, Akasaka T, Yamamuro A, *et al.* Troglitazone reduces neointimal tissue proliferation after coronary stent implantation in patients with non–insulin dependent diabetes mellitus. *J Am Coll Cardiol.* 2000;**36**:1529–1535.

35 Takagi T, Yamamuro A, Tamita K, *et al.* Impact of troglitazone on coronary stent implantation using small stents in patients with type 2 diabetes mellitus. *Am J Cardiol.* 2002;**89**:318–322.

36 Takagi T, Yamamuro A, Tamita K, *et al.* Pioglitazone reduces neointimal tissue proliferation after coronary stent implantation in patients with type 2 diabetes mellitus: an intravascular ultrasound scanning study. *Am Heart J.* 2003;**146**:1–8.

37 Choi D, Kim S, Choi S, *et al.* Preventative effects of rosiglitazone on restenosis after coronary stent implantation in patients with type 2 diabetes. *Diabetes Care.* 2004;**27**:2654–2660.

38 Marx N, Wöhrle J, Nusser T, *et al.* Pioglitazone reduces neointima volume after coronary stent implantation: a randomized, placebo-controlled, double-blind trial in nondiabetic patients. *Circulation.* 2005;**112**:2792–2798.

39 Nishio K, Sakurai M, Kusuyama T, *et al.* A randomized comparison of pioglitazone to inhibit restenosis after coronary stenting in patients with type 2 diabetes. *Diabetes Care.* 2006;**29**:101–106.

40 Osman A, Otero J, Brizolara A, *et al.* Effect of rosiglitazone on restenosis after coronary stenting in patients with type 2 diabetes. *Am Heart J.* 2004;**147**:e21–e25.

41 Katayama T, Ueba H, Tsuboi K, *et al.* Reduction of neointimal hyperplasia after coronary stenting by pioglitazone in nondiabetic patients with metabolic syndrome. *Am Heart J.* 2007;**153**:762.e1–762.e7.

42 Lindsay J, Sharma AK, Canos D, *et al.* Preprocedure hyperglycemia is more strongly associated with restenosis in diabetic patients after percutaneous coronary intervention than is hemoglobin A1C. *Cardiovasc Revasc Med.* 2007;**8**:15–20.

43 Corpus RA, George PB, House JA, *et al.* Optimal glycemic control is associated with a lower rate of target vessel revascularization in treated type II diabetic patients undergoing elective percutaneous coronary intervention. *J Am Coll Cardiol.* 2004;**43**:8–14.

CHAPTER 44

Novel pharmacotherapy in percutaneous coronary intervention

Andrew T. L. Ong
Westmead Hospital, Westmead, NSW, Australia

Introduction

Pharmacotherapy for percutaneous coronary intervention (PCI) can be divided into the following categories according to their function: (1) antiplatelet agents to prevent platelet aggregation, the first step of the coagulation cascade; (2) anticoagulants to inhibit the coagulation cascade and prevent thrombosis; (3) vasodilators to treat complications of no-reflow; and (4) agents to reduce reperfusion injury following acute myocardial infarction (AMI).

Currently in the PCI setting, heparin remains the standard anticoagulant used. Bivalirudin, a direct thrombin inhibitor, has now been shown to be equally effective as heparin in combination with a glycoprotein IIb/IIIa (GP IIb/IIIa) receptor antagonist and has replaced heparin in many institutions. The currently used intravenous antiplatelet agents are the GP IIb/IIIa receptor antagonists and include abciximab, tirofiban and eptifibatide. The oral antiplatelet agents of aspirin, together with clopidogrel (which replaced ticlopidine) are the standard dual antiplatelet agents used (1). The vasodilators, adenosine, verapamil, glyceryl trinitrate, and sodium nitroprusside are effective intracoronary agents. No agents are currently used routinely to prevent reperfusion injury.

Pharmacology in the Catheterization Laboratory. Edited by Ron Waksman and Andrew E Ajani. © 2010 Blackwell Publishing, ISBN: 978-1-4051-5704-9.

The focus on research has been the development of new and better antiplatelet agents as the currently available agents do not consistently inhibit platelet aggregation. The ideal agent should rapidly achieve full platelet inhibition, yet be reversible, show a uniform response curve, and is metabolically active in its administered form. Inhibition of this step prevents the activation of the entire cascade, leading to thrombosis. This is particularly important in PCI whereby the procedure itself is both thrombogenic and is used to treat thrombosis. Furthermore, this class of agents is particularly attractive as it has potentially widespread applicability in all areas of arterial thrombosis. The development of successful agents to reduce reperfusion injury following AMI has potential long-term implications in reducing both mortality and morbidity in this subgroup of patients.

Antiplatelet agents

Vascular injury results in release of adenosine diphosphate (ADP) from the vascular endothelium, which activates platelets, which in turn release more ADP, activating more platelets. ADP, though a second mechanism, promotes platelet activation by binding to G-protein receptors, inhibiting adenyl cyclase, and reducing levels of cAMP. This results in a conformation change in the shape of the platelet, subsequently activating GP IIb/IIIa receptors. Activated GP receptors on the surface of two adjacent platelets bind dimeric fibrinogen, which then

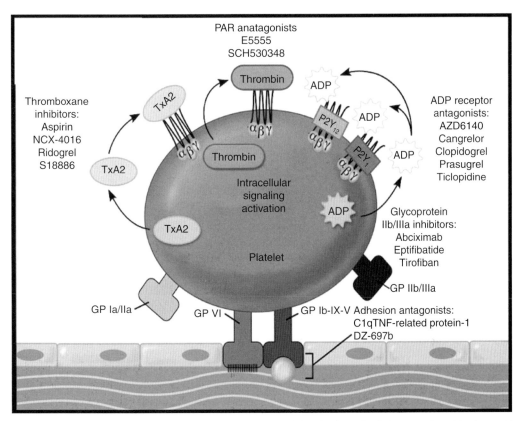

Figure 44.1 Different targets of platelet activation and targets to inhibit platelet activation. *Source*: From Meadows and Bhatt (2).

amplifies platelet aggregating via cross-linking of fibrin, eventually leads to thrombus formation (see Figure 44.1).

The three main sites that have been investigated on the platelet are the ADP receptor, the GP receptor, and the PAR receptor. Of the ADP receptors, agents that antagonize $P2Y_{12}$ have been most studied. A second target investigated are agents that antagonize the protease-activated receptor. They have the ability to modulate the platelet activation cascade via their effects on thrombin, widely considered to be the most potent platelet activator. PAR-1 and PAR-4 are the most important in platelet aggregation. PAR-1 appears to be the main thrombin receptor. Binding of thrombin to PAR-1 stimulates the release of ADP, which then subsequently binds to the P2Y receptors to further promote platelet aggregation.

Adenosine diphosphate receptor antagonist

Ticlopidine was the first commercially available ADP receptor antagonist, but in most markets has been superseded by clopidogrel due to its high side effect profile, in particular bone marrow suppression (3).

Clopidogrel binds the $P2Y_{12}$ ADP receptor as an irreversible antagonist, which results in inhibition of platelet function for the life of the platelet (5–7 days). This poses an increased bleeding risk to patients requiring urgent or emergent surgery within the first 5 days of being given the medication. More recently, there have been increasing evidence to support the concept of clopidogrel resistance with inter- and intra-individual variability seen, potentially resulting in the risk of recurrent ischemic events (4).

Prasugrel

Prasugrel (Eli Lilly) is a third generation thienopyridine which irreversibly antagonizes the $P2Y_{12}$ receptor, inhibiting ADP-induced platelet aggregation. In Phase 1 studies, prasugrel was shown to have a faster onset of action than clopidogrel, irrespective of whether a loading dose was administered. In particular, it achieved significantly higher platelet aggregation inhibition at 4 h postdose and was associated with a lower incidence of nonresponders as compared to clopidogrel-treated patients. This is because up to 85% of ingested clopidogrel is inactivated by esterases in blood, prior to undergoing hepatic metabolism by the cytochrome p450 pathway, creating the active metabolite; a feature is not seen with prasugrel (5).

The JUMBO-TIMI 26 (Joint Utilisation of Medications to Block Platelets Optimally-Thrombolysis in Myocardial Infarction 26), a double-blind, dose-ranging, Phase 2 safety trial, compared prasugrel with clopidogrel in 904 patients on aspirin undergoing elective or urgent PCI with the primary end point of clinically significant (TIMI major plus minor) non-CABG-related bleeding at 30 days (6). Patients were randomized to low (40 mg loading dose, 7.5 mg maintenance dose), intermediate (60 mg loading dose, 10 mg maintenance dose), high dose (60 mg loading dose, 15 mg maintenance) prasugrel; or to clopidogrel (300 mg loading dose, 75 mg maintenance dose). Hemorrhagic complications were infrequent, with no significant difference between patients treated with prasugrel or clopidogrel in the rate of significant bleeding (1.7% vs 1.2% respectively; hazard ratio (HR) 1.42, (95% CI 0.40–5.08)).

The PRINICPLE-TIMI 44 study was a phase 2 study that evaluated the mean inhibition of platelet aggregation (IPA) of prasugrel vs clopidogrel (7). Phase 1 compared a loading dose of prasugrel 60 mg vs clopidogrel 600 mg and assessed mean IPA at 6 h; while phase 2 was a crossover design comparing maintenance doses of prasugrel 10 mg vs clopidogrel 150 mg, assessing mean IPA at the end of 2 weeks of therapy. In all phases, prasugrel treated patients had significantly higher IPA compared with clopidogrel.

This led to the TRITON-TIMI 38 (Trial to Assess Improvement in Therapeutic Outcomes by Optimizing Platelet Inhibition with Prasugrel—TIMI 38), a Phase 3, double-blind, clinical trial of 13,608 patients with acute coronary syndrome and planned PCI, pretreated with aspirin and randomized to either prasugrel or clopidogrel for a median duration of 12 months of therapy (8,9). The primary efficacy end point was death from cardiovascular causes, nonfatal myocardial infarction, or nonfatal stroke. The key safety end point was major bleeding. A key secondary end point was the incidence of stent thrombosis. This tested the hypothesis that greater platelet inhibition resulted in better outcomes.

In this study, the primary efficacy end point occurred in 9.9% of prasugrel vs 12.1% of clopidogrel-treated patients (HR 0.81; 95% confidence interval [CI], 0.73–0.90; $P < 0.001$). Fewer myocardial infarctions were found in the prasugrel group (7.4% vs 9.7% respectively; $P < 0.001$), urgent target-vessel revascularization (2.5% vs 3.7% respectively; $P < 0.001$), and stent thrombosis (1.1% vs 2.4% respectively; $P < 0.001$).

These positive efficacy results occurred at the expense of more major bleeding in the prasugrel group (2.4% vs 1.8% respectively HR, 1.32; 95% CI, 1.03–1.68; $P = 0.03$). Also greater in the prasugrel group was the rate of life-threatening bleeding (1.4% vs 0.9% respectively; $P = 0.01$), including nonfatal bleeding (1.1% vs 0.9%; HR 1.25; $P = 0.23$) and fatal bleeding (0.4% vs 0.1% respectively; $P = 0.002$).

In assessing the balance between safety and efficacy of prasugrel, patients with a history of prior transient ischemic attack or stroke had a higher chance of developing either the primary end point or non-CABG-related, nonfatal TIMI major bleeding (23.0% for prasugrel vs 16.0% for clopidogrel, HR 1.54 (95% CI 1.02–2.32), $P = 0.04$).

In a prespecified stent subanalysis of the trial, the 12,844 patients who received at least one stent implanted (representing 94% of the trial) were divided by stent type (10). Here, 6,461 (47%) received only bare metal stents (BMS), 5,743 (42%) only drug-eluting stents (DES), while 640 (5%) received a mixture of BMS and DES. Of those that received DES, 2,766 (20%) received paclitaxel-eluting stents, 2,454 (18%) received sirolimus-eluting stents, and 523 (4%) received other or mixed stent types. Stent thrombosis was assessed according to Academic Research Consortium definitions, and the combined definition of definite or probable stent thrombosis was employed (11).

Prasugrel compared to clopidogrel reduced the primary end point in the overall stented cohort (9.7 vs 11.9%, HR 0.81, $p = 0.0001$), in DES-treated patients (9.0 vs 11.1% respectively, HR 0.82, $p = 0.019$), and in BMS-treated patients (10.0 vs 12.2% respectively, HR 0.80, $P = 0.003$). Stent thrombosis was reduced with prasugrel overall (1.13 vs 2.35% respectively, HR 0.48, $P < 0.0001$), in DES-treated patients (0.84 vs 2.31% respectively, HR 0.36, $P < 0.0001$), and in BMS-treated patients (1.27 vs 2.41% respectively, HR 0.52, $P = 0.0009$).

In the DES group, prasugrel as compared to clopidogrel reduced the incidence of both early (0–30 days) stent thrombosis (0.42 vs 1.44% respectively, HR 0.29 (0.15–0.56), $p = 0.0001$) and late (30–450 days) stent thrombosis (0.42 vs 0.91% respectively, HR 0.46 (0.22–0.97), $p = 0.04$). Interestingly, in the BMS-treated group, prasugrel reduced only early stent thrombosis (0.75 vs 1.66% respectively, HR 0.45 (0.28–0.73), $P = 0.0009$) but not late stent thrombosis (0.53 vs 0.78% respectively, HR 0.68 (0.35–1.31), $P = 0.24$).

At time of writing, prasugrel is awaiting FDA approval in the United States. Further trials are planned for the drug, including the ongoing TRILOGY ACS (TaRgeted platelet Inhibition to cLarify the Optimal strateGy to medicallY manage Acute Coronary Syndromes) trial, a 10,300 patient, multinational (35), and multicenter (>800) effort. It compares prasugrel plus aspirin against clopidogrel plus aspirin in patients with unstable angina or non-ST-elevation myocardial infarction who are medically managed, with the combined primary outcome of cardiovascular death, myocardial infarction, or stroke (ClinicalTrials.gov identifier NCT00699998).

Ticagrelor (AZD 6140)

Ticagrelor (AstraZeneca), formerly known as AZD6140, is an oral agent that is the active drug and reversibly binds to the $P2Y_{12}$ receptor. It is the first of a new class of nonthienopyridine $P2Y_{12}$ antagonists called cyclopentyltriazolopyrimidines and achieves full antiplatelet effects within 2 h of administration, possesses linear pharmacokinetics, which result in decremental levels of platelet inhibition over 24 h. It has a half-life of 12 h. Ticagrelor is a more potent and consistent inhibitor of ADP-induced platelet aggregation than clopidogrel.

The DISPERSE (Dose Confirmation Study Assessing Anti-Platelet Effects of AZD6140 vs Clopidogrel in NSTEMI) study was the first double-blinded, dose-ranging, parallel group Phase II trial to compare the safety and efficacy of ticagrelor to clopidogrel, where 200 patients with atherosclerotic disease were randomly assigned to receive one of three doses of ticagrelor (50, 100, or 200 mg b.i.d., or 400 mg q.d.) or clopidogrel 75 mg/day for 28 days (no loading dose) in addition to aspirin 75–100 mg (12). A rapid and superior platelet inhibition (>90%) was associated with ticagrelor (at doses ≥100 mg b.i.d.) treatment, whereas clopidogrel was associated with only ~60% platelet inhibition. Ticagrelor treatment was well tolerated across the dose range, with an increased bleeding time compared with clopidogrel, which was not ticagrelor-dose-related. Only one major bleeding event occurred in a patient receiving ticagrelor 400 mg once daily, whereas other bleeding events were of minor or mild-to-moderate in severity. A dose-dependent incidence of dyspnea (10% with ticagrelor 50 mg b.i.d. and 100 mg b.i.d., 16% with 200 mg b.i.d. and 20% with 400 mg b.i.d.) was observed; however, none of these events were serious and also none were associated with congestive heart failure or bronchospasm. Overall, ticagrelor treatment was well tolerated and associated with rapid, consistent, and maximum platelet inhibition throughout the treatment period in patients with atherosclerotic disease.

The DISPERSE-2 trial was designed to investigate the clinical outcomes of ticagrelor with different dosing strategies in non-ST-segment elevation acute coronary syndrome (13). A total of 990 patients were randomly assigned to receive ticagrelor 90 or 180 mg b.i.d. or clopidogrel 300-mg loading dose followed by 75-mg maintenance dose for 12 weeks. A total of 50% of the patients in the ticagrelor group received a 270-mg loading dose and all of the patients received aspirin 75–100 mg/day. Ticagrelor 180 mg was associated with a decreased incidence of MI (2.4% compared with 4.6% with clopidogrel and 3.6% with ticagrelor 90 mg). This decrease in MI was associated with superior platelet inhibition. The other end points of death, stroke, or recurrent ischemia were not different between groups.

The Phase III PLATO (a Study of Platelet Inhibition and Patient Outcomes) trial will investigate the clinical efficacy of AZD-6140 vs clopidogrel in 18,000 patients with non-ST or ST elevation acute coronary syndrome patients, with the combined primary end point of a reduction in vascular death, myocardial infarction, and stroke. This trial is due to report its results in mid- or late 2009. A dose of 180 mg as the loading dose, and 90 mg twice daily as the maintenance dose for AZD-6140, has been selected. (ClinicalTrials.gov identifier: NCT00391872).

Cangrelor (AR-C69931MX)

Cangrelor (Medicines Company) is a novel, parenteral nonthienopyridine $P2Y_{12}$ receptor antagonist known as purinoreceptor modulators and selectively and reversibly inhibits ADP-induced platelet aggregation. It is an ATP analogue that directly acts on the receptor, requiring no metabolic activation, and produces a concentration dependent inhibition of platelet aggregation. It is ultrashort-acting, with a half-life of 3–5 min, and achieves steady-state levels within 30 min. It is rapidly cleared, at 1 h post-infusion, 70% of patients had regained 60% of their baseline level of platelet aggregation (14).

The Phase 2 study was a two-part study in which the first part was a randomized, placebo-controlled dose-ranging study whereby 200 patients received either placebo or one of three doses of cangrelor 18–24 h prior to PCI, in addition to aspirin and heparin (15). At the highest dose of 4 mcg/kg/min, there was an 8% rate of major bleeding, which was not significantly higher ($p = 0.52$) compared with no bleeding in the placebo group. The second part then randomized 199 patients to either the maximum dose of cangrelor or usual dose abciximab starting 10–60 min prior to PCI. Patients who received coronary stents were then treated with ticlopidine or clopidogrel according to local practice. At 30 days follow-up, there were no significant differences in safety outcomes, with major bleeding rates of 1% and 2% in the cangrelor and abciximab group,

respectively. Thrombocytopenia was not significantly lower in the cangrelor vs the abciximab arm (1% vs 7% respectively, $p = 0.25$). The incidence of the composite end point of major adverse cardiac events (death, MI, or reintervention) was also not different (7.6% vs 5.3% in the cangrelor and abciximab arms, respectively, $p > 0.05$).

The CHAMPION-PCI (Cangrelor vs Standard Therapy to Achieve Optimal Management of Platelet Inhibition PCI) study is a 9,000-patient phase 3 randomized clinical trial which commenced enrollment in March 2006. The primary objective of this study is to demonstrate that the efficacy of cangrelor is superior, or at least noninferior, to that of clopidogrel in subjects requiring PCI as measured by a composite of all-cause mortality, myocardial infarction, and ischemia driven revascularization at 48 h. The incidence of hemorrhage by clinically relevant criteria (ACUITY, GUSTO, TIMI) and the need for blood transfusions will also be measured up to 48 h. Patients in this trial may be treated with other intravenous anticoagulants, such as bivalirudin, heparin, and GP IIb/IIIa inhibitors, at the investigator's discretion. This study is estimated to be completed by December 2009 (ClinicalTrials.gov identifier: NCT00305162).

The second trial in the phase 3 program is referred to as CHAMPION-PLATFORM, which commenced enrollment in October 2006 and is designed to enroll approximately 6,400 patients. The primary objective of this study is to demonstrate that the efficacy of cangrelor (combined with usual care) is superior to that of usual care, in subjects requiring PCI (unstable angina or non-ST elevation myocardial infarction), as measured by a composite of all-cause mortality, myocardial infarction, and ischemia-driven revascularization at 48 h. The incidence of hemorrhage by clinically relevant criteria (ACUITY, GUSTO, TIMI) and the need for blood transfusions will also be measured up to 48 h. Patients in this trial may also be treated with other intravenous anticoagulants, such as bivalirudin, heparin and GP IIb/IIIa inhibitors, at the investigator's discretion. As with the previous study, this is estimated to be completed by December 2009 (ClinicalTrials. gov identifier: NCT00385138).

Glycoprotein IIB/IIIA receptor antagonists

Initial targets were the development of oral GP IIb/IIIa inhibitor agents, however clinical trials have been unsuccessful, and as a class of agents, they have largely been abandoned (16). These agents have dose-dependent effects on platelets— at low levels of platelet inhibition function as a partial agonist by potentiating the release of CD40L, resulting in prothrombotic effects. At low levels, they also increase the inflammatory response by mediating leukocyte–platelet aggregation through the induction of P-selectin. Consequently, further development of this class of agents has ceased.

Protease-activated receptor antagonists

SCH 530348

SCH 530348 is a selective PAR 1 antagonist with a long half-life that may allow once daily oral dosing and may be an alternative to GP IIb/IIIa inhibition. The TRA-PCI (Thrombin Receptor Antagonist for Clinical Event Reduction Over Standard Concomitant Therapies PCI) trial was a 1,031-patient, double-blinded, dose-ranging, placebo-controlled trial of SCH 530348 for patients undergoing urgent or elective PCI, with the primary end point of bleeding at 60 days. Compared to standard therapy, the addition of SCH-530348 did not result in an increased bleeding rate.

This agent has entered Phase III trials as a 29,500-patient program comprising two separate trials. The first, a 10,000-patient multicenter, randomized, double-blind, placebo-controlled study called TRACER (The Safety and Efficacy of SCH 530348 in Addition to Standard of Care in Subjects With Acute Coronary Syndrome: Thrombin Receptor Antagonist for Clinical Event Reduction in Acute Coronary Syndrome). This trial will enroll patients with non-ST-elevation acute coronary syndromes with the primary efficacy end point being a composite of cardiovascular death, MI, stroke, recurrent ischemia with rehospitalization, and urgent coronary revascularization. The estimated study completion date is July 2011 (ClinicalTrials.gov identifier: NCT00527943).

The second trial is a secondary prevention trial of 19,500 patients, multicenter, randomized, double-blind, placebo-controlled known as TRA 2 P-TIMI 50 (The Safety and Efficacy of SCH 530348 in Addition to Standard of Care in Subjects with a History of Atherosclerotic Disease: Thrombin Receptor Antagonist in Secondary Prevention of Atherothrombotic Ischemic Events). The primary efficacy end point is a composite of cardiovascular death, MI, stroke, and urgent coronary revascularization and has an estimated study completion date of September 2010 (ClinicalTrials.gov identifier: NCT00526474).

Agents to reduce myocardial reperfusion injury

The acute occlusion of an epicardial coronary artery results in an AMI. The most effective strategy for reducing the size of myocardial injury and therefore improving clinical outcome is the early and successful myocardial reperfusion by primary percutaneous coronary intervention. The process of restoring blood flow to the ischemic myocardium, however, can induce injury, termed myocardial reperfusion injury, and can paradoxically reduce the benefits of myocardial reperfusion. This injury culminates in the death of cardiac myocytes that were viable immediately prior to myocardial reperfusion (17). In animal models of myocardial infarction, reperfusion injury accounts for up to 50% of the final size of myocardial infarction, however translation of strategies to improve outcomes to patients have been disappointing (18). A strategy of ischemic postconditioning, a mechanical approach whereby reperfused myocardial cells are subjected to short periods of ischemia has been shown to reduce infarct size in small studies (19–21). Most recently, several small studies have reported promising positive results with atrial natriuretic peptide (22), KAI-9803 (a protein kinase-C inhibitor) (23), and cyclosporine (24). These small studies require further confirmation with larger randomized trials to assess their safety and efficacy before they can be used routinely. Table 44.1 lists the various agents to date that have been in trials in an attempt to reduce reperfusion injury during PCI (25).

Table 44.1 Studies of agents to reduce reperfusion injury during percutaneous coronary intervention (25).

Neutral (no effect in clinical outcomes)	Contradictory results	Beneficial (improvement in clinical outcomes)
Superoxide dismutase	Nicorandil	Allopurinol
Cariporide		Edravone
MCC-135		Adenosine
Anti-CD11 antibody		Atrial natriuretic peptide (22)
Anti-CD18 antibody		KAI-9803 (Protein kinase C-delta inhibitor) (23)
Pexelizumab		Cyclosporine (24)
Glucose/Insulin/Potassium		
Magnesium		
Darbepoetin alpha (erythropoietin analogue)		

Conclusion

The ongoing search for agents to overcome the deficiencies of the currently available agent clopidogrel has resulted in the initiation of large, phase 3 trials investigating novel antiplatelet agents. Prasugrel is closest to commercialization, and with the current generation of DES and stent thrombosis, has demonstrated superior efficacy over clopidogrel. It is likely that minor subgroups identified at high bleeding risk will remain on clopidogrel, however, the majority of patients will benefit from prasugrel. Ticagrelor is the next oral agent, and its risk of unexplained dyspnea will require resolution, probably as part of the PLATO trial. Cangrelor and SCH-530348 are designed as agents to be administered in addition to usual care, so it remains to be seen whether a third agent will provide added benefit without added safety concerns. Finally, the ongoing interest in agents to reduce reperfusion injury has increased and this investigation requires large clinical trials in order to prove the safety and efficacy of the drugs investigated.

References

1 Smith SC, Jr, Feldman TE, Hirshfeld JW, Jr, et al. ACC/AHA/SCAI 2005 guideline update for percutaneous coronary intervention: a report of the American College of Cardiology/American Heart Association Task Force on Practice Guidelines (ACC/AHA/SCAI Writing Committee to Update 2001 Guidelines for Percutaneous Coronary Intervention). Circulation. 2006;**113**:e166–e286.

2 Meadows TA, Bhatt DL. Clinical aspects of platelet inhibitors and thrombus formation. Circ Res. 2007;**100**:1261–1275.

3 Bertrand ME, Rupprecht HJ, Urban P, Gershlick AH. Double-blind study of the safety of clopidogrel with and without a loading dose in combination with aspirin compared with ticlopidine in combination with aspirin after coronary stenting: the clopidogrel aspirin stent international cooperative study (CLASSICS). Circulation. 2000;**102**:624–629.

4 Gurbel PA, Bliden KP, Hiatt BL, O'Connor CM. Clopidogrel for coronary stenting: response variability, drug resistance, and the effect of pretreatment platelet reactivity. Circulation. 2003;**107**:2908–2913.

5 Angiolillo DJ, Capranzano P. Pharmacology of emerging novel platelet inhibitors. Am Heart J. 2008;**156**:S10–S15.

6 Wiviott SD, Antman EM, Winters KJ, et al. Randomized comparison of prasugrel (CS-747, LY640315), a novel thienopyridine P2Y12 antagonist, with clopidogrel in percutaneous coronary intervention: results of the Joint Utilization of Medications to Block Platelets Optimally (JUMBO)-TIMI 26 trial. Circulation. 2005;**111**:3366–3373.

7 Wiviott SD, Trenk D, Frelinger AL, et al. Prasugrel compared with high loading- and maintenance-dose clopidogrel in patients with planned percutaneous coronary intervention: the Prasugrel in Comparison to Clopidogrel for Inhibition of Platelet Activation and Aggregation-Thrombolysis in Myocardial Infarction 44 trial. Circulation. 2007;**116**:2923–2932.

8 Wiviott SD, Antman EM, Gibson CM, et al. Evaluation of prasugrel compared with clopidogrel in patients with acute coronary syndromes: design and rationale for the TRial to assess Improvement in Therapeutic Outcomes by optimizing platelet InhibitioN with prasugrel Thrombolysis In Myocardial Infarction 38 (TRITON-TIMI 38). Am Heart J. 2006;**152**:627–635.

9 Wiviott SD, Braunwald E, McCabe CH, et al. Prasugrel versus clopidogrel in patients with acute coronary syndromes. N Engl J Med. 2007;**357**:2001–2015.

10 Wiviott SD, Braunwald E, McCabe CH, *et al.* Intensive oral antiplatelet therapy for reduction of ischaemic events including stent thrombosis in patients with acute coronary syndromes treated with percutaneous coronary intervention and stenting in the TRITON-TIMI 38 trial: a subanalysis of a randomised trial. *Lancet.* 2008;**371**:1353–1363.

11 Cutlip DE, Windecker S, Mehran R, *et al.* Clinical end points in coronary stent trials: a case for standardized definitions. *Circulation.* 2007;**115**:2344–2351.

12 Husted S, Emanuelsson H, Heptinstall S, Sandset PM, Wickens M, Peters G. Pharmacodynamics, pharmacokinetics, and safety of the oral reversible P2Y12 antagonist AZD6140 with aspirin in patients with atherosclerosis: a double-blind comparison to clopidogrel with aspirin. *Eur Heart J.* 2006;**27**:1038–1047.

13 Cannon CP, Husted S, Harrington RA, *et al.* Safety, tolerability, and initial efficacy of AZD6140, the first reversible oral adenosine diphosphate receptor antagonist, compared with clopidogrel, in patients with non-ST-segment elevation acute coronary syndrome: primary results of the DISPERSE-2 trial. *J Am Coll Cardiol.* 2007;**50**:1844–1851.

14 Fugate SE, Cudd LA. Cangrelor for treatment of coronary thrombosis. *Ann Pharmacother.* 2006;**40**:925–930.

15 Greenbaum AB, Grines CL, Bittl JA, *et al.* Initial experience with an intravenous P2Y12 platelet receptor antagonist in patients undergoing percutaneous coronary intervention: results from a 2-part, phase II, multicenter, randomized, placebo- and active-controlled trial. *Am Heart J.* 2006;**151**:689e1–689e10.

16 Leebeek FW, Boersma E, Cannon CP, van de Werf FJ, Simoons ML. Oral glycoprotein IIb/IIIa receptor inhibitors in patients with cardiovascular disease: why were the results so unfavourable. *Eur Heart J.* 2002;**23**:444–457.

17 Piper HM, Garcia-Dorado D, Ovize M. A fresh look at reperfusion injury. *Cardiovasc Res.* 1998;**38**:291–300.

18 Bolli R, Becker L, Gross G, Mentzer R, Jr, Balshaw D, Lathrop DA. Myocardial protection at a crossroads: the need for translation into clinical therapy. *Circ Res.* 2004;**95**:125–134.

19 Staat P, Rioufol G, Piot C, *et al.* Postconditioning the human heart. *Circulation.* 2005;**112**:2143–2148.

20 Ma X, Zhang X, Li C, Luo M. Effect of postconditioning on coronary blood flow velocity and endothelial function and LV recovery after myocardial infarction. *J Interv Cardiol.* 2006;**19**:367–375.

21 Laskey WK. Brief repetitive balloon occlusions enhance reperfusion during percutaneous coronary intervention for acute myocardial infarction: a pilot study. *Catheter Cardiovasc Interv.* 2005;**65**:361–367.

22 Kitakaze M, Asakura M, Kim J, *et al.* Human atrial natriuretic peptide and nicorandil as adjuncts to reperfusion treatment for acute myocardial infarction (J-WIND): two randomised trials. *Lancet.* 2007;**370**: 1483–1493.

23 Bates E, Bode C, Costa M, *et al.* Intracoronary KAI-9803 as an adjunct to primary percutaneous coronary intervention for acute ST-segment elevation myocardial infarction. *Circulation.* 2008;**117**:886–896.

24 Piot C, Croisille P, Staat P, *et al.* Effect of cyclosporine on reperfusion injury in acute myocardial infarction. *N Engl J Med.* 2008;**359**:473–481.

25 Yellon DM, Hausenloy DJ. Myocardial reperfusion injury. *N Engl J Med.* 2007;**357**:1121–1135.

Appendix

Anticoagulants

Unfractionated heparin (UFH)
IV bolus and infusion
- Initial bolus 70–100 IU/kg for PCI without IIb/IIIa, to ACT 250–300 s
- Reduce bolus to 50–60 IU/kg for PCI with IIb/IIIa blocker, to ACT 200–250 s
- If procedure longer than 1 h, recheck ACT and rebolus (1,500–2,000 units) as needed
- May be reversed with protamine sulfate (1 mL = 1 mg, reverse 100 U of heparin); maximum dose 50 mg

Indications
- Treatment and prophylaxis of venous and arterial thrombosis and embolism

Contraindications
- Known hypersensitivity to heparin
- Active bleeding
- Severe thrombocytopenia
- Patients with heparin-associated antibodies
- Gastrointestinal ulcers
- Uncontrolled hypertension
- Suspected intracranial hemorrhage
- Inability to adequately monitor

Low-molecular-weight heparin (Enoxaparin)
Subcutaneous dose
- 1 mg/kg b.i.d. for 2–8 days, administered with aspirin
- Reduce to 0.5 mg/kg BID if renal insufficiency

Pharmacology in the Catheterization Laboratory. Edited by Ron Waksman and Andrew E Ajani. © 2010 Blackwell Publishing, ISBN: 978-1-4051-5704-9.

Intravenous dose for PCI
- For full anticoagulation without IIb/IIIa blocker: 1 mg/kg
- With a IIb/IIIa blocker: reduce bolus to 0.5–0.75 mg/kg for full anticoagulation
- To supplement SC dose give 8–12 h previously, 0.3 mg/kg IV bolus
- Also consider 0.3 mg/kg IV bolus if patient not at steady-state anticoagulation with SC dosing (i.e. <3 doses)
- Does not prolong ACT due to high Xa/IIa ratio
- Partial reversal with protamine: 1 mg protamine/ 1 mg enoxaparin <8 h last SC dose; 0.5 mg protamine/1 mg enoxaparin 8–12 h

Indications:
- Prophylaxis of ischemic complications in patients with unstable angina/non-STEMI
- For the prevention of deep vein thrombosis in patients undergoing/following hip replacement, knee replacement, or abdominal surgery
- For the prevention of ischemic complications of unstable angina and non-Q-wave MI administered together with aspirin and, if indicated, glycoprotein IIb/IIIa receptor antagonists
- In conjunction with warfarin—Inpatient treatment of acute deep vein thrombosis and/or pulmonary embolism; Outpatient treatment of acute deep vein thrombosis without pulmonary embolism

Contraindications:
- Active major bleeding
- Hypersensitivity to heparin or pork products
- Thrombocytopenia associated with positive antiplatelet antibody test *in vitro* induced by enoxaparin
- Hypersensitivity to the drug

Direct thrombin inhibitor: bivalirudin (Angiomax)

- Loading dose: 0.75 mg/kg intravenously
- Infusion: 1.75 mg/kg/h for the duration of PCI (Note: short half-life 25 min)
- Reduce dose to 0.25 mg/kg/h for dialysis-dependent patients
- Estimate CCr (mL/min) as $((140\text{-age}) * \text{weight (kg)})/(72 * \text{serum Cr})$ (times 0.85 for females)
- Can monitor ACT, usually >350 s after dose; no reversal agent but half-life ~25 min

Indications:

- As an anticoagulant in patients with unstable angina undergoing PTCA
- With provisional GP IIb/IIIa inhibitor as an anticoagulant in patients undergoing PCI
- For patients with, or at risk of, HIT/HITTS undergoing PCI

Contraindications:

- Active major bleeding
- Hypersensitivity to the drug or its components

Fondaparinux (Arixtra)

- 2.5 mg subcutaneously daily
- Dosing adjustment required in patients with renal dysfunction

Indications:

- In patients undergoing hip fracture surgery, including extended prophylaxis
- In patients undergoing hip replacement/knee replacement surgery
- In patients undergoing abdominal surgery who are at risk for thromboembolic complications
- The treatment of deep vein thrombosis when administered in conjunction with warfarin sodium
- The treatment of acute pulmonary embolism when administered in conjunction with warfarin sodium when initial therapy is administered in the hospital

Contraindications:

- In patients with severe renal impairment (creatinine clearance <30 mL/min)

- In patients with body weight <50 kg undergoing hip fracture, hip replacement or knee replacement surgery, and abdominal surgery
- In patients with active major bleeding or bacterial endocarditis
- In patients with thrombocytopenia associated with a positive in vitro test for antiplatelet antibody in the presence of fondaparinux sodium or in patients with known hypersensitivity to fondaparinux sodium

Antiplatelet agents

Aspirin

- 160–325 mg tablet taken as soon as possible (chewing is preferable)
- Higher doses (1,000 mg) interfere with prostacyclin production and may limit benefits

Indications:

- Analgesic
- Antipyretic
- Anti-inflammatory
- Myocardial infarction
- Transient ischemic attack
- Cerebrovascular accident

Contraindications:

- Bleeding disorders
- Children <16 years old
- Pregnancy

Thienopyridines

Clopidogrel (Plavix)

- 300 mg loading dose, given 6 h before a known procedure if possible
- 75 mg/day maintenance
- 2–4 weeks for bare metal stents; 3–6 months for drug-eluting stents; lifetime for brachytherapy

Indications:

- For patients with a history of recent MI, recent stroke, or established peripheral arterial disease
- For patients with non-ST-segment elevation acute coronary syndrome (unstable angina/non-Q-wave MI) including patients who are to be managed medically and those who are to

be managed with PCI (with or without stent), or CABG
- For patients with STEMI

Contraindications:
- Hypersensitivity to the drug substance or any component of the product
- Active pathological bleeding such as peptic ulcer or intracranial hemorrhage

Ticlopidine (Ticlid)
- 750 mg oral loading dose
- 250 mg BID oral maintenance
- Duration same as for clopidogrel
- Monitor for thrombocytopenia and neutropenia if duration more than 2 weeks
- Plavix is preferred (unless there is a clear allergy)

Indications:
- To reduce the risk of thrombotic stroke (fatal or nonfatal) in patients who have experienced stroke precursors, and in patients who have had a completed thrombotic stroke
- As adjunctive therapy with aspirin to reduce the incidence of subacute stent thrombosis in patients undergoing successful coronary stent implantation

Contraindications:
- Hypersensitivity to the drug
- Presence of hematopoietic disorders such as neutropenia and thrombocytopenia or a past history of either TTP or aplastic anemia
- Presence of a hemostatic disorder or active pathological bleeding (such as bleeding peptic ulcer or intracranial bleeding)
- In patients with severe liver impairment

Prasugrel (Effient)
- Similar mode of action to clopidogrel
- 60 mg loading dose

Indications:
- Prevention of atherothrombotic events in patients with ACS managed with PCI

Contraindications:
- In patients with a previous stroke or transient ischemic attack

IIb/IIIa Inhibitors
Abciximab (ReoPro)
- PCI or acute coronary syndrome with planned PCI within 24 h
- 0.25 mg/kg IV bolus (10–60 min before procedure) then 0.125 mcg/kg per minute (maximum of 10 mcg/min) IV infusion, × 18–24 h
- Check platelets at 4 h of infusion to monitor for thrombocytopenia

Indications:
- In patients undergoing percutaneous coronary intervention
- In patients with unstable angina not responding to conventional medical therapy when PCI is planned within 24 h

Contraindications:
- Active internal bleeding
- Recent (within 6 weeks) gastrointestinal or genitourinary bleeding of clinical significance
- History of cerebrovascular accident with 2 years, or CVA with a significant residual neurological deficit
- Bleeding diathesis
- Administration of oral anticoagulants within 7 days unless prothrombin time is ≤1.2 times control
- Thrombocytopenia (<1,00,000 cells/μL)
- Recent (within 6 weeks) major surgery or trauma
- Intracranial neoplasm, arteriovenous malformation, or aneurysm
- Severe uncontrolled hypertension
- Presumed or documented history of vasculitis
- Use of intravenous dextran before PCI, or intent to use it during an intervention

Eptifibitide (Integrilin)
For PCI
- 180 mcg/kg IV bolus
- Repeat the same dose in 10 min
- Infuse 2 mcg/kg per min for 18 h
- Reduce infusion to 1 mcg/kg/min for creatinine clearance <50 mL/min
- Maximum dose (reached at patient weight of 121 kg): 22.6 mg IV bolus × 2 then maximum infusion of 242 mcg/min

Indications:
- For the treatment of patients with acute coronary syndrome (unstable angina/non-STEMI), including patients who are to be managed medically and those undergoing PCI.
- For the treatment of patients undergoing PCI, including those undergoing intracoronary stenting

Contraindications:
- A history of bleeding diathesis, or evidence of active abnormal bleeding within the previous 30 days
- Severe hypertension (systolic blood pressure >200 mm Hg or diastolic blood pressure >110 mm Hg) not adequately controlled on antihypertensive therapy
- Major surgery within the preceding 6 weeks
- History of stroke within 30 days or any history of hemorrhagic stroke
- Current or planned administration of another parenteral GP IIb/IIIa inhibitor
- Dependency on renal dialysis
- Known hypersensitivity to any component of the product

Tirofiban (Aggrastat)

Acute coronary syndrome
- 0.4 mcg/kg per minute IV for 30 min, then 0.1 mcg/kg per minute IV infusion
- Not recommended for PCI

Indications:
- (In combination with heparin) for the treatment of acute coronary syndrome, including patients who are to be managed medically and those undergoing PTCA or atherectomy

Contraindications:
- Known hypersensitivity to any component of the product
- Active internal bleeding or a history of bleeding diathesis within the previous 30 days
- A history of intracranial hemorrhage, intracranial neoplasm, arteriovenous malformation, or aneurysm
- A history of thrombocytopenia following prior exposure to the drug
- History of stroke within 30 days or any history of hemorrhagic stroke

- Major surgical procedure or severe physical trauma within the previous month
- History, symptoms, or findings suggestive of aortic dissection
- Severe hypertension (systolic blood pressure >180 mmHg and/or diastolic blood pressure >110 mmHg)
- Concomitant use of another parenteral GP IIb/IIIa inhibitor
- Acute pericarditis

Arrhythmia

Bradycardia

Atropine sulfate

For vasovagal or symptomatic sinus bradycardia
- 0.5–1.0 mg IV every 3–5 min as needed
- Do not exceed total dose of 0.04 mg/kg

Indications:
- When excessive (or sometime normal) muscarinic effects are judged to be life-threatening or are producing symptoms severe enough to call of temporary, reversible muscarinic blockade

Contraindications:
- In patients with glaucoma, pyloric stenosis or prostatic hypertrophy, except in doses ordinarily used for preanesthetic medication

Isoproterenol

IV infusion due to bradycardia due to infranodal block with slow ventricular escape
- Mix 2 mg in 250 mL D5W
- Infuse at 2–10 mcg/min, titrated to adequate heart rate
- In torsades de pointes titrate to increase heart rate until VT rhythm is suppressed

Indications:
- For mild or transient episodes of heart block that do not require electric shock or pacemaker therapy
- For serious episodes of heart block and Adams-Stokes attacks (except when caused by ventricular tachycardia or fibrillation). For use in cardiac arrest until electric shock or pacemaker therapy, the treatments of choice, is available
- For bronchospasm occurring during anesthesia

- As an adjunct to fluid and electrolyte replacement therapy and the use of other drugs and procedures in the treatment of hypovolemic and septic shock, low cardiac output (hypoperfusion) states, congestive heart failure, and cardiogenic shock

Contraindications:
- In patients with tachyarrhythmias; tachycardia or heart block caused by digitalis intoxication; ventricular arrhythmias which require inotropic therapy; and angina pectoris

Atrial fibrillation or flutter
Dofetilide
IV infusion dose for atrial fibrillation or flutter
- Single infusion of 8 mcg/k over 30 min
- Not approved for use in the United States

Indications:
- Maintenance of normal sinus rhythm
- Conversion of atrial fibrillation/flutter

Contraindications:
- In patients with congenital oracquired long QT syndromes
- Should not be used in patients with a baseline QT interval or QTc >440 ms (500 ms in patients with ventricular conduction abnormalities)
- In patients with severe renal impairment (calculated creatinine clearance <20 mL/min)
- In patients with a known hypersensitivity to the drug

Ibutilide
IV dose for atrial fibrillation or flutter (for adults ≥60 kg)
- 1 mg (10 mL) administered IV (diluted or undiluted) over 10 min
- A second dose may be administered at the same rate 10 min after completion of the first dose

Indications:
- For the rapid conversion of atrial fibrillation or atrial flutter of recent onset to sinus rhythm

Contraindications:
- In patients who have previously demonstrated hypersensitivity to ibutilide fumarate or any of the other product components

Supraventricular tachycardia
Adenosine
IV rapid push to convert SVT
- Initial bolus of 6 mg given rapidly over 1–3 s followed by normal saline bolus of 20 mL; then elevate the extremity
- Repeat dosage of 12 mg in 1–2 min if needed
- A third dose of 12 mg may be given in 1–2 min if needed

Indications:
- Conversion to sinus rhythm of paroxysmal supraventricular tachycardia (PSVT), including that associated with accessory bypass tracts

Contraindications:
- Second- or third-degree AV block (except in patients with a functioning artificial pacemaker)
- Sinus node disease, such as sick sinus syndrome or symptomatic bradycardia (except in patients with a functioning artificial pacemaker)
- Known hypersensitivity to the drug

Ventricular
Lidocaine
For stable VT, wide-complex tachycardia or uncertain type, significant ectopy
- 1.0–1.5 mg/kg IV push
- Repeat 0.5–0.75 mg/kg every 5–10 min; maximum total dose: 3 mg/kg
- Maintenance infusion 1–4 mg/min (30–50 mcg/kg per minute)

Indications:
- For production of local or regional anesthesia by infiltration techniques including percutaneous injection, by peripheral nerve block techniques such as brachial plexus and intercostal blocks, and by central neural techniques including epidural and caudal blocks, when the accepted procedures for these techniques, as described in standard textbooks, are observed

Contraindications:
- In patients with a known history of hypersensitivity to local anesthetics of the amide type or to other components of the solution, i.e., methylparaben (multidose solutions) or sodium metabisulfite and/or citric acid in solutions containing epinephrine

Amiodarone

For VF

- IV push 300 mg
- Repeat 150 mg over 2–5 min if necessary

For VEA or stable VT

- Rapid infusion: 150 mg in 50 mL over 10 min, repeat q10 min as needed
- Slow infusion: 360 mg IV over 6 h (1 mg/min)
- Maintenance infusion: 540 mg IV over 18 h (0.5 mg/min)

Indications:

- Recurrent ventricular fibrillation
- Recurrent hemodynamically unstable ventricular tachycardia

Contraindications:

- In patients with cardiogenic shock; severe sinus-node dysfunction, causing marked sinus bradycardia; second- or third-degree atrioventricular block; and when episodes of bradycardia have caused syncope (except when used in conjunction with a pacemaker)
- In patients with a known hypersensitivity to the drug or to any of its components, including iodine

Procainamide

Recurrent VF/VT

- 20 mg/min IV infusion (maximum total dose: 17 mg/kg)
- In urgent situations, up to 50 mg/min may be administered to a total dose of 17 mg/kg
- Suspend loading infusion if one of the following occurs:
  i Arrhythmia suppression
  ii Hypotension
  iii QRS widens by >50%
- Maintenance infusion 1–4 mg/min

Indications:

- Atrial arrhythmias
- Ventricular arrhythmias

Contraindications:

- Complete heart block; second- and third-degree AV block
- Hypersensitivity to **procainamide**, procaine, or other ester-type local anesthetics

- Systemic lupus erythematosus
- Torsades de Pointes

Magnesium sulfate

Cardiac arrest (for hypomagnesemia or torsades de pointes)

- 1–2 g (2–4 mL of a 50% solution) diluted in 120 mL of D5W IV push

Torsades de Pointes (not in cardiac arrest):

- Loading dose of 1–2 g mixed in 50–100 mL of D5W, over 5–60 min IV
- Follow with 0.5–1.0 g/h IV (titrate dose to control the torsades) for up to 24 h

Indications:

- Convulsions (treatment)
- Hypomagnesemia (prophylaxis and treatment)
- To prevent or treat magnesium deficiency in patients receiving total parenteral nutrition
- Tetany, uterine (treatment)

Contraindications:

- Should not be administered parenterally in patients with heart block or myocardial damage

Sodium bicarbonate

For prolonged cardiac arrest—IV bolus

- 1 mEq/kg IV bolus
- Repeat half this dose every 10 min thereafter
- If rapidly available, use arterial blood gas analysis to guide bicarbonate therapy (calculated dose deficits or bicarbonate concentration)
- An acute change in $PaCO_2$ of 1 mmHg is associated with an increase or decrease in pH of 0.008 U (relative to normal pH of 7.4)

Indications:

- In the treatment of metabolic acidosis, which can occur in severe renal disease, uncontrolled diabetes, circulatory insufficiency due to shock, anoxia, or severe dehydration, extracorporeal circulation of blood and severe primary lactic acidosis
- In the treatment of certain drug intoxications, including barbiturates, in poisoning by salicylates or methyl alcohol, and in hemolytic reactions requiring alkalinization of the urine to diminish nephrotoxicity of blood pigments
- In severe diarrhea, which is often accompanied by a significant loss of bicarbonate

Contraindications:
- In patients with metabolic and respiratory alkalosis and in patients with hypocalcemia in which alkalosis may produce tetany

Beta-blockers

Esmolol
- 0.5 mg/kg over 1 min, followed by continuous infusion at 0.05 mg/kg per min (maximum: 0.3 mg/kg)
- Titrate to effect—note esmolol has a very short half-life (2–9 min)

Indications:
- Supraventricular tachycardia
- Intraoperative and postoperative tachycardia and/or hypertension

Contraindications:
- Hypersensitivity to beta blockers
- Asthma
- Heart block greater than first degree
- Insulin-dependent diabetics with frequent hypoglycemic episodes
- Overt heart failure/cardiogenic shock
- Severe bradycardia

Atenolol
- Initial IV dose: 5 mg slow IV (over 5 min)
- Wait 10 min, then give second dose of 5 mg slow IV (over 5 min)
- In 10 min, if well tolerated, may start PO; then give 50 mg PO twice a day

Indications:
- Hypertension
- Acute myocardial infarction
- Angina
- Arrhythmias

Contraindications:
- Hypersensitivity to beta blockers
- Asthma
- Heart block greater than first degree
- Insulin-dependent diabetics with frequent hypoglycemic episodes
- Overt heart failure/cardiogenic shock
- Severe bradycardia

Metoprolol
- Initial IV dose: 5 mg slow IV, repeat ay 5–min intervals to a total of 15 mg
- Oral regimen to follow IV dose: 50 mg BID for 24 h, then increase to 100 mg BID

Indications:
- Treatment of hypertension
- Long-term treatment of angina pectoris
- Treatment of stable, symptomatic (NYHA Class II or III) heart failure of ischemic, hypertensive, or cardiomyopathic origin

Contraindications:
- In severe bradycardia, heart block greater than first degree, cardiogenic shock, decompensated cardiac failure, sick sinus syndrome (unless a permanent pacemaker is in place), and in patients who are hypersensitive to any component of the product

Propranolol
- Total dose: 0.1 mg/kg by slow IV push, divided into 3 equal doses at 2–3 min intervals
- Do not exceed 1 mg/min watching for excessive bradycardia or hypotension
- Nonselective beta-1 and beta-2 agent (use with care in asthmatic patients)

Indications:
- Hypertension
- Angina
- Essential tremor
- Arrhythmias
- Myocardial infarction
- Migraine headache
- Hypertrophic cardiomyopathy
- Antipsychotic-induced akathisia
- Portal hypertension
- Anxiety
- Acute panic
- Preventing esophageal varices bleeding

Contraindications:
- Hypersensitivity to beta blockers
- Asthma
- Heart block greater than first degree
- Insulin-dependent diabetics with frequent hypoglycemic episodes

- Overt heart failure/cardiogenic shock
- Severe bradycardia

Labetalol

For severe hypertension
- 10 mg IV push over 1–2 min
- May repeat or double every 10 min to a maximum dose of 150 mg, or give initial bolus and start infusion at 2–8 mg/min

Indications:
- Hypertension
- Hypertensive urgency/emergency

Contraindications:
- Hypersensitivity to beta blockers
- Asthma
- Heart block greater than first degree
- Insulin-dependent diabetics with frequent hypoglycemic episodes
- Overt heart failure
- Shock
- Severe bradycardia

Calcium channel blocker
Diltiazem

Acute rate control (see vasodilator section for use in no-reflow)
- 15–20 mg (0.25 mg/kg) IV over 2 min
- May repeat in 15 min at 20–25 mg (0.35 mg/kg) over 2 min
- Maintenance infusion 5–15 mg/h, titrated to heart rate

Indications:
- Treatment of hypertension
- Management of chronic stable angina

Contraindications:
- In patients with sick sinus syndrome except in the presence of a functioning ventricular pacemaker
- In patients with second- or third-degree AV block except in the presence of a functioning ventricular pacemaker
- In patients with hypotension (<90 mmHg systolic)
- In patients with acute MI and pulmonary congestion documented by x-ray on admission

Verapamil

Acute rate control (see vasodilator section for use in no-reflow)
- 2.5–5.0 mg IV bolus over 2 min
- Second dose: 5 mg bolus every 15 min to total dose of 30 mg

Indications:
- For the management of hypertension and angina

Contraindications:
- Severe left ventricular dysfunction
- Hypotension (systolic pressure <90 mmHg) or cardiogenic shock
- Sick sinus syndrome (except in patients with a functioning artificial ventricular pacemaker)
- Second- or third-degree AV block (except in patients with a functioning artificial ventricular pacemaker)
- Patients with atrial flutter or atrial fibrillation and an accessory bypass tract
- Patients with known hypersensitivity to the drug

Conscious sedation

Fentanyl
- 25–50 mcg intravenously
- Repeat as needed every 5 min
- Monitor vital signs, oximetry, and state of consciousness as per conscious sedation guidelines

Indications:
- For the management of *persistent*, moderate to severe chronic pain that requires continuous, around-the-clock opioid administration for an extended period of time, and cannot be managed by other means such as nonsteroidal analgesics, opioid combination products, or immediate-release opioids

Contraindications:
- In patients who are not opioid-tolerant
- In the management of acute pain or in patients who require opioid analgesia for a short period of time
- In the management of postoperative pain, including use after out-patient or day surgeries
- In the management of mild paid
- In the management of intermittent pain

- In situations of significant respiratory depression, especially in unmonitored settings where there is a lack of resuscitative equipment
- In patients who have acute or severe bronchial asthma
- In patients who have or are suspected of having paralytic ileus
- In patients with known hypersensitivity to the drug or any of its components

Versed
- 0.5–1 mg intravenously
- Repeat as needed every 5 min
- Monitor vital signs, oximetry, and state of consciousness per conscious sedation guidelines

Indications:
- For preoperative sedation/anxiolysis/amnesia
- As an agent for sedation/anxiolysis/amnesia prior to or during diagnostic, therapeutic or endoscopic procedures, oncology procedures, radiologic procedures, suture of lacerations and other procedures either alone or in combination with other CNS depressants
- For induction of general anesthesia, before administration of other anesthetic agents
- Can also be used as a component of intravenous supplementation of nitrous oxide and oxygen (balanced anesthesia)
- For sedation of intubated and mechanically ventilated patients as a component of anesthesia or during treatment in a critical care setting

Contraindications:
- In patients with a known hypersensitivity to the drug
- Not intended for intrathecal or epidural administration due to the presence of the preservative benzyl alcohol in the dosage form

Morphine sulfate
- 2–4 mg IV (over 1–5 min) every 5–30 min
- Monitor vital signs, oximetry, and state of consciousness as per conscious sedation guidelines

Indications:
- For the management of moderate to severe pain when a continuous, around-the-clock opioid analgesic is needed for an extended period of time

- For the relief of pain in opioid-tolerant patients only
- For postoperative use if the patient is already receiving the drug prior to surgery or if the postoperative pain is expected to be moderate to severe and persist for an extended period of time

Contraindications:
- In patients with known hypersensitivity to morphine or in any situation where opioids are contraindicated. This includes patients with respiratory depression (in the absence of resuscitative equipment or in unmonitored settings), and in patients with acute or severe bronchial asthma or hypercarbia
- In any patient who has or is suspected of having a paralytic ileus

Reversal agents
Flumazenil (Romazicon, "Re-versed")
For oversedation with benzodiazepines
- Dosage: 0.2 to a maximum dose of 1 mg
- Administer in 0.2 mg increments over 15 s, may repeat in 1 min intervals to 1 mg
- Maximum dose: 1 mg/dose and 3 mg/h
- Monitor closely for re-sedation for at least 2 h

Indications:
- For the complete or partial reversal of the sedative effects of benzodiazepines in cases where general anesthesia has been induced and/or maintained with benzodiazepines, where sedation has been produced with benzodiazepines for diagnostic and therapeutic procedures, and for the management of benzodiazepine overdose
- For the reversal of conscious sedation induced with benzodiazepines

Contraindications:
- In patients with a known hypersensitivity to flumazenil or benzodiazepines
- In patients who have been given a benzodiazepine for control of a potentially life-threatening condition (e.g., control of intracranial pressure or status epilepticus)
- In patients who are showing signs of serious cyclic antidepressant overdose

Naloxone hydrochloride (narcan)

For oversedation with narcotics

- Dilute 0.4 mg (1 mL) with 9 mL NS (0.04 mg/mL)
- Administer 0.04 mg or 1 mL q 2–3 min PRN to increase respiratory rate and alertness
- Onset 1 min, duration 30–40 min
- Monitor closely for resedation for at least 2 h

Indications:

- For the complete or partial reversal of narcotic depression, including respiratory depression, induced by opioids including natural and synthetic narcotics, propoxyphene, methadone, and the narcotic-antagonist analgesics: nalbuphine, pentazocine, and butorphanol
- For the diagnosis of suspected acute opioid overdosage

Contraindications:

- In patients with a known hypersensitivity to the drug

"Unconscious" sedation*

*Use only with anesthesiologist

Propofol (diprivan)

Induction of general anesthesia

- Healthy adults <55 years old: 40 mg every 10 s until induction onset (2–2.5 mg/kg)
- Elderly, debilitated, ASA III/IV patients: 20 mg every 10 s until induction onset (1–1.5 mg/kg)

Maintenance of general anesthesia

- Healthy adults <55 years old: 100–200 mcg/kg/min (3–6 mg/kg/h)
- Elderly, debilitated, ASA III/IV patients: 50–100 mcg/kg/min (3–6 mg/kg/h)

Indications:

- Initiation and maintenance of monitored anesthesia care sedation
- Combined sedation and regional anesthesia
- Induction of general anesthesia
- Maintenance of general anesthesia
- Intensive care unit sedation of intubated, mechanically ventilated patients

Contraindications:

- In patients with a known hypersensitivity to the drug or any of its components

- In patients with allergies to eggs, egg products, soybeans, or soy products

Neuromuscular blocker*

*Use only with anesthesiologist

Cisatracurim besylate (nimbex)

- Dosage must be individualized
- Skeletal muscle relaxation: initial, 0.15–0.20 mg/kg IV bolus as component of a propofol/nitrous oxide/oxygen induction–intubation technique
- Skeletal muscle relaxation: maintenance, 0.03 mg/kg IV
- Skeletal muscle relaxation: maintenance, initial continuous IV infusion rate of 3 mcg/kg/min may be required to rapidly counteract spontaneous recovery from initial bolus dose; thereafter, 1–2 mcg/kg/min continuous IV infusion; in ICU, infusion range of 0.5–10.2 mcg/kg/min

Indications:

- For inpatients and outpatients as an adjunct to general anesthesia, to facilitate tracheal intubation, and to provide skeletal muscle relaxation during surgery or mechanical ventilation in the ICU

Contraindications:

- In patients known to have an allergic hypersensitivity to the drug or other bis-benzylisoquinolinium agents
- Use of Nimbex from vials containing benzyl alcohol as a preservative is contraindicated in patients with a known hypersensitivity to benzyl alcohol

Vecuronium bromide (norcuron)

- Dosage must be individualized
- Skeletal muscle relaxation: initial, 0.08–0.1 mg/kg IV bolus
- Skeletal muscle relaxation: maintenance, 0.01–0.015 mg/kg IV 25–40 min after initial dose, repeat every 12–15 min as needed
- Skeletal muscle relaxation: 1 mcg/kg/min continuous IV infusion 20–40 min after initial intubation dose, after early evidence of spontaneous recovery; then adjust to maintain 90% suppression of twitch response; range 0.8–1.2 mcg/kg/min

Indications:
- As an adjunct to general anesthesia, to facilitate endotracheal intubation and to provide skeletal muscle relaxation during surgery or mechanical ventilation

Contraindications:
- Hypersensitivity to the drug
- In pregnant and lactating women, since reproductive studies in animals have not yet been performed

Contrast toxicity

Contrast nephropathy
Hydration
For prevention of contrast-induced nephropathy
- Normal saline 1 mL/kg/h for 12 h pre- and 12 h postcontrast exposure
- Alternative normal saline 3 mL/kg over 1 h preprocedure, then 1 mL/kg/h for 6 h postprocedure
- Alternative sodium bicarbonate (154 mEq/L) in D5W
- Limit infusion and monitor closely in CHF patients
- Do not add Lasix, Mannitol, dopamine, fenodopam (systemic)
- Consider use of iodixanol (Visipaque), isoosmolar contrast; limit contrast volume

Indications:
- Patients with impaired renal function or who are at risk for developing contrast-induced nephropathy

Contraindications:
- Patients with heart failure who cannot tolerate fluid overload

N-acetylcysteine
- 600 mg orally BID, start 6 h prior to contrast exposure
- Continue for 24 h postcontrast exposure

Indications:
- As adjuvant therapy for patients with abnormal, viscid, or inspissated mucous secretions

Contraindications:
- In those patients who are sensitive to it

Contrast allergy or toxicity
Prednisone
- Pretreat 60 mg p.o. daily for 24–48 h
- May use solumedrol 100 mg IV just before procedure

Indications:
- Endocrine disorders
- Rheumatic disorders
- Collagen diseases
- Dermatologic diseases
- Allergic states
- Ophthalmic diseases
- Respiratory diseases
- Neoplastic diseases
- Edematous states
- Gastrointestinal diseases
- Nervous system

Contraindications:
- Systemic fungal infections and known hypersensitivity to components

Benadryl
- H1 blocker
- 25–50 mg p.o. before the procedure
- May also be given as 25 mg IV for intraprocedural allergic reactions

Indications:
- Temporarily relieves symptoms due to hay fever or other upper respiratory allergies
- Temporarily relieves symptoms due to the common cold

Contraindications:
- N/A

H2-blocker ranitidine (zantac)
- Needed to prevent histamine-induced vasodilation
- 150 mg p.o. prior to procedure
- Alternative, 50 mg IV, given over 5 min

Indications:
- Short-term treatment of active duodenal ulcer
- Maintenance therapy for duodenal ulcer patients at reduced dosage after healing of acute ulcers

- The treatment of pathological hypersecretory conditions
- Short-term treatment of active, benign gastric ulcer
- Maintenance therapy for gastric ulcer patients at reduced dosage after healing of acute ulcers
- Treatment of GERD
- Treatment of endoscopically diagnosed erosive esophagitis
- Maintenance of healing of erosive esophagitis

Contraindications:
- For patients known to have hypersensitivity to the drug or any of the ingredients

Ondansetron HCI (zofran)

For prevention or treatment of peri-procedural nausea and vomiting
- 2–4 mg undiluted IV over 4 min

Indications:
- Prevention of nausea and vomiting associated with initial and repeat courses of emetogenic cancer chemotherapy, including high-dose cisplatin
- Prevention of postoperative nausea and/or vomiting

Contraindications:
- For patients known to have hypersensitivity to the drug

Diruretic

Furosemide (lasix)
IV infusion
- 0.5–1.0 mg/kg given over 1–2 min
- If no response, double dose to 2.0 mg/kg, slowly over 1–2 min

Indications:
- Edema
- Hypertension

Contraindications:
- In patients with anuria and in patients with a history of hypersensitivity to furosemide

Bumetanide (bumex)
IV infusion
- Bolus 0.5–1.0 mg is equivalent to 40 mg of furosemide

Indications:
- For the treatment of edema associated with congestive heart failure, hepatic and renal disease, including the nephrotic syndrome

Contraindications:
- In anuria

Inotrope

Dobutamine (dobutrex)
IV infusion
- Dilute 500 mg (20 mL) in 250 mL D5W
- Usual infusion rate is 2–20 mcg/kg per min
- Titrate so heart rate does not increase by >10% of baseline

Indications:
- When parenteral therapy is necessary for inotropic support in the short- term treatment of patients with cardiac decompensation due to depressed contractility resulting either from organic heart disease or from cardiac surgical procedures

Contraindications:
- In patients with idiopathic hypertrophic sub-aortic stenosis and in patients who have shown previous manifestations of hypersensitivity to dobutamine

Dopamine
IV infusion
- Mix 400–800 mg in 250 mL normal saline, lactate Ringer s solution, or D5W
- Continuous infusions (titrate to patient response)
- Low dose: 1–5 mcg/kg per minute—gamma (dopaminergic) stimulation
- Moderate dose: 5–10 mcg/kg/per minute ("cardiac dose"—beta stimulation)
- High dose: 10–15 mcg/kg per minute ("vasopressor doses"—alpha stimulation)

Indications:
- For the correction of hemodynamic imbalances present in the shock syndrome due to myocardial infarctions, trauma, endotoxic septicemia, open heart surgery, renal failure, and chronic cardiac decompensation as in congestive failure

Contraindications:
- In patients with pheochromocytoma
- In the presence of uncorrected tachyarrhythmias or ventricular fibrillation

Amrinone (Inamrinone)
IV loading dose and infusion for severe pump failure
- Loading dose 0.75 mg/kg, given over 10–15 min
- Follow with infusion of 5–15 mcg/kg per minute titrated to clinical effect
- Optimal use requires hemodynamic monitoring
- Note—Amrinone and Milrinone inhibit PDE and do not depend on beta adrenergic receptors

Indications:
- For the short-term management of congestive heart failure

Contraindications:
- In patients who are hypersensitive to it
- In those patients known to be hypersensitive to bisulfites

Milrinone (Primaor)
IV loading dose and infusion for severe pump failure
- Supplied as 200 mcg/mL
- Loading dose 50 mcg/kg over 10 min
- Follow with infusion 0.5–0.75 mcg/kg/min
- Reduce infusion for renal insufficiency (i.e., 0.33 mcg/kg/min for CCr 30 mL/min)

Indications:
- For the short-term intravenous treatment of patients with acute decompensated heart failure

Contraindications:
- In patients who are hypersensitive to it

Epinephrine
Cardiac arrest
- Note: Available in 1:1,000 (1 mg/mL) and 1:10,000 (0.1 mg/mL) concentrations
- IV dose: 1 mg (10 mL of 1:10,000 solution) every 3–5 min during resuscitation
- Higher doses (up to 0.2 mg/kg) may be used if 1-mg dose fails
- Continuous infusion: 30 mg (30 mL of 1:1,000 solution) to 250 mL normal saline, run at 100 mL/h and titrate to response

Profound bradycardia or hypotension
- 2 mg in 500 mL NS
- 2–10 mcg/min infusion (add 1 mg of 1:1,000 to 500 mL NS; infuse 1–5 mL/min)

Indications:
- For temporary relief of shortness of breath, tightness of chest, and wheezing due to bronchial asthma

Contraindications:
- N/A

Glucagon
To treat excessive bradycardia from beta-blockers
- 1–5 mg over 2–5 min

Indications:
- The patient is unconscious
- The patient is unable to eat sugar or a sugar-sweetened product
- The patient is having a seizure
- Repeated administration of sugar or a sugar-sweetened product such as a regular soft drink or fruit juice does not improve the patient's condition

Contraindications:
- None

Calcium chloride
IV slow push in cardiac arrest
- 100 mg/mL in 10 mL vial (total = 1 g; a 10% solution)
- 8–16 mg/kg (usually 5–10 mL) IV for hyperkalemia and calcium channel blocker overdose—may be repeated as needed

- 2–4 mg/kg (usually mL) IV for propyhlaxis for IV calcium channel blockers

Indications:
- In the immediate treatment of hypocalcemic tetany

Contraindications:
- In cardiac resuscitation, the use of calcium chloride is contraindicated in the presence of ventricular fibrillation

Digoxin
IV infusion (for rate control in atrial fibrillation/flutter) Note: Beta or calcium channel blocker preferred
- 0.25 mg/mL or 0.1 mg/mL supplied in 1 or 2 mL ampule (totals = 0.1–0.5 mg)
- Loading doses of 10–15 mcg/kg lean body weight—therapeutic effect with minimum toxicity
- Maintenance dose is affected by body size and renal function

Indications:
- Treatment of mild to moderate heart failure
- For the control of ventricular response rate in patients with chronic atrial fibrillation

Contraindications:
- In patients with ventricular fibrillation or in patients with a known hypersensitivity to the drug

Pressor agents

Phenylephrine (neosynephrine)
For severe refractory hypotension

Bolus
- 0.04–0.1 mg IV, can be repeated in 10 min if needed

Infusion
- Mix 20 mg in 500 mL of D5W or NS (40 mcg/mL)
- Infuse 100–180 mcg/min until blood pressure stabilizes
- Reduce to 40–60 mcg/min adjusted to maintain desired blood pressure

Indications:
- To maintain blood pressure in conditions where the pressure is low
- To prolong anesthesia, or to treat certain heart rhythm problems (PSVT)

Contraindications:
- In patients with severe hypertension, ventricular tachycardia or those who are hypersensitive to it

Metaraminol (aramine)
For severe refractory hypotension
- Loading dose: 0.5–1.0 mg, IV push
- Infusion: 15 mg (1.5 mL) in 500 mL NS, adjust to maintain desired blood pressure
- Indirect acting sympathomimetic amine—mixed alpha and beta, action delayed by 5 min

Indications:
- For prevention and treatment of the acute hypotensive state occurring with spinal anesthesia
- As adjunctive treatment of hypotension due to hemorrhage, reactions to medications, surgical complications, and shock associated with brain damage due to trauma or tumor

Contraindications:
- Use of this drug with cyclopropane or halothane anesthesia should be avoided, unless clinical circumstances demand such use
- Hypersensitivity to any component of this product, including sulfites

Norepinephrine (levophed)
For severe refractory hypotension
- 4 mg in 250 mL of D5W to yield 4 mcg/mL
- Initial dose 0.5–1.0 mcg/min (usual range 0.5–30 mcg/min)

Indications:
- For blood pressure control in certain acute hypotensive states

Contraindications:
- In patients who are hypotensive from blood volume deficits except as an emergency measure to maintain coronary and cerebral artery perfusion until blood volume replacement therapy can be completed

- In patients with mesenteric or peripheral vascular thrombosis (because of the risk of increasing ischemia and extending the area of infarction) unless, in the opinion of the attending physician, the administration of norepinephrine is necessary as a life-saving procedure
- During cyclopropane and halothane, anesthesia is generally considered contraindicated because of the risk of producing ventricular tachycardia or fibrillation

Vasopressin

Doses for cardiac arrest (option to epinephrine)
- 40 U IV push × 1
- Wait 10 min before initiating epinephrine protocol

For refractory hypotension
- 20 U in 250 mL D5W
- Infuse at 0.01–0.10 U/min

Indications:
- For prevention and treatment of postoperative abdominal distention, in abdominal roentgenography to dispel interfering gas shadows, and in diabetes insipidus

Contraindications:
- Anaphylaxis or hypersensitivity to the drug or its components

Vasodilator

Systemic arterial
Nitroglycerin
IV infusion
- IV bolus: 12.5–25 mcg
- Infuse at 10–20 mcg/min
- Titrate to effect

Intracoronary (for vasospasm). Do not use for no-reflow
- Dilute to 100–200 mcg/mL
- Administer 100 mcg through guiding catheter or selectively into distal coronary
- Repeat as needed

Indications:
- For the prevention of angina pectoris due to coronary artery disease

Contraindications:
- In patients who are allergic to the drug

Nitroprusside (sodium nitroprusside)
IV infusion
- Mix 50 mg in 250 mL D5W
- Begin at 0.10 mcg/min titrated to improve blood pressure (up to 10 mcg/min)
- Do not administer in same IV line as alkaline solutions

Indications:
- For the immediate reduction of blood pressure of patients in hypertensive crises. Concomitant longer-acting antihypertensive medication should be administered so that the duration of treatment with sodium nitroprusside can be minimized
- For producing controlled hypotension in order to reduce bleeding during surgery
- For the treatment of acute congestive heart failure

Contraindications:
- In the treatment of compensatory hypertension, where the primary hemodynamic lesion is aortic coarctation or arteriovenous shunting
- Should not be used to produce hypotension during surgery in patients with known inadequate cerebral circulation, or in moribund patients (A.S.A. Class 5E) coming to emergency surgery
- For the treatment of acute congestive heart failure associated with reduced peripheral vascular resistance such as high-output heart failure that may be seen in endotoxic sepsis
- Patients with congenital (Leber's) optic atrophy or with tobacco amblyopia have unusually high cyanide thiocyanate ratios. These rare conditions are probably associated with defective or absent rhodanase, and sodium nitroprusside should be avoided in these patients

ACE inhibitors enalapril (IV = enalaprilat)
- IV: 1.25 mg IV initial dose over 5 min
- Repeat dose: 1.25–5.0 mg IV every 6 h
- IV ACEI not approved in STEMI

Indications:
- For the treatment of hypertension when oral therapy is not practical

Contraindications:
- In patients who are hypersensitive to any component of this product and in patients with a history of angioedema related to previous treatment with an angiotensin converting enzyme inhibitor and in patients with hereditary or idiopathic angioedema

Coronary
Nitroglycerin
For epicardial vasodilation or treatment of coronary spasm
- Dilute to 200 mcg/mL
- Administer 100–200 mcg intracoronary
- Note: Nitroglycerin is primarily an epicardial vasodilator and should not be used in situations like no-reflow where small vessel (arteriolar) dilation is required

Indications:
- For the prevention of angina pectoris due to coronary artery disease

Contraindications:
- In patients who are allergic to the drug

Adenosine
For measurement of fractional flow reserve
- Dilute to 10 mcg/mL
- For RCA 18–24 mcg through guiding catheter or selectively into distal coronary
- For LCA 24–36 mcg through guiding catheter or selectively into distal coronary
- Alternatively, 140–180 mcg/kg/min peripheral intravenous infusion for 3 min
For reversal of no-reflow
- 100 mcg selective into distal involved vessel

Indications:
- Conversion to sinus rhythm of paroxysmal supraventricular tachycardia, including that associated with accessory bypass tracts

Contraindications:
- Second- or third-degree AV block (except in patients with a functioning artificial pacemaker)
- Sinus node disease, such as sick sinus syndrome or symptomatic bradycardia (except in patients with a functioning artificial pacemaker)
- Known hypersensitivity to the drug

Nitroprusside (sodium nitroprusside)
For reversal of no-reflow
- Dilute to 100 mcg/mL
- Administer 100 mcg through guiding catheter or selectively into distal coronary
- Repeat as needed

Indications:
- For the immediate reduction of blood pressure of patients in hypertensive crises. Concomitant longer-acting antihypertensive medication should be administered so that the duration of treatment with sodium nitroprusside can be minimized
- For producing controlled hypotension in order to reduce bleeding during surgery
- For the treatment of acute congestive heart failure

Contraindications:
- In the treatment of compensatory hypertension, where the primary hemodynamic lesion is aortic coarctation or arteriovenous shunting
- Should not be used to produce hypotension during surgery in patients with known inadequate cerebral circulation, or in moribund patients (A.S.A. Class 5E) coming to emergency surgery
- For the treatment of acute congestive heart failure associated with reduced peripheral vascular resistance such as high-output heart failure that may be seen in endotoxic sepsis
- Patients with congenital (Leber's) optic atrophy or with tobacco amblyopia have unusually high cyanide thiocyanate ratios. These rare conditions are probably associated with defective or absent rhodanase, and sodium nitroprusside should be avoided in these patients

Nicardipine
For reversal of no reflow
- Dilute to 200 mcg/mL not C/w heparin
- Administer 200 mcg selectively into involved coronary

Indications:
- For the short-term treatment of hypertension when oral therapy is not feasible or not desirable

Contraindications:
- In patients with known hypersensitivity to the drug
- In patients with advanced aortic stenosis

Diltiazem
For reversal of no-reflow
- Dilute to 1 mg/mL
- Administer 1 mg through guiding catheter or selectively into distal coronary
- Repeat as needed up to a total of 2.5 mg

Indications:
- Treatment of hypertension
- Management of chronic stable angina

Contraindications:
- In patients with sick sinus syndrome except in the presence of a functioning ventricular pacemaker
- In patients with second- or third-degree AV block except in the presence of a functioning ventricular pacemaker
- In patients with hypotension (<90 mmHg systolic)
- In patients with acute MI and pulmonary congestion documented by x-ray on admission

Verapamil
For reversal of no reflow
- Dilute to 100 mcg/mL
- Administer 100–200 mcg through guiding catheter or selectively into distal coronary
- Repeat as needed
- Monitor for bradycardia in the right and circumflex arteries

Indications:
- For the management of hypertension and angina

Contraindications:
- Severe left ventricular dysfunction

- Hypotension (systolic pressure <90 mmHg) or cardiogenic shock
- Sick sinus syndrome (except in patients with a functioning artificial ventricular pacemaker)
- Second- or third-degree AV block (except in patients with a functioning artificial ventricular pacemaker)
- Patients with atrial flutter or atrial fibrillation and an accessory bypass tract
- Patients with a known hypersensitivity to the drug

Pulmonary arteriolar
Epoprostenol (flolan)
IV infusion for pulmonary hypertension
- Start at 2 ng/kg/min
- Increase by 2 ng/kg/min every 15 min until reduction in pulmonary resistance if dose-limiting toxicity (nausea, headache, hypotension)

Indications:
- For the long-term intravenous treatment of primary pulmonary hypertension and pulmonary hypertension associated with the scleroderma spectrum of disease in NYHA Class III and Class IV patients who do not respond adequately to conventional therapy

Contraindications:
- Chronic use in patients with congestive heart failure due to severe left ventricular systolic dysfunction
- Chronic use in patients who develop pulmonary edema during dose initiation
- In patients with known hypersensitivity to the drug or to structurally related compounds

Index